Focus on Antibiotics – New Challenges and Steps Forward in Discovery and Development

Focus on Antibiotics – New Challenges and Steps Forward in Discovery and Development

Editors

Aura Rusu
Valentina Uivarosi
Corneliu Tanase

MDPI • Basel • Beijing • Wuhan • Barcelona • Belgrade • Manchester • Tokyo • Cluj • Tianjin

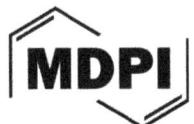

Editors

Aura Rusu
Department of Pharmaceutical
and Therapeutical Chemistry
George Emil Palade
University of Medicine,
Pharmacy, Science
and Technology
Targu Mures
Romania

Valentina Uivarosi
General and Inorganic
Chemistry Department
Carol Davila University of
Medicine and Pharmacy
Bucharest
Romania

Corneliu Tanase
Department of
Pharmaceutical Botany
George Emil Palade
University of Medicine,
Pharmacy, Science
and Technology
Targu Mures
Romania

Editorial Office
MDPI
St. Alban-Anlage 66
4052 Basel, Switzerland

This is a reprint of articles from the Special Issue published online in the open access journal *Pharmaceutics* (ISSN 1999-4923) (available at: www.mdpi.com/journal/pharmaceutics/special_issues/antibiotics_discovery).

For citation purposes, cite each article independently as indicated on the article page online and as indicated below:

LastName, A.A.; LastName, B.B.; LastName, C.C. Article Title. *Journal Name* **Year**, *Volume Number*, Page Range.

ISBN 978-3-0365-7201-7 (Hbk)
ISBN 978-3-0365-7200-0 (PDF)

© 2023 by the authors. Articles in this book are Open Access and distributed under the Creative Commons Attribution (CC BY) license, which allows users to download, copy and build upon published articles, as long as the author and publisher are properly credited, which ensures maximum dissemination and a wider impact of our publications.

The book as a whole is distributed by MDPI under the terms and conditions of the Creative Commons license CC BY-NC-ND.

Contents

About the Editors vii

Preface to "Focus on Antibiotics – New Challenges and Steps Forward in Discovery and Development" ix

Aura Rusu, Ioana-Andreea Lungu, Octavia-Laura Moldovan, Corneliu Tanase and Gabriel Hancu
Structural Characterization of the Millennial Antibacterial (Fluoro)Quinolones—Shaping the Fifth Generation
Reprinted from: *Pharmaceutics* **2021**, *13*, 1289, doi:10.3390/pharmaceutics13081289 1

Aura Rusu and Emanuela Lorena Buta
The Development of Third-Generation Tetracycline Antibiotics and New Perspectives
Reprinted from: *Pharmaceutics* **2021**, *13*, 2085, doi:10.3390/pharmaceutics13122085 39

Alexandra-Cristina Munteanu and Valentina Uivarosi
Ruthenium Complexes in the Fight against Pathogenic Microorganisms. An Extensive Review
Reprinted from: *Pharmaceutics* **2021**, *13*, 874, doi:10.3390/pharmaceutics13060874 69

Katarzyna Turecka, Agnieszka Chylewska, Michał Rychłowski, Joanna Zakrzewska and Krzysztof Waleron
Antibacterial Activity of Co(III) Complexes with Diamine Chelate Ligands against a Broad Spectrum of Bacteria with a DNA Interaction Mechanism
Reprinted from: *Pharmaceutics* **2021**, *13*, 946, doi:10.3390/pharmaceutics13070946 121

Farhan Alshammari, Bushra Alshammari, Afrasim Moin, Abdulwahab Alamri, Turki Al Hagbani and Ahmed Alobaida et al.
Ceftriaxone Mediated Synthesized Gold Nanoparticles: A Nano-Therapeutic Tool to Target Bacterial Resistance
Reprinted from: *Pharmaceutics* **2021**, *13*, 1896, doi:10.3390/pharmaceutics13111896 145

Saher Fatima, Khursheed Ali, Bilal Ahmed, Abdulaziz A. Al Kheraif, Asad Syed and Abdallah M. Elgorban et al.
Titanium Dioxide Nanoparticles Induce Inhibitory Effects against Planktonic Cells and Biofilms of Human Oral Cavity Isolates of *Rothia mucilaginosa*, *Georgenia* sp. and *Staphylococcus saprophyticus*
Reprinted from: *Pharmaceutics* **2021**, *13*, 1564, doi:10.3390/pharmaceutics13101564 159

Samir Haj Bloukh, Zehra Edis, Hamid Abu Sara and Mustafa Ameen Alhamaidah
Antimicrobial Properties of *Lepidium sativum* L. Facilitated Silver Nanoparticles
Reprinted from: *Pharmaceutics* **2021**, *13*, 1352, doi:10.3390/pharmaceutics13091352 175

Md. Amdadul Huq and Shahina Akter
Characterization and Genome Analysis of *Arthrobacter bangladeshi* sp. nov., Applied for the Green Synthesis of Silver Nanoparticles and Their Antibacterial Efficacy against Drug-Resistant Human Pathogens
Reprinted from: *Pharmaceutics* **2021**, *13*, 1691, doi:10.3390/pharmaceutics13101691 197

Mudasir Ahmad Bhat, Awdhesh Kumar Mishra, Mujtaba Aamir Bhat, Mohammad Iqbal Banday, Ommer Bashir and Irfan A. Rather et al.
Myxobacteria as a Source of New Bioactive Compounds: A Perspective Study
Reprinted from: *Pharmaceutics* **2021**, *13*, 1265, doi:10.3390/pharmaceutics13081265 217

Alistair S. Brown, Jeremy G. Owen, James Jung, Edward N. Baker and David F. Ackerley
Inhibition of Indigoidine Synthesis as a High-Throughput Colourimetric Screen for Antibiotics Targeting the Essential *Mycobacterium tuberculosis* Phosphopantetheinyl Transferase PptT
Reprinted from: *Pharmaceutics* **2021**, *13*, 1066, doi:10.3390/pharmaceutics13071066 . . . . **249**

Joonhyeok Choi, Ahjin Jang, Young Kyung Yoon and Yangmee Kim
Development of Novel Peptides for the Antimicrobial Combination Therapy against Carbapenem-Resistant *Acinetobacter baumannii* Infection
Reprinted from: *Pharmaceutics* **2021**, *13*, 1800, doi:10.3390/pharmaceutics13111800 . . . . **261**

About the Editors

Aura Rusu

Aura Rusu is currently a Professor at the Pharmaceutical and Therapeutic Chemistry Department, Faculty of Pharmacy, George Emil Palade University of Medicine, Pharmacy, Science and Technology of Târgu Mureș, Romania. Degree in Pharmacy (1994), Specialist (primary pharmacist) in Pharmaceutical Laboratory (2003), Trainer of Trainers (2008), PhD in Pharmacy (2013), Master Degree in Quality of Medicine, Food and Environment (2013), Habilitation in Pharmacy (2017), and Coordination of PhD students (2018).

She works mainly in pharmaceutical chemistry, medicinal chemistry, drug design, antibacterial agents, metal complexes, drug analysis, capillary electrophoresis, and patient–pharmacist communication.

She was involved in research projects as a director (1) or member (2) and in other institutional projects as a director (1) or member (2), all supported by the George Emil Palade University of Medicine, Pharmacy, Sciences and Technology of Targu Mures, Romania. In addition, she is the author or co-author of 10 books, 2 chapters in books, 67 articles published in international peer review journals, and 67 conference presentations.

Valentina Uivarosi

Valentina Uivarosi is currently a Professor at the General and Inorganic Chemistry, University of Medicine and Pharmacy Carol Davila in Bucharest (Faculty of Pharmacy), Romania. She graduated in Pharmacy from the University of Medicine and Pharmacy Carol Davila in 1993 and in Chemistry from the University of Bucharest in 2006. She received her PhD degree (2004) and Habilitation (2015) in Pharmacy from the University of Medicine and Pharmacy Carol Davila in Bucharest.

Her main research interests focus on the synthesis of metal complexes with biological activity (e.g., antibacterial, anticancer, and antidiabetic activity), DNA binding, protein interaction, cytotoxicity studies, and drug repositioning.

She is the author or the co-author of 10 books, 6 chapters in books, 67 articles, 8 patent applications (4 are granted), over 100 conference presentations and has conducted 4 national research grants.

Corneliu Tanase

Corneliu Tanase is currently a Professor at the Department of Pharmaceutical Botany, Faculty of Pharmacy, George Emil Palade University of Medicine, Pharmacy, Science and Technology of Târgu Mureș, Romania. Degree in Biology (2007), Master Degree in Biology (2009), PhD in Biology (2013), PhD in Chemical Engineering (2013), Habilitation in Pharmacy (2020), and Coordinator of PhD Student (2020).

He is working mainly on developing novel alternative sources of bioactive compounds using wood by-products (wood bark) or the use of bioactive compounds from plant by-products as bioregulator agents or as intermediaries in the biosynthesis of biomedical nanomaterials. He has been involved in several projects (project leader—5 projects) regarding using plant by-products and their functionalization. He is the author or co-author of 6 books, 2 chapters in books, over 80 articles, and over 50 conference presentations.

Preface to "Focus on Antibiotics – New Challenges and Steps Forward in Discovery and Development"

The design of new antibiotics is still considered the primary weapon in fighting against the growing bacterial resistance to known antibiotics. The Special Issue "Focus on Antibiotics – New Challenges and Steps Forward in Discovery and Development" covers a wide range of topics briefly presented below.

A review article was focused on new representatives of antibacterial quinolones; a new generation (the fifth) associated with higher potency, and a broad spectrum of activity arises. Additionally, the tetracycline antibiotic class has acquired new valuable members with excellent development potential. Another review article comprises the advantages and disadvantages of Ru (II/III) frameworks as antimicrobial agents. In addition, some aspects regarding the relationship between their chemical structure and mechanism of action, cellular localisation, and/or metabolism of the ruthenium complexes in bacterial and eukaryotic cells are also discussed. Synthesis and characterization of two Co(III) complexes with diamine chelate ligands were also presented; the complexes were sequentially tested against Gram-positive and Gram-negative bacteria. Nanoparticles are very attractive in multiple medical applications. Gold nanoparticles (GNPs) were synthesised by using ceftriaxone antibiotic. Titanium dioxide nanoparticles proved to induce inhibitory effects against planktonic cells and biofilms of human oral cavity isolates. *Lepidium sativum* L. and silver nanoparticles (AgNPs) were successfully combined and tested against ten reference strains of pathogens. In addition, another study targeted the characterisation and genome analysis of *Arthrobacter bangladeshi* sp. nov., applied for the green synthesis of silver nanoparticles and their antibacterial efficacy against two drug-resistant pathogens. One review has been focused on *Myxobacterial* species and assesses their ability to produce bioactive compounds. A recently validated drug target in *Mycobacterium tuberculosis* is an essential phosphopantetheinyl transferase. Newly identified tools will facilitate finding new anti-mycobacterial drug leads and guide the design of phosphopantetheinyl transferase inhibitors based on structure-activity studies. Antimicrobial peptides are very promising in their activity against drug-resistant species. Thus, a novel PapMA analogue was designed with increased anti-carbapenem-resistant *Acinetobacter baumannii* activity.

We are grateful to the authors for their contributions and hope this Special Issue will stimulate further research and discussion on antibiotics. We also thank the reviewers for their time and expertise, and the editorial team for supporting this Special Issue. Finally, we hope this Special Issue will serve as a valuable resource for researchers, clinicians, and policymakers working towards a future where antibiotics remain vital in our fight against infectious diseases.

Aura Rusu, Valentina Uivarosi, and Corneliu Tanase
Editors

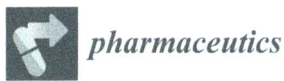

Review

Structural Characterization of the Millennial Antibacterial (Fluoro)Quinolones—Shaping the Fifth Generation

Aura Rusu [1], Ioana-Andreea Lungu [2], Octavia-Laura Moldovan [2], Corneliu Tanase [3,*] and Gabriel Hancu [1]

1. Pharmaceutical and Therapeutical Chemistry Department, Faculty of Pharmacy, George Emil Palade University of Medicine, Pharmacy, Science, and Technology of Targu Mures, 540142 Targu Mures, Romania; aura.rusu@umfst.ro (A.R.); gabriel.hancu@umfst.ro (G.H.)
2. The Doctoral School of Medicine and Pharmacy, George Emil Palade University of Medicine, Pharmacy, Science, and Technology of Targu Mures, 540142 Targu Mures, Romania; ioana-andreea.lungu@umfst.ro (I.-A.L.); octavia.moldovan@umfst.ro (O.-L.M.)
3. Pharmaceutical Botany Department, Faculty of Pharmacy, George Emil Palade University of Medicine, Pharmacy, Science, and Technology of Targu Mures, 540142 Targu Mures, Romania
* Correspondence: corneliu.tanase@umfst.ro; Tel.: +40-744-215-543

Citation: Rusu, A.; Lungu, I.-A.; Moldovan, O.-L.; Tanase, C.; Hancu, G. Structural Characterization of the Millennial Antibacterial (Fluoro)Quinolones—Shaping the Fifth Generation. *Pharmaceutics* **2021**, *13*, 1289. https://doi.org/10.3390/pharmaceutics13081289

Academic Editor: Tihomir Tomašič

Received: 9 July 2021
Accepted: 14 August 2021
Published: 18 August 2021

Publisher's Note: MDPI stays neutral with regard to jurisdictional claims in published maps and institutional affiliations.

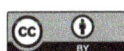

Copyright: © 2021 by the authors. Licensee MDPI, Basel, Switzerland. This article is an open access article distributed under the terms and conditions of the Creative Commons Attribution (CC BY) license (https://creativecommons.org/licenses/by/4.0/).

Abstract: The evolution of the class of antibacterial quinolones includes the introduction in therapy of highly successful compounds. Although many representatives were withdrawn due to severe adverse reactions, a few representatives have proven their therapeutical value over time. The classification of antibacterial quinolones into generations is a valuable tool for physicians, pharmacists, and researchers. In addition, the transition from one generation to another has brought new representatives with improved properties. In the last two decades, several representatives of antibacterial quinolones received approval for therapy. This review sets out to chronologically outline the group of approved antibacterial quinolones since 2000. Special attention is given to eight representatives: besifloxacin, delafoxacin, finafloxacin, lascufloxacin, nadifloxacin and levonadifloxacin, nemonoxacin, and zabofloxacin. These compounds have been characterized regarding physicochemical properties, formulations, antibacterial activity spectrum and advantageous structural characteristics related to antibacterial efficiency. At present these new compounds (with the exception of nadifloxacin) are reported differently, most often in the fourth generation and less frequently in a new generation (the fifth). Although these new compounds' mechanism does not contain essential new elements, the question of shaping a new generation (the fifth) arises, based on higher potency and broad spectrum of activity, including resistant bacterial strains. The functional groups that ensured the biological activity, good pharmacokinetic properties and a safety profile were highlighted. In addition, these new representatives have a low risk of determining bacterial resistance. Several positive aspects are added to the fourth fluoroquinolones generation, characteristics that can be the basis of the fifth generation. Antibacterial quinolones class continues to acquire new compounds with antibacterial potential, among other effects. Numerous derivatives, hybrids or conjugates are currently in various stages of research.

Keywords: fluoroquinolones; quinolones; structure-activity relationship; DNA gyrase; topoisomerase IV; antibacterial activity

1. Introduction

The historical moment of the emergence of a new class of antibacterial compounds was in 1945 when George Lesher and his team discovered the antimicrobial potential of 7-chloro-quinoline. This molecule was a compound with bactericidal action isolated during the synthesis and purification of chloroquine (antimalarial agent). Nalidixic acid, the first antibacterial quinolone (QN) derivative introduced in therapy, was discovered based on this compound (characterized by a naphthyridine nucleus) and was introduced into therapy in 1963 [1–4].

The identification of a compound which is efficient against Gram-negative bacteria led to new derivatives as pipemidic acid, piromidic acid, oxolinic acid, cinoxacin and flumequine, the first generation of antibacterial quinolones (QNs) [5]. Flumequine was the first compound with a fluorine atom in the structure [6]. This optimization proved to be valuable for the next generation of antibacterial QNs. New quinoline derivatives were synthesized with superior pharmacokinetics and pharmacodynamic properties and a broader antibacterial spectrum [7,8]. Thus, the second generation of QNs was synthesized, obtained by introducing a fluorine atom in the sixth position of the quinolinic nucleus (Figure 1). These new QNs called generically "fluoroquinolones" (FQNs) presented an improved biological activity [9]. Numerous FQNs have been synthesized and studied. New compounds with an extended antibacterial spectrum, being active on both Gram-positive and Gram-negative bacteria (including *Pseudomonas aeruginosa*), have become valuable tools in therapy. The second generation comprises of both representatives for human use (norfloxacin, ciprofloxacin, ofloxacin), and for veterinary use (enrofloxacin) [3].

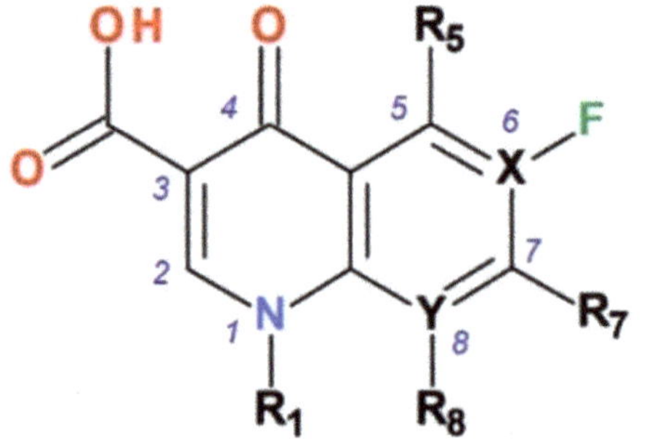

Figure 1. The general chemical structure of FQNs (1,4-quinolones) and numbering (X and Y = C or N).

More valuable representatives were included in the third generation as levofloxacin (the *L*-enantiomer of ofloxacin) and gatifloxacin, which presented increased activity against Gram-positive bacteria (*Streptococcus* sp.), increased tissue penetration and half-life. Due to severe side effects (hypoglycemia), gatifloxacin is used only topically as eye drops [3,10,11]. Fourth generation FQNs have, in addition, acquired activity against anaerobic bacteria (e.g., moxifloxacin). Also, levofloxacin and moxifloxacin were included in the therapeutic protocols used in second-line multidrug-resistant tuberculosis [12,13]. The optimization of the chemical structure also led to a long half-life in moxifloxacin (13 h) [3,11]. Data on the discovery of antibacterial QN class representatives and their approval in therapy by the U.S. Food and Drug Administration (FDA) and/or European Medicines Agency (EMA) are briefly presented in Table 1.

The aim of this review is to present the progress in FQNs class since 2000. The newest FQNs introduced in therapy are highlighted and critically analyzed. Special attention is given to eight selected representatives (besifloxacin, delafloxacin, finafloxacin, lascufloxacin, levonadifloxacin, nadifloxacin, nemonoxacin, and zabofloxacin), approached from the perspective of physicochemical properties, antibacterial activity spectrum and advantageous structural modifications which influence for antibacterial efficiency.

Table 1. The representatives of the class of antibacterial QNs and their approval in therapy.

[1] Year	Generation	Antibacterial QNs	Producer	Use and Status	References
1962	1st	Nalidixic acid	Lappin/Sterling Drug	Human and veterinary	[14,15]
1966	1st	Oxolinic acid	Warner-Lambert	Withdrawn	[14,15]
1967	1st	Piromidic acid	Dainippon	Withdrawn	[14,15]
1970	1st	Cinoxacin	Eli Lilly	Withdrawn	[14]
1973	1st	Flumequine	Riker	Veterinary	[14,15]
1974	1st	Pipemidic acid	Dainippon	Withdrawn	[14]
1978	2nd	Norfloxacin	Kyorin	Human and veterinary Approved by the FDA in 1986	[14]
1979	2nd	Pefloxacin	Roger Bellan (Rhône Poulenc)	Approved in France since 1985; approved in some EU countries	[14–17]
1980	2nd	Enoxacin	Dainippon	Withdrawn	[3,14,15]
1981	2nd	Fleroxacin	Kyorin	Introduced in therapy in 1987, withdrawn in 1990	[14,15,18]
1982	2nd	Ofloxacin [2]	Daiichi	Human and veterinary, Approved by the FDA in 1990	[14,15]
1984	2nd	Temafloxacin	Abbott Laboratories	Approved by the FDA and also withdrawn in 1992	[8,18,19]
1985	2nd	Lomefloxacin [2]	Hokuriku Pharm.	Approved by the FDA in 1992, then withdrawn	[3]
1985	2nd	Tosufloxacin	Taisho-Toyama Chemistry, Abbott	Veterinary (Japan)	[8,15,20]
1987	2nd	Ciprofloxacin	Bayer AG	Human and veterinary, Approved by the FDA in 1987	[14,15]
1987	3rd	Enrofloxacin	Bayer AG	Veterinary	[14,15,21]
1987	3rd	Sparfloxacin [3]	Dainippon	Approved by the FDA in 1996, then withdrawn	[3,14,15]
1987	4th	Prulifloxacin	Nippon	Approved only in Japan	[14,22,23]
1987	3rd	Orbifloxacin [3]	Dainippon/Schering	Veterinary	[14,24]
1989	2nd	Nadifloxacin [2]	Otsuka Pharmaceuticals	Approved in Japan in 1993 and 1998, approved by the EMA in 2000, topical use	[25–27]
1989	3rd	Grepafloxacin [2]	Warner Lambert/Glaxo Wellcome	Withdrawn in 1999	[3,15]
1990	3rd	Clinafloxacin	Parke-Davis Pharmaceutical	Withdrawn in 1999	[3,14]
1991	3rd	Danofloxacin	Pfizer	Veterinary	[14,15,28]
1992	4th	Trovafloxacin	Pfizer	Withdrawn in 2001	[3,14,15]
1994	3rd	Levofloxacin [4]	Daiichi	Approved by the FDA in 1996	[14,15,29]
1994	2nd	Sarafloxacin	Abbott Laboratories/Fort Dodge	Veterinary, withdrawn in 2001	[14,15,30,31]
1995	3rd	Balofloxacin	Choongwae Pharma	Approved by the Korean FDA in 2001	[23,32]
1995	3rd	Marbofloxacin	Vetoquinol/Pfizer	Veterinary	[14,15,33]
1995	4th	Moxifloxacin [4]	Bayer AG	Approved by the FDA in 1999	[3,29,34]
1996	2nd	Difloxacin	Fort Dodge	Veterinary	[14]
1998	3rd	Pradofloxacin	Bayer Animal Health GmbH	Approved by the EMA in 2011, and FDA in 2013; veterinary use	[35,36]

Table 1. Cont.

[1] Year	Generation	Antibacterial QNs	Producer	Use and Status	References
1999	4th	Delafloxacin	Abbott Laboratories, Melinta Therapeutics (former Rib-X Pharmaceuticals)	Approved by the FDA in 2017	[37–42]
1999	3rd	Gatifloxacin [2]	Kyorin/Bristol-Myers Squibb	Approved by the FDA in 1999, withdrawn in 2006	[3,25,43,44]
1999	4th	Gemifloxacin	Smith-Kline Beecham	Approved by the FDA in 2003 Withdrawn in 2009 (by EMA)	[3,25,29,45]
2000	4th	Besifloxacin [4]	SSP Co. Ltd., Japonia	Approved by the FDA in 2009	[46]
2000	4th	Finafloxacin [3]	Bayer HealthCare Pharmaceuticals, Byk Gulden, MerLion Pharmaceuticals	Approved by the FDA in 2017	[42,47–50]
2003	4th	Garenoxacin	Toyama Chemical Co., Ltd./Schering Plough	Approved by the FDA and EMA in 2006; withdrawn in 2007	[3,29,51,52]
2004	4th	Nemonoxacin	TaiGen Biotechnology	Approved in Taiwan in 2014	[53,54]
-	4th	Zabofloxacin	Dong Wha Pharm. Co. Ltd.	Approved in Soth Korea in 2015	[55,56]
-	4th	Sitafloxacin	Daiichi Sankyo Co., Japan	Approved in Japan in 2008, in Thailand in 2012	[57–59]

[1] first year reported, [2] racemic, [3] diastereoisomers, [4] R or S isomer.

2. Research Methodology

The literature research was conducted mainly on Clarivate Analytics and ScienceDirect databases using relevant keywords: (a) topic "fluoroquinolones", "quinolones", "antibacterials"; (b) title: "besifloxacin", "delafloxacin", "finafloxacin", "lascufloxacin", "nadifloxacin", "levonadifloxacin", "nemonoxacin", "zabofloxacin", and other relevant representatives of the FQNs class.

The articles were selected if they included relevant data regarding the aspects referred to in our review: discovery of the compound and the entities involved, data on approval in therapy, pharmaceutical formulations, infections treated by the targeted representatives, antibacterial activity spectrum, physicochemical properties, structure-activity relationships, elements of the safety profile related to chemical structure optimizations, bacterial resistance, and new QN derivatives. The manuscript contains relevant references, including those published in the first part of 2021.

Biovia Draw 2019 was used for drawing chemical structures (https://discover.3ds.com/biovia-draw-academic, accessed on 6 July 2021) [60]. MarvinSketch was used for drawing, displaying and characterizing chemical structures MarvinSketch 20.20.0, ChemAxon (https://www.chemaxon.com, accessed on 11 June 2021) [61].

3. Mechanism of Action

The FQNs mechanism of action is well known and described in the literature [62–66]. It is known that FQNs act on two bacterial DNA enzymes: gyrase and topoisomerase IV (Figure 2) [67]. Thus, due to the covalent enzyme-DNA complex stabilization, DNA is cleaved. After this interaction, depending on the concentration, the death of the bacterial cell occurs in two ways: (1) at low concentration by blocking replication and transcription [62,68] and (2) at higher concentration (over the minimum inhibitory concentration) when the DNA topoisomerase is dissociated/removed [69], the DNA strands remain free, which leads to the chromosome fragmentation [70–72]. The advantage of new representatives is the action on both target enzymes and broadening the spectrum of activity against several types of pathogens [73,74]. In general, DNA gyrase from Gram-negative bacteria is more susceptible to inhibition than topoisomerase IV. On the other hand, topoisomerase IV from Gram-positive bacteria is more susceptible to inhibition than DNA gyrase [75].

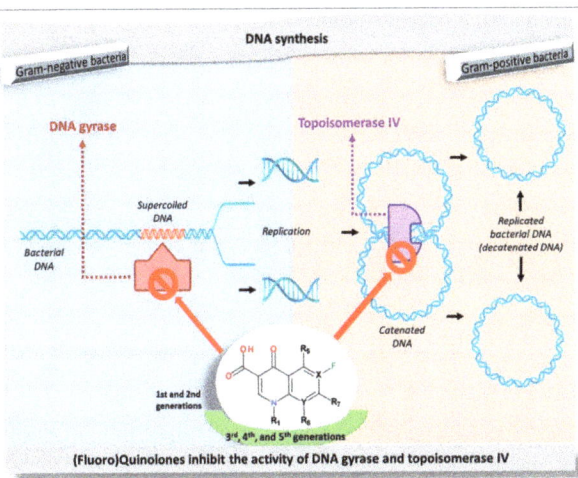

Figure 2. The mechanism of action of antibacterial (fluoro)quinolones.

Some studies have shown a correlation between FQNs lethality and reactive oxygen species (ROS) formation [76–79]. On the other hand, some issues about how do FQNs induce ROS accumulation remain unclear [80]. For example, Rodríguez-Rosado et al. (2018) studied the mechanisms of FQN-induced mutagenesis and the role of N-acetylcysteine in FQNs therapy to inhibit FQN-induced mutagenesis [81].

4. Classification into Generations of FQNs Used in Therapy

The most widely used classification of FQNs is the classification into generations based on of antibacterial activity and therapeutic use (Table 2).

Table 2. Classification into generations of the main FQNs for human use in therapy based on antibacterial spectrum and therapeutic indications (FDA and EMA approved).

Generation	Compounds	Antibacterial Spectrum	Therapeutic Indications/Pharmacokinetics, Administration	Ref.
1st	Nalidixic acid	Gram-negative pathogens—Enterobacteriaceae (without Pseudomonas species)	Uncomplicated urinary tract infections; Oral administration, low serum and tissue concentrations, renal elimination, short half-life.	[3,8,82,83]
2nd	Norfloxacin Ciprofloxacin Ofloxacin Pefloxacin	Enterobacteriaceae; Some atypical pathogens; Pseudomonas aeruginosa (ciprofloxacin only); Some Gram-positive pathogens (including Streptococcus pneumoniae), moderate activity on Staphylococcus aureus.	Uncomplicated and complicated urinary tract infections, pyelonephritis, sexually transmitted diseases, prostatitis, skin and tissue infections; Oral administration, low serum and tissue concentrations (only for norfloxacin); Oral and parenteral administration, high concentrations in serum and tissues, longer half-life.	[3,5,83–86]

Table 2. *Cont.*

Generation	Compounds	Antibacterial Spectrum	Therapeutic Indications/Pharmacokinetics, Administration	Ref.
2nd	Nadifloxacin (topical use)	Gram-positive (including methicillin-resistant Staphylococcus aureus (MRSA) and coagulase-negative staphylococci), aerobic Gram-negative, and anaerobic pathogens.	Treatment of acne vulgaris and other skin infections. Topical use, 1% cream.	[26,87–89]
3rd	Levofloxacin	Enterobacteriaceae; Atypical pathogens; Penicillin-resistant Streptococcus pneumoniae.	Acute and chronic bronchitis, exacerbated forms, acquired pneumonia (nosocomial); Oral and parenteral administration, high serum and tissue concentrations, long half-life (6–8 h). Ophthalmic use (0.5% ophthalmic solution).	[29,86,90,91]
3rd	Gatifloxacin (ophthalmic use)	Broad-spectrum including Staphylococcus aureus, Streptococcus species, and Gram-negative pathogens	Bacterial conjunctivitis, ophthalmic use (0.3% or 0.5% ophthalmic solution).	[43]
4th	Moxifloxacin	Enterobacteriaceae; Atypical pathogens; Pseudomonas aeruginosa; Streptococci; MRSA; Anaerobic pathogens. Others: Chlamydophila pneumoniae, Mycoplasma pneumonia	Sexually transmitted diseases; prostatitis, skin and tissue infections, acute and chronic bronchitis, exacerbated forms, acquired pneumonia (nosocomial), intra-abdominal infections, gynecological infections; bacterial conjunctivitis. Oral, parenteral, and ophthalmic administration (0.5%), high serum and tissue concentrations, long half-life (8–16 h).	[34,92,93]
4th	Delafloxacin	Gram-positive (including methicillin-resistant Staphylococcus aureus) and Gram-negative pathogens	Bacterial skin and skin structure infections. Oral and intravenous administration, oral bioavailability 58.8%, plasma protein binding 84%, mean half-life 4.2–8.5 h (oral), and 3.7 h (intravenous).	[39,41,94]
4th	Besifloxacin (topical, ophtalmic administration)	Streptococcus pneumonia, Staphylococcus epidermidis, Staphylococcus aureus, Haemophilus influenza, Moraxella catarrhalis, Corynebacterium spp	Bacterial conjunctivitis. Ophthalmic suspension (0.6%).	[46,95–97]
4th	Finafloxacin (topical, otic administration)	Broad-spectrum activity (very active against Pseudomonas aeruginosa, and Staphylococcus aureus)	Acute otitis externa. Otic suspension (0.3%)	[98–100]

5. Compounds in Therapy Since 2000

The class of FQNs has evolved significantly since 2000, acquiring valuable representatives for therapy, with a low risk of occurrence of antibacterial resistance (Figure 3). The fourth-generation antibacterial QNs are very active on the DNA gyrase and topoisomerase IV, enzymes involved in bacterial DNA replication, transcription, repair and recombination. Recently approved by FDA or EMA are besifloxacin (2009), finafloxacin (2014) and delafloxacin (2017). The action on the two target enzymes confers the advantage of being effective on bacteria resistant to FQNs from previous generations; the development of bacterial resistance to the fourth generation representatives with multi-target properties is more difficult [42].

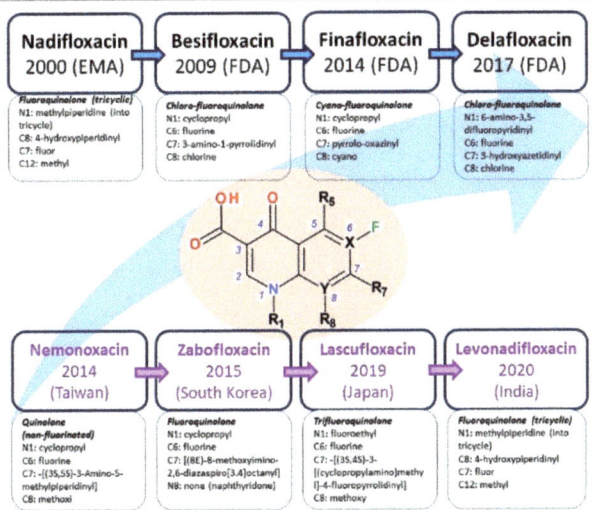

Figure 3. New FQNs chronology in therapy (since 2000) and essential structural characteristics.

The newest antibacterial 1,4-QNs used in therapy have diverse structural characteristics (Figure 4). According to the chemical structure of the base nucleus, these new compounds have a QN nucleus (besifloxacin, delafloxacin, finafloxacin, and nemonoxacin), a tricyclic ring including a QN nucleus (nadifloxacin), and naphthyridine nucleus (zabofloxacin). Regarding the presence of halogen atoms in the chemical structure, these compounds contain one fluorine atom (nadifloxacin and levonadifloxacin, finafloxacin, and zabofloxacin), one fluorine and one chlorine atom (besifloxacin), three fluorine atoms (lascufloxacin), three fluorine and one chlorine atoms (delafloxacin), but there is also an exception without any halogen atom (nemonoxacin).

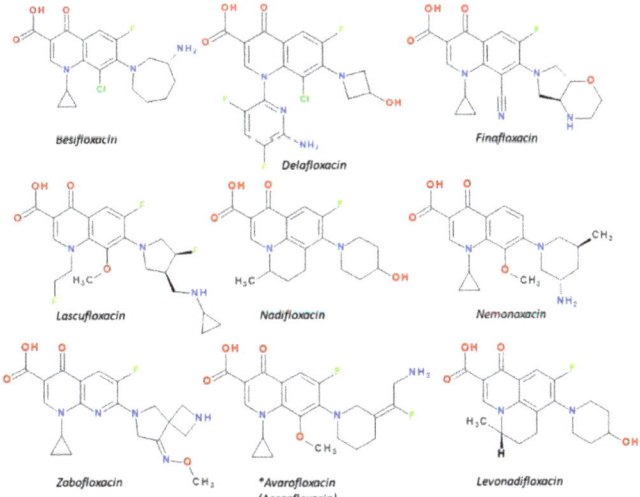

Figure 4. Chemical structures of newer approved antibacterial QNs (*final stage of approval).

Other FQNs from different generations that will be referred to for similarity to specific structural fragments, antibacterial activity or safety profile are described structurally in Figure S1—Supplementary Materials.

5.1. Besifloxacin

Besifloxacin is a chloro-FQN included in the fourth generation [101]. This new antibacterial molecule was developed for ophthalmic use by the SS Pharmaceutical SSP Co.Ltd. from Tokyo, Japan (former SS734). It has been approved by the FDA in 2009 and registered under the trade name Besivance (Bausch & Lomb Inc., Rochester, NY, USA) [46,98,101,102]. Besifloxacin is indicated for the treatment of bacterial conjunctivitis [98,103].

Besifloxacin's spectrum of activity includes various bacterial species (broad-spectrum) [104–106] described in Table S1—Supplementary Materials. As for its mechanism of action, besifloxacin inhibits the two target enzymes, DNA gyrase and topoisomerase IV, essential in DNA replication [107]. Physicochemical properties of besifloxacin are comprised in Table 3. Exclusive topical administration is a peculiarity in the class of FQNs [101]. Most ophthalmic FQNs are also systemically (e.g., ciprofloxacin, ofloxacin, levofloxacin, moxifloxacin) administered. Gatifloxacin is administered for ophthalmic use only after the withdrawal from systemic use due to its side effects (hypo- and hyperglycemia) [43,108,109]. The approved pharmaceutical formulation of besifloxacin is an ophthalmic suspension 0.6%, which contains 6.63 mg of besifloxacin hydrochloride (equivalent to 6 mg of besifloxacin) [46,95–97,107]. At present, attempts are being made to develop several ophthalmic pharmaceutical formulas with besifloxacin, such as nanoemulsions [110], positively charged liposomes [111], and for the treatment of bacterial keratitis new loaded nanofibrous ocular inserts [112].

Substitution at the N1 position in the FQN structure is essential for its antimicrobial activity. The N1 position substituent has been shown to control bacterial activity (potency) and some pharmacokinetic properties, like the increased volume of distribution and bioavailability [3]. That is why this substituent is common with other valuable FQNs such as ciprofloxacin and moxifloxacin (Figure S1—Supplementary Materials) [6,113,114]. It was considered that the cyclopropyl moiety from the N1 position of the QN nucleus confers besifloxacin activity against aerobic bacteria (Figure 5) [115].

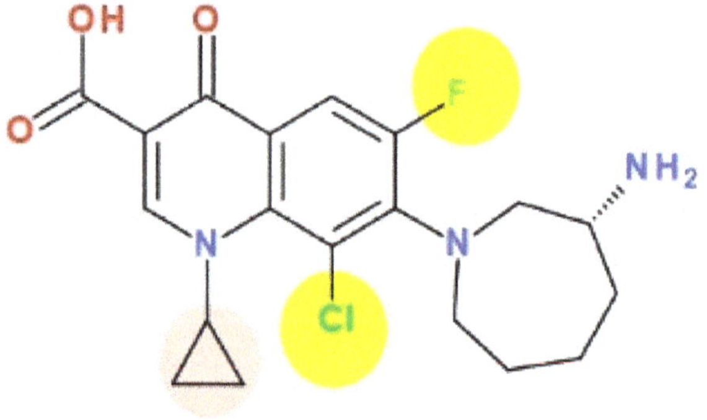

Figure 5. Chemical structure of besifloxacin.

Table 3. Physicochemical properties of besifloxacin.

Properties	Besifloxacin	Besifloxacin Hydrochloride	Ref.
Chemical name (IUPAC)	{7-[(3R)-3-aminohexahydro-1H-azepin-1-yl]-8-chloro-1-clyclopropyl-6-fluoro-1,4-dihydro-4-oxo-3-quinolinecarboxylic acid}	(+)-7-[(3R)-3-aminohexahydro-1H-azepin-1-yl]-8-chloro-1-cyclopropyl-6-fluoro-4-oxo-1,4-dihydroquinoline-3-carboxylic acid hydrochloride	[46] [97]
Chemical formula	$C_{19}H_{21}ClFN_3O_3$	$C_{19}H_{21}ClFN_3O_3 \cdot HCl$	[97]
Molecular weight	393.8 g/mol	430.40 g/mol	[116] [117]
Aspect	Not available	White to pale yellowish-white powder; white to light brown	[97,117,118]
Solubility	Insoluble in water 0.143 mg/mL (predicted values)	2 mg/mL (DMSO [1])	[46,106,116,118]
LogP	0.7; 0.54	Not available	[106]
pKa	• 6.0–7.0; 5.64—strongest acidic, 9.67—strongest basic (predicted values); • 5.45 (carboxyl), 9.84 (amino) (calculated)	Not available	[46,61,106,116]
Melting point	Not available	Over 210 °C; 270.04 °C	[117,119]
Storage	Not available	At refrigerator; −20 °C	[117,118]

[1] DMSO—Dimethyl sulfoxide.

Regarding the relationship between chemical structure and biological activity, substitution with a halogen (fluorine or chlorine) leads to decreased solubility, increased lipophilicity and increased penetration of the drug through cell membranes [120,121]. The electronic effects (inductive electron-attracting properties) are maximal for chlorine and very weak for fluorine [122]. The introduction of a fluorine atom at position C6 led to a spectacular increase in antimicrobial activity comparative to non-fluorinated QNs from the first generation. One fluorine atom in position C6 increased the degree of penetration into the bacterial cell and, at the same time, the activity against Gram-negative bacteria [6,113,114]. The fluorine atom appears to be essential in the mechanism of action.

A second substitution in the C8 position with a chlorine atom add an increased antimicrobial potency through the action on the target enzymes DNA gyrase and topoisomerase IV [46,123]. Also, C8 chlorine increases the antibacterial activity against FQN-resistant mutants of *Mycobacterium smegmatis* and *Staphylococcus aureus* [121].

Representatives of the second generation (ciprofloxacin, norfloxacin) with a piperazinyl group in the C7 position (Figure S1—Supplementary Materials) exhibit antibacterial activity against Gram-negative bacteria [6]. The C7 amino ring is a key substituent related to toxicity and solubility for analogues as clinafloxacin (with a 3-amino-1-pyrrolidinyl substituent) and sitafloxacin (with a (7S)-7-amino-5-azaspiro[2.4]heptan-5-yl) (Figure S1—Supplementary Materials). Unfortunately, clinafloxacin presented some side effects as phototoxicity and hypoglycemia. In addition, the solubility of clinafloxacin is poor and has inadequate stability in an aqueous solution [124]. Besifloxacin is administered only topically without systemic adverse reactions, being similar in terms of solubility. Assessment of besifloxacin toxicity conducted in silico presented a mutagenicity alert for two degradation products [125]. The replacement of the traditional piperazinyl group of the second generation with a hexahydro-1H-azepine cycle led to broadening the spectrum of activity on Gram-positive bacteria. The 3-aminohexahydro-1H-azepine ring contributes to specific action on the target enzyme DNA-gyrase, besifloxacin being superior to other FQNs in terms of antibacterial activity [126,127].

5.2. Delafloxacin

Delafloxacin is a recently approved FQN with an anionic chemical structure, from the fourth generation [38,128]. This new antibacterial molecule was developed for systemically use, both for oral and intravenous administration [39] by the Abbott Laboratories, Wakunaga Pharmaceutical (as ABT-492 compound or WQ-3034) and Melinta Therapeutics (former Rib-X Pharmaceuticals). It has been approved by the FDA in 2017 and registered under the trade name Baxdela for the treatment of acute bacterial skin and skin structure infections [39,129,130]. Physicochemical properties of delafloxacin are comprised in Table 4. The new product has the advantage of both oral and intravenous administration [131]. The parenteral form contains 433 mg delafloxacin meglumine (equivalent to 300 mg of delafloxacin) while the oral tablets contain 649 mg delafloxacin meglumine (equivalent to 300 mg of delafloxacin) [94]. Meglumine (1-deoxy-1-(methylamino)-D-glucitol) is a counterion used to increase the solubility of delafloxacin [132,133].

As a mechanism of action, delafloxacin inhibits the target enzymes DNA gyrase and topoisomerase IV, having a similar affinity for both [39,41]. An increased activity at acidic pH is an essential characteristic of this new chloro-FQN. Delafloxacin presents a broad spectrum of activity being active against both Gram-positive and Gram-negative bacteria, including methicillin-resistant *Staphylococcus aureus* (MRSA) and *Pseudomonas aeruginosa* (Table S1—Supplementary Materials) [130,134].

New formulations are being created to increase the effectiveness of delafloxacin. Optimized delafloxacin-loaded stearic acid (lipid) chitosan (polymer) hybrid nanoparticles proved to be superior comparative to delafloxacin standard suspension [135].

Table 4. Physicochemical properties of delafloxacin.

Delafloxacin	Properties	Ref.
Chemical name (IUPAC)	1-(6-amino-3,5-difluoropyridin-2-yl)-8-chloro-6-fluoro-7-(3-hydroxyazetidin-1-yl)-4-oxo-1,4-dihydroquinoline-3-carboxylic acid	[38,130]
Chemical formula	$C_{18}H_{12}ClF_3N_4O_4$	[38,130]
Molecular weight	440.8	[38]
Aspect	Powder, white to beige	[136]
Solubility	0.0699 mg/mL (in water); 20 mg/mL (in DMSO [1])	[136,137]
LogP	1.67 (predicted value)	[136,137]
pKa	• 5.4; 5.62 (strongest acidic); −1.3 (strongest basic); • 5.43 (carboxyl), −1.33 (piperidinic nitrogen atom), 14.77(hydroxyl)	[61,131,137]
Melting point	249.32 °C	[135,138]
Storage	Refrigerator: 2–8 °C	[136]

[1] DMSO—Dimethyl sulfoxide.

Delafloxacin differs from other FQNs by the substituent 3-hydroxyazetidinyl at the C7 position. Also, in the N1 position, delafloxacin has an unusual 6-amino-3,5-difluoropyridinyl moiety that substantially enlarges the molecule's molecular surface. This group is responsible for activity against Gram-positive bacteria [131,139]. This unique 3-hydroxyazetidinyl moiety on the C7 position confers acidic properties, and consequently, delafloxacin behaves as a weak acid (a non-zwitterion molecule with pKa 5.4) [131,139].

At acidic pH, delafloxacin is an uncharged molecule, which is favorable for its passage through biological membranes (Figure 6).

These properties give delafloxacin increased activity in an acidic pH environment with decreased minimal inhibitory concentrations (MIC). Intracellularly, at neutral pH delafloxacin will be ionized into the anionic form and thus remain inside the pathogen agent [140]. So, this drug is beneficial against abscesses produced in the infection with *Staphylococcus aureus* [131,140].

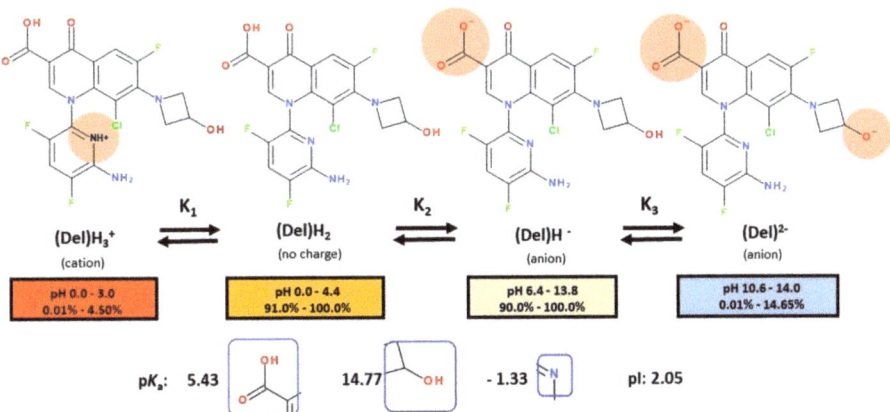

Figure 6. The macroprotonation scheme of delafloxacin and the step-wise protonation constants K_1, K_2 and K_3. The carboxylate, hydroxyl, and the pyridine ring's nitrogen atom (N1 position) are the most acidic, respectively, the most basic functions. All data were calculated with the MarvinSketch 20.20.0 version from ChemAxon [61].

In the C8 position, delafloxacin presents a chlorine substituent with an electron-withdrawing effect on the aromatic fragment of the QN nucleus (Figure 6), like besifloxacin (Figure 5). The chlorine substituent stabilizes delafloxacin molecule and could have a role in the reduction of the development of bacterial resistance. Thus, the whole polar molecule has increased activity [131,139]. C7 and C8 substitutions influence potency and spectrum of activity; both substitutions provide activity against anaerobic bacteria [139]. As a consequence, delafloxacin has proved activity against Gram-positive bacteria, especially against MRSA [139,141].

In the history of the development of FQNs, several trifluorinated molecules (e.g., fleroxacin, temafloxacin, trovafloxacin; Figure S1—Supplementary Materials) have been withdrawn due to severe side effects (Table 1). Fleroxacin (with N1-fluoroethyl, C6-fluor, C8-fluor) was the first promising trifluorinated representative but it was withdrawn due to severe phototoxic reactions [142]. Also, temafloxacin (with N1-difluorophenyl) has been withdrawn due to severe hemolysis [19]. Finally, trovafloxacin (with N1-difluorophenyl) has been withdrawn due to hepatotoxicity [142]. Unlike temafloxacin and trovafloxacin, delafloxacin contains a 6-amino-3,5-difluoropyridinyl substituent. This substituent appears to be more advantageous in reducing possible adverse reactions that have led to the withdrawal of the other trifluorinated compounds. However, the effects imprinted by the other substituents and the type of base nucleus must also be considered.

5.3. Finafloxacin

Finafloxacin (BAY35-3377) is a recent cyano-FQN included in the fourth generation. This new antibacterial molecule was developed by Bayer HealthCare Pharmaceuticals, Byk Gulden and MerLion Pharmaceuticals [42,50,99,143]. Relevant physicochemical properties are listed in Table 5. The FDA approved an otic suspension in 2014 and registered under the trade name Xtoro (developed by Novartis's division, Alcon, Geneva, Switzerland). Finafloxacin is indicated for the treatment of acute otitis externa [42,99].

At the same time, finafloxacin is in various stages of clinical trials to evaluate the efficacy of oral and intravenous formulations. These forms are intended for the treatment of uncomplicated and complicated urinary tract infections, pyelonephritis and *Helicobacter pylori* infections [99,144–147]. Finafloxacin has demonstrated broad-spectrum activity against a range of pathogens [148]. This cyano-FQN is active both in vitro and in vivo against *Pseudomonas aeruginosa* and *Staphylococcus aureus* [99].

As for the mechanism of action, similar to fourth-generation representatives, finafloxacin has a high affinity for the two target enzymes, DNA-gyrase and topoisomerase IV [99]. Antimicrobial activity of finafloxacin is enhanced in acidic conditions (pH 5.8) against multiple pathogens, including skin and urinary pathogens. Finafloxacin exhibits activity at neutral pH comparable to previous generations of FQNs. Also, a more prolonged post-antibacterial effect against multiple species was observed compared to other FQNs at acidic pH. The development of bacterial resistance to finafloxacin is less likely in acidic conditions [99,100,149,150].

Table 5. Physicochemical properties of finafloxacin.

Properties	Finafloxacin	References
Chemical name (IUPAC)	(-)-8-Cyano-1-cyclopropyl-6-fluoro-7-((4aS,7aS)-hexahydropyrrolo(3,4-b)-1,4-oxazin-6(2H)-yl)-4-oxo-1,4-dihydroquinoline-3-carboxylic acid	[49,99,151]
Chemical formula	$C_{20}H_{19}FN_4O_4$	[49]
Molecular weight	398.4	[49]
Aspect	Powder, white to beige; white to yellowish (hydrochloride salt);	[152,153]
Solubility	0.208 mg/mL (in water) 2 mg/mL (in DMSO [1]) 5.5 mg/mL (in water, hydrochloride salt)	[151–153]
LogP	−0.5; −1.1 (predicted)	[151]
pKa	5.6 (carboxylate) and 7.8 (nitrogen at C7)	[143,153]
Melting point	Not available	
Storage	−20 °C	[152]

[1] DMSO—Dimethyl sulfoxide.

The molecule optimizations include a pyrrolo-oxazinyl moiety at the C7 position and a cyano-substituent at the C8 position (Figure 7). Bearing a zwitterion chemical structure (carboxylate at C3 position and pyrrolo-oxazinyl at C7 position) finafloxacin presents two dissociation constants (Table 5) [143]. The voluminous C7 substituent confers to the molecule's unique characteristic of not being recognized by efflux transporters, the key to decreased bacterial resistance development [48]. The C7 pyrrolo-oxazinyl fragment emerged from the C7 azabicycle (pyrrolidine-piperidine) fragment of moxifloxacin and pradofloxacin (Figure 7), which confers the ability to remain longer in the bacterial cell (difficult to efflux molecules) [154,155].

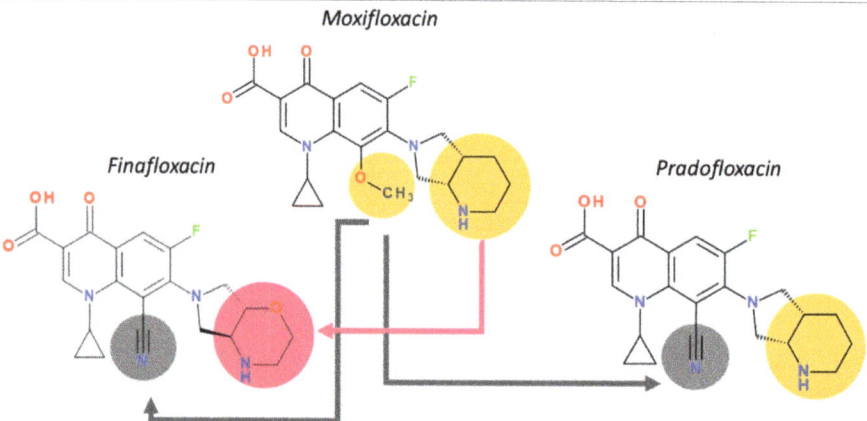

Figure 7. Relevant structural elements to the antibacterial activity of moxifloxacin (C7—pyrrolo-piperidinyl, C8—methoxi), pradofloxacin (C7—pyrrolo-piperidinyl, C8—cyano) and finafloxacin (C7—pyrrolo-oxazinyl, C8—cyano).

A cyano-substituent at C8 is also present in the chemical structure of pradofloxacin, a veterinary-approved FQN classified in the third generation. This compound can be considered an analogue of moxifloxacin (fourth generation) due to the methoxy group at the C8 position which has been replaced by a cyano group. Pradofloxacin is more active against Gram-positive bacteria comparative to previous generations. Also, pradofloxacin exhibits good activity against anaerobic bacteria, similar to moxifloxacin, and an equal or lower activity against Gram-negative bacteria [36,156,157]. The C8 cyano group appears to play an essential role in activity against Gram-positive when comparing finafloxacin with pradofloxacin (Figure 7).

At the N1 position, finafloxacin has a cyclopropyl substituent similar to second-generation ciprofloxacin and fourth-generation besifloxacin.

Finafloxacin and delafloxacin in acidic conditions (pH 5.0–6.0 and respectively pH ≤ 5.5) are more active than other FQNs, but for different reasons. In the key C7 position of delafloxacin, the 3-hydroxyazetidine without a basic group is the substituent that confers acidic properties. In finafloxacin, the nitrogen atom from the oxazine fragment is responsible for the great activity in acidic conditions (can accept protons) [42,61]. In acidic conditions, finafloxacin is very active against *Staphylococcus aureus* due to an increased uptake in the bacteria [48].

5.4. Lascufloxacin

Lascufloxacin (KRP-AM1977) is a new FQN (Figure 8) developed in Japan by Kyorin Pharmaceutical Co., Ltd. [158]. Some physicochemical properties of lascufloxacin are comprised in Table 6.

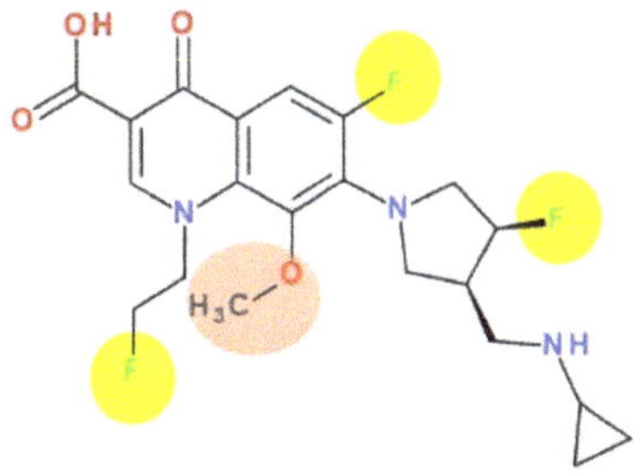

Figure 8. Chemical structure of lascufloxacin.

Table 6. Physicochemical properties of lascufloxacin.

Lascufloxacin	Properties	References
Chemical name (IUPAC)	7-[(3S,4S)-3-[(cyclopropylamino)methyl]-4-fluoropyrrolidin-1-yl]-6-fluoro-1-(2-fluoroethyl)-8-methoxy-4-oxoquinoline-3-carboxylic acid	[159]
Chemical formula	$C_{21}H_{24}F_3N_3O_4$	[159]
Molecular weight	439.4 g/mol	[159]
Aspect	White to off-white solid powder	[160]
Solubility	Slightly soluble in chloroform, very slightly soluble in DMSO [1], insoluble in water	[160,161]
LogP	1.79 (nonionic species)	[61]
pKa	5.64 (carboxyl), 9.75 (secondary amino group)—calculated	[61]
Melting point	Not available	
Storage	0–4 °C (short term, days to weeks); −20 °C (long term, months), dry and dark conditions	[162]

[1] DMSO—Dimethyl sulfoxide.

This new antibacterial agent was approved recently in Japan (2019) as a hydrochloride salt (oral formulation, Lasvic® 75 mg tablets) for the treatment of respiratory infections (including community-acquired pneumonia (CAP)) and ear, nose and throat infections [163,164]. Lascufloxacin acts by binding to the target enzymes, DNA gyrase and topoisomerase IV (inhibiting DNA synthesis), similar to other antibacterial FQNs [165]. Also, lascufloxacin demonstrated a high binding capacity to phosphatidylserine (a component of human cell membranes; primary surfactant of alveolar epithelial fluid). Lascufloxacin is superior in tissue penetration (head and neck infections) compared with levofloxacin, garenoxacin, and moxifloxacin [158].

Lascufloxacin proved to be very active against Gram-positive bacteria, including resistant species (Table S1—Supplementary Materials). Also, lascufloxacin is very promising against FQN-resistant pathogens located in the respiratory tract [166–168]. For example, a potent activity of lascufloxacin was proved against first-step mutants of *Streptococcus pneumoniae*. Being a new FQN, lascufloxacin has a significant potential to fight against the installation of bacterial resistance in pneumococcal infections [169].

Another formulation for parenteral administration (KRPAM1977Y) was recently approved in Japan (November 2020) [56,163,164]. Lasvic® is the generic brand and contains lascufloxacin hydrochloride 150 mg [163]. A phase I clinical study of lascufloxacin was recently performed in Japan. The pharmacokinetic and safety profile was assessed in non-elderly healthy men comparative to elderly healthy men. The obtained results proved that lascufloxacin has a safe pharmacokinetic profile without dose adjustments for the two groups of men [170]. The average half-life of lascufloxacin is about 16.1 h after 100 mg (orally administered) [168]. This new FQN presented an extensive distribution into the lungs [171].

The substitution with a fluoroethyl of the N1 position is similar to the fleroxacin, the first trifluorinated antibacterial QN, whose use has been limited by the severe phototoxicity [142]. The fluoroethyl substituent was correlated with the photosensitising effect [172,173]. However, according to the data published so far lascufloxacin has a good safety profile [170].

In the C7 position, FQNs usually have nitrogen heterocycles (five or six atoms), aminopyrrolidines and piperazines. In lascufloxacin chemical structure, an unusual structural fragment is present in the C7 position, a main pyrrolidine heterocycle substituted with a (cyclopropylamino)methyl moiety. This position is essential for interaction with DNA gyrase or topoisomerase IV [114,174,175]. Also, an aminopyrrolidine improves Gram-positive activity, proven by the clinafloxacin representative [176]. Thus, clinafloxacin (with a C8 chlorine atom) was associated with severe side effects (phototoxicity hypoglycaemia) [18]. Sitafloxacin, a FQN approved in Japan (2008) and Thailand (2012) contains in the C7 position a pyrrolidinyl fragment included in a spiro substituent, [(7S)-7-amino-5-azaspiro[2.4]heptanyl] [57,177]. This FQN produces mild to moderate adverse reactions (mostly gastrointestinal disorders and laboratory abnormalities, phototoxicity potential) [178,179]. Another pyrrolidinyl fragment is found in the structure of zabofloxacin, also included in a spiro substituent, [(8Z)-8-methoxyimino-2,6-diazaspiro[3.4]octanyl] (chapter 5.7). Unlike sitafloxacin, zabofloxacin is considered a well-tolerated FQN with acceptable side effects [143].

The methoxy substituent in the C8 position improves activity and enhances antimicrobial potency, especially against anaerobic bacteria [158], similar to moxifloxacin and pradofloxacin [34,36,114].

5.5. Nadifloxacin and Levonadifloxacin

Nadifloxacin is the first FQN approved for dermatological use, being classified in the second generation. This new antibacterial molecule was developed by the Otsuka Pharmaceuticals from Japan (former OPC-7251) [27]. The physicochemical properties of nadifloxacin are comprised in Table 7. It has been approved in Japan in 1993 (Aqutim) and in several countries in the European Union (2000). Nadifloxacin was initially approved for the treatment of acne vulgaris, and then for other skin infections (1998) [26,89,180,181]. The approved topical formulation is a cream containing 1% nadifloxacin [89,180].

Nadifloxacin proved to be effective against Gram-positive (including MRSA and coagulase-negative staphylococci), aerobic Gram-negative, and anaerobic bacteria (Table S1—Supplementary Materials) [88]. Superior antibacterial activity of nadifloxacin has been reported comparative with ciprofloxacin, clindamycin and erythromycin against *Propionibacterium acnes*, *Staphylococcus epidermidis*, methicillin-susceptible *Staphylococcus aureus* (MSSA), and MRSA. Moreover, nadifloxacin did not have an additional effect on resistance [182].

Regarding the mechanism of action, nadifloxacin inhibits the enzyme DNA gyrase, involved in the synthesis and replication of bacterial DNA [180,183]. Also, nadifloxacin proved to have inhibitory effects upon activated T cells and keratinocytes, as a part of the mechanism involved in its effect against inflammatory acne [87].

Table 7. Physicochemical properties of nadifloxacin.

Nadifloxacin	Properties	References
Chemical name (IUPAC)	7-fluoro-8-(4-hydroxypiperidin-1-yl)-12-methyl-4-oxo-1-azatricyclo[7.3.1.0^{5,13}]trideca-2,5,7,9(13)-tetraene-3-carboxylic acid	[184]
Chemical formula	$C_{19}H_{21}FN_2O_4$	[184]
Molecular weight	360.4 g/mol	[184]
Aspect	White; light yellow powder	[185,186]
Solubility	25 mg/mL (in DMF [1]), 20 mg/mL (in DMSO [2]), 0.25 mg/mL (in ethanol), insoluble in water	[185–188]
LogP	2.47; 1.77 (calculated)	[61,187]
pKa	5.94 (carboxyl), 0.44 (piperidinic nitrogen atom), 15.18 (hydroxyl)	[61]
Melting point	245–247 °C (decomposition)	[87,189]
Storage	−20 °C	[188,189]

[1] DMF—Dimethylformamide, [2] DMSO—Dimethyl sulfoxide.

Nadifloxacin (Figure 9) is a tricyclic FQN very similar to ofloxacin (Figure S1—Supplementary Materials) [184,190]. The essential modification is the replacement in the C8 position of the methyl-piperazine moiety from the ofloxacin structure with a 4-hydroxypiperidine moiety. Nadifloxacin is considered a lipophilic compound compared to ofloxacin (logP = −0.39) [191,192]. In therapy, nadifloxacin is used as a racemic [26]. However, the two enantiomers have different biological activities. Thus, it is known that the levorotatory (S)-isomer is 64- to 256-times more potent than the (R)-isomer. Also, the levorotatory (S)-isomer is approximately twice as active as the racemate against Gram-positive and Gram-negative pathogens [180]. This stereoisomer is under study as an arginine salt for intravenous administration (WCK 771) and is known as levonadifloxacin [193]. In general, the introduction of hydroxyl groups into the structure of a compound will produce analogues with increased hydrophilicity and low solubility in lipids. The hydroxyl group into the chemical structure provides a new center for hydrogen bonding, which can influence the binding of the analogue to the active center of the target, the biological activity, and metabolism [120]. The introduction of a hydroxyl group on the piperidine heterocycle at position C8 confers a slight increase of the hydrophilic character of nadifloxacin and an increase of acidic properties. However, the molecule has a LogP 2.47, which denotes increased lipophilia and low aqueous solubility. This structural optimization is present in the structure of delafloxacin, but on an azetidine heterocycle on C7 position. Nevertheless, the LogP value of delafloxacin is lower (1.67—predicted value) than that of nadifloxacin.

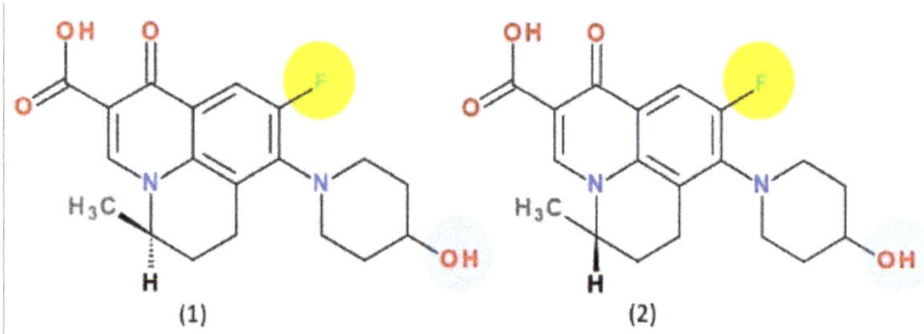

Figure 9. Chemical structures of nadifloxacin (**1**) and levonadifloxacin (**2**).

Levonadifloxacin ((12S)-7-fluoro-8-(4-hydroxypiperidin-1-yl)-12-methyl-4-oxo-1-azatricyclo[7.3.1.05,13]trideca-2,5,7,9(13)-tetraene-3-carboxylic acid) is the active $S(-)$ isomer of nadifloxacin recently approved in India (Figure 9) [194,195]. The $S(-)$ isomer of nadifloxacin, has been shown to be more potent than the $R(+)$ isomer and twice as active as the racemic form of nadifloxacin against Gram-positive and Gram-negative bacteria. It is a new broad-spectrum anti-MRSA agent belonging to the benzoquinolizine subclass of QN [180,195].

Levonadifloxacin (WCK 771) (S-(−)-9-fluoro-6,7-dihydro-8-(4-hydroxypiperidin-1-yl)-5-methyl-1-oxo-1H,5H-benzo[i,j] quinolizine-2-carboxylic acid L-arginine salt tetrahydrate) is administered parenterally (intravenous) in the form of an L-arginine salt while its prodrug alalevonadifloxacin (WCK 2349) ((S)-(−)-9-fluoro-8-(4-L-alaninyl oxypiperidin-1-yl)-5-methyl-6,7-dihydro-1-oxo-1H,5H-benzo[i,j] quinolizine-2-carboxylic acid, methane sulfonic acid salt) in the form developed of an L-alanine ester mesylate salt can be administered orally. Both substances are being developed by Wockhardt Limited (India) [193,196].

Both levonadifloxacin and alalevonadifloxacin have successfully completed phase II and phase III trials, indicating that they are clinically appealing therapeutic alternatives for infections caused by multidrug-resistant Gram-positive pathogens. Due to simultaneous inhibition of DNA gyrase and topoisomerase IV, both representatives exhibit significant antibacterial activity against Gram-negative and Gram-positive bacteria, with an emphasis on MRSA [193,197,198]. Levonadifloxacin has the advantage of being potent against resistant pathogens with a very low frequency of mutation [199,200]. Both substances have been studied for the treatment of acute skin and skin structure bacterial infections, community-acquired bacterial pneumonia, and other infections in both non-clinical and clinical studies [193,197,199].

Because of its non-basic hydroxy piperidine side chain, levonadifloxacin remains un-ionized at acidic pH, allowing it to enter the bacterial cell more easily. As a result, levonadifloxacin's efficacy in acidic conditions increases significantly; this characteristic might be helpful for intracellular activity and antibacterial action [197]. Various in vitro and in vivo investigations have established levonadifloxacin's antibacterial spectrum against Gram-positive, Gram-negative, atypical, and anaerobic pathogens [201].

The excellent bioavailability of oral formulations can be helpful in the smooth switch from parenteral to oral therapy. Both medication forms have well-established pharmacokinetics and safety; in the phase I trial, there were no notable severe or unfavourable clinical or laboratory side effects, indicating that both formulations are well tolerated [193].

5.6. Nemonoxacin

Nemonoxacin is a new non-fluorinated QN chemotherapeutic (Figure 10). Nemonoxacin (TG-873870) was developed by TaiGen Biotechnology under the commercial name of Taigexyn® for the treatment of CAP, both orally and intravenously as well as the treatment of diabetic foot ulcer infections and skin and soft tissue infections [202]. Procter & Gamble initially developed nemonoxacin, and TaiGen Biotechnology was granted a worldwide license in October 2004. In March 2014, it gained its first global approval in Taiwan to treat CAP in adults. TaiGen Biotechnology holds the nemonoxacin patent portfolio, which protects the drug's use, composition, and manufacturing techniques until 2029 [53,54].

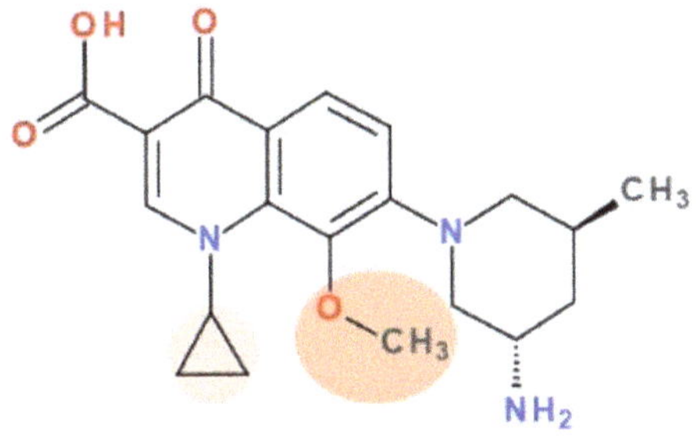

Figure 10. Chemical structure of nemonoxacin.

A clinical study (phase II) regarding the safety and efficacy of nemonoxacin in diabetic foot infections was completed [203,204]. As a result, the FDA authorized oral administration of nemonoxacin to treat CAP and bacterial skin infections [166,205,206].

Taigexyn product contains nemonoxacin malate hemihydrate salt [207,208]. The understudy intravenously administered formula contains nemonoxacin malate sodium chloride [209]. Physicochemical properties of nemonoxacin are comprised in Table 8.

Table 8. Physico-chemical properties of nemonoxacin.

Nemonoxacin	Properties	References
Chemical name (IUPAC)	7-[(3S,5S)-3-Amino-5-methylpiperidin-1-yl]-1-cyclopropyl-8-methoxy-4-oxo-1,4-dihydroquinoline-3-carboxylic acid	[210,211]
Chemical formula	$C_{20}H_{25}N_3O_4$	[210,211]
Molecular weight	371.4 g/mol	[210,211]
Aspect	Not available	
Solubility	Insoluble in water 0.453 mg/mL (predicted values)	[212]
LogP	0.32; −0.44	[212]
pKa	• 5.73—strongest acidic, 9.66—strongest basic (predicted values); • 5.53 (carboxyl), 0.28 (piperidinic atom nitrogen), 9.83 (amino)	[212] [61]
Melting point	Not available	
Storage	Not available	

The QN ring's C8 methoxy substituent improves antibacterial efficacy against Gram-positive bacteria and lowers the selection of resistant variants. The fluorine substituent absence may reduce the frequency of dangerous side effects [143]. The addition of a methoxy group at position C8 allows nemonoxacin to target both DNA gyrase and topoisomerase IV, resulting in a broader spectrum of activity and less mutant selection [213,214].

Nemonoxacin is similar to gatifloxacin (a fourth-generation FQN) (Figure S1—Supplementary Materials), except for the lack of C6 substitutions of fluorine and the 5′-methyl piperidinyl ring at C7 position of the QN ring [215,216]. Gatifloxacin proved to be more active against *Streptococcus pneumoniae* than second generation ciprofloxacin or the third generation levofloxacin [34,216]. This increased activity against *Streptococcus pneumoniae* is similar to moxifloxacin, another fourth-generation FQN with a methoxy group at C8 [34]. The C8 methoxy group of nemonoxacin probably potentiates the same level of inhibition of DNA gyrase and topoisomerase IV in *Streptococcus pneumoniae* cells, and confers low mutant selectivity [216].

The introduction of a piperidine substituent to C7 has not been common in the past. Few representatives were obtained with a piperidine substituent in the C7 position. Among them is balofloxacin (Figure S1—Supplementary Materials), developed by Choongwae Pharma and approved only in Korea to treat urinary tract infections [32]. At the C7 position, balofloxacin exhibits a 3-(methylamino)piperidinyl moiety [217]. Balofloxacin did not have the expected success. This FQN from the third generation reported total adverse drug reaction rates of 5.4% compared to levofloxacin (1.3%). The side effects reported were gastrointestinal, CNS and skin-related [18,23,218]. Shankar et al. (2018) published the predicted toxicity of balofloxacin and its metabolites (*in silico* study); most of the metabolites are found to be immunotoxic [219]. Avarofloxacin (acorafloxacin, JNJ-Q2) is a new promising FQN in development with a piperidine substituent in the C7 (discussed in a later chapter) [143,220].

In vitro investigations have shown that nemonoxacin has broad-spectrum antibacterial activity, including activity against microorganisms resistant to other antibacterial drugs, including multidrug-resistant *Streptococcus pneumoniae* and MRSA [221,222]. It is used to treat Gram-positive and Gram-negative bacterial infections, including MSSA and MRSA, with once-daily oral and intravenous preparations. Nemonoxacin presented higher activity than levofloxacin and ciprofloxacin against a variety of Gram-positive bacteria, including resistant species. For Gram-negative bacteria such as *Escherichia coli, Hemophilus influenzae, Klebsiella pneumoniae,* and *Pseudomonas aeruginosa,* nemonoxacin activity was equivalent to levofloxacin and ciprofloxacin [223]. In vitro testing of nemonoxacin against 2440 clinical isolates revealed that it had better efficacy against most Gram-positive species than levofloxacin and moxifloxacin [224]. In the murine model of systemic, pulmonary, or ascending urinary tract infection, nemonoxacin outperforms the most commonly used FQNs [225]. Compared to other FQNs, nemoxacin has a low predisposition for generating resistant infections because bacteria develop resistance to nemonoxacin only when three distinct mutations happen in the QN resistance-determining region of the relevant gene [214].

Nemonoxacin has a favourable pharmacokinetic profile, being rapidly absorbed, having a high bioavailability, and a large distribution volume; it has a relatively long elimination half-life of more than 10 h and achieves maximum concentration (C_{max}) 1–2 h after oral administration. Approximately 60–75% of the given dosage is excreted in an unaltered state; only a minor metabolite (5%) was identified due to metabolic processes [213,226]. Nemonoxacin is well tolerated, the gastrointestinal and neurological system-related are the most prevalent side effects of oral administration, with a frequency equivalent to that of levofloxacin therapy [227].

Nemonoxacin may play a significant role in the treatment of many infectious illnesses due to its equivalent or higher potency against Gram-positive bacteria and similar activity against Gram-negative pathogens when compared with other classic FQNs.

5.7. Zabofloxacin

Zabofloxacin is a FQN approved in 2015 only in South Korea [55,56]. The new compound (PB-101, DW224a, DW224aa) was developed by Dong Wha Pharm. Co. Ltd. (Seoul, Korea) [56]. There were two salts in development: DW224a as zabofloxacin hydrochloride, and DW224aa as zabofloxacin aspartate [228]. The physicochemical properties of zabofloxacin are comprised in Table 9. Zabofloxacin is marketed under the name Zabolante to treat acute bacterial exacerbation of chronic obstructive pulmonary disease by oral administration. Zabolante contains 512.98 mg zabofloxacin aspartate hydrate (equivalent to 366.69 mg of zabofloxacin) [56,229].

Zabofloxacin activity is mainly against Gram-negative and Gram-positive respiratory pathogens, especially against *Streptococcus pneumoniae,* and drug-resistant *Neisseria gonorrhoeae* (Table S1—Supplementary Materials) [230–232]. In Phase III clinical trial zabofloxacin

(367 mg once daily; 5 days) proved to be as efficient as moxifloxacin (400 mg once daily; 7 days) in treating chronic obstructive pulmonary disease exacerbations [92].

Zabofloxacin mechanism of action is similar to other FQNs with a broad spectrum against respiratory pathogens [233].

Table 9. Physicochemical properties of zabofloxacin.

Zabofloxacin	Properties	References
Chemical name (IUPAC)	1-cyclopropyl-6-fluoro-7-[(8E)-8-methoxyimino-2,6-diazaspiro[3.4]octan-6-yl]-4-oxo-1,8-naphthyridine-3-carboxylic acid	[234]
Chemical formula	$C_{19}H_{20}FN_5O_4$	[234]
Molecular weight	401.4 g/mol	[234]
Aspect	Not available	
Solubility	0.196 mg/mL in water (calculated)	[235]
LogP	−0.89 (calculated); 2.43 for non ionic species	[61,235]
pKa	• 5.53—strongest acidic, 9.41—strongest basic; • 5.34 (carboxyl), 2.66 (N8 atom), 0.30 (N imino), 9.50 (N6' from spiro heterocycle) (calculated)	[61,235]
Melting point	155 °C	[236]
Storage	Not available	

Unlike previous compounds in the class of new antibacterial QNs, zabofloxacin is a fluoronaphthyridone (Figure 11) [56].

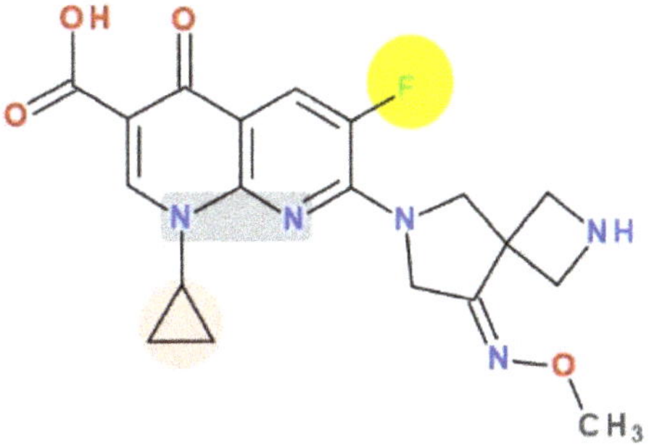

Figure 11. Chemical structure of zabofloxacin.

At the C7 position, zabofloxacin has an unusual heterocycle, a spiro substituent (2,6-diazaspiro[3.4]octan) substituted in C8' with an imino methoxy group. This new compound could be considered an analogue of gemifloxacin (from the fourth-generation) by optimizing the heterocycle from position C7 (Figure S1—Supplementary Materials) [34]. Although the antibacterial activity of gemifloxacin was superior to moxifloxacin, unfortunately, due to side effects (mainly rash), it was withdrawn [34,45]. Increasing the volume of the C7 heterocycle by maintaining the substituted methoxy-imino pyrrolidine ring resulted in a compound with acceptable side effects [228]. Various spiro compounds with antibacterial activity have been published [237–240].

6. Is the Fifth Generation of Antibacterial FQNs Outlined?

The therapeutic value of the newer FQNs discussed in this review is undeniable. This recent evolution in the class of FQNs is based on several essential elements of the chemical structure, which are further analyzed (Table 10).

Table 10. Essential moieties on the QN nucleus for the newer compounds.

Position (Atom)	Substituent	Moieties' Chemical Structure	Antibacterial QN
1 (C)	Cyclopropyl	(cyclopropyl structure)	Besifloxacin, Finafloxacin, Nemonoxacin, Zabofloxacin
	6-Amino-3,5-difluoropyridinyl	(6-amino-3,5-difluoropyridinyl structure)	Delafloxacin
6 (C)	Fluor	–F	All compounds, except nemonoxacin
7 (C)	3-Aminoazepane	(3-aminoazepane structure)	Besifloxacin
	3-Hydroxyazetidinyl	(3-hydroxyazetidinyl structure)	Delafloxacin
	Pyrrolo-oxazinyl	(pyrrolo-oxazinyl structure)	Finafloxacin
	3-Amino-5-methylpiperidinyl	(3-amino-5-methylpiperidinyl structure)	Nemonoxacin
	2,6-Diazaspiro[3.4]octanyl	(2,6-diazaspiro[3.4]octanyl structure)	Zabofloxacin
	[(Cyclopropylamino)methyl]-4-fluoropyrrolidinyl	(structure)	Lascufloxacin
8 (7 [1]) (C)	4-Hydroxypiperidinyl	(4-hydroxypiperidinyl structure)	Nadifloxacin [2] and levonadifloxacin

20

Table 10. *Cont.*

Position (Atom)	Substituent	Moieties' Chemical Structure	Antibacterial QN
8 (C)	Chloride	–Cl	Besifloxacin
			Delafloxacin
	Cyano group	–CN	Finafloxacin
	Methoxy	–O–CH$_3$	Nemonoxacin
8 (N)	Lack of substituent	none	Zabofloxacin
9 (8 [3])	Condensation of quinolone nucleus with methylpiperidine		Nadifloxacin

[1] Similar to C7 on QN nucleus; [2] Tricyclic structure; [3] Similar to C8 on QN nucleus.

The substituent at the N1 position increased potency, antibacterial activity and pharmacokinetic properties [241]. Cyclopropyl is known as the most potent optimization at the N1 position [113]. Thus, the substitution to N1 with cyclopropyl was preferred in four chemical structures of new FQNs (Table 10). An interesting issue is that in the past difluorophenyl in the N1 position was associated with several side effects (temafloxacin, trovafloxacin) [177]. This substitution is optimized in the chemical structure of delafloxacin with a 6-amino-3,5-difluoropyridinyl moiety. Basic groups are known to form salts in biological media. Substitution with basic groups will produce analogues with lower lipophilia and increased solubility in water. The more basic is the optimized molecule, the more likely it is to form salts and the less likely it is to be transported through a lipid membrane. The introduction of an amino group is likely to increase the binding of delafloxacin to target enzymes via hydrogen bonds [120]. The substituted pyridine residue proved to be more advantageous for the safety profile of delafloxacin comparative to older FQNs [134]. However, it should be noted that the incorporation of an aromatic amine (considered a toxophore) into the structure of a compound is avoided because aromatic amines are often highly toxic and carcinogenic [120].

The fluorine atom has an essential role in medicinal chemistry. Comparative to hydrogen, fluorine atom has small size, van der Waals radius of 1.47 Å versus van der Waals radius of 1.20 Å. In addition, the fluorine atom is highly electron-withdrawing (with impact on pK_a), the C-F bond is more stable than the C-H bond, and the lipophilicity of the fluorinated molecule is higher than the non-fluorinated version. Also, substitution with a fluorine atom confers metabolic stability, influences the metabolic pathways and pharmacokinetic properties, increases the permeability of the molecule through cell membranes and the binding affinity to the target proteins [242,243]. Changes in potency produced by the introduction of a halogen-containing substituent or halogen group depend on the substitution position [120]. In the C6 position, the fluorine substituent increased the potency of FQNs versus non-fluorinated QNs. The fluorine atom increased the bacterial cell penetration and the affinity to the DNA-gyrase [113,241]. Over time, most synthesized compounds retain fluoride substitution at C6. All new compounds discussed in this review have a fluorine atom in position 6 (respectively 7 for nadifloxacin), except nemonoxacin. The other structural optimizations in the case of nemonoxacin compensated for the effect that the fluorine atom would have brought.

The substituent from the C7 position increased potency, the spectrum of antibacterial activity, safety profile, and pharmacokinetic properties. This position on the QN nucleus was most often targeted for structural optimizations. Advantageous optimizations for antibacterial activity were a five or six-membered nitrogen heterocycle, four-membered heterocycle, piperazinyl, fluorine or chlorine atoms, substituted hydrazine fragment or bicyclic substitution [241].

A C7 pyrrolidine substituent increases the activity against Gram-positive bacteria. An attempt to optimize the structure of FQNs with a C7 pyrrolidine substituent was clinafloxacin [244,245]. Although it had potential antibacterial clinafloxacin was associated with phototoxicity and hypoglycaemia [18].

Lascufloxacin contains an optimized pyrrolidine nucleus which confers great potential for treating respiratory infections (including CAP) and ear, nose and throat infections [158,246]. Regarding the new compounds, the pyrrolidine nucleus is found condensed with another heterocycle (morpholine) in finafloxacin's chemical structure. In zabofloxacin's chemical structure, the pyrrolidine nucleus is part of a spiro fragment.

A potential increase of antibacterial activity may appear with C7 and C8 cyclization. C8 substituents are essential for target affinity, because of the planar configuration of the molecule. Fluorine or chlorine, methyl or methoxy substituents proved to enhance antibacterial potency [247]. Out of these, the methoxy substituent is found in the structure of the representatives with potent anaerobic activity (e.g., moxifloxacin). Furthermore, the carbon atom at the C8 position can be replaced with nitrogen in naphthyridonic representatives with broad-spectrum activity (gemifloxacin, zabofloxacin) [244].

The third generation levofloxacin, and fourth generation moxifloxacin, are used against *Mycobacterium tuberculosis* [12,13]. The fourth generation exhibits broad-spectrum activity against Gram-positive and Gram-negative bacteria. Also, these representatives are active against anaerobes and atypical bacteria [243].

Jones et al. (2016) consider that avarofloxacin (acorafloxaxin, JNJ-Q2) is a new FQN from the fifth generation (chapter 8). This new compound is highly active against drug-resistant pathogens as MRSA, ciprofloxacin-resistant MRSA, and drug-resistant *Streptococcus pneumoniae* [248].

Although the mechanism of action of new FQNs(QNs) is based on the activity on the two target enzymes, DNA gyrase and topoisomerase IV, some particular aspects emerge from the structural and biological properties of the new compounds:

- the majority of the new representatives have a broad spectrum of activity, including activity against anaerobic bacteria (except nemonoxacin);
- the new representatives are active against many resistant bacteria (including resistant to FQNs); this is the main advantage of the newly approved compounds;
- some representatives are very active in the environment with acidic pH (delafloxacin, finafloxacin), this being an advantage over previous generations' representatives;
- some representatives were approved only for a specific type of administration (topic); these are very effective in the treatment of targeted infections (besifloxacin, finafloxacin); for these compounds, there are numerous ongoing clinical trials for oral or parenteral administration;
- lascufloxacin has superior tissue penetration due to its high binding capacity to phosphatidylserine.

Given these aspects, we believe that there' are premises to classify these new compounds in a new generation (the fifth). However, these new representatives still require supervision and further studies considering the fate of the many representatives withdrawn from previous generations due to the severe side-effects.

7. Antimicrobial Resistance to the Newer FQNs

Bacterial resistance to FQNs is a worldwide growing phenomenon; new resistant strains to FQNs have emerged in the last twenty years. The enhancement of bacterial resistance to FQNs will change patient management. This threatening phenomenon will produce changes in the therapeutic guidelines [249].

In this context, the newer FQNs aimed to reduce bacterial resistance in both humans and animals. However, the increase in bacterial resistance to FQNs has led to researchers' efforts to understand resistance mechanisms and to identify new FQNs to combat the growing resistance. Mainly, the mechanisms of bacterial resistance to FQNs include: (1) mutations in topoisomerase II; (2) decreased drug absorption by upregulation of efflux pumps; and (3) plasmid-mediated resistance [62,63].

Mutations cause the most significant form of antimicrobial resistance in DNA gyrase and DNA topoisomerase IV. These mutations affect the interactions between FQNs and DNA enzymes [63]. Plasmid-mediated resistance encodes proteins that disrupt FQNs-enzyme interactions, increase FQNs efflux, or alter FQNs metabolism [250]. Chromosome-mediated resistance affects cellular efflux pumps, decreasing cellular concentrations of FQNs [251,252].

It is known that older FQNs act on a single target enzyme [253]. On the other hand, it is currently considered that newer FQNs drugs, such as besifloxacin [105], delafloxacin or zabofloxacin [254] can act on both DNA topoisomerases [255,256]. Thus, antimicrobial activity increases and the spontaneous occurrence of FQNs resistance is reduced [257]. For example, some studies on *Staphylococus pneumoniae* have concluded that besifloxacin has a higher inhibitory activity against DNA gyrase and DNA topoisomerase IV than ciprofloxacin and moxifloxacin. In the case of DNA gyrase, the inhibitory concentration of besifloxacin against *Staphylococus pneumoniae* was up to eight times lower comparing with moxifloxacin and 15 times lower comparing with ciprofloxacin [126]. These results suggest that besifloxacin is less affected by target enzymes mutations than earlier FQNs [258]. The same conclusion was presented by Roychoudhury et al., following in vitro study with nemonoxacin on resistant *Streptococcus pneumoniae* [259].

It was shown that drug efflux pumps do not contribute significantly to antibiotic resistance for newer FQNs, such as besifloxacin [260]. Besifloxacin is administered only ophthalmically. This can be considered an advantage due to the less likely risk of the development of microbial resistance [101].

Other in vitro studies have also shown that MRSA is less likely to develop resistance to delafloxacin compared to older FQNs. Regarding nadifloxacin, Alba et al. [182] demonstrated no increase in resistance of *Propionibacterium acnes*, *Staphylococcus aureus* (MRSA and MSSA) and *Staphylococcus epidermidis*, showing much better antimicrobial activity compared to other antibiotics. The reduction in resistance to nadifloxacin appears probably because it is not influenced by overexpression of the NorA efflux pump on the bacterial cell membrane [88].

Predicting resistance potential is based on some essential aspects. Among them are determinants of bacterial resistance, dual activity on target enzymes, and effects on bacterial efflux systems. In addition, the newer FQNs seem to have the advantage to maintain concentrations higher than MIC of first-step resistant mutants. The detection of all gyrA mutations which confer resistance is helpful in rapid molecular diagnosis of FQN resistance [261]. Mismatch amplification mutation assay-polymerase chain reaction (MAMA PCR) technique may serve as a tool to identify the multiple point mutations in the FQN resistance in Gram-negative bacteria [262].

Therefore, the double targeting and low resistance of bacteria are specific features of the new FQNs. Future studies are needed to complete the description of the resistance mechanism of new FQNs.

8. Compounds in Development Based on Antibacterial QNs Structures

There are numerous compounds in development that have been included in several recently published review articles [247,263]. The discovery of new potential drugs is in continuous progress. Below are briefly presented some relevant compounds under development.

8.1. Avarofloxacin (Acorafloxacin)

Avarofloxacin (acorafloxacin, JNJ-Q2) or (7-[3-[2-Amino-1(*E*)-fluoroethylidene]piperidin-1-yl]-1-cyclopropyl-6-fluoro-8-methoxy-4-oxo-1,4-dihydroquinoline-3-carboxylic acid) [143,220] is a new FQN with a zwitterionic aminoethylidenylpiperidine structure [233]. It is currently undergoing clinical testing (phase III) to treat acute bacterial skin and skin-structure infections, CAP. It has shown improved antibacterial effectiveness against pathogens resistant to current FQNs [143].

It has antibacterial activity against a wide range of Gram-positive bacteria, including *Streptococcus pneumoniae*, MRSA, *Enterococcus* sp., *Escherichia coli*, *Klebsiella* spp., *Haemophilus influenzae* and *Pseudomonas aeruginosa* making it more potent than previously used FQNs [264].

Avarofloxacin can be administered orally and parenterally; the bioavailability is around 65% in parenteral oral administration. The fact that avarofloxacin is accessible in both parenteral and oral formulations sets it apart from several other MRSA treatments that are only available via injection [265].

In vitro investigations show that avarofloxacin has significant efficacy against pathogens including *Staphylococcus aureus* and *Streptococcus pneumoniae*, which cause acute bacterial skin and skin structure infections and community-acquired bacterial pneumonia; it was also demonstrated to have a more considerable resistance barrier than other drugs in the class, and it is still effective against drug-resistant organisms like MRSA, ciprofloxacin-resistant MRSA. Avarofloxacin was found to be as effective as linezolid for bacterial skin and skin structure infections and moxifloxacin for community-acquired bacterial pneumonia in two Phase II investigations [248]. Avarofloxacin has been granted Qualified Infectious Disease Product and Fast Track designations from the FDA [266].

8.2. Other Derivatives of Antibacterial QNs

Darehkordi et al. (2011) used N-substituted trifluoroacetimidoyl chlorides to synthesize piperazinyl QN derivatives. Out of the obtained compounds, two exhibited superior antibacterial activity against strains of *Escherichia coli*, *Klebsiella pneumonia* (compared to ciprofloxacin) and *Staphylococcus aureus* (compared to vancomycin) [267].

Sweelmeen et al. (2019) synthesized a novel derivative with antimicrobial potential (7-chloro-1-alkyl-6-fluoro-8-nitro-4-oxo-1,4-dihydroquinoline-3-carboxylic acid). This compound has been shown to be active against *Pseudomonas aeruginosa*, *Staphylococcus aureus*, and *Streptococcus agalactiae* [268]. In a review article, Zhang Bo (2014) highlighted different series of QN derivatives with antifungal potential in terms of structure-activity relationship: 2-quinolone, 4-quinolone, and FQN derivatives and FQN-metal complexes [263]. Lapointe et al. (2021) recently published the discovery and optimization of a novel series of compounds that inhibit the two bacterial target enzymes and stabilize the DNA cleavage complexes [269].

8.3. Hybrids

Numerous studies have aimed to obtain hybrid compounds that combine the properties of FQN with other types of active molecules [237,241,270,271]. In addition to broadening the spectrum of activity, the decrease in susceptibility to the installation of bacterial resistance is also pursued. Several hybrids were obtained with other antibiotics (e.g., oxazolidinones, tetracyclines, and aminoglycosides).

Gordeev et al. (2003) synthesized several compounds that incorporated pharmacophore structures of FQNs and oxazolidinones and demonstrated superior potency to linezolid against Gram-positive and Gram-negative bacteria, even for linezolid and ciprofloxacin-resistant strains of *Staphylococcus aureus* and *Enterococcus faecium*. The mechanism of action combined the inhibition of protein synthesis but also of DNA gyrase and topoisomerase IV [272]. Sriram et al. (2007) combined representatives from the tetracyclines class (tetracycline, oxytetracycline, and minocycline) with the secondary amino (piperazine) function of FQNs (norfloxacin, lomefloxacin, ciprofloxacin, and gatifloxacin). The results revealed anti-HIV and antitubercular activities, most significant for one of the compounds (minocycline-lomefloxacin derivative), making it a promising candidate in treating patients with HIV-1, co-infected with *Mycobacterium tuberculosis* [273].

Pokrovskaya et al. (2009) synthesized a series of hybrids with ciprofloxacin and neomycin. The antibacterial activity of most of the synthesized compounds was significantly higher on *Escherichia coli* and *Bacillus subtilis*, compared to that of the two free antibiotics. This case also showed that the combinations presented a dual mechanism of action, namely the inhibition of protein synthesis and target enzymes of FQNs [274]. Gorityala et al. (2016) studied an antibacterial hybrid consisting of moxifloxacin and tobramycin that acts against multidrug-resistant strains of *Pseudomonas aeruginosa*, by improving membrane permeability and reducing efflux [275]. Shavit et al. (2017) synthesized a series of hybrids composed of ciprofloxacin and kanamycin A, which showed superior action on Gram-negative bacteria. These hybrids delayed the emergence of resistance for strains of *Escherichia coli* and *Bacillus subtilis* compared to the 1:1 mixture of the two antibiotics [276].

In addition to the hybridization of antibacterial QNs with other antibiotics, several studies have included different types of drugs with biological potential in the design of hybrids. For example, Chugunova et al. (2016) synthesized a series of FQN hybrids with benzofuroxane derivatives. Some combinations showed superior antibacterial activity on *Bacillus cereus* 8035 strains compared to the free FQN [270]. Wang YN et al. (2018) synthesized a series of hybrids between QN derivatives and benzimidazole. One of the compounds showed unusual activity on the resistant strains of *Pseudomonas aeruginosa* and *Candida tropicalis* strains. It also caused a decrease in the resistance of *Pseudomonas aeruginosa*, compared to norfloxacin [277].

A series of 34 clinafloxacin-azole conjugates were synthesized and tested in vitro against *Mycobacterium tuberculosis* (H37Rv) and other Gram-negative and Gram-positive bacteria. A particular conjugate (TM2l) has been the most promising delimited in terms of a great activity against *Mycobacterium tuberculosis* (MIC = 0.29 µM), good safety predicted profile, and good drug-likeness values [124].

Yi-Lei Fan et al. (2018) review the numerous FQN derivatives as antituberculosis agents. Among them are FQN-isatin hybrids, FQN-azole hybrids, FQN-amide/azetidinone derivatives, FQN-quinoline/phenanthridine hybrids, FQN-hydrazone/hydrazide hybrids, dimeric FQN derivatives, FQN-oxime hybrids, FQN-sugar/coumarin/dihydroartemisinin/ tetracycline hybrids, and other FQN derivatives [241].

A whole decade has been reviewed from the perspective of hybrid compounds and dual-action molecules by Fedorowicz and Sączewski (2018) [271].

9. Concerning Side Effects

Currently, FQNs are a valuable class of drugs used to treat infections with Gram-positive and Gram-negative bacteria (Table S1—Supplementary Material). However, the new generations of FQNs have a broad spectrum of activity, including drug-resistant bacterial species (see recent authorized FQNs previously discussed). Unfortunately, this antibacterial class has been overused in therapy over time. It is known that FQNs could produce a series of severe side effects, which vary from one representative to another, mainly if they are not used judiciously [18,278–283]. These side effects occur at the gastrointestinal tract level (nausea and diarrhea), central nervous system (headache, dizziness, confusion, seizures, and insomnia), joints (Achilles tendon rupture), and muscles (neuromuscular blocking activity), cardiovascular system (QT prolongation and arrhythmias). Also, the FQNs could produce dysglycemia, hepatotoxicity, renal toxicity, phototoxicity, rush, anaphylactoid reactions, and anaphylaxis [11,18,282,284–287].

FDA has approved labeling changes of FQNs (black box warning) [288,289] and has issued a series of warnings about FQNs side effects [290], as tendinopathy and tendon rupture [291], aortic rupture or tears [292], and the negative impact on mental health and glucose homeostasis (dysglycemia) [293]. EMA has also issued similar warnings, suspensions, or restrictions of FQNs due to their potentially permanent side effects [294–298].

However, FQNs proved to be a beneficial antibacterial class, safe in the low doses and short course [281]; these drugs have potential side effects, especially in long or high doses, limiting their use. Therefore, FQNs of the new generations must be used responsibly, only in severe life-threatening infections with no alternative treatment options [281,288,299,300].

10. Conclusions

Antibacterial QNs had developed spectacularly over time, many compounds being approved and used successfully in therapy. Therefore, identifying novel antibacterial compounds has been a priority in recent years to produce effective treatments against bacteria that have gained resistance to classic FQNs. However, more information on efficacy against multidrug-resistant organisms is still needed, as these new medications are primarily aimed at these resistant strains.

Structure-activity relationship investigations were crucial in identifying substituents with a high affinity for binding to two target enzymes, the DNA gyrase and the topoisomerase IV enzymes. We have critically analyzed the structural changes in the new compounds compared to analogues from previous generations. Substitutes and combinations of substituents on the QN nucleus proved to confer to these new FQNs an acceptable safety profile by exceeding the possible side-effects identified in older compounds. These new representatives were highlighted by a broad spectrum of activity, including activity against anaerobic bacteria (except nemonoxacin). Many resistant bacteria (including resistant to FQNs) are susceptible to these compounds. Delafloxacin and finafloxacin have the advantage of being very active in an environment with acidic pH. Lascufloxacin has superior tissue penetration due to its high binding capacity to phosphatidylserine. Besifloxacin and finafloxacin were approved only for topic administration and are very effective in treating targeted infections. Thus, several positive aspects are added to the fourth generation FQNs, characteristics that can be the basis of a new generation (the fifth).

New molecules are in different phases of research, derivatives of FQNs (e.g., levonadifloxacin, avarofloxacin), and their conjugates or hybrids. This class of antimicrobials remains in the attention of researchers focused on developing new drugs efficient against resistant pathogens. However, the maximum therapeutic potential of this antimicrobials class has not been reached yet.

Supplementary Materials: The following are available online at https://www.mdpi.com/article/10.3390/pharmaceutics13081289/s1, Figure S1: Chemical structures of other FQNs from different generations, Table S1: Activity spectrum of major QNs approved for use in therapy after 2000.

Author Contributions: Conceptualization: A.R.; methodology, A.R., writing—original draft preparation, A.R., G.H., C.T., O.-L.M. and I.-A.L.; writing—review and editing, A.R., C.T., G.H. and I.-A.L.; visualization O.-L.M., I.-A.L. and A.R.; supervision, A.R.; All authors have read and agreed to the published version of the manuscript.

Funding: This research received no external funding.

Institutional Review Board Statement: Not applicable.

Informed Consent Statement: Not applicable.

Conflicts of Interest: The authors declare no conflict of interest.

References

1. Sheehan, G.; Chew, N.S.Y. The history of quinolones. In *Fluoroquinolone Antibiotics*; Milestones in Drug Therapy; Ronald, A.R., Low, D.E., Eds.; Birkhäuser: Basel, Switzerland, 2003; pp. 1–10. ISBN 978-3-0348-8103-6.
2. Oliphant, C.M.; Green, G.M. Quinolones: A Comprehensive Review. *Am. Fam. Physician* 2002, *65*, 455–464.
3. Pham, T.D.M.; Ziora, Z.M.; Blaskovich, M.A.T. Quinolone Antibiotics. *Medchemcomm* 2019, *10*, 1719–1739. [CrossRef]
4. Lesher, G.Y.; Froelich, E.J.; Gruett, M.D.; Bailey, J.H.; Brundage, R.P. 1,8-Naphthyridine derivatives. A new class of chemotherapeutic agents. *J. Med. Pharm. Chem.* 1962, *91*, 1063–1065. [CrossRef]
5. Ball, P. Chapter 1-The Quinolones: History and Overview. In *The Quinolones*, 3rd ed.; Andriole, V.T., Ed.; Academic Press: San Diego, CA, USA, 2000; pp. 1–31. ISBN 978-0-12-059517-4.
6. Emami, S.; Shafiee, A.; Foroumadi, A. Quinolones: Recent Structural and Clinical Developments. *Iran. J. Pharm. Res.* 2005, *3*, 123–136. [CrossRef]
7. Bisacchi, G.S. Origins of the Quinolone Class of Antibacterials: An Expanded "Discovery Story". *J. Med. Chem.* 2015, *58*, 4874–4882. [CrossRef] [PubMed]
8. Ball, P. Quinolone Generations: Natural History or Natural Selection? *J. Antimicrob. Chemother.* 2000, *46*, 17–24. [CrossRef] [PubMed]

9. Beale, J.M., Jr.; Block, J.H. (Eds.) *Wilson and Gisvold's Textbook of Organic Medicinal and Pharmaceutical Chemistry*, 12th ed.; Wolters Kluwer Health: Baltimore, MD, USA, 2010; ISBN 978-0-7817-7929-6.
10. Scoper, S.V. Review of Third-and Fourth-Generation Fluoroquinolones in Ophthalmology: In-Vitro and in-Vivo Efficacy. *Adv. Ther.* **2008**, *25*, 979–994. [CrossRef] [PubMed]
11. Bolon, M.K. The Newer Fluoroquinolones. *Infect. Dis. Clin. N. Am.* **2009**, *23*, 1027–1051. [CrossRef] [PubMed]
12. WHO Operational Handbook on Tuberculosis, Module 4: Treatment—Drug-Resistant Tuberculosis Treatment. Available online: https://www.who.int/publications-detail-redirect/9789240006997 (accessed on 30 June 2021).
13. Pranger, A.D.; van der Werf, T.S.; Kosterink, J.G.W.; Alffenaar, J.W.C. The Role of Fluoroquinolones in the Treatment of Tuberculosis in 2019. *Drugs* **2019**, *79*, 161–171. [CrossRef]
14. Sukul, P.; Spiteller, M. Fluoroquinolone Antibiotics in the Environment. *Rev. Environ. Contam. Toxicol.* **2007**, *191*, 131–162. [CrossRef] [PubMed]
15. Ware, G. *Reviews of Environmental Contamination and Toxicology 191*; Springer Science & Business Media: Berlin/Heidelberg, Germany, 2008; ISBN 978-0-387-69163-3.
16. Simon, J.; Guyot, A. Pefloxacin: Safety in Man. *J. Antimicrob. Chemother.* **1990**, *26* (Suppl. B), 215–218. [CrossRef]
17. List of Nationally Authorised Medicinal Products EMA/116496/2021 09 April 2021. Available online: https://www.ema.europa.eu/en/documents/psusa/pefloxacin-list-nationally-authorised-medicinal-products-psusa/00002322/202008_en.pdf (accessed on 6 August 2021).
18. Rubinstein, E. History of Quinolones and Their Side Effects. *Chemotherapy* **2001**, *47*, 3–8. [CrossRef]
19. Blum, M.D.; Graham, D.J.; McCloskey, C.A. Temafloxacin Syndrome: Review of 95 Cases. *Clin. Infect. Dis.* **1994**, *18*, 946–950. [CrossRef] [PubMed]
20. Takahama, H.; Tazaki, H. Tosufloxacin Tosilate-Induced Thrombocytopenic Purpura. *J. Derm.* **2007**, *34*, 465–467. [CrossRef]
21. Trouchon, T.; Lefebvre, S. A Review of Enrofloxacin for Veterinary Use. *Open J. Vet. Med.* **2016**, *6*, 40–58. [CrossRef]
22. Yang, Z.; Wang, X.; Qin, W.; Zhao, H. Capillary Electrophoresis–Chemiluminescence Determination of Norfloxacin and Prulifloxacin. *Anal. Chim. Acta* **2008**, *623*, 231–237. [CrossRef] [PubMed]
23. Deep, A.; Chaudhary, U.; Sikka, R. In the Quest of Drugs for Bad Bugs: Are Newer Fluoroquinolones Any Better? *J. Lab. Physicians* **2011**, *3*, 130–131. [CrossRef]
24. Cazedey, E.C.L.; Salgado, H.R.N. Orbifloxacin: A Review of Properties, Its Antibacterial Activities, Pharmacokinetic/Pharmacodynamic Characteristics, Therapeutic Use, and Analytical Methods. *Crit. Rev. Anal. Chem.* **2013**, *43*, 79–99. [CrossRef]
25. Martindale, W.; Sweetman, S.C. (Eds.) *Martindale: The Complete Drug Reference*, 36th ed.; Pharmaceuticale Press, PhP: London, UK; Chicago, IL, USA,, 2009; ISBN 978-0-85369-840-1.
26. Nenoff, P. Acne Vulgaris and Bacterial Skin Infections: Review of the Topical Quinolone Nadifloxacin. *Expert. Rev. Dermatol.* **2006**, *1*, 643–654. [CrossRef]
27. Morita, S.; Otsubo, K.; Uchida, M.; Kawabata, S.; Tamaoka, H.; Shimizu, T. Synthesis and Antibacterial Activity of the Metabolites of 9-Fluoro-6,7-Dihydro-8-(4-Hydroxy-1-Piperidyl)-5-Methyl-1-Oxo-1H,5H- Benzo[i,j]Quinolizine-2-Carboxylic Acid (OPC-7251). *Chem. Pharm. Bull.* **1990**, *38*, 2027–2029. [CrossRef]
28. Grimshaw, W.T.; Giles, C.J.; Cooper, A.C.; Shanks, D.J. The Efficacy of Danofloxacin in the Therapy of Pneumonia Associated with Pasteurella Species in Housed Calves. *Dtsch. Tierarztl. Wochenschr.* **1990**, *97*, 529–532.
29. Limberakis, C. Quinolone Antibiotics: Levofloxacin (Levaquin®), Moxifloxacin (Avelox®), Gemifloxacin (Factive®), and Garenoxacin (T-3811). In *The Art of Drug Synthesis*; John Wiley & Sons, Ltd.: Hoboken, NJ, USA, 2007; pp. 39–69. ISBN 978-0-470-13497-9.
30. Yu, Y.; Zhou, Y.F.; Sun, J.; Shi, W.; Liao, X.P.; Liu, Y.H. Pharmacokinetic and Pharmacodynamic Modeling of Sarafloxacin against Avian Pathogenic Escherichia Coli in Muscovy Ducks. *BMC Vet. Res.* **2017**, *13*, 47. [CrossRef] [PubMed]
31. Abbott Laboratories' Sarafloxacin for Poultry; Withdrawal of Approval of NADAs. Available online: https://www.federalregister.gov/documents/2001/04/30/01-10067/abbott-laboratories-sarafloxacin-for-poultry-withdrawal-of-approval-of-nadas (accessed on 8 June 2021).
32. Alksne, L. Balofloxacin Choongwae. *Curr. Opin. Investig. Drugs* **2003**, *4*, 224–229. [PubMed]
33. Shen, J.; Qian, J.-J.; Gu, J.-M.; Hu, X.-R. Marbofloxacin. *Acta Crystallogr. Sect. E Struct. Rep. Online* **2012**, *68*, o998–o999. [CrossRef] [PubMed]
34. Saravolatz, L.D.; Leggett, J. Gatifloxacin, Gemifloxacin, and Moxifloxacin: The Role of 3 Newer Fluoroquinolones. *Clin. Infect. Dis.* **2003**, *37*, 1210–1215. [CrossRef] [PubMed]
35. EMA/CVMP/411755/2010-Rev.1 Summary of Opinion, Veraflox. European Medicines Agency 2011. Available online: https://www.ema.europa.eu/en/documents/smop-initial/cvmp-summary-positive-opinion-veraflox_en.pdf (accessed on 25 May 2021).
36. Sykes, J.E.; Blondeau, J.M. Pradofloxacin: A Novel Veterinary Fluoroquinolone for Treatment of Bacterial Infections in Cats. *Vet. J.* **2014**, *201*, 207–214. [CrossRef] [PubMed]
37. Hanselmann, R.; Johnson, G.; Reeve, M.M.; Huang, S.-T. Identification and Suppression of a Dimer Impurity in the Development of Delafloxacin. *Org. Process Res. Dev.* **2009**, *13*, 54–59. [CrossRef]
38. PubChem Delafloxacin. Available online: https://pubchem.ncbi.nlm.nih.gov/compound/487101 (accessed on 1 June 2021).
39. Markham, A. Delafloxacin: First Global Approval. *Drugs* **2017**, *77*, 1481–1486. [CrossRef]
40. Haight, A.R.; Ariman, S.Z.; Barnes, D.M.; Benz, N.J.; Gueffier, F.X.; Henry, R.F.; Hsu, M.C.; Lee, E.C.; Morin, L.; Pearl, K.B.; et al. Synthesis of the Quinolone ABT-492: Crystallizations for Optimal Processing. *Org. Process Res. Dev.* **2006**, *10*, 751–756. [CrossRef]

41. Van Bambeke, F. Delafloxacin, a Non-Zwitterionic Fluoroquinolone in Phase III of Clinical Development: Evaluation of Its Pharmacology, Pharmacokinetics, Pharmacodynamics and Clinical Efficacy. *Future Microbiol.* **2015**, *10*, 1111–1123. [CrossRef]
42. Wetzel, C.; Lonneman, M.; Wu, C. Polypharmacological Drug Actions of Recently FDA Approved Antibiotics. *Eur. J. Med. Chem.* **2021**, *209*, 112931. [CrossRef]
43. Cervantes, L.J.; Mah, F.S. Clinical Use of Gatifloxacin Ophthalmic Solution for Treatment of Bacterial Conjunctivitis. *Clin. Ophthalmol.* **2011**, *5*, 495–502. [CrossRef] [PubMed]
44. Fish, D.N.; North, D.S. Gatifloxacin, an Advanced 8-Methoxy Fluoroquinolone. *Pharmacother. J. Hum. Pharmacol. Drug Ther.* **2001**, *21*, 35–59. [CrossRef] [PubMed]
45. Factive: Withdrawal of the Marketing Authorisation Application. Available online: https://www.ema.europa.eu/en/medicines/human/withdrawn-applications/factive (accessed on 1 June 2021).
46. Totoli, E.G.; Nunes Salgado, H.R. Besifloxacin: A Critical Review of Its Characteristics, Properties, and Analytical Methods. *Crit. Rev. Anal. Chem.* **2018**, *48*, 132–142. [CrossRef] [PubMed]
47. Higgins, P.G.; Stubbings, W.; Wisplinghoff, H.; Seifert, H. Activity of the Investigational Fluoroquinolone Finafloxacin against Ciprofloxacin-Sensitive and -Resistant Acinetobacter Baumannii Isolates. *Antimicrob. Agents Chemother.* **2010**, *54*, 1613–1615. [CrossRef]
48. Lemaire, S.; Van Bambeke, F.; Tulkens, P.M. Activity of Finafloxacin, a Novel Fluoroquinolone with Increased Activity at Acid PH, towards Extracellular and Intracellular Staphylococcus Aureus, Listeria Monocytogenes and Legionella Pneumophila. *Int. J. Antimicrob. Agents* **2011**, *38*, 52–59. [CrossRef] [PubMed]
49. PubChem Finafloxacin. Available online: https://pubchem.ncbi.nlm.nih.gov/compound/11567473 (accessed on 25 May 2021).
50. Hong, J.; Zhang, Z.; Lei, H.; Cheng, H.; Hu, Y.; Yang, W.; Liang, Y.; Das, D.; Chen, S.-H.; Li, G. A Novel Approach to Finafloxacin Hydrochloride (BAY35-3377). *Tetrahedron Lett.* **2009**, *50*, 2525–2528. [CrossRef]
51. Takagi, H.; Tanaka, K.; Tsuda, H.; Kobayashi, H. Clinical Studies of Garenoxacin. *Int. J. Antimicrob. Agents* **2008**, *32*, 468–474. [CrossRef]
52. Andersson, M.I.; MacGowan, A.P. Development of the Quinolones. *J. Antimicrob. Chemother.* **2003**, *51* (Suppl. 1), 1–11. [CrossRef]
53. Newman, D.J.; Cragg, G.M. Natural Products as Sources of New Drugs over the Nearly Four Decades from 01/1981 to 09/2019. *J. Nat. Prod.* **2020**, *83*, 770–803. [CrossRef]
54. Poole, R.M. Nemonoxacin: First Global Approval. *Drugs* **2014**, *74*, 1445–1453. [CrossRef]
55. Kocsis, B.; Szabo, D. Zabofloxacin for Chronic Bronchitis. *Drugs Today* **2016**, *52*, 495–500. [CrossRef] [PubMed]
56. Butler, M.S.; Paterson, D.L. Antibiotics in the Clinical Pipeline in October 2019. *J. Antibiot.* **2020**, *73*, 329–364. [CrossRef]
57. Ghebremedhin, B. Bacterial Infections in the Elderly Patient: Focus on Sitafloxacin. *Clin. Med. Insights Ther.* **2012**, *4*, CMT-S7435. [CrossRef]
58. Chen, C.-K.; Cheng, I.-L.; Chen, Y.-H.; Lai, C.-C. Efficacy and Safety of Sitafloxacin in the Treatment of Acute Bacterial Infection: A Meta-Analysis of Randomized Controlled Trials. *Antibiotics* **2020**, *9*, 106. [CrossRef] [PubMed]
59. Czyrski, A. Analytical Methods for Determining Third and Fourth Generation Fluoroquinolones: A Review. *Chromatographia* **2017**, *80*, 181–200. [CrossRef]
60. Systèmes, D. BIOVIA Draw for Academics. Available online: https://discover.3ds.com/biovia-draw-academic (accessed on 6 July 2021).
61. ChemAxon-Software Solutions and Services for Chemistry & Biology. Available online: https://chemaxon.com/ (accessed on 11 June 2021).
62. Bush, N.G.; Diez-Santos, I.; Abbott, L.R.; Maxwell, A. Quinolones: Mechanism, Lethality and Their Contributions to Antibiotic Resistance. *Molecules* **2020**, *25*, 5662. [CrossRef]
63. Aldred, K.J.; Kerns, R.J.; Osheroff, N. Mechanism of Quinolone Action and Resistance. *Biochem.* **2014**, *53*, 1565–1574. [CrossRef]
64. Hooper, D.C. Mechanisms of Action and Resistance of Older and Newer Fluoroquinolones. *Clin. Infect. Dis.* **2000**, *31*, S24–S28. [CrossRef]
65. Hooper, D.C. Mechanisms of Action of Antimicrobials: Focus on Fluoroquinolones. *Clin. Infect. Dis.* **2001**, *32*, S9–S15. [CrossRef]
66. Hooper, D.C.; Jacoby, G.A. Topoisomerase Inhibitors: Fluoroquinolone Mechanisms of Action and Resistance. *Cold Spring Harb. Perspect. Med.* **2016**, *6*, a025320. [CrossRef] [PubMed]
67. Fàbrega, A.; Madurga, S.; Giralt, E.; Vila, J. Mechanism of Action of and Resistance to Quinolones. *Microb. Biotechnol.* **2009**, *2*, 40–61. [CrossRef] [PubMed]
68. Jeong, K.S.; Xie, Y.; Hiasa, H.; Khodursky, A.B. Analysis of Pleiotropic Transcriptional Profiles: A Case Study of DNA Gyrase Inhibition. *PLoS Genet.* **2006**, *2*, e152. [CrossRef] [PubMed]
69. Chen, C.R.; Malik, M.; Snyder, M.; Drlica, K. DNA Gyrase and Topoisomerase IV on the Bacterial Chromosome: Quinolone-Induced DNA Cleavage. *J. Mol. Biol.* **1996**, *258*, 627–637. [CrossRef]
70. Drlica, K.; Malik, M.; Kerns, R.J.; Zhao, X. Quinolone-Mediated Bacterial Death. *Antimicrob. Agents Chemother.* **2008**, *52*, 385–392. [CrossRef]
71. Malik, M.; Zhao, X.; Drlica, K. Lethal Fragmentation of Bacterial Chromosomes Mediated by DNA Gyrase and Quinolones. *Mol. Microbiol.* **2006**, *61*, 810–825. [CrossRef]
72. Andryukov, B.G.; Somova, L.M.; Timchenko, N.F. Molecular and Genetic Characteristics of Cell Death in Prokaryotes. *Mol. Genet. Microbiol. Virol.* **2018**, *33*, 73–83. [CrossRef]

73. Correia, S.; Poeta, P.; Hébraud, M.; Capelo, J.L.; Igrejas, G. Mechanisms of Quinolone Action and Resistance: Where Do We Stand? *J. Med. Microbiol.* **2017**, *66*, 551–559. [CrossRef]
74. Redgrave, L.S.; Sutton, S.B.; Webber, M.A.; Piddock, L.J.V. Fluoroquinolone Resistance: Mechanisms, Impact on Bacteria, and Role in Evolutionary Success. *Trends Microbiol.* **2014**, *22*, 438–445. [CrossRef]
75. Solano-Gálvez, S.G.; Valencia-Segrove, M.F.; Prado, M.J.O.; Boucieguez, A.B.L.; Álvarez-Hernández, D.A.; Vázquez-López, R. Mechanisms of Resistance to Quinolones; IntechOpen: London, UK, 2020; ISBN 978-1-83962-433-9.
76. Hong, Y.; Li, Q.; Gao, Q.; Xie, J.; Huang, H.; Drlica, K.; Zhao, X. Reactive Oxygen Species Play a Dominant Role in All Pathways of Rapid Quinolone-Mediated Killing. *J. Antimicrob. Chemother.* **2020**, *75*, 576–585. [CrossRef]
77. Hong, Y.; Zeng, J.; Wang, X.; Drlica, K.; Zhao, X. Post-Stress Bacterial Cell Death Mediated by Reactive Oxygen Species. *Proc. Natl. Acad. Sci. USA* **2019**, *116*, 10064–10071. [CrossRef] [PubMed]
78. Dwyer, D.J.; Kohanski, M.A.; Hayete, B.; Collins, J.J. Gyrase Inhibitors Induce an Oxidative Damage Cellular Death Pathway in Escherichia Coli. *Mol. Syst. Biol.* **2007**, *3*, 91. [CrossRef]
79. Pan, X.; Qin, P.; Liu, R.; Li, J.; Zhang, F. Molecular Mechanism on Two Fluoroquinolones Inducing Oxidative Stress: Evidence from Copper/Zinc Superoxide Dismutase. *RSC Adv.* **2016**, *6*, 91141–91149. [CrossRef]
80. Michalak, K.; Sobolewska-Włodarczyk, A.; Włodarczyk, M.; Sobolewska, J.; Woźniak, P.; Sobolewski, B. Treatment of the Fluoroquinolone-Associated Disability: The Pathobiochemical Implications. *Oxidative Med. Cell. Longev.* **2017**, *2017*, e8023935. [CrossRef]
81. Rodríguez-Rosado, A.I.; Valencia, E.Y.; Rodríguez-Rojas, A.; Costas, C.; Galhardo, R.S.; Blázquez, J.; Rodríguez-Beltrán, J. Reactive Oxygen Species Are Major Contributors to SOS-Mediated Mutagenesis Induced by Fluoroquinolones. *BioRxiv* **2018**, 428961. [CrossRef]
82. Loganathan, R.; Ganeshpandian, M.; Bhuvanesh, N.S.P.; Palaniandavar, M.; Muruganantham, A.; Ghosh, S.K.; Riyasdeen, A.; Akbarsha, M.A. DNA and Protein Binding, Double-Strand DNA Cleavage and Cytotoxicity of Mixed Ligand Copper(II) Complexes of the Antibacterial Drug Nalidixic Acid. *J. Inorg. Biochem.* **2017**, *174*, 1–13. [CrossRef]
83. Dearden, J.C. The History and Development of Quantitative Structure-Activity Relationships (QSARs). Available online: www.igi-global.com/article/the-history-and-development-of-quantitative-structure-activity-relationships-qsars/144688 (accessed on 14 June 2020).
84. Refat, M.S. Synthesis and Characterization of Norfloxacin-Transition Metal Complexes (Group 11, IB): Spectroscopic, Thermal, Kinetic Measurements and Biological Activity. *Spectrochim. Acta Mol Biomol. Spectrosc.* **2007**, *68*, 1393–1405. [CrossRef]
85. Clardy, J.; Fischbach, M.; Currie, C. The Natural History of Antibiotics. *Curr. Biol.* **2009**, *19*, R437–R441. [CrossRef]
86. Van, T.T.; Minejima, E.; Chiu, C.A.; Butler-Wu, S.M. Don't Get Wound Up: Revised Fluoroquinolone Breakpoints for Enterobacteriaceae and Pseudomonas Aeruginosa. *J. Clin. Microbiol.* **2019**, *57*, e02072-18. [CrossRef] [PubMed]
87. Kuwahara, K.; Kitazawa, T.; Kitagaki, H.; Tsukamoto, T.; Kikuchi, M. Nadifloxacin, an Antiacne Quinolone Antimicrobial, Inhibits the Production of Proinflammatory Cytokines by Human Peripheral Blood Mononuclear Cells and Normal Human Keratinocytes. *J. Dermatol. Sci.* **2005**, *38*, 47–55. [CrossRef]
88. Narayanan, V.; Motlekar, S.; Kadhe, G.; Bhagat, S. Efficacy and Safety of Nadifloxacin for Bacterial Skin Infections: Results from Clinical and Post-Marketing Studies. *Dermatol. Ther.* **2014**, *4*, 233–248. [CrossRef]
89. EMA EMA/150639/2017 Nadifloxacin, List of Nationally Authorised Medicinal Products. Available online: https://www.ema.europa.eu/en/documents/psusa/nadifloxacin-list-nationally-authorised-medicinal-products-psusa/0000 2102/201605_en.pdf (accessed on 11 June 2021).
90. Fish, D.N.; Chow, A.T. The Clinical Pharmacokinetics of Levofloxacin. *Clin. Pharm.* **1997**, *32*, 101–119. [CrossRef]
91. Keating, G.M. Levofloxacin 0.5% Ophthalmic Solution A Review of Its Use in the Treatment of External Ocular Infections and in Intraocular Surgery. *Drugs* **2009**, *69*, 1267–1286. [CrossRef]
92. Rhee, C.K.; Chang, J.H.; Choi, E.G.; Kim, H.K.; Kwon, Y.-S.; Kyung, S.Y.; Lee, J.-H.; Park, M.J.; Yoo, K.H.; Oh, Y.M. Zabofloxacin versus Moxifloxacin in Patients with COPD Exacerbation: A Multicenter, Double-Blind, Double-Dummy, Randomized, Controlled, Phase III, Non-Inferiority Trial. *Int. J. Chronic Obstr. Pulm. Dis.* **2015**, *10*. [CrossRef]
93. Al Omari, M.M.H.; Jaafari, D.S.; Al-Sou'od, K.A.; Badwan, A.A. Chapter Seven-Moxifloxacin Hydrochloride. In *Profiles of Drug Substances, Excipients and Related Methodology*; Brittain, H.G., Ed.; Academic Press: Cambridge, MA, USA, 2014; Volume 39, pp. 299–431.
94. Baxdela (Delafloxacin) Tablets and Injection. Available online: https://www.accessdata.fda.gov/drugsatfda_docs/nda/2017/2 08610Orig1s000,208611Orig1s000TOC.cfm (accessed on 5 June 2021).
95. Singh, C.L.; Singh, A.; Kumar, S.; Majumdar, D.K. Besifloxacin the fourth generation fluoroquinolone: A review. *J. Drug Deliv. Ther.* **2014**, *4*, 39–44. [CrossRef]
96. DeCory, H.H.; Sanfilippo, C.M.; Proskin, H.M.; Blondeau, J.M. Characterization of Baseline Polybacterial versus Monobacterial Infections in Three Randomized Controlled Bacterial Conjunctivitis Trials and Microbial Outcomes with Besifloxacin Ophthalmic Suspension 0.6%. *PLoS ONE* **2020**, *15*, e0237603. [CrossRef] [PubMed]
97. BESIVANCE®(Besifloxacin Ophthalmic Suspension) 0.6%, for Topical Ophthalmic Use. 9. Available online: https://www.accessdata.fda.gov/drugsatfda_docs/label/2018/022308s013lbl.pdf (accessed on 28 May 2021).
98. FDA Drug Approval Package Xtoro (Finafloxacin) Otic Suspension. Available online: https://www.accessdata.fda.gov/drugsatfda_docs/nda/2014/206307Orig1s000TOC.cfm (accessed on 7 June 2021).

99. McKeage, K. Finafloxacin: First Global Approval. *Drugs* **2015**, *75*, 687–693. [CrossRef] [PubMed]
100. Barnes, K.B.; Zumbrun, S.D.; Halasohoris, S.A.; Desai, P.D.; Miller, L.L.; Richards, M.I.; Russell, P.; Bentley, C.; Harding, S.V. Demonstration of the Broad-Spectrum In Vitro Activity of Finafloxacin against Pathogens of Biodefense Interest. *Antimicrob. Agents Chemother.* **2019**, *63*, e01470-19. [CrossRef] [PubMed]
101. Khimdas, S.; Visscher, K.L.; Hutnik, C.M.L. Besifloxacin Ophthalmic Suspension: Emerging Evidence of Its Therapeutic Value in Bacterial Conjunctivitis. *Ophthalmol. Eye Dis.* **2011**, *3*, 7–12. [CrossRef] [PubMed]
102. Liu, K.K.-C.; Sakya, S.M.; O'Donnell, C.J.; Flick, A.C.; Li, J. Synthetic Approaches to the 2009 New Drugs. *Bioorganic. Med. Chem.* **2011**, *19*, 1136–1154. [CrossRef]
103. FDA. N. 22308/S-013 Besifloxacin Label. Available online: https://www.accessdata.fda.gov/drugsatfda_docs/label/2009/0223081bl.pdf (accessed on 6 May 2021).
104. Haas, W.; Pillar, C.M.; Zurenko, G.E.; Lee, J.C.; Brunner, L.S.; Morris, T.W. Besifloxacin, a Novel Fluoroquinolone, Has Broad-Spectrum in Vitro Activity against Aerobic and Anaerobic Bacteria. *Antimicrob. Agents Chemother.* **2009**, *53*, 3552–3560. [CrossRef]
105. Mah, F.S.; Sanfilippo, C.M. Besifloxacin: Efficacy and Safety in Treatment and Prevention of Ocular Bacterial Infections. *Ophthalmol. Ther.* **2016**, *5*, 1–20. [CrossRef]
106. Besifloxacin. Available online: https://go.drugbank.com/drugs/DB06771 (accessed on 1 June 2021).
107. O'Brien, T.P. Besifloxacin Ophthalmic Suspension, 0.6%: A Novel Topical Fluoroquinolone for Bacterial Conjunctivitis. *Adv. Ther.* **2012**, *29*, 473–490. [CrossRef]
108. Watanabe, R.; Nakazawa, T.; Yokokura, S.; Kubota, A.; Kubota, H.; Nishida, K. Fluoroquinolone Antibacterial Eye Drops: Effects on Normal Human Corneal Epithelium, Stroma, and Endothelium. *Clin. Ophthalmol.* **2010**, *4*, 1181–1187. [CrossRef]
109. Kovoor, T.A.; Kim, A.S.; McCulley, J.P.; Cavanagh, H.D.; Jester, J.V.; Bugde, A.C.; Petroll, W.M. Evaluation of the Corneal Effects of Topical Ophthalmic Fluoroquinolones Using In Vivo Confocal Microscopy. *Eye Contact Lens.* **2004**, *30*, 90–94. [CrossRef]
110. Kassaee, S.N.; Mahboobian, M.M. Besifloxacin-Loaded Ocular Nanoemulsions: Design, Formulation and Efficacy Evaluation. *Drug Deliv. Transl. Res.* **2021**. [CrossRef]
111. Dos Santos, G.A.; Ferreira-Nunes, R.; Dalmolin, L.F.; dos Santos Re, A.C.; Vieira Anjos, J.L.; Mendanha, S.A.; Aires, C.P.; Lopez, R.F.V.; Cunha-Filho, M.; Gelfuso, G.M.; et al. Besifloxacin Liposomes with Positively Charged Additives for an Improved Topical Ocular Delivery. *Sci. Rep.* **2020**, *10*, 19285. [CrossRef]
112. Polat, H.K.; Pehlivan, S.B.; Ozkul, C.; Calamak, S.; Ozturk, N.; Aytekin, E.; Firat, A.; Ulubayram, K.; Kocabeyoglu, S.; Irkec, M.; et al. Development of Besifloxacin HCl Loaded Nanofibrous Ocular Inserts for the Treatment of Bacterial Keratitis: In Vitro, Ex Vivo and In Vivo Evaluation. *Int. J. Pharm.* **2020**, *585*, 119552. [CrossRef]
113. Peterson, L.R. Quinolone Molecular Structure-Activity Relationships: What We Have Learned about Improving Antimicrobial Activity. *Clin. Infect. Dis.* **2001**, *33*, S180–S186. [CrossRef]
114. Asif, M. Study of Antimicrobial Quinolones and Structure Activity Relationship of Anti-Tubercular Compounds. *Res. Rev. J. Chem.* **2015**, *4*, 28–70.
115. Schaumann, R.C.; Rodloff, A.C. Activities of Quinolones Against Obligately Anaerobic Bacteria. *Anti-Infect. Agents Med. Chem.* **2006**, *6*, 49–56. [CrossRef]
116. PubChem Besifloxacin. Available online: https://pubchem.ncbi.nlm.nih.gov/compound/10178705 (accessed on 28 May 2021).
117. PubChem Besifloxacin Hydrochloride. Available online: https://pubchem.ncbi.nlm.nih.gov/compound/10224595 (accessed on 28 May 2021).
118. Besifloxacin Hydrochloride SML1608. Available online: https://www.sigmaaldrich.com/catalog/product/sigma/sml1608 (accessed on 1 June 2021).
119. Attia, A.K.; Abdel-Moety, M.M.; Abdel-Hamid, S.G. Thermal Analyses of Some Fluoroquinolone Pharmaceutical Compounds in Comparison with Molecular Orbital Calculations. *New J. Chem.* **2017**, *41*, 10189–10197. [CrossRef]
120. Thomas, G. *Medicinal Chemistry: An Introduction*; John Wiley & Sons: Hoboken, NJ, USA, 2011; ISBN 978-1-119-96542-8.
121. Lu, T.; Zhao, X.; Li, X.; Drlica-Wagner, A.; Wang, J.-Y.; Domagala, J.; Drlica, K. Enhancement of Fluoroquinolone Activity by C-8 Halogen and Methoxy Moieties: Action against a Gyrase Resistance Mutant of Mycobacterium Smegmatis and a Gyrase-Topoisomerase IV Double Mutant of Staphylococcus Aureus. *Antimicrob. Agents Chemother.* **2001**, *45*, 2703–2709. [CrossRef]
122. Wermuth, C.G. Preface to the Third Edition. In *The Practice of Medicinal Chemistry*, 4th ed.; Wermuth, C.G., Aldous, D., Raboisson, P., Rognan, D., Eds.; Academic Press: San Diego, CA, USA, 2015; p. xvii. ISBN 978-0-12-417205-0.
123. Haas, W.; Sanfilippo, C.M.; Hesje, C.K.; Morris, T.W. Contribution of the R8 Substituent to the in Vitro Antibacterial Potency of Besifloxacin and Comparator Ophthalmic Fluoroquinolones. *Clin. Ophthalmol.* **2013**, *7*, 821–830. [CrossRef] [PubMed]
124. Liu, J.; Ren, Z.; Fan, L.; Wei, J.; Tang, X.; Xu, X.; Yang, D. Design, Synthesis, Biological Evaluation, Structure-Activity Relationship, and Toxicity of Clinafloxacin-Azole Conjugates as Novel Antitubercular Agents. *Bioorganic Med. Chem.* **2019**, *27*, 175–187. [CrossRef] [PubMed]
125. Salunke, N.; Kharkar, P.S.; Pandita, N. Study of Degradation Behavior of Besifloxacin, Characterization of Its Degradation Products by LC-ESI-QTOF-MS and Their in Silico Toxicity Prediction. *Biomed. Chromatogr.* **2019**, *33*, e4489. [CrossRef]
126. Cambau, E.; Matrat, S.; Pan, X.-S.; Roth Dit Bettoni, R.; Corbel, C.; Aubry, A.; Lascols, C.; Driot, J.-Y.; Fisher, L.M. Target Specificity of the New Fluoroquinolone Besifloxacin in Streptococcus Pneumoniae, Staphylococcus Aureus and Escherichia Coli. *J. Antimicrob. Chemother.* **2009**, *63*, 443–450. [CrossRef]

127. Haas, W.; Pillar, C.M.; Hesje, C.K.; Sanfilippo, C.M.; Morris, T.W. In Vitro Time-Kill Experiments with Besifloxacin, Moxifloxacin and Gatifloxacin in the Absence and Presence of Benzalkonium Chloride. *J. Antimicrob. Chemother.* **2011**, *66*, 840–844. [CrossRef]
128. Hoover, R.; Alcorn, H.; Lawrence, L.; Paulson, S.K.; Quintas, M.; Cammarata, S.K. Pharmacokinetics of Intravenous Delafloxacin in Patients With End-Stage Renal Disease. *J. Clin. Pharmacol.* **2018**, *58*, 913–919. [CrossRef]
129. Scott, L.J. Delafloxacin: A Review in Acute Bacterial Skin and Skin Structure Infections. *Drugs* **2020**, *80*, 1247–1258. [CrossRef]
130. Tulkens, P.M.; Van Bambeke, F.; Zinner, S.H. Profile of a Novel Anionic FluoroquinoloneDelafloxacin. *Clin. Infect. Dis.* **2019**, *68*, S213–S222. [CrossRef]
131. Mogle, B.T.; Steele, J.M.; Thomas, S.J.; Bohan, K.H.; Kufel, W.D. Clinical Review of Delafloxacin: A Novel Anionic Fluoroquinolone. *J. Antimicrob. Chemother.* **2018**, *73*, 1439–1451. [CrossRef]
132. Meglumine-Brief Profile-ECHA. Available online: https://echa.europa.eu/brief-profile/-/briefprofile/100.025.916 (accessed on 5 June 2021).
133. Meglumine Active Pharmaceutical Ingredient | Small Molecule Pharmaceuticals | Merck. Available online: https://www.merckmillipore.com/RO/ro/products/small-molecule-pharmaceuticals/formulation/solid-dosage-form/meglumine/mwub.qB.gf0AAAFSBHgEZXop,nav?ReferrerURL=https%3A%2F%2Fwww.google.com%2F&gclid=EAIaIQobChMI_rKg7pHT8QIV44ODBx1C3QiFEAMYASAAEgL54PD_BwE (accessed on 8 July 2021).
134. Cho, J.C.; Crotty, M.P.; White, B.P.; Worley, M.V. What Is Old Is New Again: Delafloxacin, a Modern Fluoroquinolone. *Pharmacotherapy* **2018**, *38*, 108–121. [CrossRef]
135. Anwer, M.K.; Iqbal, M.; Muharram, M.M.; Mohammad, M.; Ezzeldin, E.; Aldawsari, M.F.; Alalaiwe, A.; Imam, F. Development of Lipomer Nanoparticles for the Enhancement of Drug Release, Anti-Microbial Activity and Bioavailability of Delafloxacin. *Pharmaceutics* **2020**, *12*, 252. [CrossRef]
136. Delafloxacin SML1869. Available online: https://www.sigmaaldrich.com/catalog/product/sigma/sml1869 (accessed on 3 June 2021).
137. Delafloxacin. Available online: https://go.drugbank.com/drugs/DB11943 (accessed on 3 June 2021).
138. Hanselmann, R.; Reeve, M.M. Crystalline Forms of D-Glucitol, 1-Deoxy-1-(Methylamino)-, 1-(6-Amino-3,5-Difluoropyridine-2-Yl)-8-Chloro-6-Fluoro-1,4-Dihydro-7-(3-Hydroxyazetidin-1-Yl)-4-Oxo-3-Quinolinecarboxylate. U.S. Patent Application 14/773,655, 18 February 2016.
139. Saravolatz, L.D.; Stein, G.E. Delafloxacin: A New Anti-Methicillin-Resistant Staphylococcus Aureus Fluoroquinolone. *Clin. Infect. Dis.* **2019**, *68*, 1058–1062. [CrossRef]
140. Lemaire, S.; Tulkens, P.M.; Van Bambeke, F. Contrasting Effects of Acidic PH on the Extracellular and Intracellular Activities of the Anti-Gram-Positive Fluoroquinolones Moxifloxacin and Delafloxacin against Staphylococcus Aureus. *Antimicrob. Agents Chemother.* **2011**, *55*, 649–658. [CrossRef]
141. Ocheretyaner, E.R.; Park, T.E. Delafloxacin: A Novel Fluoroquinolone with Activity against Methicillin-Resistant Staphylococcus Aureus (MRSA) and Pseudomonas Aeruginosa. *Expert Rev. Anti-Infect. Ther.* **2018**, *16*, 523–530. [CrossRef] [PubMed]
142. Emmerson, A.M. The Quinolones: Decades of Development and Use. *J. Antimicrob. Chemother.* **2003**, *51*, 13–20. [CrossRef] [PubMed]
143. Kocsis, B.; Domokos, J.; Szabo, D. Chemical Structure and Pharmacokinetics of Novel Quinolone Agents Represented by Avarofloxacin, Delafloxacin, Finafloxacin, Zabofloxacin and Nemonoxacin. *Ann. Clin. Microbiol. Antimicrob.* **2016**, *15*, 34. [CrossRef] [PubMed]
144. Taubert, M.; Lueckermann, M.; Vente, A.; Dalhoff, A.; Fuhr, U. Population Pharmacokinetics of Finafloxacin in Healthy Volunteers and Patients with Complicated Urinary Tract Infections. *Antimicrob. Agents Chemother.* **2018**, *62*, e02328-17. [CrossRef] [PubMed]
145. Vente, A.; Bentley, C.; Lueckermann, M.; Tambyah, P.; Dalhoff, A. Early Clinical Assessment of the Antimicrobial Activity of Finafloxacin Compared to Ciprofloxacin in Subsets of Microbiologically Characterized Isolates. *Antimicrob. Agents Chemother.* **2018**, *62*, e02325-17. [CrossRef]
146. Wagenlehner, F.; Nowicki, M.; Bentley, C.; Lueckermann, M.; Wohlert, S.; Fischer, C.; Vente, A.; Naber, K.; Dalhoff, A. Explorative Randomized Phase II Clinical Study of the Efficacy and Safety of Finafloxacin versus Ciprofloxacin for Treatment of Complicated Urinary Tract Infections. *Antimicrob. Agents Chemother.* **2018**, *62*, e02317-17. [CrossRef]
147. Lee, J.W.; Kim, N.; Nam, R.H.; Kim, J.M.; Park, J.Y.; Lee, S.M.; Kim, J.S.; Lee, D.H.; Jung, H.C. High Efficacy of Finafloxacin on Helicobacter Pylori Isolates at PH 5.0 Compared with That of Other Fluoroquinolones. *Antimicrob. Agents Chemother.* **2015**, *59*, 7629–7636. [CrossRef] [PubMed]
148. Barnes, K.B.; Richards, M.; Laws, T.R.; Nunez, A.; Thwaite, J.E.; Bentley, C.; Harding, S. Finafloxacin Is an Effective Treatment for Inhalational Tularemia and Plague in Mouse Models of Infection. *Antimicrob. Agents Chemother.* **2021**, *65*, e02294-20. [CrossRef] [PubMed]
149. Chalhoub, H.; Harding, S.V.; Tulkens, P.M.; Van Bambeke, F. Influence of PH on the Activity of Finafloxacin against Extracellular and Intracellular Burkholderia Thailandensis, Yersinia Pseudotuberculosis and Francisella Philomiragia and on Its Cellular Pharmacokinetics in THP-1 Monocytes. *Clin. Microbiol. Infect.* **2020**, *26*. [CrossRef] [PubMed]
150. Patel, H.; Andresen, A.; Vente, A.; Heilmann, H.-D.; Stubbings, W.; Seiberling, M.; Lopez-Lazaro, L.; Pokorny, R.; Labischinski, H. Human Pharmacokinetics and Safety Profile of Finafloxacin, a New Fluoroquinolone Antibiotic, in Healthy Volunteers. *Antimicrob. Agents Chemother.* **2011**, *55*, 4386–4393. [CrossRef]
151. Finafloxacin. Available online: https://go.drugbank.com/drugs/DB09047 (accessed on 7 June 2021).

152. Finafloxacin ≥95% (HPLC) | Sigma-Aldrich. Available online: http://www.sigmaaldrich.com/ (accessed on 7 June 2021).
153. Wohlert, S.-E.; Jaetsch, T.; Gallenkamp, B.; Knops, H.J.; Lui, N.; Preiss, M.; Haebich, D.; Labischinski, H. New Fluoroquinolone Finafloxacin HCl (FIN): Route of Synthesis, Physicochemical Characteristics and Activity under Neutral and Acid Conditions. In Proceedings of the 48th Annual ICAAC/IDSA 46th Annual Meeting 2008, Washington DC, USA, 25–28 October 2008.
154. Wise, R. A Review of the Clinical Pharmacology of Moxifloxacin, a New 8-Methoxyquinolone, and Its Potential Relation to Therapeutic Efficacy. *Clin. Drug Investig.* **1999**, *17*, 365–387. [CrossRef]
155. Miravitlles, M. Moxifloxacin in the Management of Exacerbations of Chronic Bronchitis and COPD. *Int. J. Chron. Obs. Pulmon Dis.* **2007**, *2*, 191–204.
156. Vardanyan, R.; Hruby, V. Chapter 31-Antibacterial Drugs. In *Synthesis of Best-Seller Drugs*; Vardanyan, R., Hruby, V., Eds.; Academic Press: Boston, MA, USA, 2016; pp. 645–667. ISBN 978-0-12-411492-0.
157. Silley, P.; Stephan, B.; Greife, H.A.; Pridmore, A. Comparative Activity of Pradofloxacin against Anaerobic Bacteria Isolated from Dogs and Cats. *J. Antimicrob. Chemother.* **2007**, *60*, 999–1003. [CrossRef]
158. Tanaka, K.; Vu, H.; Hayashi, M. In Vitro Activities and Spectrum of Lascufloxacin (KRP-AM1977) against Anaerobes. *J. Infect. Chemother.* **2021**, *27*, 1265–1269. [CrossRef]
159. PubChem Lascufloxacin. Available online: https://pubchem.ncbi.nlm.nih.gov/compound/71528768 (accessed on 25 June 2021).
160. THE BioTek: Recombinant Proteins, Antibodies, Antigens, Enzymes, Peptides, Inhibitors. Available online: https://www.thebiotek.com/ (accessed on 29 June 2021).
161. 848416-07-9 | Lascufloxacin | 7-[(3S,4S)-3-[(Cyclopropylamino)Methyl]-4-Fluoro-1-Pyrrolidinyl]-6-Fluoro-1-(2-Fluoroethyl)-1,4-Dihydro-8-Methoxy-4-Oxo-3-Quinolinecarboxylic Acid | $C_{21}H_{24}F_3N_3O_4$ | TRC. Available online: https://www.trc-canada.com/product-detail/?L176205 (accessed on 29 June 2021).
162. Lascufloxacin | Targetmol. Available online: https://www.targetmol.com/compound/Lascufloxacin (accessed on 29 June 2021).
163. Ogihara, S. NHI Drug Price Listing and Release of Oral Quinolone Antibacterial Agent "Lasvic®Tablets 75mg." 2. Available online: https://www.kyorin-pharm.co.jp/en/news/a329f0ae64024c1173f40660eede0efb37f1cbb0.pdf (accessed on 25 June 2021).
164. Lascufloxacin-Kyorin Pharmaceutical-AdisInsight. Available online: https://adisinsight.springer.com/drugs/800035339 (accessed on 29 June 2021).
165. Cornick, J.E.; Bentley, S.D. Streptococcus Pneumoniae: The Evolution of Antimicrobial Resistance to Beta-Lactams, Fluoroquinolones and Macrolides. *Microbes Infect.* **2012**, *14*, 573–583. [CrossRef]
166. Koulenti, D.; Xu, E.; Yin Sum Mok, I.; Song, A.; Karageorgopoulos, D.E.; Armaganidis, A.; Lipman, J.; Tsiodras, S. Lefamulin. Comment on: "Novel Antibiotics for Multidrug-Resistant Gram-Positive Microorganisms. Microorganisms, 2019, 7, 270". *Microorganisms* **2019**, *7*, 386. [CrossRef]
167. Thakare, R.; Singh, S.; Dasgupta, A.; Chopra, S. Lascufloxacin Hydrochloride to Treat Bacterial Infection. *Drugs Today* **2020**, *56*, 365–376. [CrossRef]
168. Kishii, R.; Yamaguchi, Y.; Takei, M. In Vitro Activities and Spectrum of the Novel Fluoroquinolone Lascufloxacin (KRP-AM1977). *Antimicrob. Agents Chemother.* **2017**, *61*, e00120-17. [CrossRef] [PubMed]
169. Murata, M.; Kosai, K.; Yamauchi, S.; Sasaki, D.; Kaku, N.; Uno, N.; Morinaga, Y.; Hasegawa, H.; Miyazaki, T.; Izumikawa, K.; et al. In Vitro Activity of Lascufloxacin against Streptococcus Pneumoniae with Mutations in the Quinolone Resistance-Determining Regions. *Antimicrob. Agents Chemother.* **2018**, *62*, e01971-17. [CrossRef] [PubMed]
170. Totsuka, K.; Sesoko, S.; Fukase, H.; Ikushima, I.; Odajima, M.; Niwayama, Y. Pharmacokinetic Study of Lascufloxacin in Non-Elderly Healthy Men and Elderly Men. *J. Infect. Chemother.* **2020**, *26*, 231–239. [CrossRef] [PubMed]
171. Furuie, H.; Tanioka, S.; Shimizu, K.; Manita, S.; Nishimura, M.; Yoshida, H. Intrapulmonary Pharmacokinetics of Lascufloxacin in Healthy Adult Volunteers. *Antimicrob. Agents Chemother.* **2018**, *62*, e02169-17. [CrossRef]
172. Hayashi, N.; Nakata, Y.; Yazaki, A. New Findings on the Structure-Phototoxicity Relationship and Photostability of Fluoroquinolones with Various Substituents at Position 1. *Antimicrob. Agents Chemother.* **2004**, *48*, 799–803. [CrossRef]
173. Balfour, J.A.; Todd, P.A.; Peters, D.H. Fleroxacin. A Review of Its Pharmacology and Therapeutic Efficacy in Various Infections. *Drugs* **1995**, *49*, 794–850. [CrossRef]
174. Ahmed, A.; Daneshtalab, M. Nonclassical Biological Activities of Quinolone Derivatives. *J. Pharm. Pharm. Sci.* **2012**, *15*, 52–72. [CrossRef]
175. Domagala, J.M.; Hagen, S.E. Structure-Activity Relationships of the Quinolone Antibacterials in the New Millennium: Some Things Change and Some Do Not. In *Quinolone Antimicrobial Agents*, 3rd ed.; Hooper, D.C., Rubinstein, E., Eds.; ASM Press: Washington DC, USA, 2003; pp. 3–18. [CrossRef]
176. Piddock, L.J.; Johnson, M.; Ricci, V.; Hill, S.L. Activities of New Fluoroquinolones against Fluoroquinolone-Resistant Pathogens of the Lower Respiratory Tract. *Antimicrob. Agents Chemother.* **1998**, *42*, 2956–2960. [CrossRef] [PubMed]
177. PubChem Sitafloxacin. Available online: https://pubchem.ncbi.nlm.nih.gov/compound/461399 (accessed on 1 July 2021).
178. Keating, G.M. Sitafloxacin: In Bacterial Infections. *Drugs* **2011**, *71*, 731–744. [CrossRef] [PubMed]
179. Anderson, D.L. Sitafloxacin Hydrate for Bacterial Infections. *Drugs Today* **2008**, *44*, 489–501. [CrossRef] [PubMed]
180. Jacobs, M.R.; Appelbaum, P.C. Nadifloxacin: A Quinolone for Topical Treatment of Skin Infections and Potential for Systemic Use of Its Active Isomer, WCK 771. *Expert Opin. Pharmacother.* **2006**, *7*, 1957–1966. [CrossRef]
181. Schofer, H.; Gollner, A.; Kusche, W.; Schwantes, U. Effectiveness and Tolerance of Topical Nadifloxacin in the Therapy of Acne Vulgaris (Grade I-II): Results of a Non-Interventional Trial in 555 Patients. *J. Appl. Res.* **2009**, *9*, 44.

182. Alba, V.; Urban, E.; Angeles Dominguez, M.; Nagy, E.; Nord, C.-E.; Palacín, C.; Vila, J. In Vitro Activity of Nadifloxacin against Several Gram-Positive Bacteria and Analysis of the Possible Evolution of Resistance after 2 Years of Use in Germany. *Int. J. Antimicrob. Agents* **2009**, *33*, 272–275. [CrossRef]
183. Takei, M.; Fukuda, H.; Kishii, R.; Hosaka, M. Target Preference of 15 Quinolones against Staphylococcus Aureus, Based on Antibacterial Activities and Target Inhibition. *Antimicrob Agents Chemother.* **2001**, *45*, 3544–3547. [CrossRef]
184. PubChem Nadifloxacin. Available online: https://pubchem.ncbi.nlm.nih.gov/compound/4410 (accessed on 11 June 2021).
185. [Hot Item] Manufacturers Supply Top Quality High Purity Apis Powder Nadifloxacin CAS No. 124858-35-1. Available online: https://dgpeptides.en.made-in-china.com/product/bjZnRINJksWv/China-Manufacturers-Supply-Top-Quality-High-Purity-Apis-Powder-Nadifloxacin-CAS-No-124858-35-1.html (accessed on 11 June 2021).
186. Nadifloxacin | ≥99%(HPLC) | Selleck | Antibiotics Chemical. Available online: https://www.selleckchem.com/products/nadifloxacin.html (accessed on 11 June 2021).
187. Shinde, U.; Pokharkar, S.; Modani, S. Design and Evaluation of Microemulsion Gel System of Nadifloxacin. *Indian J. Pharm. Sci.* **2012**, *74*, 237–247. [CrossRef]
188. Nadifloxacin (CAS 124858-35-1). Available online: https://www.caymanchem.com/product/20252 (accessed on 11 June 2021).
189. 124858-35-1 CAS MSDS (Nadifloxacin) Melting Point Boiling Point Density CAS Chemical Properties. Available online: https://www.chemicalbook.com/ChemicalProductProperty_US_CB3301560.aspx (accessed on 11 June 2021).
190. Kumar, A.; Bhashkar, B.; Bhavsar, J. New Approach for the Preparation of Key Intermediates of Nadifloxacin. *J. Chem. Pharm. Res.* **2016**, *8*, 609–613.
191. Martin, Y.C. Exploring QSAR: Hydrophobic, Electronic, and Steric Constants, C. Hansch, A. Leo, and D. Hoekman. American Chemical Society, Washington, DC. 1995. Xix + 348 Pp. 22 × 28.5 Cm. Exploring QSAR: Fundamentals and Applications in Chemistry and Biology. C. Hansch and A. Leo. American Chemical Society, Washington, DC. 1995. Xvii + 557 Pp. 18.5 × 26 Cm. ISBN 0-8412-2993-7 (Set). $99.95 (Set). *J. Med. Chem.* **1996**, *39*, 1189–1190. [CrossRef]
192. PubChem Ofloxacin. Available online: https://pubchem.ncbi.nlm.nih.gov/compound/4583 (accessed on 13 June 2021).
193. Bhagwat, S.S.; Nandanwar, M.; Kansagara, A.; Patel, A.; Takalkar, S.; Chavan, R.; Periasamy, H.; Yeole, R.; Deshpande, P.K.; Bhavsar, S.; et al. Levonadifloxacin, a Novel Broad-Spectrum Anti-MRSA Benzoquinolizine Quinolone Agent: Review of Current Evidence. *Drug Des. Devel. Ther.* **2019**, *13*, 4351–4365. [CrossRef]
194. Bakthavatchalam, Y.D.; Shankar, A.; Muniyasamy, R.; Peter, J.V.; Marcus, Z.; Triplicane Dwarakanathan, H.; Gunasekaran, K.; Iyadurai, R.; Veeraraghavan, B. Levonadifloxacin, a Recently Approved Benzoquinolizine Fluoroquinolone, Exhibits Potent In Vitro Activity against Contemporary Staphylococcus Aureus Isolates and Bengal Bay Clone Isolates Collected from a Large Indian Tertiary Care Hospital. *J. Antimicrob. Chemother.* **2020**, *75*, 2156–2159. [CrossRef]
195. Baliga, S.; Mamtora, D.K.; Gupta, V.; Shanmugam, P.; Biswas, S.; Mukherjee, D.N.; Shenoy, S. Assessment of Antibacterial Activity of Levonadifloxacin against Contemporary Gram-Positive Clinical Isolates Collected from Various Indian Hospitals Using Disk-Diffusion Assay. *Indian J. Med. Microbiol.* **2020**, *38*, 307–312. [CrossRef]
196. Rodvold, K.A.; Gotfried, M.H.; Chugh, R.; Gupta, M.; Yeole, R.; Patel, A.; Bhatia, A. Intrapulmonary Pharmacokinetics of Levonadifloxacin Following Oral Administration of Alalevonadifloxacin to Healthy Adult Subjects. *Antimicrob. Agents Chemother.* **2018**, *62*, e02297-17. [CrossRef]
197. Lautre, C.; Sharma, S.; Sahu, J.K. Chemistry, Biological Properties and Analytical Methods of Levonadifloxacin: A Review. *Crit. Rev. Anal. Chem.* **2020**, *2020*, 1855412. [CrossRef]
198. Bhatia, A.; Mastim, M.; Shah, M.; Gutte, R.; Joshi, P.; Kumbhar, D.; Periasamy, H.; Palwe, S.R.; Chavan, R.; Bhagwat, S.; et al. Efficacy and Safety of a Novel Broad-Spectrum Anti-MRSA Agent Levonadifloxacin Compared with Linezolid for Acute Bacterial Skin and Skin Structure Infections: A Phase 3, Openlabel, Randomized Study. *J. Assoc. Physicians India* **2020**, *68*, 30–36. [PubMed]
199. Saxena, D.; Kaul, G.; Dasgupta, A.; Chopra, S. Levonadifloxacin Arginine Salt to Treat Acute Bacterial Skin and Skin Structure Infection Due to S. Aureus Including MRSA. *Drugs Today* **2020**, *56*, 583–598. [CrossRef]
200. Kongre, V.; Bhagwat, S.; Bharadwaj, R.S. Resistance Pattern among Contemporary Gram Positive Clinical Isolates and in Vitro Activity of Novel Antibiotic, Levonadifloxacin (WCK 771). *Int. J. Infect. Dis.* **2020**, *101*, 30. [CrossRef]
201. Tellis, M.; Joseph, J.; Khande, H.; Bhagwat, S.; Patel, M. In Vitro Bactericidal Activity of Levonadifloxacin (WCK 771) against Methicillin- and Quinolone-Resistant Staphylococcus Aureus Biofilms. *J. Med. Microbiol.* **2019**, *68*, 1129–1136. [CrossRef] [PubMed]
202. Lai, C.-C.; Lee, K.-Y.; Lin, S.-W.; Chen, Y.-H.; Kuo, H.-Y.; Hung, C.-C.; Hsueh, P.-R. Nemonoxacin (TG-873870) for Treatment of Community-Acquired Pneumonia. *Expert Rev. Anti. Infect. Ther.* **2014**, *12*, 401–417. [CrossRef] [PubMed]
203. Safety and Efficacy Study of TG-873870 (Nemonoxacin) in Diabetic Foot Infections. Available online: https://clinicaltrials.gov/ct2/show/results/NCT00685698 (accessed on 21 June 2021).
204. Liapikou, A.; Cilloniz, C.; Mensa, J.; Torres, A. New Antimicrobial Approaches to Gram Positive Respiratory Infections. *Pulm. Pharmacol. Ther.* **2015**, *32*, 137–143. [CrossRef]
205. Chang, L.-W.; Hsu, M.-C.; Zhang, Y.-Y. *Nemonoxacin (Taigexyn®): A New Non-Fluorinated Quinolone*; IntechOpen: London, UK, 2019; ISBN 978-1-78984-473-3.
206. Jean, S.-S.; Chang, L.-W.; Hsueh, P.-R. Tentative Clinical Breakpoints and Epidemiological Cut-off Values of Nemonoxacin for Streptococcus Pneumoniae and Staphylococcus Aureus Isolates Associated with Community-Acquired Pneumonia. *J. Glob. Antimicrob. Resist.* **2020**, *23*, 388–393. [CrossRef]

207. Lin, L.; Chang, L.-W.; Tsai, C.-Y.; Hsu, C.-H.; Chung, D.T.; Aronstein, W.S.; Ajayi, F.; Kuzmak, B.; Lyon, R.A. Dose Escalation Study of the Safety, Tolerability, and Pharmacokinetics of Nemonoxacin (TG-873870), a Novel Potent Broad-Spectrum Nonfluorinated Quinolone, in Healthy Volunteers. *Antimicrob. Agents Chemother.* **2010**, *54*, 405–410. [CrossRef] [PubMed]
208. NCATS Inxight: Drugs-Nemonoxacin Malate Hemihydrate. Available online: https://drugs.ncats.io/drug/Y97F3051FH (accessed on 22 June 2021).
209. Wu, X.-J.; Zhang, J.; Guo, B.-N.; Zhang, Y.-Y.; Yu, J.-C.; Cao, G.-Y.; Yuan-cheng, C.; Zhu, D.-M.; Ye, X.-Y.; Wu, J.-F.; et al. Pharmacokinetics and Pharmacodynamics of Multiple-Dose Intravenous Nemonoxacin in Healthy Chinese Volunteers. *Antimicrob. Agents Chemother.* **2014**, *59*. [CrossRef]
210. PubChem Nemonoxacin. Available online: https://pubchem.ncbi.nlm.nih.gov/compound/11993740 (accessed on 22 June 2021).
211. NCATS Inxight: Drugs-NEMONOXACIN. Available online: https://drugs.ncats.io/drug/P94L0PVO94 (accessed on 22 June 2021).
212. Nemonoxacin. Available online: https://go.drugbank.com/drugs/DB06600 (accessed on 22 June 2021).
213. Arjona, A. Nemonoxacin Quinolone Antibiotic. *Drug Future* **2009**, *34*, 196–203. [CrossRef]
214. Qin, X.; Huang, H. Review of Nemonoxacin with Special Focus on Clinical Development. *Drug Des. Dev. Ther.* **2014**, *8*, 765–774. [CrossRef]
215. Gatifloxacin. Available online: https://go.drugbank.com/drugs/DB01044 (accessed on 22 June 2021).
216. Kishii, R.; Takei, M.; Fukuda, H.; Hayashi, K.; Hosaka, M. Contribution of the 8-Methoxy Group to the Activity of Gatifloxacin against Type II Topoisomerases of Streptococcus Pneumoniae. *Antimicrob. Agents Chemother.* **2003**, *47*, 77–81. [CrossRef] [PubMed]
217. PubChem Balofloxacin. Available online: https://pubchem.ncbi.nlm.nih.gov/compound/65958 (accessed on 28 June 2021).
218. Ball, P.; Mandell, L.; Niki, Y.; Tillotson, G. Comparative Tolerability of the Newer Fluoroquinolone Antibacterials. *Drug Saf.* **1999**, *21*, 407–421. [CrossRef]
219. Shankar, G.; Borkar, R.M.; Udutha, S.; Anagoni, S.P.; Srinivas, R. Identification and Structural Characterization of in Vivo Metabolites of Balofloxacin in Rat Plasma, Urine and Feces Samples Using Q-TOF/LC/ESI/MS/MS: In Silico Toxicity Studies. *J. Pharm. Biomed. Anal.* **2018**, *159*, 200–211. [CrossRef]
220. PubChem Acorafloxacin. Available online: https://pubchem.ncbi.nlm.nih.gov/compound/11546234 (accessed on 28 June 2021).
221. Chen, Y.-H.; Liu, C.-Y.; Lu, J.-J.; King, C.-H.R.; Hsueh, P.-R. In Vitro Activity of Nemonoxacin (TG-873870), a Novel Non-Fluorinated Quinolone, against Clinical Isolates of Staphylococcus Aureus, Enterococci and Streptococcus Pneumoniae with Various Resistance Phenotypes in Taiwan. *J. Antimicrob. Chemother.* **2009**, *64*, 1226–1229. [CrossRef]
222. Li, Z.; Liu, Y.; Wang, R.; Li, A. Antibacterial Activities of Nemonoxacin against Clinical Isolates of Staphylococcus Aureus: An in Vitro Comparison with Three Fluoroquinolones. *World J. Microbiol. Biotechnol.* **2014**, *30*, 2927–2932. [CrossRef]
223. Lauderdale, T.-L.; Shiau, Y.-R.; Lai, J.-F.; Chen, H.-C.; King, C.-H.R. Comparative In Vitro Activities of Nemonoxacin (TG-873870), a Novel Nonfluorinated Quinolone, and Other Quinolones against Clinical Isolates. *Antimicrob. Agents Chemother.* **2010**, *54*, 1338–1342. [CrossRef]
224. Adam, H.J.; Laing, N.M.; King, C.R.; Lulashnyk, B.; Hoban, D.J.; Zhanel, G.G. In Vitro Activity of Nemonoxacin, a Novel Nonfluorinated Quinolone, against 2,440 Clinical Isolates. *Antimicrob. Agents Chemother.* **2009**, *53*, 4915–4920. [CrossRef]
225. Li, C.-R.; Li, Y.; Li, G.-Q.; Yang, X.-Y.; Zhang, W.-X.; Lou, R.-H.; Liu, J.-F.; Yuan, M.; Huang, P.; Cen, S.; et al. In Vivo Antibacterial Activity of Nemonoxacin, a Novel Non-Fluorinated Quinolone. *J. Antimicrob. Chemother.* **2010**, *65*, 2411–2415. [CrossRef] [PubMed]
226. Van Rensburg, D.J.J.; Perng, R.-P.; Mitha, I.H.; Bester, A.J.; Kasumba, J.; Wu, R.-G.; Ho, M.-L.; Chang, L.-W.; Chung, D.T.; Chang, Y.-T.; et al. Efficacy and Safety of Nemonoxacin versus Levofloxacin for Community-Acquired Pneumonia. *Antimicrob. Agents Chemother.* **2010**, *54*, 4098–4106. [CrossRef]
227. Liang, W.T.; Chen, Y.; Cao, Y.; Liu, X.; Huang, J.; Hu, J.; Zhao, M.; Guo, Q.; Zhang, S.; Wu, X.; et al. Pharmacokinetics and Pharmacodynamics of Nemonoxacin against Streptococcus Pneumoniae in an In Vitro Infection Model. *Antimicrob. Agents Chemother.* **2013**, *57*, 2942–2947. [CrossRef]
228. Han, H.; Kim, S.E.; Shin, K.-H.; Lim, C.; Lim, K.S.; Yu, K.-S.; Cho, J.-Y. Comparison of Pharmacokinetics between New Quinolone Antibiotics: The Zabofloxacin Hydrochloride Capsule and the Zabofloxacin Aspartate Tablet. *Curr. Med. Res. Opin.* **2013**, *29*, 1349–1355. [CrossRef] [PubMed]
229. DONG WHA PHARMACEUTICAL CO., LTD. Available online: https://www.dong-wha.co.kr/english/product/content.asp?t_idx=545&t_page=1&d=&b=10&s=11 (accessed on 24 June 2021).
230. Park, H.-S.; Oh, S.-H.; Kim, H.-S.; Choi, D.-R.; Kwak, J.-H. Antimicrobial Activity of Zabofloxacin against Clinically Isolated Streptococcus Pneumoniae. *Molecules* **2016**, *21*, 1562. [CrossRef] [PubMed]
231. Park, H.-S.; Kim, H.-J.; Seol, M.-J.; Choi, D.-R.; Choi, E.-C.; Kwak, J.-H. In Vitro and In Vivo Antibacterial Activities of DW-224a, a New Fluoronaphthyridone. *Antimicrob. Agents Chemother.* **2006**, *50*, 2261–2264. [CrossRef] [PubMed]
232. Jones, R.N.; Biedenbach, D.J.; Ambrose, P.G.; Wikler, M.A. Zabofloxacin (DW-224a) Activity against Neisseria Gonorrhoeae Including Quinolone-Resistant Strains. *Diagn. Microbiol. Infect. Dis.* **2008**, *62*, 110–112. [CrossRef]
233. Sellarès-Nadal, J.; Burgos, J.; Falcó, V.; Almirante, B. Investigational and Experimental Drugs for Community-Acquired Pneumonia: The Current Evidence. *J. Exp. Pharm.* **2020**, *12*, 529–538. [CrossRef] [PubMed]
234. PubChem Zabofloxacin. Available online: https://pubchem.ncbi.nlm.nih.gov/compound/9952872 (accessed on 19 June 2021).
235. Zabofloxacin. Available online: https://go.drugbank.com/drugs/DB12479 (accessed on 23 June 2021).

236. Jin, H.E.; Kang, I.H.; Shim, C.K. Fluorescence Detection of Zabofloxacin, a Novel Fluoroquinolone Antibiotic, in Plasma, Bile, and Urine by HPLC: The First Oral and Intravenous Applications in a Pharmacokinetic Study in Rats. *J. Pharm. Pharm. Sci.* **2011**, *14*, 291–305. [CrossRef] [PubMed]
237. Benadallah, M.; Talhi, O.; Nouali, F.; Choukchou-Braham, N.; Bachari, K.; Silva, A.M.S. Advances in Spirocyclic Hybrids: Chemistry and Medicinal Actions. *Curr. Med. Chem.* **2018**, *25*, 3748–3767. [CrossRef] [PubMed]
238. Yang, Y.-T.; Zhu, J.-F.; Liao, G.; Xu, H.-J.; Yu, B. The Development of Biologically Important Spirooxindoles as New Antimicrobial Agents. *Curr. Med. Chem.* **2018**, *25*, 2233–2244. [CrossRef] [PubMed]
239. Zhou, L.; Zhao, J.; Shan, T.; Cai, X.; Peng, Y. Spirobisnaphthalenes from Fungi and Their Biological Activities. *Mini Rev. Med. Chem.* **2010**, *10*, 977–989. [CrossRef] [PubMed]
240. Chen, C.; He, L. Advances in Research of Spirodienone and Its Derivatives: Biological Activities and Synthesis Methods. *Eur. J. Med. Chem.* **2020**, *203*, 112577. [CrossRef]
241. Fan, Y.-L.; Wu, J.-B.; Cheng, X.-W.; Zhang, F.-Z.; Feng, L.-S. Fluoroquinolone Derivatives and Their Anti-Tubercular Activities. *Eur. J. Med. Chem.* **2018**, *146*, 554–563. [CrossRef]
242. Shah, P.; Westwell, A.D. The Role of Fluorine in Medicinal Chemistry: Review Article. *J. Enzym. Inhib. Med. Chem.* **2007**, *22*, 527–540. [CrossRef]
243. Gillis, E.P.; Eastman, K.J.; Hill, M.D.; Donnelly, D.J.; Meanwell, N.A. Applications of Fluorine in Medicinal Chemistry. *J. Med. Chem.* **2015**, *58*, 8315–8359. [CrossRef]
244. Sharma, P.C.; Jain, A.; Jain, S. Fluoroquinolone Antibacterials: A Review on Chemistry, Microbiology and Therapeutic Prospects. *Acta Pol. Pharm.* **2009**, *66*, 587–604.
245. Zhanel, G.G.; Walkty, A.; Vercaigne, L.; Karlowsky, J.A.; Embil, J.; Gin, A.S.; Hoban, D.J. The New Fluoroquinolones: A Critical Review. *Canadian J. Infect. Dis.* **1999**, *10*, 207–238. [CrossRef]
246. Yamagishi, Y.; Matsukawa, Y.; Suematsu, H.; Mikamo, H. In Vitro Activity of Lascufloxacin, a Novel Fluoroquinolone Antibacterial Agent, against Various Clinical Isolates of Anaerobes and Streptococcus Anginosus Group. *Anaerobe* **2018**, *54*, 61–64. [CrossRef] [PubMed]
247. Suaifan, G.A.R.Y.; Mohammed, A.A.M. Fluoroquinolones Structural and Medicinal Developments (2013–2018): Where Are We Now? *Bioorganic Med. Chem.* **2019**, *27*, 3005–3060. [CrossRef]
248. Jones, T.M.; Johnson, S.W.; DiMondi, V.P.; Wilson, D.T. Focus on JNJ-Q2, a Novel Fluoroquinolone, for the Management of Community-Acquired Bacterial Pneumonia and Acute Bacterial Skin and Skin Structure Infections. *Infect. Drug Resist.* **2016**, *9*, 119–128. [CrossRef] [PubMed]
249. Dalhoff, A. Global Fluoroquinolone Resistance Epidemiology and Implictions for Clinical Use. *Interdiscip. Perspect. Infect. Dis.* **2012**, *2012*, e976273. [CrossRef]
250. Yamane, K.; Wachino, J.; Suzuki, S.; Kimura, K.; Shibata, N.; Kato, H.; Shibayama, K.; Konda, T.; Arakawa, Y. New Plasmid-Mediated Fluoroquinolone Efflux Pump, QepA, Found in an Escherichia Coli Clinical Isolate. *Antimicrob. Agents Chemother.* **2007**, *51*, 3354–3360. [CrossRef]
251. Li, X.-Z.; Nikaido, H. Efflux-Mediated Drug Resistance in Bacteria: An Update. *Drugs* **2009**, *69*, 1555–1623. [CrossRef]
252. Grkovic, S.; Brown, M.H.; Skurray, R.A. Regulation of Bacterial Drug Export Systems. *Microbiol. Mol. Biol. Rev.* **2002**, *66*, 671–701. [CrossRef]
253. Blondeau, J.M. Fluoroquinolones: Mechanism of Action, Classification, and Development of Resistance. *Surv. Ophthalmol.* **2004**, *49*, S73–S78. [CrossRef]
254. Park, H.S.; Jung, S.J.; Kwak, J.-H.; Choi, D.-R.; Choi, E.-C. DNA Gyrase and Topoisomerase IV Are Dual Targets of Zabofloxacin in Streptococcus Pneumoniae. *Int. J. Antimicrob. Agents* **2010**, *36*, 97–98. [CrossRef] [PubMed]
255. Fisher, L.M.; Heaton, V.J. Dual Activity of Fluoroquinolones against Streptococcus Pneumoniae. *J. Antimicrob. Chemother.* **2003**, *51*, 463–464. [CrossRef]
256. Remy, J.M.; Tow-Keogh, C.A.; McConnell, T.S.; Dalton, J.M.; Devito, J.A. Activity of Delafloxacin against Methicillin Resistant Staphylococcus Aureus: Resistance Selection and Characterization. *J. Antimicrob. Chemother.* **2012**, *67*, 2814–2820. [CrossRef]
257. Smith, H.J.; Nichol, K.A.; Hoban, D.J.; Zhanel, G.G. Dual Activity of Fluoroquinolones against Streptococcus Pneumoniae: The Facts behind the Claims. *J. Antimicrob. Chemother.* **2002**, *49*, 893–895. [CrossRef] [PubMed]
258. Sanfilippo, C.M.; Hesje, C.K.; Haas, W.; Morris, T.W. Topoisomerase Mutations That Are Associated with High-Level Resistance to Earlier Fluoroquinolones in Staphylococcus Aureus Have Less Effect on the Antibacterial Activity of Besifloxacin. *Chemotherapy* **2011**, *57*, 363–371. [CrossRef] [PubMed]
259. Roychoudhury, S.; Makin, K.; Twinem, T.; Leunk, R.; Hsu, M.C. In Vitro Resistance Development to Nemonoxacin in Streptococcus Pneumoniae: A Unique Profile for a Novel Nonfluorinated Quinolone. *Microb. Drug Resist.* **2016**, *22*, 578–584. [CrossRef] [PubMed]
260. Shinabarger, D.L.; Zurenko, G.E.; Hesje, C.K.; Sanfilippo, C.M.; Morris, T.W.; Haas, W. Evaluation of the Effect of Bacterial Efflux Pumps on the Antibacterial Activity of the Novel Fluoroquinolone Besifloxacin. *J. Chemother.* **2011**, *23*, 80–86. [CrossRef]
261. Avalos, E.; Catanzaro, D.; Catanzaro, A.; Ganiats, T.; Brodine, S.; Alcaraz, J.; Rodwell, T. Frequency and Geographic Distribution of GyrA and GyrB Mutations Associated with Fluoroquinolone Resistance in Clinical Mycobacterium Tuberculosis Isolates: A Systematic Review. *PLoS ONE* **2015**, *10*, e0120470. [CrossRef]

262. Deekshit, V.K.; Jazeela, K.; Chakraborty, G.; Rohit, A.; Chakraborty, A.; Karunasagar, I. Mismatch Amplification Mutation Assay-Polymerase Chain Reaction: A Method of Detecting Fluoroquinolone Resistance Mechanism in Bacterial Pathogens. *Indian J. Med. Res.* **2019**, *149*, 146–150. [CrossRef]
263. Zhang, B. Quinolone Derivatives and Their Antifungal Activities: An Overview. *Arch. Pharm.* **2019**, *352*, e1800382. [CrossRef]
264. Morrow, B.J.; He, W.; Amsler, K.M.; Foleno, B.D.; Macielag, M.J.; Lynch, A.S.; Bush, K. In Vitro Antibacterial Activities of JNJ-Q2, a New Broad-Spectrum Fluoroquinolone. *Antimicrob. Agents Chemother.* **2010**, *54*, 1955–1964. [CrossRef]
265. Davenport, J.M.; Covington, P.; Gotfried, M.; Medlock, M.; Watanalumlerd, P.; McIntyre, G.; Turner, L.; Almenoff, J. Summary of Pharmacokinetics and Tissue Distribution of a Broad-Spectrum Fluoroquinolone, JNJ-Q2. *Clin. Pharm. Drug Dev.* **2012**, *1*, 121–130. [CrossRef]
266. Avarofloxacin (Furiex), Has Been Granted QIDP and Fast-Track Designations for Treatment of Acute Bacterial Skin and Skin-Structure Infections. *Formulary* **2013**, *48*, 135.
267. Darehkordi, A.; Javanmiri, M.; Ghazi, S.; Assar, S. Synthesis of N-Aryl-2,2,2-Trifluoroacetimidoyl Piperazinylquinolone Derivatives and Their Antibacterial Evaluations. *J. Fluor. Chem.* **2011**, *132*, 263–268. [CrossRef]
268. Swellmeen, L.; Uzrail, A.; Shahin, R.; AL-Hiari, Y. Synthesis of Fluoroquinolones Derivatives as Antimicrobial Agents. *Orient. J. Chem.* **2019**, *35*, 1248–1253. [CrossRef]
269. Lapointe, G.; Skepper, C.K.; Holder, L.M.; Armstrong, D.; Bellamacina, C.; Blais, J.; Bussiere, D.; Bian, J.; Cepura, C.; Chan, H.; et al. Discovery and Optimization of DNA Gyrase and Topoisomerase IV Inhibitors with Potent Activity against Fluoroquinolone-Resistant Gram-Positive Bacteria. *J. Med. Chem.* **2021**, *64*, 6329–6357. [CrossRef] [PubMed]
270. Chugunova, E.; Akylbekov, N.; Bulatova, A.; Gavrilov, N.; Voloshina, A.; Kulik, N.; Zobov, V.; Dobrynin, A.; Syakaev, V.; Burilov, A. Synthesis and Biological Evaluation of Novel Structural Hybrids of Benzofuroxan Derivatives and Fluoroquinolones. *Eur. J. Med. Chem.* **2016**, *116*, 165–172. [CrossRef] [PubMed]
271. Fedorowicz, J.; Sączewski, J. Modifications of Quinolones and Fluoroquinolones: Hybrid Compounds and Dual-Action Molecules. *Mon. Chem.Chem. Mon.* **2018**, *149*, 1199–1245. [CrossRef] [PubMed]
272. Gordeev, M.F.; Hackbarth, C.; Barbachyn, M.R.; Banitt, L.S.; Gage, J.R.; Luehr, G.W.; Gomez, M.; Trias, J.; Morin, S.E.; Zurenko, G.E.; et al. Novel Oxazolidinone-Quinolone Hybrid Antimicrobials. *Bioorgan. Med. Chem.* **2003**, *13*, 4213–4216. [CrossRef] [PubMed]
273. Sriram, D.; Yogeeswari, P.; Senchani, G.; Banerjee, D. Newer Tetracycline Derivatives: Synthesis, Anti-HIV, Antimycobacterial Activities and Inhibition of HIV-1 Integrase. *Bioorganic. Med. Chem. Lett.* **2007**, *17*, 2372–2375. [CrossRef]
274. Pokrovskaya, V.; Belakhov, V.; Hainrichson, M.; Yaron, S.; Baasov, T. Design, Synthesis, and Evaluation of Novel Fluoroquinolone–Aminoglycoside Hybrid Antibiotics. *J. Med. Chem.* **2009**, *52*, 2243–2254. [CrossRef]
275. Gorityala, B.K.; Guchhait, G.; Goswami, S.; Fernando, D.M.; Kumar, A.; Zhanel, G.G.; Schweizer, F. Hybrid Antibiotic Overcomes Resistance in P. Aeruginosa by Enhancing Outer Membrane Penetration and Reducing Efflux. *J. Med. Chem.* **2016**, *59*, 8441–8455. [CrossRef] [PubMed]
276. Shavit, M.; Pokrovskaya, V.; Belakhov, V.; Baasov, T. Covalently Linked Kanamycin-Ciprofloxacin Hybrid Antibiotics as a Tool to Fight Bacterial Resistance. *Bioorganic Med. Chem.* **2017**, *25*, 2917–2925. [CrossRef] [PubMed]
277. Wang, Y.-N.; Bheemanaboina, R.R.Y.; Gao, W.-W.; Kang, J.; Cai, G.-X.; Zhou, C.-H. Discovery of Benzimidazole-Quinolone Hybrids as New Cleaving Agents toward Drug-Resistant Pseudomonas Aeruginosa DNA. *Chem. Med. Chem.* **2018**, *13*, 1004–1017. [CrossRef] [PubMed]
278. Bertino, J.; Fish, D. The Safety Profile of the Fluoroquinolones. *Clin. Ther.* **2000**, *22*, 798–817. [CrossRef]
279. Briasoulis, A.; Agarwal, V.; Pierce, W.J. QT Prolongation and Torsade de Pointes Induced by Fluoroquinolones: Infrequent Side Effects from Commonly Used Medications. *Cardiology* **2011**, *120*, 103–110. [CrossRef]
280. Daneman, N.; Lu, H.; Redelmeier, D.A. Fluoroquinolones and Collagen Associated Severe Adverse Events: A Longitudinal Cohort Study. *BMJ Open* **2015**, *5*, e010077. [CrossRef]
281. Raini, M. Fluoroquinolones Antibiotics: Benefit and Side Effects. *Media Penelit. Pengemb. Kesehat.* **2016**, *26*, 163–174.
282. Roberts, J.R. InFocus: Fluoroquinolone Side Effects Just Got Scarier. *Emerg. Med. News* **2018**, *40*, 26–27. [CrossRef]
283. Tandan, M.; Cormican, M.; Vellinga, A. Adverse Events of Fluoroquinolones vs. Other Antimicrobials Prescribed in Primary Care: A Systematic Review and Meta-Analysis of Randomized Controlled Trials. *Int. J. Antimicrob. Agents* **2018**, *52*, 529–540. [CrossRef]
284. Lewis, T.; Cook, J. Fluoroquinolones and Tendinopathy: A Guide for Athletes and Sports Clinicians and a Systematic Review of the Literature. *J. Athl. Train.* **2014**, *49*, 422–427. [CrossRef]
285. Gorelik, E.; Masarwa, R.; Perlman, A.; Rotshild, V.; Abbasi, M.; Muszkat, M.; Matok, I. Fluoroquinolones and Cardiovascular Risk: A Systematic Review, Meta-Analysis and Network Meta-Analysis. *Drug Saf.* **2019**, *42*, 529–538. [CrossRef] [PubMed]
286. Haiping, L.; Ziqiang, J.; Qina, Z.; Yuhua, D. Adverse Reactions of Fluoroquinolones to Central Nervous System and Rational Drug Use in Nursing Care. *Pak. J. Pharm. Sci.* **2019**, *32*, 427–432. [PubMed]
287. Gatti, M.; Bianchin, M.; Raschi, E.; De Ponti, F. Assessing the Association between Fluoroquinolones and Emerging Adverse Drug Reactions Raised by Regulatory Agencies: An Umbrella Review. *Eur. J. Intern. Med.* **2020**, *75*, 60–70. [CrossRef] [PubMed]
288. FDA. Approves Safety Labeling Changes for Fluoroquinolones. FDA. 2019. Available online: https://www.fda.gov/drugs/information-drug-class/fda-approves-safety-labeling-changes-fluoroquinolones (accessed on 12 August 2021).
289. Aschenbrenner, D.S. The FDA Revises Boxed Warning For Fluoroquinolones-Again. *Am. J. Nurs.* **2016**, *116*, 22–23. [CrossRef] [PubMed]

290. FDA Updates Warnings for Fluoroquinolone Antibiotics. Available online: https://www.fda.gov/news-events/press-announcements/fda-updates-warnings-fluoroquinolone-antibiotics (accessed on 12 August 2021).
291. FDA. Drug Safety Communication: FDA Advises Restricting Fluoroquinolone Antibiotic Use for Certain Uncomplicated Infections. Warns about Disabling Side Effects That Can Occur Together. FDA. 2019. Available online: https://www.fda.gov/drugs/drug-safety-and-availability/fda-drug-safety-communication-fda-advises-restricting-fluoroquinolone-antibiotic-use-certain (accessed on 12 August 2021).
292. FDA Warns about Increased Risk of Ruptures or Tears in the Aorta Blood Vessel with Fluoroquinolone Antibiotics in Certain Patients.7. Available online: https://www.fda.gov/media/119532/download (accessed on 12 August 2021).
293. FDA Updates Warnings for Fluoroquinolone Antibiotics on Risks of Mental Health and Low Blood Sugar Adverse Reactions. Available online: https://www.fda.gov/news-events/press-announcements/fda-updates-warnings-fluoroquinolone-antibiotics-risks-mental-health-and-low-blood-sugar-adverse (accessed on 12 August 2021).
294. Francisco, E.M. Fluoroquinolone and Quinolone Antibiotics: PRAC Recommends New Restrictions on Use Following Review of Disabling Potentially Long-Lasting Side Effects. Available online: https://www.ema.europa.eu/en/news/fluoroquinolone-quinolone-antibiotics-prac-recommends-new-restrictions-use-following-review (accessed on 12 August 2021).
295. Francisco, E.M. Meeting Highlights from the Pharmacovigilance Risk Assessment Committee (PRAC) 1-4 October 2018. Available online: https://www.ema.europa.eu/en/news/meeting-highlights-pharmacovigilance-risk-assessment-committee-prac-1-4-october-2018 (accessed on 12 August 2021).
296. Quinolone- and Fluoroquinolone-Containing Medicinal Products. Available online: https://www.ema.europa.eu/en/medicines/human/referrals/quinolone-fluoroquinolone-containing-medicinal-products (accessed on 12 August 2021).
297. EMA/175398/2019, Disabling and Potentially Permanent Side Effects Lead to Suspension or Restrictions of Quinolone and Fluoroquinolone Antibiotics. 2019. Available online: https://www.ema.europa.eu/en/documents/referral/quinolone-fluoroquinolone-article-31-referral-disabling-potentially-permanent-side-effects-lead_en.pdf (accessed on 12 August 2021).
298. EMA/413844/2018, Summary of the EMA Public Hearing on Quinolone and Fluoroquinolone Antibiotics. 2018. Available online: https://www.ema.europa.eu/en/documents/report/summary-ema-public-hearing-quinolone-luoroquinolone-antibiotics_en.pdf (accessed on 12 August 2021).
299. Majalekar, P.P.; Shirote, P.J. Fluoroquinolones: Blessings or Curses. *Curr. Drug Targets* **2020**, *21*, 1354–1370. [CrossRef]
300. Richards, G.A.; Brink, A.J.; Feldman, C. Rational Use of the Fluoroquinolones. *SAMJ S. Afr. Med. J.* **2019**, *109*, 378–381. [CrossRef] [PubMed]

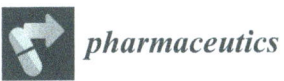

Review

The Development of Third-Generation Tetracycline Antibiotics and New Perspectives

Aura Rusu * and Emanuela Lorena Buta

Pharmaceutical and Therapeutical Chemistry Department, Faculty of Pharmacy, George Emil Palade University of Medicine, Pharmacy, Science and Technology of Targu Mures, 540142 Targu Mures, Romania; lorrenush@yahoo.com
* Correspondence: aura.rusu@umfst.ro; Tel.: +40-766-600-898

Abstract: The tetracycline antibiotic class has acquired new valuable members due to the optimisation of the chemical structure. The first modern tetracycline introduced into therapy was tigecycline, followed by omadacycline, eravacycline, and sarecycline (the third generation). Structural and physicochemical key elements which led to the discovery of modern tetracyclines are approached. Thus, several chemical subgroups are distinguished, such as glycylcyclines, aminomethylcyclines, and fluorocyclines, which have excellent development potential. The antibacterial spectrum comprises several resistant bacteria, including those resistant to old tetracyclines. Sarecycline, a narrow-spectrum tetracycline, is notable for being very effective against *Cutinebacterium acnes*. The mechanism of antibacterial action from the perspective of the new compound is approached. Several severe bacterial infections are treated with tigecycline, omadacycline, and eravacycline (with parenteral or oral formulations). In addition, sarecycline is very useful in treating acne vulgaris. Tetracyclines also have other non-antibiotic properties that require in-depth studies, such as the anti-inflammatory effect effect of sarecycline. The main side effects of modern tetracyclines are described in accordance with published clinical studies. Undoubtedly, this class of antibiotics continues to arouse the interest of researchers. As a result, new derivatives are developed and studied primarily for the antibiotic effect and other biological effects.

Keywords: tetracyclines; structure-activity relationship; mechanism; antibacterial activity; resistance; fluorocycline; aminomethylcycline; glycylcycline

Citation: Rusu, A.; Buta, E.L. The Development of Third-Generation Tetracycline Antibiotics and New Perspectives. *Pharmaceutics* 2021, 13, 2085. https://doi.org/10.3390/pharmaceutics13122085

Academic Editor: Teresa Cerchiara

Received: 29 October 2021
Accepted: 3 December 2021
Published: 5 December 2021

Publisher's Note: MDPI stays neutral with regard to jurisdictional claims in published maps and institutional affiliations.

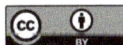

Copyright: © 2021 by the authors. Licensee MDPI, Basel, Switzerland. This article is an open access article distributed under the terms and conditions of the Creative Commons Attribution (CC BY) license (https://creativecommons.org/licenses/by/4.0/).

1. Introduction

Tetracyclines are an important class of broad-spectrum antibiotics that prevent bacterial growth by inhibiting protein biosynthesis. This large family includes compounds with bacteriostatic activity and a wide range of uses, from Gram-positive and Gram-negative bacterial infections to those caused by a protozoan parasite and intracellular organisms [1]. Sarecycline is unique, being the only narrow-spectrum antibiotic in the tetracycline-class family. The basic structure of tetracyclines consists of four linearly condensed benzene rings in a hydronaphtacene nucleus. The essential differences between the analogues of this class are given by the C5, C6, C7, and C9 substituents (Figure 1) [2].

1.1. Brief History of Tetracycline Antibiotics

The emergence of tetracycline development is due to the contribution of hundreds of dedicated researchers, scientists, and clinicians over more than 60 years [3]. Since their discovery (1948, aureomycin), tetracyclines have played an essential role in treating bacterial infections [4]. Stimulated by the extraordinary success of penicillins, several companies and academic institutions have focused on discovering new antibiotics produced by microorganisms, analysing numerous samples of soil sent from different parts of the world. It was observed that actinomycete bacteria produced a yellow colony, with a remarkable inhibitory effect against many pathogenic strains, including rickettsia and Gram-positive and Gram-negative bacteria. This actinomycete bacteria became famous for its broad-spectrum antibiotic. The first tetracycline was extracted from *Streptomyces aureofaciens* and was named aureomycin (syn. chlortetracycline) [5–8]. Professor Benjamin Minge Duggar supervised the discovery of the first tetracycline. After the Food and Drug Administration (FDA) approval in 1948, aureomycin saved many lives and brought fame and profit to the Cyanamid (Lederle Laboratories Division) manufacturing company, being successfully marketed [3,7,9,10]. After Pfizer isolated *Streptomyces rimosus*, the aureomycin and terramycin (syn. oxytetracycline) were discovered [7]. This new compound was the second representative of this class of antibiotics, similar in chemical structure but with superior bioavailability and water solubility. The FDA approved Terramycin in 1950 [3,9,11].

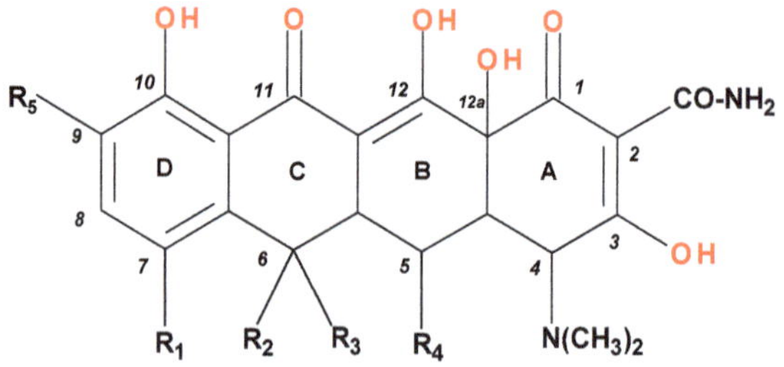

Figure 1. Tetracyclines—the general chemical structure and conventional numbering of the condensed rings and key positions.

Tetracycline was discovered in 1953, on the basis of the chemical structure of chlortetracycline, by catalitic hidrogenation (with palladium and hydrogen). The new antibiotic agent presented and improved the pharmacokinetic profile, which quickly became a favourite in therapy [12,13]. This remarkable success has proven for the first time in history that other biologically active and valuable antibiotics can be obtained by operating changes on the basic structure (molecule optimisations) [3,14]. After discovering chlortetracycline, oxytetracycline, and tetracycline (first generation of tetracyclines), the chemists of Pfizer and Lederle Laboratories began the development of new tetracyclines, with superior pharmacokinetic properties, wider antimicrobial spectrum, and lower toxicity [15]. Among the discovered representatives were methacycline (1966), doxycycline (1967), and minocycline (1972) [13,16]. Doxycycline is a semisynthetic analogue based on the chemical structure of the metacycline, approved in 1967 by the FDA. These tetracyclines are classified in the second generation (Table S1—Supplementary Materials) [3,14,17].

The further development of semisynthetic analogues of the second generation, and, more recently, of the third generation (Table 1), reveals the evolution of this class. The modern tetracyclines had acquired high potency and an increased efficacy, even against bacteria resistant to tetracyclines [18–20]. Therefore, biochemical mutants of *Streptomycetes* strains have been created for a higher production yield and to discover novel tetracyclines [3,15].

Table 1. Tetracyclines—classification into generations [14,21–24].

Generations	Obtaining Method	Representatives
First	Biosynthesis	Chlortetracycline, oxytetracycline, tetracycline, demeclocycline
Second	Semisynthesis	Doxycycline, minocycline, lymecycline, meclocycline, methacycline, rolitetracycline
Third	Semisynthesis Total synthesis	Tigecycline, omadacycline, sarecycline Eravacycline

Therefore, compounds such as demeclocycline were discovered, being later converted in 1971 to a C7-amino-derivative known as minocycline. Some authors classified minocycline as the last tetracycline in the second generation. Moreover, demeclocycline was a precursor of sancycline (obtained by reduction), a tetracycline with a simplified chemical structure and retained biological activity [1,25]. Thus, the main advantage of minocycline is a broader spectrum of activity compared to previously representatives. Furthermore, minocycline presented a better pharmacokinetic profile and was the most potent representative at the time, being the last introduced on the market in the next three decades [3,17,26].

1.2. The Discovery of Modern Tetracyclines

The growing occurrence of bacterial resistance to antibiotics has once again aroused the interest of scientists in the development of new tetracyclines. Thus, at the end of the 1980s, the programs were reopened for the synthesis of new compounds that could be classified into a new generation (the third one), re-evaluating the compounds already synthesised (Table S2—Supplementary Materials) [3]. The main interest was about the modification of C7 and C9 positions of the D ring in the sancycline structure (Figure 2, Table S3—Supplementary Materials). These steps have led to the discovery of a novel class of C9-aminotetracyclines, which bear a glycyl moiety known as *glycylcycline* [3,27–29].

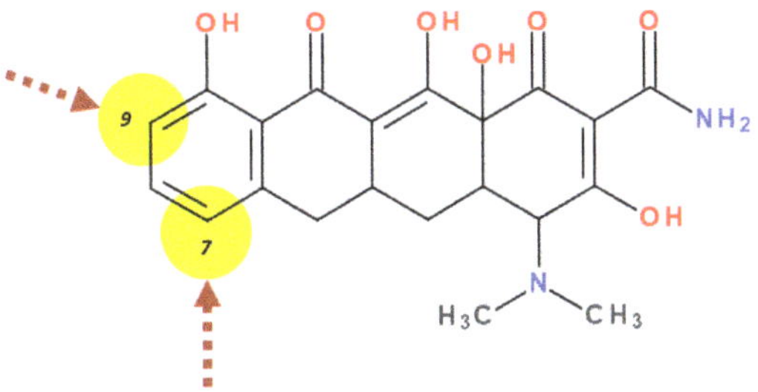

Figure 2. The chemical structures of sancycline; key positions highlighted C7 and C9 for structural design optimisation to obtain new derivatives.

Modern tetracyclines include derivatives with more or less similar chemical structures: a glycylglicine (tigecycline), an aminomethylcycline (omadacycline), a fluorocycline (eravacycline), and a 7-[(methoxy-(methyl)-amino)-methyl]methyl derivative (sarecycline) (Figure 3).

Tigecycline is a synthetic derivative of minocycline discovered in 1993. Tigecycline was the first tetracycline introduced in therapy after more than 30 years. Thus, tigecycline could be considered the prototype of a new subclass of tetracyclines [27,29]. This new tetracycline has the advantage of a superior potency over Gram-positive and Gram-negative multidrug-resistant bacteria (multiple drug resistance, MDR) [26,30]. Tigecycline was discovered by Wyeth Pharmaceuticals Inc. and approved by the FDA in 2005 [31] and later by the European Medicine Agency (EMA) in 2006, under the trade name Tygacil [32]. Tygacil received approval for complicated intra-abdominal and complicated skin and soft tissue infections [33,34]. Likewise, in 2008, the FDA approved the use of tigecycline to treat community-acquired pneumonia [35,36]. Once placed in the market, several other uses have been investigated: nosocomial pneumonia, diabetic foot infections, emergency therapy for MDR pathogens, nosocomial urinary tract infections, and *Clostridium difficile* infections [26]. A disadvantage of tigecycline is its exclusive parenteral use due to its poor bioavailability [37].

Omadacycline is one of the newest and most popular tetracyclines and the first in the aminomethylcycline subclass [3,38]. It has a broad spectrum of activity, proving in vitro effects against Gram-positive and Gram-negative bacteria, anaerobic bacteria, and atypical bacteria. In addition, the activity of this compound extends to methicillin-resistant *Staphylococcus aureus* (MRSA); penicillin-resistant, MDR *Streptococcus pneumoniae*; and vancomycin-resistant enterococci [22]. Unlike tigecycline, omadacycline is available for both oral and parenteral administration. Both forms were approved in 2018 by the

FDA for the treatment of complicated intra-abdominal and complicated skin and soft tissue infections and community-acquired pneumonia. Currently, omadacycline is in phase II of clinical trials to treat urinary tract infections, such as acute pyelonephritis and cystitis [38]. The pharmaceutical product Nuzyra was approved in the United States of America (USA) [39].

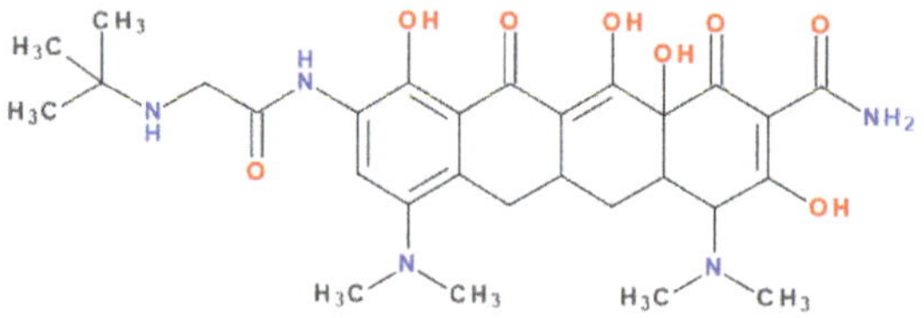

Figure 3. The chemical structure of the representatives of the third-generation tetracyclines.

Eravacycline is a synthetic fluorocycline, obtained by total synthesis, that contains a basic chemical structure of the tetracyclines class [40,41]. In addition, particular modifications on the D ring of the naphtacen nucleus were introduced. Those chemical optimisations give it a remarkable activity against Gram-positive and Gram-negative bacteria that developed specific resistance mechanisms to the tetracycline antibiotic class to treat complicated intra-abdominal infections in adults. It is available for parenteral administration in many countries in Europe, as well as in the USA [41].

Sarecycline is an analogue of tetracycline specifically designed for the treatment of acne [42]. It is available as an oral formulation to treat inflammatory lesions of moderate to severe non-nodular acne vulgaris. The main advantage of this new tetracycline is a higher selective activity against *Cutinebacterium acnes* comparative to older tetracyclines (doxycycline and minocycline) used in acne therapy. Due to this selectivity, the probability of developing antibiotic resistance is lower than minocycline and doxycycline [43]. Sarecycline was developed by Paratek Pharmaceuticals and Allergan but acquired by Almirall S.A by purchasing the dermatological portfolio [44]. The FDA approved sarecycline in 2018 under the trade name Seysara [45,46].

2. Research Methodology

The relevant primary data were found on Clarivate Analytics and ScienceDirect databases using the following keywords: (i) topic: "tetracyclines", "antibacterials"; (ii) title: "tigecycline", "omadacycline", "eravacycline", "sarecycline", and other classic derivatives of the tetracycline class. In the second stage, the articles were selected if they comprised development of tetracyclines class, physicochemical properties, aspects related to structure–activity relationships, new tetracyclines design, mechanism of action, antibacterial spectrum, therapeutical value, safety profile, bacterial resistance, and new derivatives in development. The paper includes significant references, including the latest articles published in 2021.

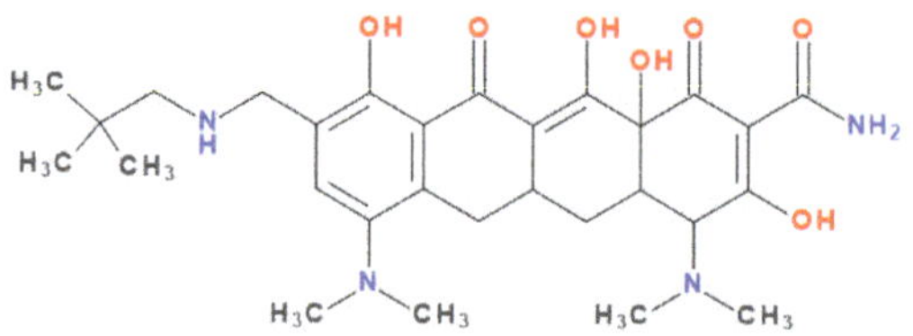

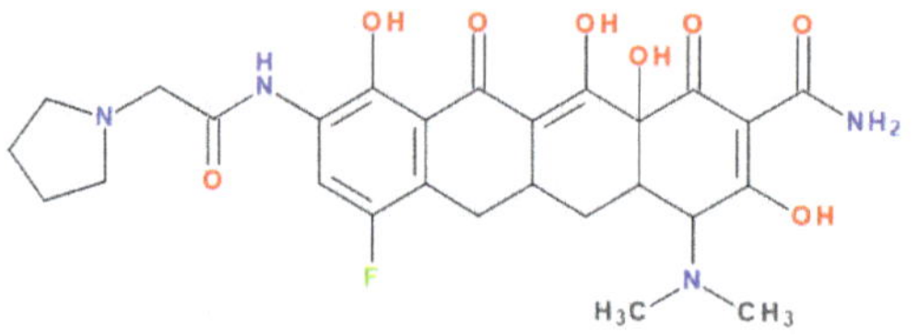

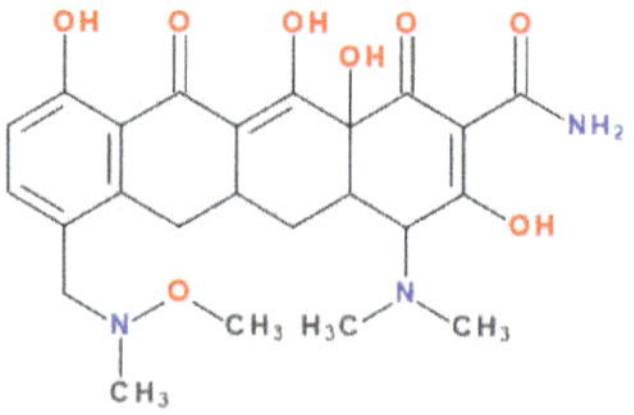

All chemical structures were drowned with Biovia Draw 2019 (San Diego, CA, USA) [47].

3. Overview of Modern Tetracyclines

This paper's primary targeted the new tetracyclines classified as the third generation: tigecycline, omadacycline, eravacycline, and sarecycline.

3.1. Considerations Regarding the Chemical Structure and Physicochemical Properties of the New Tetracyclines

Recently introduced compounds in the tetracycline class contain the basic chemical structure specific to this class, four condensed rings (A, B, C, and D) into a naphtacen-carboxamide system. Other common structural elements are a dimethyl-amino group at the C4 position, an amidic group at the C2 position, a keto–enol alternation system (C11, C12, and 12a positions), and asymmetric carbons at the junction of rings A-B (stereochemical configurations) (Figures 1 and 3) [21,48,49]. X-ray crystallography of tetracycline, doxycycline, and sancycline revealed that the C2 amide group is oriented to form an intramolecular hydrogen bond with oxygen atom from C3 position [50]. The above elements are considered the minimum pharmacophore (6-deoxy-dimethyltetracycline) required for antimicrobial activity and a start point for inserting other substituents [21,48,49].

Depending on the radicals grafted on the tetracyclic system, these new molecules introduced on the market after 2000 present different physicochemical and pharmacological characteristics and changes in the antimicrobial spectrum [13,21,38,41,44]. The optimisation of the basic structure consisted of C7 and C9 substitutions. Position C7 is subject to substitution with electron acceptor or donor groups [40]. Thus, tigecycline and omadacycline have a dimethyl-amino group in this position. Eravacycline has a fluorine atom at the C7 position, being an electron-withdrawing substituent [40,51]. In the same place, sarecycline has a more voluminous radical, methoxy-methyl-amino-methyl [42]. The radicals in the C9 position are distinct for each of the new representatives. Tigecycline and eravacycline are synthetic analogues that contain a glycyl-amide substituent [40,52].

Tigecycline was synthesised by adding a *tert*-butyl-glycyl-amide substituent, while in eravacycline this group was replaced with a pyrrolidinyl-acetamide group [32,40]. However, tigecycline is an analogue of minocycline formed by adding the *tert*-butyl-glycyl-amide substituent at the C9 position (Figure 4). It is the first glycylcycline tetracycline discovered [29,31]. Currently, tigecycline is manufactured as a lyophilised powder form because it undergoes a degradation process. Tigecycline is commercialised under the trade name Tygacil (pharmaceutical form for intravenous infusion). The recommended doses regimen is 100 mg initial dose, followed by 50 mg every 12 h [31].

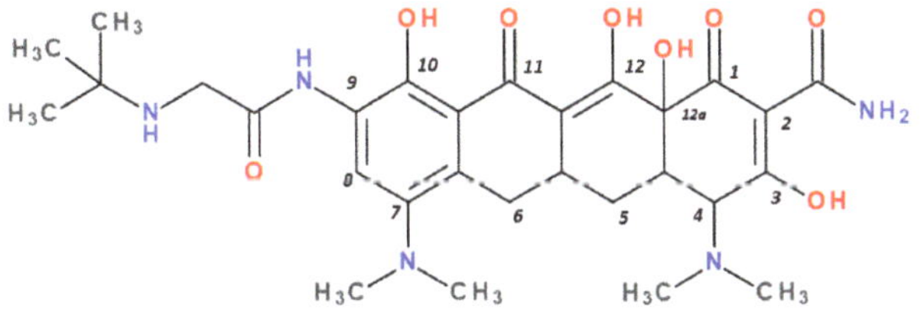

Figure 4. The chemical structures of the tigecycline and conventional numbering.

Omadacycline (sin. amadacycline) is the first aminomethylcycline of this new subclass, for which the glycyl-amide group was changed to an alkyl-amino-methyl group [38,53,54]. The optimisation at the C9 atom was based on a methyl(2,2-dimethylpropylamino) fragment that replaces the glycylamide group present in the case of its homologues (tigecycline and eravacycline) (Figure 5) [52]. Omadacycline is formulated as tosylate salt for intravenous or oral administration under the trade name Nuzyra [38].

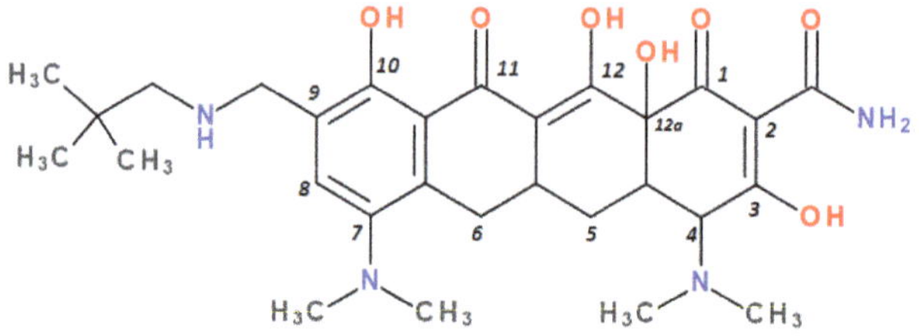

Figure 5. The chemical structures of the omadacycline and conventional numbering.

The primary structure of tetracyclines is maintained in the chemical structure of eravacycline, which is an analogue of tigecycline, with two changes on the D ring: the addition of a fluorine atom in the C7 position and the substitution of the *tert*-butyl-aminoacetamide group in the C9 position with a pyrrolidin-acetamido group (Figure 6) [41]. Pharmaceutical formulation under the trade name Xerava contains eravacycline, powder for concentrate for solution for infusion (50 mg and 100 mg) for intravenous use [55].

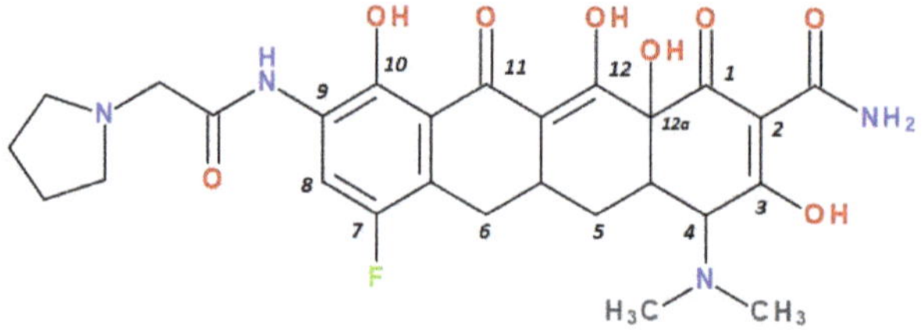

Figure 6. The chemical structures of the eravacycline and conventional numbering.

Sarecycline has no substitute in the C9 position [56]. Sarecycline is chemically distinguishable from other tetracycline-class antibiotics by the 7 [[methoxy(methyl)amino]methyl] group attached at the C7 position of the ring D. This stable modification represents the longest and the largest C7 moiety among all of the tetracyclines (Figure 7). Sarecycline inhibits bacterial ribosomes through interactions with the mRNA as a consequence of C7 optimisation. This new tetracycline blocks accommodation into the A site of the first aminoacyl transfer RNA and appears to be a more potent initiation inhibitor comparative to previous analogues [57]. Sarecycline is manufactured as hydrochloride salt [42]. Pharmaceutical formula Seysara tablets for oral use contains sarecycline (60 mg, 100 mg, 150 mg) [46].

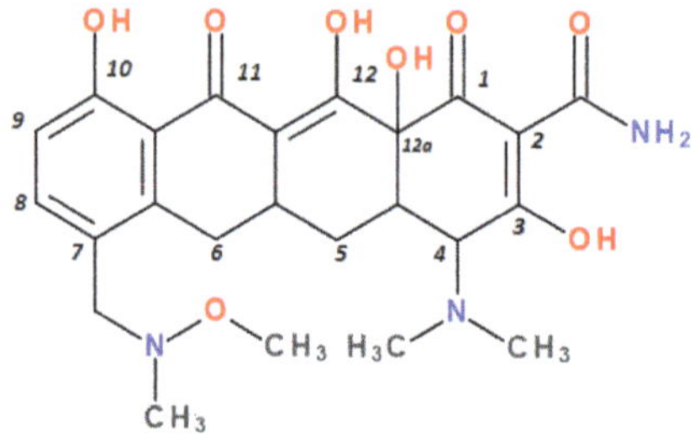

Figure 7. The chemical structures of the sarecycline and conventional numbering.

Essential physicochemical properties of the third generation tetracyclines are shown in Table S4 (Supplementary Materials).

Tetracyclines are optically active substances. The X-ray diffraction analysis (XRD) established the stereochemistry of the basic structure of these compounds. Depending on substitution, several chiral atoms are C4, C4*a*, C5, C5*a*, C6, and C12*a* (Figure 8a). Some derivatives, such as oxytetracycline and doxycycline, have six chiral carbon atoms, due to the C5α-hydroxyl substituent. Moreover, a conjugated system is known in the naphtacene nucleus (C10 to C12; C1 to C3) [58].

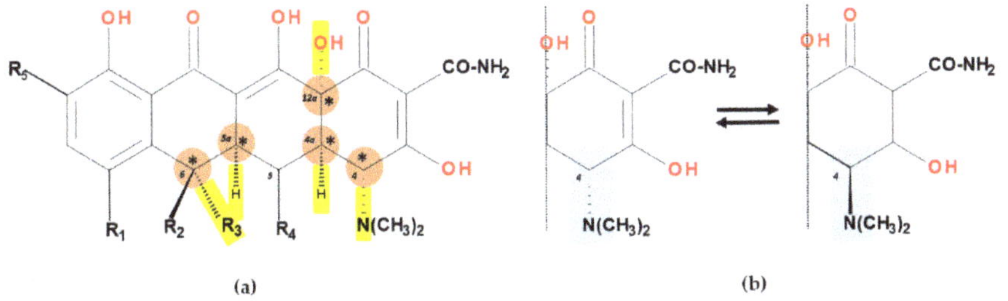

Figure 8. The chiral atoms on the chemical structure of tetracyclines and conventional numbering (**a**); epimerisation of tetracyclines (**b**); *—chiral centers.

In acidic conditions, tetracyclines epimerase reversibly at the C4 position (Figure 8b). The resulted isomers are known as "epitetracyclines", founded in equal amounts after establishing the equilibrium. The formation of 4-epitetracyclines is notable because they are less active than non-epimerised isomers [58,59].

Tetracyclines are amphoteric compounds due to the characteristic structural elements (hydroxyls and dimethylamino substituents and the conjugated keto-enolic system). In reaction with an acid or a base, tetracyclines form salts. In pharmaceutical formulations, tetracyclines are most commonly used in the form of hydrochloric salts (e.g., eravacycline, sarecycline). Depending on the solvent, the tetracyclines' structure changes from an ionised to a non-ionised state (protonation–deprotonation equilibria). At the neutral pH, tetracyclines mainly adopt the zwitterion form. It is known that acid salts of tetracyclines exhibit a minimum of three acidity constants in aqueous solutions [14,50,59,60].

The main protonation sites of tetracyclines are the tricarbonyl system (C1-C2-C3), phenolic diketone-system (C10-C11-C12), and dimethylamino group (C4) (Figure 9) [58,61–63]. Depending on the substituents on the basic chemical structure, the protonation state of the compound also changes [64]. Tetracyclines are multiprotic compounds. Put simply, tetracyclines can be considered to behave similar to triprotic acids [63]. Other authors have suggested that tetracyclines have four ionisation equilibria and four correspondent pKa values (at pH values of 3.2, 7.6, 9.6, and 12) and five protonation states [63].

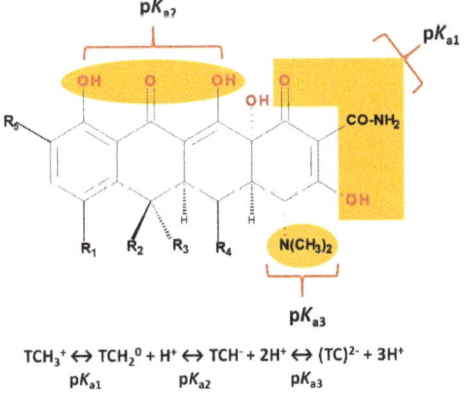

$$TCH_3^+ \leftrightarrow TCH_2^0 + H^+ \leftrightarrow TCH^- + 2H^+ \leftrightarrow (TC)^{2-} + 3H^+$$
$$pK_{a1} \qquad pK_{a2} \qquad pK_{a3}$$

Figure 9. The tetracycline (TC) structural sites and the correspondent acidic dissociation constants [61–65].

Thus, tigecycline poses five main ionisation groups, specifically, five values of pK_a (at pH values of 2.8, 4.4, 7.4, 8.9, and 9.5), an important role having the substitutes from C7 and C9 [65]. Using MarvinSketck (ChemAxon, Budapest, Hungary) for sarecycline, researchers found 17 possible microspecies depending on the pH value. Table 2 comprises the predicted microspecies and the highest value of ionisation (%) at a specific pH; additionally, the degree of ionisation at the physiologic pH (7.4) was highlighted. The highest ionisation percentages of the microspecies were identified as follows: no. 3 at pH 0–1 (98.15%), no. 6 at pH 4 (98.66%), no. 14 at pH 11 (96.30%), no. 17 at pH 14 (95.55%), and no. 7 at pH 8.6 (49.38%). At the physiologic pH (7.4), no. 2 was 21.59%, the highest ionisation percentage.

Table 2. Sarecycline microspecies and the degree of ionisation as a function of pH (calculated) [66].

No.	Microspecies	No.	Microspecies	No.	Microspecies
1	pH 6.60 (32.92%; highest) pH 7.40 (17.87%)	2	pH 7.60 (22.31%; highest) pH 7.40 (21.59%)	4	pH 7.60 (12.59%; highest) pH 7.40 (12.19%)
3	pH 4.00 (98.86%; highest) pH 7.40 (2.11%)	5	pH 7.60 (3.84%; highest) pH 7.40 (3.72%)	6	pH 0.00 (98.16%; highest) pH 7.40 (0.00%)
7	pH 8.60 (49.38%; highest) pH 7.40 (11.90%)	8	pH 6.80 (24.07%; highest) pH 7.40 (13.10%)	9	pH 8.80 (17.75%; highest) pH 7.40 (4.50%)
10	pH 8.80 (17.75%; highest) pH 7.40 (4.50%)	11	pH 6.60 (2.80%; highest) pH 7.40 (1.52%)	12	pH 6.60-6.80 (0.81%; highest) pH 7.40 (0.44%)

Table 2. Cont.

No.	Microspecies	No.	Microspecies	No.	Microspecies
13	pH 7.60 (7.85%; highest) pH 7.40 (7.60%)	14	pH 11.00 (96.30%; highest) pH 7.40 (0.26%)	15	pH 7.60 (2.82%; highest) pH 7.40 (2.73%)
16	pH 8.60 (0.69%; highest) pH 7.40 (0.17%)	17	pH 14.00 (95.55%; highest) pH 7.40 (0.00%)		

Protonation equilibria and formed microspecies play an essential role in the bioavailability of tetracyclines [63]. The protonated state of tetracyclines is also essential in the analysis. For example, in electrospray mass spectrometry, both protonated molecules of tigecycline (MH+ and MH_2^{2+}) are predominantly formed [67].

Electron-rich functional groups depending on pH can be protonated or deprotonated. Consequently, the tetracyclines have excellent chelating properties with several bivalent or trivalent metal cations [60]. Thus, tetracyclines form stable complexes with metal ions due to the characteristic substituents (Table S3—Supplementary Materials) [60].

First-generation tetracyclines form insoluble complexes with metal ions (Ca^{2+}, Mg^{2+}, Fe^{3+}, and Al^{3+}) and consequently present reduced absorption [49]. Doxycycline and minocycline (second generation) are known for their excellent ability to chelate Fe^{3+}. Both doxycycline and minocycline absorption are impaired by ferrous sulphate; bismuth; and other antacids containing aluminium, calcium, and magnesium salts, such as co-administration of pharmaceuticals with Fe^{3+} and antacids (rich in Ca^{2+}, Mg^{2+}) [49,68].

Minocycline (second generation) and tigecycline (third generation) are more chelated by Ca^{2+} than tetracycline due to the C7 dimethylamino group. This moiety increased the electron density at the Ca^{2+} coordination site for the two studied tetracyclines. In addition, it was observed that tigecycline formed a different higher-order complex comparative to minocycline through the C9 N-t-butylglycylamido substituent in Ca^{2+} coordination [65]. Complexes with magnesium ions inhibit bacterial growth by impairing protein synthesis; these tetracycline complexes with magnesium act by binding to the 30S ribosomal subunits [69]. In plasma, tetracyclines are mainly chelated with Ca^{2+} and Mg^{2+} ions. A known mechanism of bacterial resistance to tetracyclines involves metal complexation. A possible strategy to combat bacterial resistance is to use in therapy the metal complexes of tetracycline (e.g., Pt^{2+} or Pd^{2+} complexes) [69,70].

3.2. Structure-Activity Relationships

As a result of studies of the relationship between chemical structure and biological activity, several aspects related to the class of tetracyclines are already known [3,13,48,49,71]. Next, the structural elements with an impact on the biological properties of the new tetracyclines are targeted.

Tigecycline was discovered as a result of chemical structure–activity studies [72]. Due to structural modifications made to C9 position (Figure 10), tigecycline has an affinity for the ribosomal target five times higher than tetracycline or minocycline. Therefore, this change is responsible for broadening the antibacterial spectrum and combating ribosomal protection, one of the two mechanisms of bacterial resistance specific to tetracycline [29,73,74]. Moreover, this radical is a bulky steric hindrance that prevents the expulsion of the substance out of the bacterial cell by effluent tet proteins, thus reducing the susceptibility of developing antibiotic resistance [28,75].

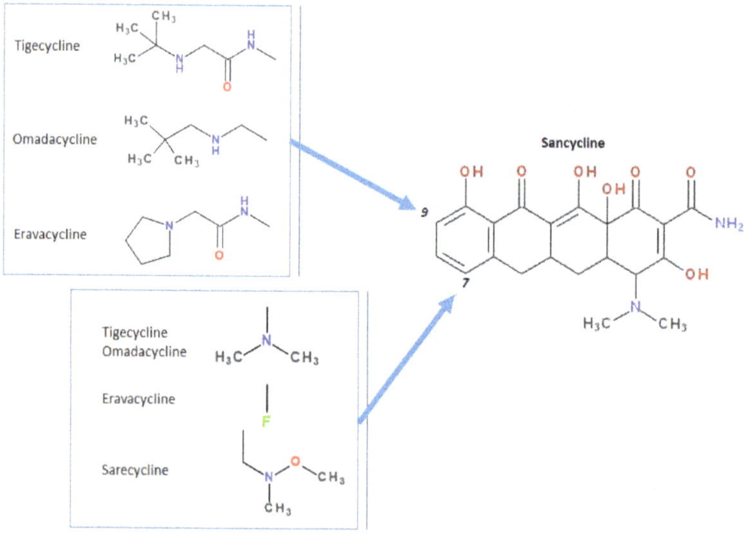

Figure 10. Optimisation of C7 and C9 positions in the development of new tetracyclines.

Researchers observed some structural features of glycylcyclines that are essential in maintaining biological activity [13]. A critical element is the basic nitrogen atom from the glycyl unit; derivatives containing low volume alkyl-amino or cyclic amine groups have shown optimal results. Attempts to replace the radical from the C9 position with other amino acids such as alanine, phenylalanine, and leucine failed because the resulting compounds were much less effective [72]. Similarly, substitutions with smaller groups than the *tert*-butyl-amino group led to compounds with low potency, while the attempt to substitute the amine with n-propyl, n-butyl, and n-hexyl has not brought improvements [76]. The antimicrobial activity and the pharmacokinetics of tigecycline are considerably influenced by the ability to form complexes with metal ions (calcium, magnesium, and iron). The target of the cations is the keto–enol system (C11 and C12 positions), the enol in position C1, and the carboxamide in position C2. Therefore, water-insoluble chelates are formed with a low absorption [13].

Chemical modulations performed to obtain omadacycline on C9 led to an increase in antimicrobial potency by overcoming the resistance to the efflux mechanisms and overcoming ribosomal protection [22,77]. Furthermore, the aminomethyl moiety from C9 position provides improved pharmacokinetic parameters, such as dose reduction (high doses cause side effects such as nausea and vomiting, often encountered in C9 glycylcyclines), and, in particular, oral bioavailability [78]. Due to these changes, omadacycline has a pharmacokinetic profile (absorption, distribution, metabolism, and excretion, ADME) that distinguishes it from the glycylcycline subgroup [77].

A study was conducted on aminomethycyclines with in vitro potency (with a minimum inhibitory concentration (MIC) $\leq$ 0.06–2.0 µg/mL) against Gram-negative bacteria with different mechanisms of resistance by ribosomal protection (Tet(M)): *Staphylococcus aureus*, *Enterococcus faecalis*, and *Streptococcus pneumoniae*, and on the efflux mechanisms Tet(K) in *Staphylococcus aureus*, Tet(L) in *Enterococcus faecalis*) [51]. Compounds with lipophilia-enhancing or benzyl substitutions in the aminomethyl side group showed the highest potency against ribosomal alteration and efflux of resistant strains. However, high-polarity analogues or electrically charged groups, as well as acyl derivatives, showed a significant decrease in antibacterial activity. Although alkyl substituents (e.g., *tert*-butyl group) showed moderate potency, they were chosen for further optimisation and screening. It was found that analogues with the alkyl group, which extend with at least three carbon atoms to the aminomethyl group; those with branched alkyl chains; and piperidine analogues have superior activity. The ramification in the alkyl chain from position 1 has a detrimental impact due to steric hindrance. The introduction of two methyl groups in position 2 showed a significant improvement in antibacterial activity. Finally, residues containing more than five carbon atoms had reduced activity in the presence of plasma, indicating a high percentage binding to plasma proteins [38,51].

Therefore, following classical studies on the chemical structure–biological activity relationships, omadacycline, a compound containing a neopentyl moiety in the aminomethyl group, has been identified as the most valuable aminomethylcycline in this series, becoming a new subclass of tetracyclines [77].

It has been observed on fluorocyclines that as the substituents attached to the carbon atom at the C9 positions are more polar or more basic, the microbiological activity of the compound will increase, especially on Gram-negative bacteria. A study conducted in 2012 examined the behaviour of analogues of 7-fluoro-9-amino-acetamido-6-demethyl-6-deoxytetracyclines on various Gram-negative and Gram-positive bacteria, but also on gene isolates resistant to tetracycline class [79]. In general, less voluminous secondary or tertiary amine analogues from C9 position were found to have a lower MIC compared to analogues with substituents such as aromatic amines or alkylamines with lower basicity. Compared to tertiary alkylamine, dimethyl, azetidine, and piperidine analogues, eravacycline, a compound bearing a pyrrolidine nucleus, showed a 8 to 16 times higher potency against *K. pneumoniae* (tet(A)) and 4 to 8 times higher potency against *E. coli* (tet(A)). In addition, eravacycline is 4 to 64 times more potent than piperidine and azetidine omologues against bacterial isolates that have been tested (except for *S. pneumoniae* expressing or not expressing tet(M) protein, were it showing an equivalent response). The addition of polar substituents, fluorine atoms, or pyrrolidine bicycles produced no improvements, but neither did negative influence on the activity against pneumococcal bacteria when compared to unsubstitued pyrrolidine analogues [40,80]. The pyrrolidine substituent at the C9 the fluoro substituent at C7, the main optimisations in eravacycline, positively influenced the potency and the antibacterial spectrum [19].

Unlike other tetracyclines, the chemical structure of sarecycline includes a unique modification at the C7 position (the longest and most voluminous of the whole class), a 7-[(methoxy-(methyl)-amino)-methyl]methyl group (Figure 10). As a result of this chemical optimisation, the activity of this compound is enhanced, binding to the codon of the A site, interfering with the movement of messenger RNA (mRNA) along the channel, or disrupting the codon A-anticodon interaction [42].

The substituted tetracycline system at positions C7 and C9 is the basis of compounds with increased antibacterial activity, while any modification made at the C1-C4, C10-C12, C-11a, and C-12a will have a negative consequence on their action. Other important aspects regarding the relationship between chemical structure and biological activity are presented in Figure 11 [3,38,40,51].

In addition, tetracyclines contain a 4S(α)-dimethyl-amino group in the C4 position, an absolute necessity for optimal antibacterial activity. On the other hand, the epimerisation of the 4R(β) isomer will lead to a decrease in antibacterial activity, especially against Gram-negative bacteria. The epimerisation process from position C4 takes place during harsh chemical reactions, in vivo metabolism phenomenon, but also under changes in the pH values [25].

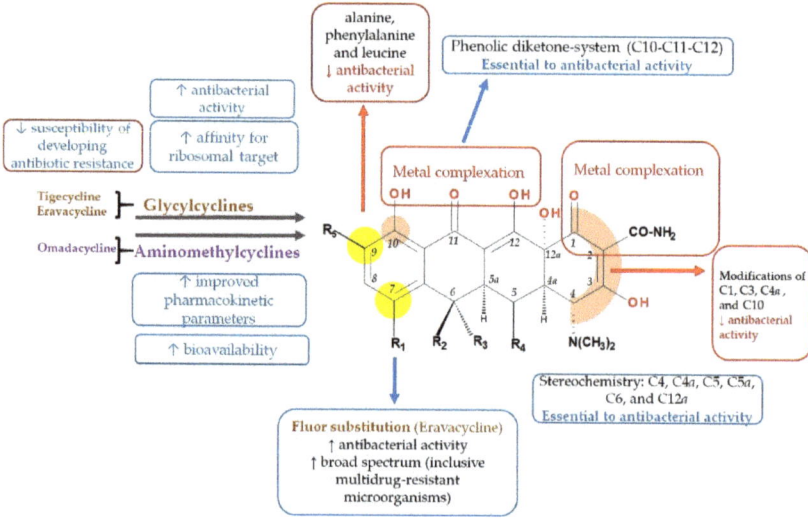

Figure 11. The essential relationship between chemical structure and biological activity of modern tetracyclines.

The C4 β-epimers have noticeably different properties from those of compounds with a normal configuration. The most significant difference is observed in antibacterial activity manifested in vitro. β-Epimers have been found to be responsible for approximately 5% of normal tetracycline activity. It has been observed that the epimerisation phenomenon takes place in different solvent systems, at variations of pH between 2 and 6 [14]. Tetracyclines are prone to epimer formation, particularly under weak acidic conditions. The epimers have distinct toxicological and antibacterial properties, and therefore selective biosynthesis is a major challenge. This is due to the fact that the epimers are isobars with the parent compound, having very similar physico-chemical properties. Epimerisation can occur in vivo, even in the bladder [59].

3.3. Mechanism of Action

Tetracyclines inhibit protein synthesis by inhibiting the association of aminoacyl-tRNA with bacterial ribosome [49,75]. Tetracyclines bind with high affinity to a specific locus (16S) on the 30S ribosomal unit during translation. In this way, the penetration of aminoacyl transporter RNA (tRNA) into the acceptor site (A) on the bacterial ribosome is blocked, the consequence being the cessation in the incorporation of amino acids residues in the process of elongation of the polypeptide chain. Thus, the protein synthesis is stopped (Figure 12) [18,81,82]. Commonly, at therapeutic concentrations, tetracyclines are consider bacteriostatic antibiotics [18], but late studies have described their bactericidal effects in vitro, especially in the case of tigecycline (studies on mice) [83].

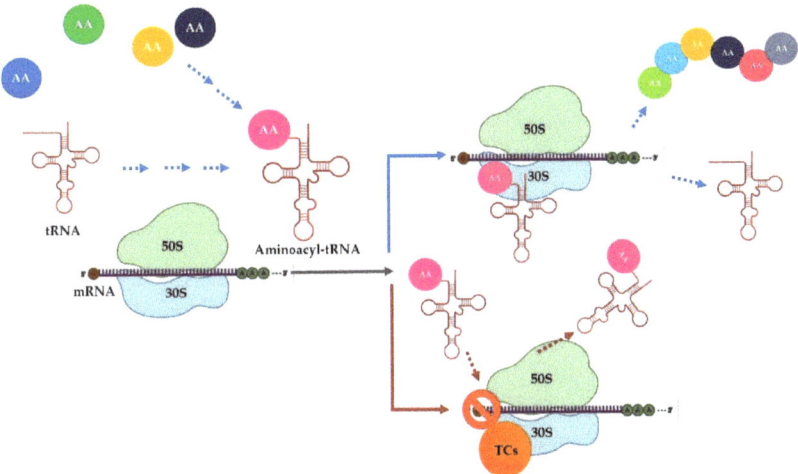

Figure 12. Scheme of the tetracyclines' mechanism of action, where AA—aminoacids, TCs—tetracyclines, tRNA—transfer ribonucleic acid, mRNA—messenger ribonucleic acid, 30S and 50S—ribosomal subunits (created with BioRender.com (accessed on 30 September 2021) [84].

It is well known that tetracyclines cross the membranes of Gram-negative bacteria through a cationic complex with Mg^{2+}, using the OmpF and OmpC porins in the outer membrane [38,85]. Later on, the Donnan potential generated along the outer membrane causes the accumulation of the complex in the periplasmic space, where the dissociation from the Mg^{2+} ion of tetracycline takes place and there is a release of an electrically uncharged molecule that is lipophilic enough to diffuse through the inner membrane into the cytoplasm [86]. The uptake of tetracyclines in the cytoplasm is partially energy-dependent, involving, in addition to passive diffusion, the proton-motive force and the hydrolysis of phosphate bonds [18]. For Gram-positive bacteria, it has been reported that these agents reach the cytoplasm by passive diffusion and/or active transport. In the cytoplasm, tetracyclines chelate Mg^{2+} ions again and, in this form, attack the ribosomal target [75]. Hence, bivalent ions are a vital element in the transport and efficiency of these compounds [85].

Tigecycline is not affected by most common antibiotic resistance mechanisms because it binds to the 30S subunit (five times stronger than tetracyclines) [28], even in the presence of ribosomal protection, being excepted from membrane efflux [87]. This is due to the voluminous substituent in the C9 position of the naphtacenic nucleus, representing a steric hindrance [88,89]. Tigecycline's activity was evaluated by a study on *Escherichia coli* derivatives containing plasmids expressing different specific efflux genes (tet[B], tet[C], and tet[K]). An unchanged MIC value confirmed tigecycline's protection against these efflux genes [90]. Moreover, glycylcyclines also manifest resistance to less common mechanisms, such as altered target site conformation, enzymatic degradation, and mutations in DNA gyrase [87].

Similar to tigecycline, omadacycline possesses excellent activity against bacterial isolates carrying a wide variety of resistance mechanisms, including both tet[K] and tet[O] genes simultaneously [22,91]. Due to the reversible binding of tetracyclines to ribosomes, they act as bacteriostatic agents. Instead, in vitro omadacycline has demonstrated bactericidal activity against *Haemophilus influenzae*, *Streptococcus penumoniae*, and *Moraxella catarrhalis* [78]. Omadacycline has no significant effect on the synthesis of RNA, DNA, and peptidoglycan. Like tigecycline, omadacycline binds to the 30S subunit of the bacterial ribosome with enhanced binding based on other molecular interactions [77]. Having a D-ring modified with a pyrrolidinacetamide side chain, eravacycline was designed to maintain its activity against resistant bacteria (e.g., carbapenem-resistant, MDR, and extended-spectrum cephalosporin-resistant Enterobacteriaceae and extended-spectrum, β-lactamase-producing Enterobacteriaceae) [41,92]. Eravacycline has 10 times the affinity for the ribosomal target in vitro and inhibits translation at four times lower concentrations than tetracycline [93]. A study conducted by *Batool* et al. in 2020 concluded that sarecycline differs slightly from other tetracycline derivatives in terms of mechanism of action, emphasising its unique role in this large family, a role that clinicians should take into account when evaluating its therapeutic potential. By analysing the crystal structure of sarecycline related to the bacterial initiation complex, it has demonstrated that in addition to binding to the same site of the small ribosomal subunit, sarecycline, due to the C7 moiety, expands and establishes uncommon interactions with mRNA. This contact leads to the stabilisation of the substance on the ribosome and an increased inhibitory effect. Thus, sarecycline overcome the mechanisms of bacterial resistance to tetracyclines [42,57].

Other Biological Effects

In addition to the approved therapeutical uses as antibiotics, tetracyclines have other biological effects, which have been investigated and exploited. These non-antibiotic properties comprise anti-inflammatory effects; anti-apoptotic activity; immunomodulatory properties; inhibitory effects on proteolysis, angiogenesis, and tumour metastasis; and a neuroprotector effect [17].

The anti-inflammatory activity of this class is mediated by a large number of mechanisms such as inhibition of neutrophil activation and migration; T lymphocyte activation and proliferation; inhibition of phospholipase, angiogenesis, nitric oxide synthesis, and granuloma formation; suppression of inflammatory cytokine release (TNFα, IL-1β, IL-6, IL-8); and decrease of reactive oxygen species [94,95]. However, the best-known mechanism of anti-inflammatory action is the inhibition of matrix metalloproteinases (MMPs). This mechanism occurs both directly and indirectly by inhibiting the MMPs synthesis [96]. Therefore, tetracyclines, such as doxycycline, minocycline, and sarecycline, are frequently prescribed for acne vulgaris when topical treatment is unsuccessful [94]. In a study using the carrageenan-induced rat paw oedema inflammation model, sarecycline presented an anti-inflammatory effect comparable to doxycycline and minocycline at all the tested doses [42]. Moreover, sarecycline has been proven to be a valuable alternative for treating papulopustular rosacea in terms of efficiency, safety, and tolerability [97].

The non-antibiotic properties of tetracyclines and their analogues were studied in both dermatological and non-dermatological diseases, as presented in Table 3 [98].

Table 3. Other therapeutical uses of tetracyclines related to their non-antibiotic properties.

Dermatological Conditions	Reference	Non-Dermatological Conditions	Reference
Acne	[99,100]	Rheumatoid arthritis	[101,102]
Rosacea	[103,104]	Scleroderma	[105]
Bullous dermatitis	[106]	Cancer	[107]
Kaposi's sarcoma	[108]	Aortic aneurysm	[109]
Sarcoidosis	[110]	Acute myocardial infarction	[111]
Pyoderma gangrenosum	[112]	Periodontitis	[113]
Hidradenitis suppurativa	[114]		
Sweet's syndrome	[115]		
Alpha-1-antitrypsin deficiency panniculitis	[116]		
Pityriasis lichenoides chronica (PLC)	[117]		

Research has shown that minocycline has several non-antibiotic biological effects that are beneficial in experimental models of various inflammatory diseases. These include dermatitis, periodontitis, atherosclerosis, and autoimmune diseases such as rheumatoid arthritis and inflammatory bowel disease. Due to its high lipophilicity, minocycline readily penetrates the blood–brain barrier and achieves high concentrations in the brain; hence, it has been effective in neuroprotection. However, because of its lipophilicity, vestibular side effects such as dizziness and vertigo have been associated with minocycline therapy. This outcome has been confirmed by experimental studies of ischemia, traumatic brain injury, and neuropathic pain, as well as several neurodegenerative diseases (e.g., Parkinson's disease, Huntington's disease, Alzheimer's disease, amyotrophic lateral sclerosis, spinal cord injury, and multiple sclerosis). In addition, other pre-clinical studies have shown the ability of minocycline to inhibit malignant cell growth and activation, HIV replication, and prevent bone resorption [17].

3.4. Spectrum of Antibacterial Activity

Detailed antibacterial spectrum of the new generation of tetracyclines is shown in Table S5 (Supplementary Materials).

Tigecycline presents activity against MDR pathogens, such as MRSA; *Staphylococcus epidermidis*; vancomycin-resistant Enterococcus; *Acinetobacter* spp.; *Stenotrophomonas maltophilia*; penicillin-resistant *Streptococcus pneumoniae*; and Enterobacteriaceae resistant to aminoglycosides, carbapenems, fluoroquinolones, and β-lactamase producers [118,119]. Tigecycline is very active against *Neisseria gonorhoae* and *Eikenella corrodens*, as well as on rapidly growing species of mycobacteria (*M. chelonae*, *M. abscessus*, *M. fortuitum*) [120]. Although against most of tigecycline's action is bacteriostatic, there are pathogens on which it acts bactericidally, such as *Legionella pneumophila* and *Streptococcus pneumoniae*. However, tigecycline is not effective against *Pseudomonas aeruginosa*, *Proteus mirabilis*, *Providencia* spp., or *Morganella morganii* [121].

Omadacycline is very potent against atypical bacteria, as well as Gram-positive and Gram-negative aerobic pathogens [22,122,123], and further against anaerobic bacteria that cause infections from dog or cat bites (except *Eikenella corrodens*); however, omadacycline is not effective on the species of *Proteus*, *Providencia*, *Morganella*, and *Pseudomonas* [124]. Generally, omadacycline acts as bacteriostatic agent, but against *Escherichia coli*, *Streptococcus pneumoniae*, and *Haemophilus influenzae* acts bactericidal [125]. This new tetracycline is more active than tigecycline and acts similar to eravacycline against Gram-positive pathogens [40].

Eravacycline is a broad-spectrum tetracycline that has showed a great activity against aerobic and anaerobic Gram-negative and Gram-positive bacteria, except *P. aeruginosa* and *Burkholderia cenocepacia*. Eravacycline also shows good activity against MDR bacteria, including Enterobacteriaceae and *A. baumannii*, expressing extended spectrum β-lactamases, carbapenem resistance, and mechanisms conferring resistance to other antibiotic classes [18]. Eravacycline is more effective than omadacycline against Gram-negative and broad-spectrum beta-lactamase-producing bacteria. Eravacycline is two to four times more active than tigecycline on clinically relevant Gram-positive species [40].

The spectrum of sarecycline is narrow, with little activity against aerobic and anaerobic Gram-negative bacteria and microflora commonly found in the gastrointestinal tract. The activity of this compound specifically targets *Cutinebacterium acnes*, but also some clinically relevant Gram-positive bacteria, including MRSA [126]. It is noteworthy that the prolonged and intermittent use of broad-spectrum antibiotics such as doxycycline and minocycline in acne vulgaris has been associated with the development of antimicrobial resistance and permanent perturbation of the gut and cutaneous microbiome. Although no causal relationship has been definitively established, the use of doxycycline in patients with acne was found to be associated with a 2.25-fold greater risk of developing Crohn's disease [127,128].

3.5. Bacterial Resistance to New Tetracyclines

The widespread use of these antibacterial agents has unavoidably led to the development of bacterial resistance through plasmid-encoded tetracycline resistance genes (tet), conjugated transposons and integrons, which allow tet genes to be transmitted from one species/generation to another species/generation through conjugation [13,72,129]. The four main types of tetracycline resistance are outlined in Table 4 [18,27,38].

Table 4. Mechanisms of resistance and resistance determinants of tetracyclines.

Resistance Determinants	Resistance Mechanisms			
	Efflux Pump	Ribosomal Protection	Chemical Inactivation	rRNA Mutations
Gram-positive bacteria	tetK, tetL, tetV, tetY, tetZ, tetAP, tet 33, tet 38, tet40, tet 45, otrB otrC, ter3	tetM, tetO, tetP, tetQ, tetS, tetT, tetW, tetZ, tetB(P), tet32, tet36, otrA	-	G1058C
Gram negative bacteria	tetA, tetB, tetC, tetD, tetE, tetG, tetH, tetJ, tetK, tetL, tetY, tet30, tet31, tet34, tet 35, tet39, tet41, tet42	tetM, tetO, tetQ, tetS, tetW, tet36, tet44	tetX, tet34, tet37	A926T, A928C, G927T, ΔG942, G966U

The expression of these genes leads to the production of proteins that contribute to the two primary mechanisms of resistance: ribosomal protection by dissociating tetracyclines from their target (e.g., tet[M], tet[O]) and the efflux of the substance out of the cell by active transport (e.g., tet[A], tet[B]) [28,118]. The efflux pumps are located in the cytoplasmic membrane and act through the antiport of a proton in exchange with a tetracycline–magnesium monocationic complex. Thus, the intracellular concentration of tetracyclines decreases [13]. The most common pumps are part of the Major Facilitator Superfamily of carriers [75]. In contrast to efflux pumps, for which the mechanism is elucidated, the ribosomal protection mechanism is not fully known. However, studies suggest that genes involved (e.g., tet[M], tet[O], and tet[S]) alter the conformation of ribosomes and displace the drug from the active site [38,85,130]. These genes are protein molecules GTPases (guanosine triphosphatases) that have structures and sequences similar to elongation factors (EF-G and EF-Tu) [131].

The other two less common mechanisms include two distinct genes that modify tetracyclines, leading to their degradation and mutations of the ribosomal 16S subunit, decreasing the affinity of the compounds for the ribosomal target [27]. The first of the mechanisms, chemical inactivation, is caused by a FAD-monooxygenase encoded by the tet[X] and tet [37] genes. These hydroxylate the C11 position, altering its structure and coordination with the magnesium ion, and therefore the affinity for the ribosome [38,132]. Moreover, the hydroxylated version degrades even in the absence of enzymes [133]. Because monooxygenase uses NADPH and O_2 in its activity, this resistance occurs only in aerobic organisms [27]. The second mechanism of resistance, the site-binding mutation, is found predominantly in bacteria with a small number of copies of rRNA [18]. The first case was described by Ross et al. (1998) on a bacterial strain of *Propionibacterium acnes*. In addition, there are innate resistance mechanisms, with some bacteria being more immune to the tetracycline class due to differences in membrane permeability. For example, Gram-negative bacteria are more resistant due to the outer wall containing lipopolysaccharide molecules [27].

Although tigecycline is not affected by the main resistance mechanisms, since its introduction in the clinic (2005), the number of pathogens that have developed resistance is continuously increasing. In Gram-negative bacteria, most cases were caused by overexpression of resistance-nodulation-cell division (RND) pumps. For example, MexXY-OprM for *Pseudomonas aeruginosa* strains and AdeIJK/AdeABC for *Acinetobacter baumannii* [134–137]. Something similar occurs for some Gram-positive bacteria by overexpressing the Multidrug and Toxic Compound Extrusion (MATE) (case of MepA pump for Staphylococcus aureus) [138]. Other mechanisms also decrease the susceptibility of tigecycline to other microorganisms: mutations in ribosomal protein genes, mutations in the 16S subunit of rRNA [139], inactivation by FAD-dependent monooxygenase [140], and tetX gene-carrying plasmids [141]. A recent study on *Acinetobacter baumannii* found a resistance plasmid containing the tet(X5) gene, with similarity regarding structure and function of other tet(X) variants, probably using the same transfer elements for spreading [142].

The antimicrobial activity of omadacycline is not disturbed by the two significant resistance mechanisms in therapy [143]. This aspect is due to the functional groups in the C7 (dimethylamino) and C9 (aminomethyl) positions, which prevent the expulsion of the antibiotic by the efflux pumps and the ribosomal protection, respectively [22]. Omadacycline has demonstrated in vitro activity against bacterial strains containing efflux and ribosomal protection genes (*Staphylococcus aureus* expressing the tet(K) and tet(M) genes, *Enterococcus faecalis* expressing the tet(L) and tet(M) genes) [125]. However, the activity of omadacycline is decreased by mutations in the ribosomal RNA of some microorganisms. According to a study conducted by Heidrich et al. (2016), the MIC for tetracycline, tigecycline, and omadacycline on species containing mutations (G1055C, G996U) of the 16S ribosomal subunit increased four to eightfold, suggesting that they are susceptible to these changes, regardless to their affinity for the target [27,144]. The omadacycline's action and the action of glycylcyclines, in general, are also affected by chemical inactivation [27].

Eravacycline avoids tet(A) efflux pumps, maintains activity against staphylococci-containing tet(K) genes, and successfully binds to bacterial ribosomes modified by tet(M) proteins [98,145]. However, eravacycline remains vulnerable to overexpression of MDR efflux pumps belonging to Gram-negative bacteria, change in ribosomal target (16S or 10S), and enzymatic degradation sometimes encountered in Bacterioides spp. The resistance to eravacycline has also been observed in mutant species of Enterococcus, mutations encoded by the rpsJ gene [41,146,147].

In the case of sarecycline, the probability of inducing bacterial resistance is low due to the narrow spectrum of activity and the unique structural modifications at the C7 position. The rate of spontaneous mutations varies from 10^{-9} to 10^{-11} in *Cutinebacterium acnes*, and 10^{-9} and 10^{-8} in *Staphylococcus aureus* and *Staphylococcus epidermidis*, respectively (at increases in MIC values between four and eight times) [126,148].

4. Therapeutic Use of the New Tetracyclines

In the past, tetracyclines have been widely used for various genitourinary, gastrointestinal, respiratory tract, and dermatological diseases. However, the tremendous onset of bacterial resistance, as well as the emergence of new antibacterial agents, has diminished the area of infections for which tetracyclines are considered the first therapeutic option [1,18,27].

The activity of tigecycline has been evaluated in several in vivo clinical trials in human subjects, following which the three FDA-approved indications were formulated. In the treatment of hospitalised patients with complicated skin and soft tissue infections, tigecycline has not only been shown to be effective but has also shown a favourable pharmacokinetic profile [149]. In another phase 2 open-label clinical trial, which included patients with complicated intra-abdominal infections (gangrenous perforated appendicitis, cholecystitis, diverticulitis, peritonitis), tigecycline was a safe and effective treatment [120]. Last but not least, tigecycline is indicated and approved in the treatment of community-acquired pneumonia. For all research, tigecycline met all non-inferiority criteria [31,150].

Omadacycline, unlike tigecycline or eravacycline, brings an advantage through oral formulation, facilitating patient compliance and hospitalisation costs [38]. Omadacycline is recommended in treating complicated skin and soft tissue infections and community-acquired pneumonia, but there are ongoing studies for its use in urinary tract infections [39,151–153].

Eravacycline, due to its broad antibacterial spectrum, in vitro activity, and superior tolerability in comparison with tigecycline, is an appropriate solution for treating complicated intra-abdominal infections in adults, especially when the pathogen possesses resistance mechanisms to other tetracyclines or classes of antibiotics [41]. Infection, for which the efficacy of eravacycline has been studied by comparison with the beta-lactam antibiotics meropenem or ertapenem, include: appendicitis, cholecystitis, diverticulitis, gastric or duodenal perforation, intra-abdominal abscess, intestinal perforation, and peritonitis [145].

The FDA-approved sarecycline is used for treating acne vulgaris in patients aged nine years or above, demonstrating efficacy against moderate-to-severe, inflammatory, or non-inflammatory (comedones) forms. In addition, due to its targeted action on *Cutinebacterium acnes* and low blood–brain penetration, sarecycline has a good safety profile (minimal side effects), low potential to induce bacterial resistance, and also potentially low impact on the gut microbiota when compared to the broad-spectrum doxycycline and minocycline [154,155].

Pharmacokinetic properties. Tigecycline is highly bound to plasma proteins and has a large volume of distribution (above plasmatic volume), which indicates its concentration in tissues. Moreover, tigecycline is rapidly distributed in tissues; the highest concentrations were observed in the bone marrow, thyroid gland, salivary glands, spleen, and kidneys. Tigecycline metabolises independent of cytochrome P450 enzymes, but not extensively. Consequently, tigecycline does not interfere with the metabolism of other substances mediated by the six cytochrome P450 isoforms (1A2, 2C8, 2C9, 2C19, 2D6, and 3A4) [31]. The pharmacokinetics of tigecycline is linear—this may be influenced by the coadministration of P-glycoprotein inhibitors or inducers; tigecycline acts as a substrate of these [156]. Similarly, omadacycline presented a low probability of interactions through transport mechanisms [133]. The omadacycline rate of absorption decreases if a high-fat meal is consumed two hours earlier. Thus, omadacycline must be taken after a fasting period of at least 4 h, followed by 2 h without ingestion of drinks and food (apart from water), as well as 4 h without administration of antacids, multivitamins, and dairy products [157]. The liver metabolises eravacycline, but none of the metabolites are pharmacologically active. Therefore, caution is required in CYP3A4 inducers to increase the extent of eravacycline metabolism to a clinically relevant rate [41]. Sarecycline inhibits P-glycoprotein in vitro. Consequently, decreasing dose and toxicity examination is required when it is coadministered with substrate substances [56]. Generally, the pharmacokinetics of modern tetracyclines are not remarkably influenced by age, sex, or renal function (including renal failure and haemodialysis) [29,39,158]. The pharmacokinetic parameters of the four modern tetracyclines are shown in Table S6 (Supplementary Materials).

5. Side Effects of the Third-Generation Tetracyclines

As an antibiotic class, tetracyclines are generally well tolerated. However, there is a diversity of side effects and contraindications, with these compounds affecting several systems of the human body. For example, tetracyclines often cause gastrointestinal disorders such as abdominal discomfort, nausea, vomiting, and epigastric pain. Moreover, typical side effects are photosensitivity, manifested by erythema and skin blisters, discolouration of the teeth, and inhibition of bone growth in children. Rarely, tetracyclines may cause increased intracranial pressure (pseudotumor cerebri), renal toxicity, hepatotoxicity, and *Clostridium difficile* infections [159].

Similar to tetracyclines in the first generations, the most common side effects of modern tetracyclines are those of the gastrointestinal tract [75,160–162]. Other side effects of the tetracycline new generation are shown in Table 5. Nausea and vomiting may occur in the first two days of treatment and are usually mild to moderate. In the case of tigecycline, these effects are correlated with the dose administered, the highest tolerated doses being 100 mg for healthy subjects without fasting, 200 mg postprandial [156]. Diarrhoea has been reported, and is associated, in the vast majority of cases, with *Clostridium difficile* superinfection, ranging from mild forms to severe or fatal colitis. Other less common side effects are constipation, anorexia, dyspepsia, dry mouth, acute pancreatitis, and pancreatic necrosis [1,31,39,46,145]. Regarding the pharmacotoxicology of sarecycline, due to its narrower spectrum, it does not affect the intestinal flora as much, and therefore adverse effects such as diarrhoea and fungal infections have been observed less clinically [126].

Table 5. Other side effects of modern tetracyclines [31,33,38,39,46,145,152,154,160,163,164].

No.	Affected Level/Disorders	Side Effects	Representatives (Frequency)
1	Nervous system	lethargy, dizziness, dysgeusia, tinitus, vertigo	Sarecycline (<1%)
2	Metabolism	hypocalcemia	Tigecycline (<2%)
			Eravacycline (<1%)
		hyponatremia, hypoglycemia	Tigecycline (<2%)
			Eravacycline (<1%)
3	Psychiatric disorders	anxiety, insomnia, depression	Tigecycline, omadacycline (insomnia only)
4	Urogenital disorders	vulvovaginal fungal infections, vulvovaginal candidiasis	Sarecycline, omadacycline (no data available)
		vaginal moniliasis, vaginitis, leukorrhea	Tigecycline (<2%)
5	Respiratory system	vaginal moniliasis, vaginitis, leukorrhea oropharyngeal pain	Omadacycline (<2%)
		pleurisy, dyspnea	Eravacycline (<1%)
6	Others	vertigo	Omadacycline (<2%)
		abdominal pain	Tigecycline (>2%), omadacycline (<2%)

Tetracyclines affect teeth and bones by forming stable complexes with calcium ions, accumulating in deposits at these levels. Thus, the teeth may acquire a yellow to brown colour, sometimes even permanent, due to the formation of chelates of tetracycline-calcium orthophosphate, which darkens after exposure to the sun [126]. This phenomenon has effects from an aesthetic point of view but can be aggravated, leading to demineralisation and hypoplasia of tooth enamel with decreased resistance to caries attack [165]. Tooth staining is more common in long-term treatment with tetracycline derivatives but has also been observed with repeated short-term administrations. Children who receive tetracyclines in the first part of life and children whose mothers have used them since the second trimester of pregnancy tend to have tetracyclines deposited at the level of baby teeth. There was also a decrease in the rate of fibula growth and ossification processes for the foetus exposed in utero due to accumulation in the tissues [39,46,145].

Another subgroup of side effects is skin damage. Tetracyclines may cause allergic-type side effects with pruritus, transient rash, or itchy skin and hyperhidrosis [31,145]. These reactions are due to the increased sensitivity of the skin to light during systemic tetracycline therapy. Therefore, patients undergoing treatment should avoid excessive exposure to natural or artificial sunlight (ultraviolet radiation) [46]. Hypersensitivity reactions (Stevens–Johnson syndrome, anaphylaxis), sepsis, and death have been reported with low frequency when using tigecycline [166].

Hepatobiliary disorders due to tetracyclines are not very common in this class but are reflected in increased plasma concentrations of aspartate aminotransferase (AST), alanine aminotransferase (ALT), bilirubin, and hepatic transaminases (TGP, TGO). Other laboratory parameters that may change are increased amylase, lipase, gamma-glutamyltransferase, urea nitrogen (class effect), creatinine phosphokinase, alkaline phosphatase, and decreased creatinine clearance. These reactions occur relatively infrequently, with a frequency <2% for tigecycline and omadacycline, and <1% for eravacycline (following clinical trials) [31,39,145]. Cases of cholestatic jaundice and mild pancreatitis induced by tigecycline have been reported [73,167]. At the vascular level, forms intended for the intravenous route produce reactions at the site of administration. With the exception of sarecycline (orally administration), cases of extravasation of the infusion solution, hypoesthesia, pain, erythema, swelling, inflammation, irritation, phlebitis, and thrombophlebitis have been reported [29,39,145,168]. Other side effects that may occur with omadacycline are cardiovascular, with grouped clinical trials showing a frequency of over 2% of hypertension and <2% of tachycardia and atrial fibrillation. No adverse cardiovascular reactions are known for tigecycline. A study in healthy subjects showed that this compound has no significant effect on the QT interval [169].

At the haematological and lymphatic levels, tigecycline and omadacycline may lead to anaemia but have opposite effects on platelets, with tigecycline decreasing their number (thrombocytopenia) [170], compared to omadacycline, which may cause thrombocytosis [157]. Other common side effects of tigecycline are prolongation of partially activated thromboplastin time (aPTT) and prothrombin time. However, an increase in the international normalised ratio (INR) is less common [31].

The primary concern with tigecycline is the increased mortality due to its use, compared with other anti-infective agents [73]. The results obtained in phases 3 and 4 of 13 clinical trials alerted the FDA, which issued a black box warning about the increased risk of mortality of patients treated with this drug [171]. Consequently, several meta-analyses of all controlled and randomised clinical trials were performed, concluding that tigecycline is not indicated in severe infections and should only be reserved for use in situations where alternative treatments are not appropriate [170,172–174]. Because these studies also found higher rates of clinical failure, superinfections, and septic shock compared to the comparator group, several hypotheses were postulated in an attempt to find a cause. These could be low efficacy, low plasma concentrations (could explain persistent bacteremia), and low alveolar concentrations (partly explains the low efficacy in patients with pneumonia associated with mechanical ventilation) [175,176]. In addition, on the basis of animal studies (rats), eravacycline and omadacycline have been shown to have undesirable effects on fertility, affecting sperm production, maturation, morphology, and motility [39,145].

During pregnancy, tetracyclines are not recommended, due to fetotoxicity and teratogenicity (tigecycline, according to the recommendations given by the FDA is classified as risk category D). Tetracyclines are used only when the benefit to the mother outweighs the potential risk for the foetus [171]. The results of animal studies indicate that tetracyclines cross the placenta, reach therapeutic concentrations in the foetal circulation, and may have toxic effects on foetal growth (often related to delayed skeletal development) [43,177]. Cases of embryotoxicity in animal models treated at the beginning of pregnancy were also highlighted. In addition, tetracyclines are excreted in human milk. Although the rate of absorption for infants is unknown, it is recommended that they not be used in breastfeeding either to avoid the risk of tooth discolouration and damage to osteogenesis [31,39,46,145].

The absorption of modern oral tetracyclines (omadacycline, sarecycline), similar to older members of this class, may be affected by the concomitant use of multivitamins; antacids (containing aluminium, calcium); or those in the composition of which magnesium, iron, and/or zinc are found. In these situations, non-absorbable chelating complexes are formed. Tetracyclines may also increase the anticoagulant effect of warfarin [13]. Several reports note decreased coagulation efficiency and bleeding in some patients after starting tetracycline therapy [38]. In a pharmacokinetic-pharmacodynamic study, tigecycline decreased the clearance of warfarin, and therefore careful monitoring of anticoagulant levels is indicated by more frequent international normalised ratio (INR) and prothrombin time (PT) [31,52,178]. The use of tetracyclines may decrease the effectiveness of oral contraceptives, but this interaction is quite controversial due to limited information [38,179]. There is no clinically significant effect of sarecycline on the efficacy of oral contraceptives containing ethinyl estradiol and norethindrone acetate [46]. Other interactions recorded in the literature are increased serum digoxin concentration, interference with penicillin activity, and a synergistic effect with oral retinoids on increased intracranial pressure [38,46].

6. New Compounds under Development

Sriram et al. (2007) synthesised tetracycline derivatives with anti-HIV, antimycobacterial, and HIV-1 integrase inhibitory properties. This was achieved by the reaction between certain tetracyclines (minocycline, tetracycline, and oxytetracycline), formaldehyde, and the secondary amine function (piperazine) of some fluoroquinolones (norfloxacin, lomefloxacin, ciprofloxacin, gatifloxacin), with the help of microwave radiation. Compound no. 10 (a tetracycline hybrid with lomefloxacin) represented in Figure 13 demonstrated the most potent effect on HIV-1 replication. These studies show that the combination of tetracyclines with fluoroquinolones has resulted in both anti-HIV and anti-tuberculosis activity (*Mycobacterium tuberculosis*) and has a promising prospect in treating AIDS [180,181].

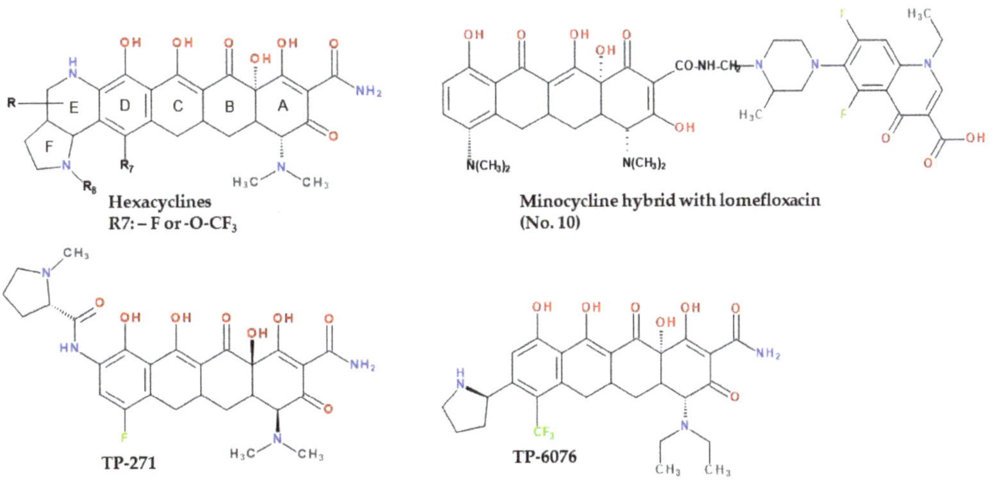

Figure 13. Promising derivatives of tetracyclines.

Using total synthesis, Sun et al. (2015) projected a series of tetracycline analogues with six fused rings called hexacyclines. Their structure consists of the classical skeleton of tetracyclines, having attached a bicyclic ring EF at the level of ring D (Figure 13) [170].

The relationships between chemical structure and antibacterial activity were tested, with substitutions in positions C7, N8, C9, and C10, evaluating the efficacy of various analogues on a wide range of Gram-positive and Gram-negative bacteria, including tetracycline-resistant or multidrug-resistant strains. Of all the compounds studied, the best results were recorded for C7-fluorohexacycline and C7-trifluoromethoxyhexacycline, with a broad antibacterial activity in vitro and good activity in vivo on *Pseudomonas aeruginosa*. The promising data extracted from this study support the optimisation of this type of skeleton to discover and obtain in the future some new tetracyclines that are clinically valuable [182].

Currently, Tetraphase Pharmaceuticals holds two compounds, phase I of clinical trials, TP-271 and TP-6076, whose structures are represented in Figure 13 [183–186]. Thanks to a research program opened in the mid-1990s, synthetic routes with increased scalability and efficacy of obtaining tetracycline analogues have been discovered. To date, more than 3000 analogues have been synthesised using these methods, including the two previously mentioned [187]. TP-271 is a new, clinically developing fluorocycline with promising activity against bacteria that cause respiratory infections, community-acquired pneumonia, anthrax, bubonic plague, and tularemia [187]. Following both in vivo studies and in vivo evaluations, TP-271 has shown an increased potential against susceptible and multidrug-resistant pathogens associated with moderate to severe community-acquired pneumonia. These include key bacteria in respiratory infections, *Streptococcus pneumoniae* (MIC_{90} = 0.03 µg/mL), methicillin-sensitive *Staphylococcus aureus* (MIC_{90} = 0.25 µg/mL), methicillin-resistant *Staphylococcus aureus* (MIC_{90} = 0.12 µg/mL), *Streptococcus pyogenes* (MIC_{90} = 0.03 µg/mL), *Moraxella catarrhalis* ($MIC_{90} \leq$ 0.016 µg/mL), and *Haemophilus influenzae* (MIC_{90} = 0.12 µg/mL) [185]. TP-271 has also shown strong activity against important pathogens: *Yersinia pestis*, *Bacillus anthracis*, *Francisella tularensis*, *Burkholderia mallei*, and *Burkholderia pseudomallai* [188]. Furthermore, TP-271 has been shown to be effective in animal studies of immunocompetent pneumonia and neutropenia with *Streptococcus pneumoniae*, MRSA, and *Haemophilus influenzae*. Regarding the mechanism of action, this compound binds to the 30S ribosomal subunit and maintains its activity, even in the presence of the ribosomal protective protein Tet (M). Therefore, due to the positive results obtained on animal models and the broad spectrum, TP-271 is a promising candidate for treating moderate to severe community-acquired pneumonia [185].

Tetraphase Pharmaceuticals investigated analogues of C4, C7, and C8 trisubstituted tetracyclines. Thereby, some of these tetracyclines have demonstrated increased in vitro potency against clinically significant pathogens, including *Acinetobacter baumannii* (MIC_{90} = 0.063 μg/mL) and carbapenem-resistant Enterobacteriaceae (MIC_{90} = 0.5 μg/mL). The C4-positioned diethyl-amine analogue, TP-6076 (Figure 13), currently in phase I of clinical trials, showed the highest activity of all the three-substituted compounds analysed. The phase I clinical trial is focused on pharmacokinetics and safety studies to assess the bronchopulmonary disposition of intravenous TP-6076 in healthy subjects, in order to assess the potential utility in *Acinetobacter baumannii* pneumonia. According to Tetraphase, TP-6076 is in development for the treatment of serious and life-threatening bacterial infections. The potency of this compound on Gram-negative, multidrug-resistant bacteria is 2 to 64 times higher than that of tigecycline. TP-6076 also retains a high efficacy against isolates with intrinsic resistance mechanisms that generally affect the tetracycline class (e.g., carbapanemase-producing Enterobacteriaceae and carbapanemase-producing *Acinetobacter baumannii*). Antibacterial activity was not affected by the type of carbapenem resistance determinant or international clone. The increased in vitro potency also resulted in high in vivo efficiency in models of mice infected with resistant Gram-negative multi-drug isolates [185,189,190].

7. Conclusions

The evolution of the tetracycline class is remarkable, through its development of semisynthetic analogues of the second generation, and, more recently, of the third generation. The new tetracyclines had acquired high potency and increased efficacy, even against resistant bacteria to tetracyclines. On the basis of the classical method of production, biosynthesis, and semi-synthesis, we are able to obtain the new compounds by total chemical synthesis, such as eravacycline.

The main focus in optimising the chemical structure was on modifying the C7 and C9 positions of the D ring in the simplest tetracycline with biological activity (sancycline). Thus, a new tetracycline class was discovered, based on C9-aminotetracyclines, which bear a glycyl moiety known as glycylcyclines. First in class was the tigecycline representative. Recently approved tetracyclines include beside tigecycline, omadacycline (an aminomethylcycline), eravacycline (a fluorocycline), and sarecycline (a 7-[(methoxy)-(methyl)-amino)-methyl]methyl] derivative).

Tigecycline has the advantage of a superior potency over Gram-positive and Gram-negative MDR bacteria; its pharmaceutical formulation is only parenteral. Omadacycline has a broad spectrum of activity, including MRSA, penicillin-resistant, MDR *Streptococcus pneumoniae* and vancomycin-resistant enterococci. This new tetracycline drug is more advantageous in therapy than tigecycline because it can be administered orally and parenterally. Eravacycline is a synthetic fluorocycline with a great activity against Gram-positive and Gram-negative bacteria that developed specific resistance mechanisms to tetracyclines. Similar to tigecycline, eravacycline is administered exclusively parenterally. The main advantage of sarecycline is the narrow-spectrum activity and the higher selective activity against *Cutinebacterium acnes*. Sarecycline is available as an oral formulation to treat inflammatory lesions of moderate-to-severe non-nodular acne vulgaris.

Although tetracyclines currently act bacteriostatically, omadacycline has demonstrated bactericidal activity in vitro against some bacterial agents. It was proven that glycylcyclines manifest resistance to less common mechanisms, such as altered target site conformation, enzymatic degradation, and mutations in DNA gyrase. Therefore, eravacycline was designed to maintain its activity against resistant bacteria. Sarecycline expands and establishes uncommon interactions with mRNA.

Currently, some studies confirm other biological effects in tetracyclines class that require in-depth future studies. Therefore, through its newly acquired members, this class of antibiotics arouses the interest of researchers in the field. Consequently, new derivatives have been already developed, and many are in development. These are studied primarily studied for the antibiotic effect and also for other biological effects.

Supplementary Materials: The following are available online at https://www.mdpi.com/article/10.3390/pharmaceutics13122085/s1, Table S1. The representatives of tetracyclines class from first and second generations and their approval in therapy (FDA—USA Food and Drug Administration, EMA—European Medicine Agency, MHRA—UK Medicines and Healthcare Products Regulatory Agency). Table S2. Modern tetracyclines of the third generation introduced in therapy. Table S3. Essential structural features of tetracycline antibiotics. Table S4. Physicochemical properties of third-generation tetracyclines. Table S5. The antibacterial spectrum of the newly approved tetracyclines. Table S6. Pharmacokinetics parameters of modern tetracyclines.

Author Contributions: Conceptualisation, methodology, writing—review and editing, supervision, A.R.; writing—original draft preparation, visualisation, E.L.B. All authors have read and agreed to the published version of the manuscript.

Funding: This research received no external funding.

Conflicts of Interest: The authors declare no conflict of interest.

References

1. Moffa, M.; Brook, I. 26—Tetracyclines, Glycylcyclines, and Chloramphenicol. In *Mandell, Douglas, and Bennett's Principles and Practice of Infectious Diseases*, 8th ed.; Bennett, J.E., Dolin, R., Blaser, M.J., Eds.; W.B. Saunders: Philadelphia, PA, USA, 2015; pp. 2607–2618.e2, ISBN 9781455748013. [CrossRef]
2. Klein, N.C.; Cunha, B.A. Tetracyclines. *Med. Clin. N. Am.* **1995**, *79*, 789–801. [CrossRef]
3. Nelson, M.L.; Levy, S.B. The history of the tetracyclines. *Ann. N. Y. Acad. Sci.* **2011**, *1241*, 17–32. [CrossRef]
4. Duggar, B.M. Aureomycin; a product of the continuing search for new antibiotics. *Ann. N. Y. Acad. Sci.* **1948**, *51*, 177–181. [CrossRef]
5. Dubos, R.J.; Hotchkiss, R.D. The production of bactericidal substances by aerobic sporulating bacilli. *J. Exp. Med.* **1941**, *73*, 629–640. [CrossRef] [PubMed]
6. Waksman, S.A.; Schatz, A.; Reynolds, D.M. Production of antibiotic substances by actinomycetes. *Ann. N. Y. Acad. Sci.* **2010**, *1213*, 112–124. [CrossRef] [PubMed]
7. Finland, M. Twenty-fifth anniversary of the discovery of Aureomycin: The place of the tetracyclines in antimicrobial therapy. *Clin. Pharmacol. Ther.* **1974**, *15*, 3–8. [CrossRef] [PubMed]
8. Raistrick, H. Aureomycin, a New Antibiotic. *Nature* **1949**, *163*, 159–160. [CrossRef] [PubMed]
9. The Tetracyclines; Hlavka, J.J.; Boothe, J.H. (Eds.) *Handbook of Experimental Pharmacology*; Springer: Berlin/Heidelberg, Germany, 1985; ISBN 978-3-642-70306-5.
10. Griffin, M.O.; Fricovsky, E.; Ceballos, G.; Villarreal, F. Tetracyclines: A pleitropic family of compounds with promising therapeutic properties. Review of the literature. *Am. J. Physiol. Physiol.* **2010**, *299*, C539–C548. [CrossRef]
11. Lombardino, J.G. A brief history of pfizer central research. *Bull. Hist. Chem.* **2000**, *25*, 6.
12. Stephens, C.R.; Conover, L.H.; Hochstein, F.A.; Regna, P.P.; Pilgrim, F.J.; Brunings, K.J.; Woodward, R.B. Terramycin. VIII. structure of aureomycin and terramycin. *J. Am. Chem. Soc.* **1952**, *74*, 4976–4977. [CrossRef]
13. Zhanel, G.G.; Homenuik, K.; Nichol, K.; Noreddin, A.; Vercaigne, L.; Embil, J.; Gin, A.; Karlowsky, J.A.; Hoban, D.J. The Glycylcyclines: A Comparative Review with the Tetracyclines. *Drugs* **2004**, *64*, 63–88. [CrossRef]
14. Rogalski, W. Chemical Modification of the Tetracyclines. In *The Tetracyclines*; Handbook of Experimental Pharmacology; Hlavka, J.J., Boothe, J.H., Eds.; Springer: Berlin/Heidelberg, Germany, 1985; pp. 179–316, ISBN 978-3-642-70304-1.
15. McCormick, J.R.D.; Sjolander, N.O.; Hirsch, U.; Jensen, E.R.; Doerschuk, A.P. A new family of antibiotics: The demethyltetracyclines. *J. Am. Chem. Soc.* **1957**, *79*, 4561–4563. [CrossRef]
16. NCATS Inxight Drugs—Methacycline. Available online: https://drugs.ncats.io/substance/IR235I7C5P (accessed on 29 October 2021).
17. Garrido-Mesa, N.; Zarzuelo, A.; Galvez, J. Minocycline: Far beyond an antibiotic. *Br. J. Pharmacol.* **2013**, *169*, 337–352. [CrossRef]
18. Grossman, T.H. Tetracycline Antibiotics and Resistance. *Cold Spring Harb. Perspect. Med.* **2016**, *6*, a025387. [CrossRef]
19. Lee, Y.R.; Burton, C.E. Eravacycline, a newly approved fluorocycline. *Eur. J. Clin. Microbiol. Infect. Dis.* **2019**, *38*, 1787–1794. [CrossRef]
20. Moore, A.Y.; Charles, J.E.M.; Moore, S. Sarecycline: A narrow spectrum tetracycline for the treatment of moderate-to-severe acne vulgaris. *Futur. Microbiol.* **2019**, *14*, 1235–1242. [CrossRef]
21. Fuoco, D. Classification Framework and Chemical Biology of Tetracycline-Structure-Based Drugs. *Antibiotics* **2012**, *1*, 1. [CrossRef]

22. Villano, S.; Steenbergen, J.; Loh, E. Omadacycline: Development of a novel aminomethylcycline antibiotic for treating drug-resistant bacterial infections. *Futur. Microbiol.* **2016**, *11*, 1421–1434. [CrossRef]
23. Giovanni, P.; Eugenio, C.; Giuseppe, M.; Brenner, M.; Lu, R.; Huang, S.; Armstrong, W.P.; Gajanan, J.; Seyedi, F.; Johnston, S. Process for Making Sarecycline Hydrochloride. U.S. Patent 17/043,017, 21 January 2021.
24. Ramachanderan, R.; Schaefer, B. Tetracycline antibiotics. *ChemTexts* **2021**, *7*, 1–42. [CrossRef]
25. Nelson, M.L.; Ismail, M.Y.; McIntyre, L.; Bhatia, B.; Viski, P.; Hawkins, P.; Rennie, G.; Andorsky, D.; Messersmith, D.; Stapleton, K.; et al. Versatile and Facile Synthesis of Diverse Semisynthetic Tetracycline Derivatives via Pd-Catalyzed Reactions. *J. Org. Chem.* **2003**, *68*, 5838–5851. [CrossRef]
26. Stein, G.E.; Babinchak, T. Tigecycline: An update. *Diagn. Microbiol. Infect. Dis.* **2013**, *75*, 331–336. [CrossRef]
27. Nguyen, F.; Starosta, A.L.; Arenz, S.; Sohmen, D.; Dönhöfer, A.; Wilson, D.N. Tetracycline antibiotics and resistance mechanisms. *Biol. Chem.* **2014**, *395*, 559–575. [CrossRef]
28. Doan, T.-L.; Fung, H.B.; Mehta, D.; Riska, P.F. Tigecycline: A glycylcycline antimicrobial agent. *Clin. Ther.* **2006**, *28*, 1079–1106. [CrossRef]
29. Greer, N.D. Tigecycline (Tygacil): The First in the Glycylcycline Class of Antibiotics. *Bayl. Univ. Med. Cent. Proc.* **2006**, *19*, 155–161. [CrossRef]
30. Olson, M.W.; Ruzin, A.; Feyfant, E.; Rush, T.S.; O'Connell, J.; Bradford, P.A. Functional, Biophysical, and Structural Bases for Antibacterial Activity of Tigecycline. *Antimicrob. Agents Chemother.* **2006**, *50*, 2156–2166. [CrossRef]
31. FDA. Drug Approval Package: Tygacil (Tigecycline) NDA #021821. Available online: https://www.accessdata.fda.gov/drugsatfda_docs/nda/2005/21-821_Tygacil.cfm (accessed on 4 October 2021).
32. EMA Tygacil. Available online: https://www.ema.europa.eu/en/medicines/human/EPAR/tygacil (accessed on 29 September 2021).
33. Babinchak, T.; Ellis-Grosse, E.; Dartois, N.; Rose, G.M.; Loh, E.; Tigecycline 301 Study Group; Tigecycline 306 Study Group. The Efficacy and Safety of Tigecycline for the Treatment of Complicated Intra-Abdominal Infections: Analysis of Pooled Clinical Trial Data. *Clin. Infect. Dis.* **2005**, *41* (Suppl. S5), S354–S367. [CrossRef] [PubMed]
34. Breedt, J.; Teras, J.; Gardovskis, J.; Maritz, F.J.; Vaasna, T.; Ross, D.P.; Gioud-Paquet, M.; Dartois, N.; Ellis-Grosse, E.J.; Loh, E. Safety and Efficacy of Tigecycline in Treatment of Skin and Skin Structure Infections: Results of a Double-Blind Phase 3 Comparison Study with Vancomycin-Aztreonam. *Antimicrob. Agents Chemother.* **2005**, *49*, 4658–4666. [CrossRef]
35. Tanaseanu, C.; Bergallo, C.; Teglia, O.; Jasovich, A.; Oliva, M.E.; Dukart, G.; Dartois, N.; Cooper, C.A.; Gandjini, H.; Mallick, R. Integrated results of 2 phase 3 studies comparing tigecycline and levofloxacin in community-acquired pneumonia. *Diagn. Microbiol. Infect. Dis.* **2008**, *61*, 329–338. [CrossRef]
36. Falagas, M.E.; Metaxas, E.I. Tigecycline for the treatment of patients with community-acquired pneumonia requiring hospitalization. *Expert Rev. Anti-Infect. Ther.* **2009**, *7*, 913–923. [CrossRef]
37. Tigecycline | DrugBank Online. Available online: https://go.drugbank.com/drugs/DB00560 (accessed on 2 August 2021).
38. Zhanel, G.G.; Esquivel, J.; Zelenitsky, S.; Lawrence, C.K.; Adam, H.J.; Golden, A.; Hink, R.; Berry, L.; Schweizer, F.; Zhanel, M.A.; et al. Omadacycline: A Novel Oral and Intravenous Aminomethylcycline Antibiotic Agent. *Drugs* **2020**, *80*, 285–313. [CrossRef]
39. FDA Drug Approval Package: Nuzyra. Available online: https://www.accessdata.fda.gov/drugsatfda_docs/nda/2018/209816Orig1s000,209817Orig1s000TOC.cfm (accessed on 4 October 2021).
40. Zhanel, G.G.; Cheung, D.; Adam, H.; Zelenitsky, S.; Golden, A.; Schweizer, F.; Gorityala, B.; Lagacé-Wiens, P.R.S.; Walkty, A.; Gin, A.S.; et al. Review of Eravacycline, a Novel Fluorocycline Antibacterial Agent. *Drugs* **2016**, *76*, 567–588. [CrossRef] [PubMed]
41. Scott, L.J. Eravacycline: A Review in Complicated Intra-Abdominal Infections. *Drugs* **2019**, *79*, 315–324. [CrossRef]
42. Bunick, C.G.; Keri, J.; Tanaka, S.K.; Furey, N.; Damiani, G.; Johnson, J.L.; Grada, A. Antibacterial Mechanisms and Efficacy of Sarecycline in Animal Models of Infection and Inflammation. *Antibiotics* **2021**, *10*, 439. [CrossRef]
43. Haidari, W.; Bruinsma, R.; Cardenas-de La Garza, J.A.; Feldman, S.R. Sarecycline Review. *Ann. Pharmacother.* **2019**, *54*, 164–170. [CrossRef]
44. Deeks, E.D. Sarecycline: First Global Approval. *Drugs* **2019**, *79*, 325–329. [CrossRef]
45. Kaul, G.; Saxena, D.; Dasgupta, A.; Chopra, S. Sarecycline hydrochloride for the treatment of acne vulgaris. *Drugs Today* **2019**, *55*, 615–625. [CrossRef]
46. FDA. Drug Approval Package: Seysara (Sarecycline). Available online: https://www.accessdata.fda.gov/drugsatfda_docs/nda/2018/209521Orig1s000TOC.cfm (accessed on 7 October 2021).
47. Systèmes, D. BIOVIA Draw for Academics. Available online: https://discover.3ds.com/biovia-draw-academic (accessed on 6 July 2021).
48. Bahrami, F.; Morris, D.L.; Pourgholami, M.H. Tetracyclines: Drugs with Huge Therapeutic Potential. *Mini-Rev. Med. Chem.* **2012**, *12*, 44–52. [CrossRef]
49. Rizvi, S.F.A.; Tariq, S.; Anwar, U. Tetracycline: Classification, Structure Activity Relationship and Mechanism of Action as a Theranostic Agent for Infectious Lesions-A Mini Review. *Biomed. J. Sci. Tech. Res.* **2018**, *7*, 001–010. [CrossRef]
50. Heinemann, F.W.; Leypold, C.F.; Roman, C.R.; Schmitt, M.O.; Schneider, S. X-Ray Crystallography of Tetracycline, Doxycycline and Sancycline. *J. Chem. Crystallogr.* **2013**, *43*, 213–222. [CrossRef]

51. Honeyman, L.; Ismail, M.; Nelson, M.L.; Bhatia, B.; Bowser, T.E.; Chen, J.; Mechiche, R.; Ohemeng, K.; Verma, A.K.; Cannon, E.P.; et al. Structure-Activity Relationship of the Aminomethylcyclines and the Discovery of Omadacycline. *Antimicrob. Agents Chemother.* **2015**, *59*, 7044–7053. [CrossRef]
52. Zhanel, G.G.; Karlowsky, J.A.; Rubinstein, E.; Hoban, D.J. Tigecycline: A novel glycylcycline antibiotic. *Expert Rev. Anti-Infect. Ther.* **2006**, *4*, 9–25. [CrossRef]
53. Omadacycline. Available online: https://go.drugbank.com/drugs/DB12455 (accessed on 7 October 2021).
54. PubChem Omadacycline. Available online: https://pubchem.ncbi.nlm.nih.gov/compound/54697325 (accessed on 5 October 2021).
55. European Medicines Agency Xerava. Available online: https://www.ema.europa.eu/en/medicines/human/EPAR/xerava (accessed on 3 August 2021).
56. PubChem Sarecycline. Available online: https://pubchem.ncbi.nlm.nih.gov/compound/54681908 (accessed on 4 October 2021).
57. Batool, Z.; Lomakin, I.B.; Polikanov, Y.S.; Bunick, C.G. Sarecycline interferes with tRNA accommodation and tethers mRNA to the 70S ribosome. *Proc. Natl. Acad. Sci. USA* **2020**, *117*, 20530–20537. [CrossRef]
58. John, M.; Beale, J.H.B. *Wilson and Giswold's Organic Medicinal and Pharmaceutical Chemistry*, 12th ed.; Lippincott Williams & Wilkins, Wolters Kluwer Health: Baltimore, MD, USA, 2011; pp. 301–307.
59. Bayliss, M.A.J.; Rigdova, K.; Kyriakides, M.; Grier, S.; Lovering, A.M.; Ellery, K.; Griffith, D.C.; MacGowan, A. Challenges in the bioanalysis of tetracyclines: Epimerisation and chelation with metals. *J. Chromatogr. B* **2019**, *1134–1135*, 121807. [CrossRef]
60. Pulicharla, R.; Hegde, K.; Brar, S.K.; Surampalli, R.Y. Tetracyclines metal complexation: Significance and fate of mutual existence in the environment. *Environ. Pollut.* **2017**, *221*, 1–14. [CrossRef]
61. Sanli, S.; Şanli, N.; Alsancak, G. Determination of Protonation Constants of Some Tetracycline Antibiotics by Potentiometry and Lc Methods in Water and Acetonitrile-Water Binary Mixtures. *J. Braz. Chem. Soc.* **2009**, *20*, 939–946. [CrossRef]
62. Zhao, Y.; Geng, J.; Wang, X.; Gu, X.; Gao, S. Tetracycline adsorption on kaolinite: pH, metal cations and humic acid effects. *Ecotoxicology* **2011**, *20*, 1141–1147. [CrossRef]
63. Schmitt, M.O.; Schneider, S. Novel Insight into the Protonation–Deprotonation Equilibria of Tetracycline, Sancycline and 10-Propoxy-Sancycline in Aqueous Solution. I. Analysis of the pH-Dependent UV/vis Absorption Spectra by the SVD Technique. *Z. Phys. Chem.* **2006**, *220*, 441–475. [CrossRef]
64. Jin, L.; Amaya-Mazo, X.; Apel, M.E.; Sankisa, S.S.; Johnson, E.; Zbyszynska, M.A.; Han, A. Ca2+ and Mg2+ bind tetracycline with distinct stoichiometries and linked deprotonation. *Biophys. Chem.* **2007**, *128*, 185–196. [CrossRef]
65. Arias, K.; Robinson, S.G.; Lyngaas, S.S.; Cherala, S.S.; Hartzell, M.; Mei, S.; Vilic, A.; Girel, J.K.; Kuemmell, A.; Vrettos, J.S.; et al. Minocycline and tigecycline form higher-order Ca2+ complexes of stronger affinity than tetracycline. *Inorg. Chim. Acta* **2016**, *441*, 181–191. [CrossRef]
66. Marvin|ChemAxon. Available online: https://chemaxon.com/products/marvin (accessed on 11 October 2021).
67. Tu, Y.-P. Dissociative protonation and long-range proton migration: The chemistry of singly- and doubly-protonated tigecycline. *Int. J. Mass Spectrom.* **2018**, *434*, 164–171. [CrossRef]
68. Grenier, D.; Huot, M.-P.; Mayrand, D. Iron-Chelating Activity of Tetracyclines and Its Impact on the Susceptibility of Actinobacillus actinomycetemcomitans to These Antibiotics. *Antimicrob. Agents Chemother.* **2000**, *44*, 763–766. [CrossRef]
69. Guerra, W.; Silva-Caldeira, P.P.; Terenzi, H.; Pereira-Maia, E.C. Impact of metal coordination on the antibiotic and non-antibiotic activities of tetracycline-based drugs. *Coord. Chem. Rev.* **2016**, *327–328*, 188–199. [CrossRef]
70. Rocha, D.P.; Pinto, G.F.; Ruggiero, R.; De Oliveira, C.A.; Guerra, W.; Fontes, A.P.S.; Tavares, T.T.; Marzano, I.M.; Pereira-Maia, E.C. Coordenação de metais a antibióticos como uma estratégia de combate à resistência bacteriana. *Quím. Nova* **2011**, *34*, 111–118. [CrossRef]
71. *Wilson and Gisvold's Textbook of Organic Medicinal and Pharmaceutical Chemistry*, 12th ed.; Beale, J.M., Jr.; Block, J.H. (Eds.) Wolters Kluwer Health: Baltimore, MD, USA, 2010; ISBN 978-0-7817-7929-6.
72. Sum, P.-E.; Petersen, P. Synthesis and structure-activity relationship of novel glycylcycline derivatives leading to the discovery of GAR-936. *Bioorg. Med. Chem. Lett.* **1999**, *9*, 1459–1462. [CrossRef]
73. Kaewpoowat, Q.; Ostrosky-Zeichner, L. Tigecycline: A critical safety review. *Expert Opin. Drug Saf.* **2014**, *14*, 335–342. [CrossRef]
74. Jenner, L.; Starosta, A.L.; Terry, D.S.; Mikolajka, A.; Filonava, L.; Yusupov, M.; Blanchard, S.C.; Wilson, D.N.; Yusupova, G. Structural basis for potent inhibitory activity of the antibiotic tigecycline during protein synthesis. *Proc. Natl. Acad. Sci. USA* **2013**, *110*, 3812–3816. [CrossRef]
75. Chopra, I.; Roberts, M. Tetracycline Antibiotics: Mode of Action, Applications, Molecular Biology, and Epidemiology of Bacterial Resistance. *Microbiol. Mol. Biol. Rev.* **2001**, *65*, 232–260. [CrossRef]
76. Bronson, J.; Barrett, J.F. Quinolone, Everninomycin, Glycylcycline, Carbapenem, Lipopeptide and Cephem Antibacterials in Clinical Development. *Curr. Med. Chem.* **2001**, *8*, 1775–1793. [CrossRef] [PubMed]
77. Tanaka, S.K.; Steenbergen, J.; Villano, S. Discovery, pharmacology, and clinical profile of omadacycline, a novel aminomethylcycline antibiotic. *Bioorg. Med. Chem.* **2016**, *24*, 6409–6419. [CrossRef]
78. Burgos, R.M.; Rodvold, K.A. Omadacycline: A novel aminomethylcycline. *Infect. Drug Resist.* **2019**, *12*, 1895–1915. [CrossRef]
79. Xiao, X.-Y.; Hunt, D.K.; Zhou, J.; Clark, R.B.; Dunwoody, N.; Fyfe, C.; Grossman, T.H.; O'Brien, W.J.; Plamondon, L.; Rönn, M.; et al. Fluorocyclines. 1. 7-Fluoro-9-pyrrolidinoacetamido-6-demethyl-6-deoxytetracycline: A Potent, Broad Spectrum Antibacterial Agent. *J. Med. Chem.* **2012**, *55*, 597–605. [CrossRef]

80. Clark, R.B.; Hunt, D.K.; He, M.; Achorn, C.; Chen, C.-L.; Deng, Y.; Fyfe, C.; Grossman, T.H.; Hogan, P.C.; O'Brien, W.J.; et al. Fluorocyclines. 2. Optimization of the C-9 Side-Chain for Antibacterial Activity and Oral Efficacy. *J. Med. Chem.* **2012**, *55*, 606–622. [CrossRef] [PubMed]
81. Brodersen, D.E.; Clemons, W.M.; Carter, A.P.; Morgan-Warren, R.J.; Wimberly, B.T.; Ramakrishnan, V. The Structural Basis for the Action of the Antibiotics Tetracycline, Pactamycin, and Hygromycin B on the 30S Ribosomal Subunit. *Cell* **2000**, *103*, 1143–1154. [CrossRef]
82. Maxwell, I.H. Partial removal of bound transfer RNA from polysomes engaged in protein synthesis in vitro after addition of tetracycline. *Biochim. Biophys. Acta (BBA) Nucleic Acids Protein Synth.* **1967**, *138*, 337–346. [CrossRef]
83. Tessier, P.R.; Nicolau, D.P. Tigecycline Displays In Vivo Bactericidal Activity against Extended-Spectrum-β-Lactamase-Producing Enterobacteriaceae after 72-Hour Exposure Period. *Antimicrob. Agents Chemother.* **2012**, *57*, 640–642. [CrossRef] [PubMed]
84. BioRender. Available online: https://biorender.com/ (accessed on 30 September 2021).
85. Thaker, M.; Spanogiannopoulos, P.; Wright, G.D. The tetracycline resistome. *Cell. Mol. Life Sci.* **2009**, *67*, 419–431. [CrossRef] [PubMed]
86. Schnappinger, D.; Hillen, W. Tetracyclines: Antibiotic action, uptake, and resistance mechanisms. *Arch. Microbiol.* **1996**, *165*, 359–369. [CrossRef]
87. Peterson, L.R. A review of tigecycline—The first glycylcycline. *Int. J. Antimicrob. Agents* **2008**, *32*, S215–S222. [CrossRef]
88. Pankey, G.A. Tigecycline. *J. Antimicrob. Chemother.* **2005**, *56*, 470–480. [CrossRef]
89. Projan, S.J. Preclinical Pharmacology of GAR-936, a Novel Glycylcycline Antibacterial Agent. *Pharmacother. J. Hum. Pharmacol. Drug Ther.* **2000**, *20*, 219S–223S; discussion 224S–228S. [CrossRef] [PubMed]
90. Hirata, T.; Saito, A.; Nishino, K.; Tamura, N.; Yamaguchi, A. Effects of Efflux Transporter Genes on Susceptibility of Escherichia coli to Tigecycline (GAR-936). *Antimicrob. Agents Chemother.* **2004**, *48*, 2179–2184. [CrossRef]
91. Macone, A.B.; Caruso, B.K.; Leahy, R.G.; Donatelli, J.; Weir, S.; Draper, M.P.; Tanaka, S.K.; Levy, S.B. In Vitro and In Vivo Antibacterial Activities of Omadacycline, a Novel Aminomethylcycline. *Antimicrob. Agents Chemother.* **2013**, *58*, 1127–1135. [CrossRef] [PubMed]
92. Heaney, M.; Mahoney, M.V.; Gallagher, J.C. Eravacycline: The Tetracyclines Strike Back. *Ann. Pharmacother.* **2019**, *53*, 1124–1135. [CrossRef]
93. Grossman, T.H.; Starosta, A.L.; Fyfe, C.; O'Brien, W.; Rothstein, D.M.; Mikolajka, A.; Wilson, D.N.; Sutcliffe, J.A. Target- and Resistance-Based Mechanistic Studies with TP-434, a Novel Fluorocycline Antibiotic. *Antimicrob. Agents Chemother.* **2012**, *56*, 2559–2564. [CrossRef] [PubMed]
94. Farrah, G.; Tan, E. The use of oral antibiotics in treating acne vulgaris: A new approach. *Dermatol. Ther.* **2016**, *29*, 377–384. [CrossRef]
95. Mays, R.M.; Gordon, R.A.; Wilson, J.M.; Silapunt, S. New antibiotic therapies for acne and rosacea. *Dermatol. Ther.* **2012**, *25*, 23–37. [CrossRef] [PubMed]
96. Perret, L.J.; Tait, C.P. Non-antibiotic properties of tetracyclines and their clinical application in dermatology. *Australas. J. Dermatol.* **2013**, *55*, 111–118. [CrossRef]
97. Rosso, J.Q.; Draelos, Z.D.; Effron, C.; Kircik, L.H. Oral Sarecycline for Treatment of Papulopustular Rosacea: Results of a Pilot Study of Effectiveness and Safety. *J. Drugs Dermatol.* **2021**, *20*, 426–431. [CrossRef] [PubMed]
98. Sapadin, A.N.; Fleischmajer, R. Tetracyclines: Nonantibiotic properties and their clinical implications. *J. Am. Acad. Dermatol.* **2006**, *54*, 258–265. [CrossRef]
99. Esterly, N.B.; Koransky, J.S.; Furey, N.L.; Trevisan, M. Neutrophil chemotaxis in patients with acne receiving oral tetracycline therapy. *Arch. Dermatol.* **1984**, *120*, 1308–1313. [CrossRef]
100. Skidmore, R.; Kovach, R.; Walker, C.; Thomas, J.; Bradshaw, M.; Leyden, J.; Powala, C.; Ashley, R. Effects of Subantimicrobial-Dose Doxycycline in the Treatment of Moderate Acne. *Arch. Dermatol.* **2003**, *139*, 459–464. [CrossRef] [PubMed]
101. Tilley, B.C.; Alarcón, G.S.; Heyse, S.P.; Trentham, D.E.; Neuner, R.; Kaplan, D.A.; Clegg, D.O.; Leisen, J.C.C.; Buckley, L.; Cooper, S.M.; et al. Minocycline in Rheumatoid Arthritis: A 48-Week, Double-Blind, Placebo-Controlled Trial. *Ann. Intern. Med.* **1995**, *122*, 81–89. [CrossRef]
102. O'Dell, J.R.; Elliott, J.R.; Mallek, J.A.; Mikuls, T.R.; Weaver, C.A.; Glickstein, S.; Blakely, K.M.; Hausch, R.; Leff, R.D. Treatment of early seropositive rheumatoid arthritis: Doxycycline plus methotrexate versus methotrexate alone. *Arthritis Rheum.* **2006**, *54*, 621–627. [CrossRef]
103. Macdonald, A.; Feiwel, M. Perioral dermatitis: Aetiology and treatment with tetracycline. *Br. J. Dermatol.* **1972**, *87*, 315–319. [CrossRef]
104. Jansen, T.; Plewig, G. Rosacea: Classification and Treatment. *J. R. Soc. Med.* **1997**, *90*, 144–150. [CrossRef]
105. Le, C.H.; Morales, A.; Trentham, D.E. Minocycline in early diffuse scleroderma. *Lancet* **1998**, *352*, 1755–1756. [CrossRef]
106. Chaidemenos, G.C. Tetracycline and niacinamide in the treatment of blistering skin diseases. *Clin. Dermatol.* **2001**, *19*, 781–785. [CrossRef]
107. Lokeshwar, B.L.; Selzer, M.G.; Zhu, B.-Q.; Block, N.L.; Golub, L.M. Inhibition of cell proliferation, invasion, tumor growth and metastasis by an oral non-antimicrobial tetracycline analog (COL-3) in a metastatic prostate cancer model. *Int. J. Cancer* **2001**, *98*, 297–309. [CrossRef] [PubMed]

108. Cianfrocca, M.; Cooley, T.P.; Lee, J.Y.; Rudek, M.A.; Scadden, D.T.; Ratner, L.; Pluda, J.M.; Figg, W.D.; Krown, S.E.; Dezube, B.J. Matrix Metalloproteinase Inhibitor COL-3 in the Treatment of AIDS-Related Kaposi's Sarcoma: A Phase I AIDS Malignancy Consortium Study. *J. Clin. Oncol.* **2002**, *20*, 153–159. [CrossRef]
109. Mosorin, M.; Juvonen, J.; Biancari, F.; Satta, J.; Surcel, H.-M.; Leinonen, M.; Saikku, P.; Juvonen, T. Use of doxycycline to decrease the growth rate of abdominal aortic aneurysms: A randomized, double-blind, placebo-controlled pilot study. *J. Vasc. Surg.* **2001**, *34*, 606–610. [CrossRef]
110. Bachelez, H.; Senet, P.; Cadranel, J.; Kaoukhov, A.; Dubertret, L. The Use of Tetracyclines for the Treatment of Sarcoidosis. *Arch. Dermatol.* **2001**, *137*, 69–73. [CrossRef]
111. Takeshita, S.; Ono, Y.; Kozuma, K.; Suzuki, M.; Kawamura, Y.; Yokoyama, N.; Furukawa, T.; Isshiki, T. Modulation of oxidative burst of neutrophils by doxycycline in patients with acute myocardial infarction. *J. Antimicrob. Chemother.* **2002**, *49*, 411–413. [CrossRef]
112. Mrcp, J.B.-J.; Tan, S.V.; Graham-Brown, R.A.C.; Pembroke, A.C. The successful use of minocycline in pyoderma gangrenosum—A report of seven cases and review of the literature. *J. Dermatol. Treat.* **1989**, *1*, 23–25. [CrossRef]
113. Wennström, J.L.; Newman, H.N.; MacNeill, S.R.; Killoy, W.J.; Griffiths, G.S.; Gillam, D.G.; Krok, L.; Needleman, I.G.; Weiss, G.; Garrett, S. Utilisation of locally delivered doxycycline in non-surgical treatment of chronic periodontitis. A Comparative Multi-Centre Trial of 2 Treatment Approaches. *J. Clin. Periodontol.* **2001**, *28*, 753–761. [CrossRef] [PubMed]
114. Jemec, G.B.; Wendelboe, P. Topical clindamycin versus systemic tetracycline in the treatment of hidradenitis suppurativa. *J. Am. Acad. Dermatol.* **1998**, *39*, 971–974. [CrossRef]
115. Joshi, R.K.; Atukorala, D.N.; Abanmi, A.; Al Khamis, O.; Haleem, A. Successful treatment of Sweet's syndrome with doxycycline. *Br. J. Dermatol.* **1993**, *128*, 584–586. [CrossRef]
116. Humbert, P.; Faivre, B.; Gibey, R.; Agache, P. Use of anti-collagenase properties of doxycycline in treatment of alpha 1-antitrypsin deficiency panniculitis. *Acta Derm. Venereol.* **1991**, *71*, 189–194.
117. Piamphongsant, T. Tetracycline for the treatment of pityriasis lichenoides. *Br. J. Dermatol.* **1974**, *91*, 319–322. [CrossRef]
118. Da Silva, L.M.; Salgado, H.R.N. Tigecycline: A Review of Properties, Applications, and Analytical Methods. *Ther. Drug Monit.* **2010**, *32*, 282–288. [CrossRef]
119. Pillar, C.M.; Draghi, D.C.; Dowzicky, M.J.; Sahm, D.F. In Vitro Activity of Tigecycline against Gram-Positive and Gram-Negative Pathogens as Evaluated by Broth Microdilution and Etest. *J. Clin. Microbiol.* **2008**, *46*, 2862–2867. [CrossRef]
120. Noskin, G.A. Tigecycline: A New Glycylcycline for Treatment of Serious Infections. *Clin. Infect. Dis.* **2005**, *41*, S303–S314. [CrossRef]
121. Petersen, P.J.; Jacobus, N.V.; Weiss, W.J.; Sum, P.E.; Testa, R.T. In Vitro and In Vivo Antibacterial Activities of a Novel Glycylcycline, the 9- t -Butylglycylamido Derivative of Minocycline (GAR-936). *Antimicrob. Agents Chemother.* **1999**, *43*, 738–744. [CrossRef]
122. Karlowsky, J.A.; Steenbergen, J.; Zhanel, G.G. Microbiology and Preclinical Review of Omadacycline. *Clin. Infect. Dis.* **2019**, *69*, S6–S15. [CrossRef]
123. Pfaller, M.A.; Rhomberg, P.R.; Huband, M.D.; Flamm, R.K. Activities of Omadacycline and Comparator Agents against Staphylococcus aureus Isolates from a Surveillance Program Conducted in North America and Europe. *Antimicrob. Agents Chemother.* **2017**, *61*, e02411-16. [CrossRef] [PubMed]
124. Goldstein, E.J.C.; Citron, D.M.; Tyrrell, K.L.; Leoncio, E.; Merriam, C.V. Comparative In Vitro Activity of Omadacycline against Dog and Cat Bite Wound Isolates. *Antimicrob. Agents Chemother.* **2018**, *62*, e02551-17. [CrossRef] [PubMed]
125. Antimicrobial Drugs Advisory Committee (AMDAC) Briefing Book. Omadacycline P-Toluenesulfonate Tablets and Injection. Available online: https://www.fda.gov/media/115100/download (accessed on 10 June 2021).
126. Zhanel, G.; Critchley, I.; Lin, L.-Y.; Alvandi, N. Microbiological Profile of Sarecycline, a Novel Targeted Spectrum Tetracycline for the Treatment of Acne Vulgaris. *Antimicrob. Agents Chemother.* **2019**, *63*, e01297-18. [CrossRef] [PubMed]
127. Thompson, K.G.; Rainer, B.M.; Antonescu, C.; Florea, L.; Mongodin, E.F.; Kang, S.; Chien, A.L. Minocycline and Its Impact on Microbial Dysbiosis in the Skin and Gastrointestinal Tract of Acne Patients. *Ann. Dermatol.* **2020**, *32*, 21–30. [CrossRef]
128. Graber, E.M. Treating acne with the tetracycline class of antibiotics: A review. *Dermatol. Rev.* **2021**, 1–10. [CrossRef]
129. Chopra, I. Glycylcyclines: Third-generation tetracycline antibiotics. *Curr. Opin. Pharmacol.* **2001**, *1*, 464–469. [CrossRef]
130. Draper, M.P.; Weir, S.; Macone, A.; Donatelli, J.; Trieber, C.A.; Tanaka, S.K.; Levy, S.B. Mechanism of Action of the Novel Aminomethylcycline Antibiotic Omadacycline. *Antimicrob. Agents Chemother.* **2013**, *58*, 1279–1283. [CrossRef]
131. Kobayashi, T.; Nonaka, L.; Maruyama, F.; Suzuki, S. Molecular Evidence for the Ancient Origin of the Ribosomal Protection Protein That Mediates Tetracycline Resistance in Bacteria. *J. Mol. Evol.* **2007**, *65*, 228–235. [CrossRef]
132. Yang, W.; Moore, I.F.; Koteva, K.P.; Bareich, D.C.; Hughes, D.W.; Wright, G.D. TetX Is a Flavin-dependent Monooxygenase Conferring Resistance to Tetracycline Antibiotics. *J. Biol. Chem.* **2004**, *279*, 52346–52352. [CrossRef] [PubMed]
133. Dougherty, J.A.; Sucher, A.J.; Chahine, E.B.; Shihadeh, K.C. Omadacycline: A New Tetracycline Antibiotic. *Ann. Pharmacother.* **2018**, *53*, 486–500. [CrossRef] [PubMed]
134. Dean, C.R.; Visalli, M.A.; Projan, S.J.; Sum, P.-E.; Bradford, P.A. Efflux-Mediated Resistance to Tigecycline (GAR-936) in Pseudomonas aeruginosa PAO1. *Antimicrob. Agents Chemother.* **2003**, *47*, 972–978. [CrossRef] [PubMed]
135. Visalli, M.A.; Murphy, E.; Projan, S.J.; Bradford, P.A. AcrAB Multidrug Efflux Pump Is Associated with Reduced Levels of Susceptibility to Tigecycline (GAR-936) in Proteus mirabilis. *Antimicrob. Agents Chemother.* **2003**, *47*, 665–669. [CrossRef]

136. Peleg, A.Y.; Adams, J.; Paterson, D.L. Tigecycline Efflux as a Mechanism for Nonsusceptibility in *Acinetobacter baumannii*. *Antimicrob. Agents Chemother.* **2007**, *51*, 2065–2069. [CrossRef]
137. Damier-Piolle, L.; Magnet, S.; Breémont, S.; Lambert, T.; Courvalin, P. AdeIJK, a Resistance-Nodulation-Cell Division Pump Effluxing Multiple Antibiotics in *Acinetobacter baumannii*. *Antimicrob. Agents Chemother.* **2008**, *52*, 557–562. [CrossRef] [PubMed]
138. McAleese, F.; Petersen, P.; Ruzin, A.; Dunman, P.M.; Murphy, E.; Projan, S.J.; Bradford, P.A. A Novel MATE Family Efflux Pump Contributes to the Reduced Susceptibility of Laboratory-Derived Staphylococcus aureus Mutants to Tigecycline. *Antimicrob. Agents Chemother.* **2005**, *49*, 1865–1871. [CrossRef]
139. Beabout, K.; Hammerstrom, T.G.; Perez, A.M.; Magalhaes, B.D.F.; Prater, A.G.; Clements, T.P.; Arias, C.A.; Saxer, G.; Shamoo, Y. The Ribosomal S10 Protein Is a General Target for Decreased Tigecycline Susceptibility. *Antimicrob. Agents Chemother.* **2015**, *59*, 5561–5566. [CrossRef]
140. Moore, I.F.; Hughes, D.W.; Wright, G.D. Tigecycline Is Modified by the Flavin-Dependent Monooxygenase TetX. *Biochemistry* **2005**, *44*, 11829–11835. [CrossRef]
141. He, T.; Wang, R.; Liu, D.; Walsh, T.R.; Zhang, R.; Lv, Y.; Ke, Y.; Ji, Q.; Wei, R.; Liu, Z.; et al. Emergence of plasmid-mediated high-level tigecycline resistance genes in animals and humans. *Nat. Microbiol.* **2019**, *4*, 1450–1456. [CrossRef]
142. Wang, L.; Liu, D.; Lv, Y.; Cui, L.; Li, Y.; Li, T.; Song, H.; Hao, Y.; Shen, J.; Wang, Y.; et al. Novel Plasmid-Mediated tet (X5) Gene Conferring Resistance to Tigecycline, Eravacycline, and Omadacycline in a Clinical *Acinetobacter baumannii* Isolate. *Antimicrob. Agents Chemother.* **2019**, *64*, e01326-19. [CrossRef]
143. Roberts, M.C. Update on acquired tetracycline resistance genes. *FEMS Microbiol. Lett.* **2005**, *245*, 195–203. [CrossRef]
144. Heidrich, C.G.; Mitova, S.; Schedlbauer, A.; Connell, S.R.; Fucini, P.; Steenbergen, J.N.; Berens, C. The Novel Aminomethylcycline Omadacycline Has High Specificity for the Primary Tetracycline-Binding Site on the Bacterial Ribosome. *Antibiotics* **2016**, *5*, 32. [CrossRef]
145. XERAVA (Eravacycline) for Injection. Available online: https://www.accessdata.fda.gov/drugsatfda_docs/label/2018/211109lbl.pdf (accessed on 6 June 2021).
146. Alosaimy, S.; Abdul-Mutakabbir, J.C.; Kebriaei, R.; Jorgensen, S.C.J.; Rybak, M.J. Evaluation of Eravacycline: A Novel Fluorocycline. *Pharmacother. J. Hum. Pharmacol. Drug Ther.* **2020**, *40*, 221–238. [CrossRef]
147. Abdallah, M.; Olafisoye, O.; Cortes, C.; Urban, C.; Landman, D.; Quale, J. Activity of Eravacycline against Enterobacteriaceae and *Acinetobacter baumannii*, Including Multidrug-Resistant Isolates, from New York City. *Antimicrob. Agents Chemother.* **2014**, *59*, 1802–1805. [CrossRef]
148. Robertsen, H.L.; Musiol-Kroll, E.M. Actinomycete-Derived Polyketides as a Source of Antibiotics and Lead Structures for the Development of New Antimicrobial Drugs. *Antibiotics* **2019**, *8*, 157. [CrossRef]
149. Postier, R.G.; Green, S.L.; Klein, S.R.; Ellis-Grosse, E.J.; Loh, E.; Tigecycline 200 Study Group. Results of a multicenter, randomized, open-label efficacy and safety study of two doses of tigecycline for complicated skin and skin-structure infections in hospitalized patients. *Clin. Ther.* **2004**, *26*, 704–714. [CrossRef]
150. Li, L.; Hassan, K.A.; Tetu, S.G.; Naidu, V.; Pokhrel, A.; Cain, A.K.; Paulsen, I.T. The Transcriptomic Signature of Tigecycline in *Acinetobacter baumannii*. *Front. Microbiol.* **2020**, *11*, 565438. [CrossRef]
151. Durães, F.; Sousa, M.E. Omadacycline: A Newly Approved Antibacterial from the Class of Tetracyclines. *Pharmaceuticals* **2019**, *12*, 63. [CrossRef]
152. Stets, R.; Popescu, M.; Gonong, J.R.; Mitha, I.; Nseir, W.; Madej, A.; Kirsch, C.; Das, A.F.; Garrity-Ryan, L.; Steenbergen, J.N.; et al. Omadacycline for Community-Acquired Bacterial Pneumonia. *N. Engl. J. Med.* **2019**, *380*, 517–527. [CrossRef]
153. O'Riordan, W.; Green, S.; Overcash, J.S.; Puljiz, I.; Metallidis, S.; Gardovskis, J.; Garrity-Ryan, L.; Das, A.F.; Tzanis, E.; Eckburg, P.B.; et al. Omadacycline for Acute Bacterial Skin and Skin-Structure Infections. *N. Engl. J. Med.* **2019**, *380*, 528–538. [CrossRef]
154. Moore, A.Y.; Del Rosso, J.; Johnson, J.L.; Grada, A. Sarecycline: A Review of Preclinical and Clinical Evidence. *Clin. Cosmet. Investig. Dermatol.* **2020**, *13*, 553–560. [CrossRef]
155. Pariser, D.M.; Green, L.J.; Lain, E.L.; Schmitz, C.; Chinigo, A.S.; McNamee, B.; Berk, D.R. Safety and Tolerability of Sarecycline for the Treatment of Acne Vulgaris: Results from a Phase III, Multicenter, Open-Label Study and a Phase I Phototoxicity Study. *J. Clin. Aesthet. Dermatol.* **2019**, *12*, E53–E62. [CrossRef]
156. Muralidharan, G.; Micalizzi, M.; Speth, J.; Raible, D.; Troy, S. Pharmacokinetics of Tigecycline after Single and Multiple Doses in Healthy Subjects. *Antimicrob. Agents Chemother.* **2005**, *49*, 220–229. [CrossRef]
157. Markham, A.; Keam, S.J. Omadacycline: First Global Approval. *Drugs* **2018**, *78*, 1931–1937. [CrossRef]
158. FDA Drug Approval Package: XERAVA (Eravacycline). Available online: https://www.accessdata.fda.gov/drugsatfda_docs/nda/2018/211109Orig1s000TOC.cfm (accessed on 30 November 2021).
159. Shutter, M.C.; Akhondi, H. Tetracycline. In *StatPearls*; StatPearls Publishing: Treasure Island, FL, USA, 2021.
160. Overcash, J.S.; Bhiwandi, P.; Garrity-Ryan, L.; Steenbergen, J.; Bai, S.; Chitra, S.; Manley, A.; Tzanis, E. Pharmacokinetics, Safety, and Clinical Outcomes of Omadacycline in Women with Cystitis: Results from a Phase 1b Study. *Antimicrob. Agents Chemother.* **2019**, *63*, e02083-18. [CrossRef] [PubMed]
161. Efimova, E.; Olesky, M.; Izmailyan, S.; Tsai, L. 1976. Pooled Analysis of Safety Data from Phases 2 and 3 Clinical Trials Evaluating Eravacycline in Complicated Intra-Abdominal Infections. *Open Forum Infect. Dis.* **2018**, *5*, S573–S574. [CrossRef]
162. Moore, T.J.; Zhang, H.; Anderson, G.; Alexander, G.C. Estimated Costs of Pivotal Trials for Novel Therapeutic Agents Approved by the US Food and Drug Administration, 2015–2016. *JAMA Intern. Med.* **2018**, *178*, 1451–1457. [CrossRef]

163. Solomkin, J.S.; Ramesh, M.K.; Cesnauskas, G.; Novikovs, N.; Stefanova, P.; Sutcliffe, J.A.; Walpole, S.M.; Horn, P.T. Phase 2, Randomized, Double-Blind Study of the Efficacy and Safety of Two Dose Regimens of Eravacycline versus Ertapenem for Adult Community-Acquired Complicated Intra-Abdominal Infections. *Antimicrob. Agents Chemother.* **2014**, *58*, 1847–1854. [CrossRef]
164. Moore, A.; Green, L.J.; Bruce, S.; Sadick, N.; Tschen, E.; Werschler, P.; Cook-Bolden, F.E.; Dhawan, S.S.; Forsha, D.; Gold, M.H.; et al. Once-Daily Oral Sarecycline 1.5 mg/kg/day Is Effective for Moderate to Severe Acne Vulgaris: Results from Two Identically Designed, Phase 3, Randomized, Double-Blind Clinical Trials. *J. Drugs Dermatol.* **2018**, *17*, 987–996. [CrossRef]
165. Witkop, C.J., Jr.; Wolf, R.O. Hypoplasia and Intrinsic Staining of Enamel Following Tetracycline Therapy. *JAMA* **1963**, *185*, 1008–1011. [CrossRef]
166. Kadoyama, K.; Sakaeda, T.; Tamon, A.; Okuno, Y. Adverse Event Profile of Tigecycline: Data Mining of the Public Version of the U.S. Food and Drug Administration Adverse Event Reporting System. *Biol. Pharm. Bull.* **2012**, *35*, 967–970. [CrossRef]
167. Marot, J.-C.; Jonckheere, S.; Munyentwali, H.; Belkhir, L.; Vandercam, B.; Yombi, J.C. Tigecycline-induced acute pancreatitis: About two cases and review of the literature. *Acta Clin. Belg.* **2012**, *67*, 229–232. [CrossRef]
168. Berg, J.K.; Tzanis, E.; Garrity-Ryan, L.; Bai, S.; Chitra, S.; Manley, A.; Villano, S. Pharmacokinetics and Safety of Omadacycline in Subjects with Impaired Renal Function. *Antimicrob. Agents Chemother.* **2018**, *62*, e02057-17. [CrossRef]
169. Korth-Bradley, J.M.; McGovern, P.C.; Salageanu, J.; Matschke, K.; Plotka, A.; Pawlak, S. Tigecycline Does Not Prolong Corrected QT Intervals in Healthy Subjects. *Antimicrob. Agents Chemother.* **2013**, *57*, 1895–1901. [CrossRef]
170. Yahav, D.; Lador, A.; Paul, M.; Leibovici, L. Efficacy and safety of tigecycline: A systematic review and meta-analysis. *J. Antimicrob. Chemother.* **2011**, *66*, 1963–1971. [CrossRef]
171. FDA Drug Safety Communication: Increased Risk of Death with Tygacil (Tigecycline) Compared to Other Antibiotics Used to Treat Similar Infections. Available online: https://www.fda.gov/drugs/drug-safety-and-availability/fda-drug-safety-communication-increased-risk-death-tygacil-tigecycline-compared-other-antibiotics (accessed on 22 October 2021).
172. Cai, Y.; Wang, R.; Liang, B.; Bai, N.; Liu, Y. Systematic Review and Meta-Analysis of the Effectiveness and Safety of Tigecycline for Treatment of Infectious Disease. *Antimicrob. Agents Chemother.* **2011**, *55*, 1162–1172. [CrossRef]
173. Tasina, E.; Haidich, A.-B.; Kokkali, S.; Arvanitidou, M. Efficacy and safety of tigecycline for the treatment of infectious diseases: A meta-analysis. *Lancet Infect. Dis.* **2011**, *11*, 834–844. [CrossRef]
174. Prasad, P.; Sun, J.; Danner, R.L.; Natanson, C. Excess Deaths Associated with Tigecycline After Approval Based on Noninferiority Trials. *Clin. Infect. Dis.* **2012**, *54*, 1699–1709. [CrossRef]
175. Powers, J.H. Editorial Commentary: Asking the Right Questions: Morbidity, Mortality, and Measuring What's Important in Unbiased Evaluations of Antimicrobials. *Clin. Infect. Dis.* **2012**, *54*, 1710–1713. [CrossRef]
176. Burkhardt, O.; Rauch, K.; Kaever, V.; Hadem, J.; Kielstein, J.T.; Welte, T. Tigecycline possibly underdosed for the treatment of pneumonia: A pharmacokinetic viewpoint. *Int. J. Antimicrob. Agents* **2009**, *34*, 101–102. [CrossRef]
177. Briggs, G.G.; Freeman, R.K.; Yaffe, S.J. *Drugs in Pregnancy and Lactation: A Reference Guide to Fetal and Neonatal Risk*, 9th ed.; Lippincott Williams & Wilkins: Philadelphia, PA, USA, 2011; ISBN 978-1-60831-708-0.
178. Zimmerman, J.J.; Raible, D.G.; Harper, D.M.; Matschke, K.; Speth, J.L. Evaluation of a Potential Tigecycline-Warfarin Drug Interac. *Pharmacother. J. Hum. Pharmacol. Drug Ther.* **2008**, *28*, 895–905. [CrossRef]
179. Zhanel, G.G.; Siemens, S.; Slayter, K.; Mandell, L. Antibiotic and Oral Contraceptive Drug Interactions: Is There a Need for Concern? *Can. J. Infect. Dis.* **1999**, *10*, 429–433. [CrossRef]
180. Sriram, D.; Yogeeswari, P.; Senchani, G.; Banerjee, D. Newer tetracycline derivatives: Synthesis, anti-HIV, antimycobacterial activities and inhibition of HIV-1 integrase. *Bioorg. Med. Chem. Lett.* **2007**, *17*, 2372–2375. [CrossRef]
181. Castro, W.; Navarro, M.; Biot, C. Medicinal potential of ciprofloxacin and its derivatives. *Futur. Med. Chem.* **2013**, *5*, 81–96. [CrossRef]
182. Sun, C.; Hunt, D.K.; Chen, C.-L.; Deng, Y.; He, M.; Clark, R.B.; Fyfe, C.; Grossman, T.H.; Sutcliffe, J.A.; Xiao, X.-Y. Design, Synthesis, and Biological Evaluation of Hexacyclic Tetracyclines as Potent, Broad Spectrum Antibacterial Agents. *J. Med. Chem.* **2015**, *58*, 4703–4712. [CrossRef]
183. Tetraphase. Pipeline. Available online: https://www.tphase.com/products/pipeline/ (accessed on 6 October 2021).
184. PubChem TP-271. Available online: https://pubchem.ncbi.nlm.nih.gov/compound/54726193 (accessed on 24 October 2021).
185. Grossman, T.H.; Fyfe, C.; O'Brien, W.; Hackel, M.; Minyard, M.B.; Waites, K.B.; Dubois, J.; Murphy, T.M.; Slee, A.M.; Weiss, W.J.; et al. Fluorocycline TP-271 Is Potent against Complicated Community-Acquired Bacterial Pneumonia Pathogens. *mSphere* **2017**, *2*, e00004-17. [CrossRef] [PubMed]
186. Sun, C.; Deng, Y.; Hunt, D.; Fyfe, C.; Kerstein, K.; Xiao, X. *TP-6076, A Fully Synthetic Tetracycline Antibacterial Agent, Is Highly Potent against a Broad Range of Pathogens, Including Carbapenem-Resistant Enterobacteriaceae*; ASM Microbe: New Orleans, LA, USA, 2017.
187. Liu, F.; Myers, A.G. Development of a platform for the discovery and practical synthesis of new tetracycline antibiotics. *Curr. Opin. Chem. Biol.* **2016**, *32*, 48–57. [CrossRef]
188. Grossman, T.; Hunt, D.; Iii, H.H.; Sutcliffe, J. TP-271, a Novel Oral Fluorocycline for Community-Acquired Respiratory and Biothreat Pathogens. In Proceedings of the 50th Annual Interscience Conference of Antimicrobial Agents and Chemotherapy, Boston, MA, USA, 12–15 September 2010; p. 1.

189. Seifert, H.; Stefanik, D.; Olesky, M.; Higgins, P.G. In vitro activity of the novel fluorocycline TP-6076 against carbapenem-resistant *Acinetobacter baumannii*. *Int. J. Antimicrob. Agents* **2019**, *55*, 105829. [CrossRef]
190. Tetraphase Pharmaceuticals, Inc. A Phase 1, Open-Label, Randomized, PK and Safety Study to Assess Bronchopulmonary Disposition of Intravenous TP-6076 in Healthy Men and Women; ClinicalTrials.gov. Available online: https://clinicaltrials.gov/ct2/show/NCT03691584 (accessed on 28 November 2021).

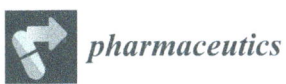

Review

Ruthenium Complexes in the Fight against Pathogenic Microorganisms. An Extensive Review

Alexandra-Cristina Munteanu * and Valentina Uivarosi *

Department of General and Inorganic Chemistry, Faculty of Pharmacy, "Carol Davila" University of Medicine and Pharmacy, 020956 Bucharest, Romania
* Correspondence: alexandra.ticea@umfcd.ro (A.-C.M.); valentina.uivarosi@umfcd.ro (V.U.)

Abstract: The widespread use of antibiotics has resulted in the emergence of drug-resistant populations of microorganisms. Clearly, one can see the need to develop new, more effective, antimicrobial agents that go beyond the explored 'chemical space'. In this regard, their unique modes of action (e.g., reactive oxygen species (ROS) generation, redox activation, ligand exchange, depletion of substrates involved in vital cellular processes) render metal complexes as promising drug candidates. Several Ru (II/III) complexes have been included in, or are currently undergoing, clinical trials as anticancer agents. Based on the in-depth knowledge of their chemical properties and biological behavior, the interest in developing new ruthenium compounds as antibiotic, antifungal, antiparasitic, or antiviral drugs has risen. This review will discuss the advantages and disadvantages of Ru (II/III) frameworks as antimicrobial agents. Some aspects regarding the relationship between their chemical structure and mechanism of action, cellular localization, and/or metabolism of the ruthenium complexes in bacterial and eukaryotic cells are discussed as well. Regarding the antiviral activity, in light of current events related to the Covid-19 pandemic, the Ru (II/III) compounds used against SARS-CoV-2 (e.g., BOLD-100) are also reviewed herein.

Keywords: ruthenium; antimicrobial; antibacterial; antiviral; antiparasitic; COVID-19

Citation: Munteanu, A.-C.; Uivarosi, V. Ruthenium Complexes in the Fight against Pathogenic Microorganisms. An Extensive Review. *Pharmaceutics* 2021, *13*, 874. https://doi.org/10.3390/pharmaceutics13060874

Academic Editor: Carlos Alonso-Moreno

Received: 1 May 2021
Accepted: 9 June 2021
Published: 13 June 2021

Publisher's Note: MDPI stays neutral with regard to jurisdictional claims in published maps and institutional affiliations.

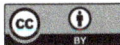

Copyright: © 2021 by the authors. Licensee MDPI, Basel, Switzerland. This article is an open access article distributed under the terms and conditions of the Creative Commons Attribution (CC BY) license (https://creativecommons.org/licenses/by/4.0/).

1. Introduction

The alarming pace at which microorganisms are evading antibiotics constitutes a challenge for modern medicine [1]. The phenomenon of multidrug resistance has generated a sense of urgency around the development of new classes of antibiotics. Yet most of the drugs under clinical development for the treatment of bacterial infections are organic derivatives of currently used antibiotics, which suggests that these molecules are susceptible to in place mechanisms of bacterial resistance [2].

Although the pipeline for new antibiotics is running dry, the coordination chemistry field is still largely underexplored for antibacterial drug development, with limited clinical use for bismuth and silver-based antimicrobials. Bismuth compounds, for instance, are used for the treatment of *H. pylori* infections and diarrhea and in wound dressings [3], while silver compounds are used for wound healing applications and management of topical infections [4]. The focus of current research is directed towards the development of metal-based nanoparticles (NPs), with special interest being given to AgNPs following their introduction to the U.S. market in 2016 [5].

It is rather unfortunate that less attention is being given to metal complexes. It should be noted that metal-based compounds offer a vast structural diversity of three-dimensional (3D) scaffolds due to the variety of metal ions, ligands, and possible geometries [2,6,7]. While most organic fragments have linear (1D) or planar (2D) shapes, more complex 3D fragments are desirable for the molecular recognition by biomolecules and optimal interaction with intracellular targets [6]. Furthermore, increasing the 3D chemical topology of molecules has been correlated with a broader activity spectrum [7,8]. Therefore, metal complexes are ideal candidates for future drug discovery pursuits meant to access the underexplored 3D chemical space [6]. In addition, metal complexes possess unique mechanisms of action that are not readily available to organic compounds: ROS generation, redox activation, ligand exchange, and depletion of substrates involved in vital cellular processes [2,9,10]. When compared with solely organic molecules, metal-based compounds were found to display a significantly higher hit-rate against critical antibiotic-resistant pathogens (0.87% vs. 9.9%). Moreover, the percentages of toxic to healthy eukaryotic cells and/or hemolytic compounds in the two groups were found to be nearly identical. Therefore, a generally higher degree of toxicity cannot explain the remarkably high antimicrobial activity of the metal-based set of compounds compared with the organic molecules [2].

The potential of metal complexes has been acknowledged over the last two decades through several platinum-, ruthenium-, copper-, iron-, and gallium-based drugs, which have reached different stages in clinical trials for the treatment of cancer, neurodegenerative diseases, and malaria [11,12]. Several ruthenium (Ru) complexes have been evaluated in clinical trials for the treatment of cancer, namely NAMI-A [13,14], KP1019 [15,16] and its water-soluble sodium salt IT-139 (formerly KP1339) [17], and, more recently, TLD-1433 [18]. Previous knowledge of their chemical properties and biological behavior, gained from the research directed towards the development of novel anticancer compounds, has led to increased focus on tailoring ruthenium complexes as antimicrobial agents [1]. Moreover, a recent study screening 906 metal-containing compounds for antimicrobial activity identified ruthenium as the most frequent element found in active compounds that are nontoxic to eukaryotic cells, followed by silver, palladium, and iridium [2]. Therefore, ruthenium-based compounds hold promise for potential antimicrobial applications, which will be extensively reviewed in this paper.

In order to clarify the use of the terms 'antibacterial', 'antibiotic', and 'antimicrobial' in this manuscript, definitions are given below. The term antibacterial refers to substances, materials, or assemblies that kill or inhibit the growth of bacteria. WHO defines an antibiotic as a substance with a direct action on bacteria that is used for the treatment or prevention of infections or infectious diseases [19]. Although we recognize the distinction between these two terms, in order to avoid repetition, we have occasionally used the terms 'antibiotic' and 'antibacterial' interchangeably. Antimicrobials, on the other hand, will be used generically for compounds or materials that act against microorganisms (bacteria, fungi, viruses, protozoa, parasites, etc.). Consequently, antimicrobials will include antibacterials, antifungals, antivirals, antiprotozoals, and antiparasitics.

2. General Remarks on Bacterial Cell Structure. Gram-Positive vs. Gram-Negative Strains

The bacterial cell structure comes as a result of the extreme conditions they must survive in, which are inhospitable for eukaryotes. For instance, the rigid cell wall that covers the cell membrane is vital for protection from physical, chemical, and mechanical stressors. Based on the Gram staining procedure, bacteria are classified into two groups: Gram-positive and Gram-negative bacteria [1].

Gram-positive strains retain the Crystal Violet stain due to the presence of a thick layer of peptidoglycan in their cell walls, which is densely embedded with negatively charged glycopolymers called wall teichoic acids (Figure 1). The fairly porous cell wall structure generally allows for passage for exogenous molecules into the bacterial cells [20].

Gram-negative bacteria, however, have more complex cell wall structures (Figure 1). Due to the absence of inlaid teichoic acid molecules, their layer of peptidoglycan is thin, yet bound to an outer membrane coated with lipopolysaccharides (LPSs). LPSs are amphiphiles, consisting of a hydrophobic lipidic domain (lipid A) covalently bound to a polysaccharide, which comprises the O antigen and the inner and outer cores; these negatively charged (due to the presence of the phosphate and acid groups) macromolecules are stabilized by divalent cations such as calcium and magnesium. LPSs greatly decrease bacterial permeability to antibiotics and play a crucial role in the development of resistance mechanisms for many pathogenic Gram-negative bacteria [1,20].

Additionally, on the cell surface of some bacteria (e.g., *Streptococcus pneumoniae*) a slime layer or a capsule can offer additional protection against desiccation or phagocytosis by host cells. Flagella, fimbriae, and pili are external filamentous appendages that serve as organelles of locomotion or assist with bacterial attachment and adhesion to a surface or genetic exchange [1,21].

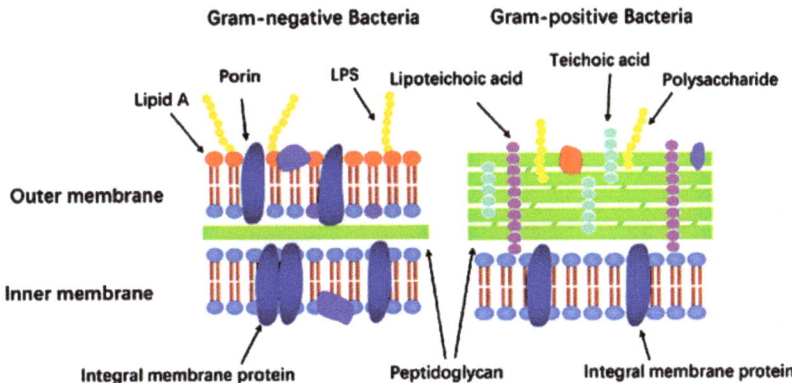

Figure 1. Comparison between Gram-negative and Gram-positive bacteria cell walls. Adapted from [22] with permission. Copyright © 2020 Huan, Kong, Mou and Yi.

At physiological pH, the high content of zwitterionic phosphatidylcholine confers an overall neutral charge to the eukaryotic cell membranes. In contrast, bacterial outer cell walls and membranes are usually negatively charged due to the presence of negatively charged components (phospholipids, teichoic acids, and lipopolysaccharides) [1,23]. Hence, in order to increase selectivity, new antibacterial drugs (including ruthenium complexes) are generally designed so as to possess a cationic component.

3. Mechanisms of Action of Current Drugs

Antibiotics are classified into four major groups (Figure 2), based on their intracellular target and mechanism of action: (1) inhibition of bacterial cell wall synthesis (penicillin and its derivatives, cephalosporins, carbapenems, and glycopeptides—these drugs are more active against Gram-positive bacteria); (2) disruption of bacterial membranes (polymyxins—these are active against Gram-negative bacteria and considered a last-line therapy against Gram-negative 'superbugs'); (3) inhibition of nucleic acid synthesis (quinolones, rifampicin, and sulphonamidesare—these are broad-spectrum synthetic antibiotics); and (4) inhibition of protein synthesis (tetracycline, aminoglycosides, chloramphenicol, and macrolides—these inhibit protein synthesis by targeting the RNA-rich surfaces of ribosomes) [1].

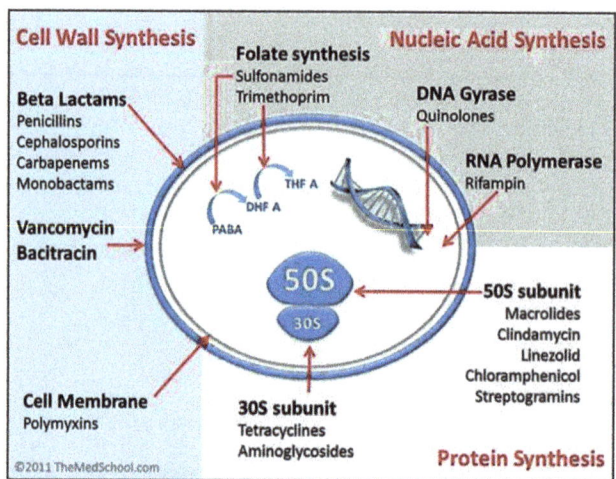

Figure 2. Mechanisms of action of currently used antibiotics (Image by Kendrick Johnson, licensed under the Creative Commons Attribution-Share Alike 3.0 Unported license).

Several new classes of antibiotics have been discovered over the last two decades. Gepotidacin, for instance, belongs to a new chemical class of antibiotics called triazaacenaphthylene. It is a topoiosomerase inhibitor, which is currently being investigated in a phase III clinical study in patients with uncomplicated urinary tract infection and urogenital gonorrhoea [24]. Other current strategies include the use of phages (viruses that kill specific bacterial strains) [25], various types of engineered nanoparticles [25], and cationic materials, including cationic polypeptides, polymers, copolymers, and dendrimers [26]. Furthermore, several natural products, e.g., teixobactin, have been identified as lead compounds in the fight against antimicrobial resistance [27].

4. Mechanisms of Resistance to Antibiotics

Bacterial resistance to antibiotics can result from intrinsic or acquired antibiotic-resistant mechanisms. *P. aeruginosa* and other Gram-negative pathogens are intrinsically more resistant to antibiotics due to the reduced permeability of their outer membranes. These bacterial strains have porins of unusually low permeability. In addition, the outer membranes of mycobacteria have a high lipid content that allows for hydrophobic drugs such as fluoroquinolones to enter the cell but limits the access of hydrophilic drugs.

Acquired bacterial resistance is caused by alterations in microorganisms that result in drug inactivation or a decrease in therapeutic efficacy. Improper prescribing and overuse of antibiotics are factors that have contributed to the growing issue of microbial resistance. Consequently, infections have become increasingly difficult or even impossible to treat [28].

Bacterial resistance can emerge as a result of various biochemical mechanisms, including decreased drug uptake, modification of a specific bacterial target, enzymatic inactivation of the drug, and modifications to the bacterial efflux systems [1,28]. For instance, a common resistance mechanism is the alteration of the bacterial membrane permeability, resulting in limited uptake of an antibiotic. Modification of the drug's target can involve mutations in DNA gyrase and topoisomerase IV or alterations in the structure and/or number of penicillin-binding proteins [5]. Drug inactivation occurs via mutations in genes coding for key enzymes, such as β-lactamases, acetyltransferases, adenylyltransferases, and aminoglycoside-3′-phosphotransferase. These mutations can occur either inside the bacterial chromosomal DNA or as a result of foreign genetic material acquisition. Acquisition of genetic material that confers resistance is possible through horizontal gene transfer, which is mediated either by plasmids or bacteriophages [28].

Another common mechanism of resistance used by many pathogens involves the association of multiple bacterial cells in matrices called biofilms. The bacterial cells within the biofilm have a slow metabolism rate and slow cell division. Therefore, antimicrobials targeting growing and dividing bacterial cells are rendered ineffective. Moreover, the thick biofilm extracellular matrix consists of bacterial polysaccharides, proteins, and DNA, which hinder access of the antimicrobial agent to the bacteria. It is also likely that the proximity of the bacterial cells facilitates horizontal gene transfer. Therefore, the antimicrobial resistance genes can be shared between the cells forming the biofilm [28–30].

Nosocomial infections or hospital-acquired infections are a growing threat worldwide and are often caused by multidrug-resistant bacteria. Interestingly, a small group of microorganisms, known as ESKAPE pathogens, are responsible for most antibiotic-resistant infections. These pathogens include: *Enterococcus faecium, Staphylococcus aureus, Klebsiella pneumoniae, Acinetobacter baumannii, Pseudomonas aeruginosa*, and *Enterobacter* spp., which possess innate resistance or can acquire resistance against multiple antibiotics [31].

5. Antibacterial and Antifungal Activities of Ruthenium Complexes

Based upon their chemical stability, Ru complexes can be classified as either stable, relatively inert compounds, and prodrugs. A metal complex is inert when the ligand framework remains unaltered in biological media. The ruthenium ion in these compounds acts merely as a central scaffold that carries the bioactive ligands to their target. Consequently, the properties of the coordinated ligands are essential to the antibacterial activity [32]. The presence of the ruthenium ion, however, provides the molecule with a positive charge, which aids in targeting the negatively charged cell wall structures of bacteria. The antibacterial activity of these complexes depends on their lipophilicity and charge, which in turn shape their ability to interact with specific targets (e.g., DNA, RNA, proteins, bacterial membranes).

Prodrugs are labile complexes that release the ligand/s when exposed to solvents and/or media and generate species that can bind to various biological targets or photoactivated drugs. The latter become active upon light irradiation and act as photosensitizers. Since this behavior is somewhat unconventional for the general understanding of the term 'prodrug' in the traditional medicinal chemistry sense, 'prodrug-like molecules' seems more appropriate to describe this type of metal complex. In the case of labile complexes, active species are released as a result of either partial or total ligand exchange in biological media. These active species are either ruthenium species resulting from ligand exchange with media components or the released ligands. In the latter case, the ruthenium compounds are called 'carrier' complexes; one such example is the Ru(II) chelate–chloroquine complex, $[RuCl_2(CQ)]_2$, where CQ = chloroquine (see 6. Antiparasitic activity of ruthenium complexes). In the following sections, ruthenium complexes will be classified based on their structure. Details and comments with regard to their mechanisms of action will be provided wherever such information is available.

5.1. Mononuclear Ruthenium (II) Complexes

Mononuclear polypyridylruthenium (II) complexes with antimicrobial activities were first reported in the 1950s and 1960s by Dwyer et al. [33,34]. With the general interest shifting towards discovering new analogues of existing classes of antibiotics, their impressive seminal work was unfortunately not further pursued. However, the advancement into clinical trials of NAMI-A, KP1019, and TLD1433 for the treatment of cancer and the urge to develop new classes of antibiotics have led, over the last two decades, to an increased focus on research and development of ruthenium-based antimicrobials [35].

Dwyer et al. made the first steps towards the development of kinetically inert Ru(II) complexes and the study of their in vitro and in vivo antimicrobial activities. The addition of methyl groups to the phenanthroline ligands enhanced lipophilicity and increased the activity of $[Ru(Me_4phen)_3]^{2+}$ (Figure 3) against Gram-positive bacteria, as compared with $[Ru(phen)_3]^{2+}$ (Figure 3) [36]. More recent studies [37,38], however, have shown that these complexes are much less active against various antibiotic-resistant ESKAPE pathogens. Additionally, their activity in vivo has been proven to be unsatisfactory, as they caused severe neurotoxic effects when injected into mice [39].

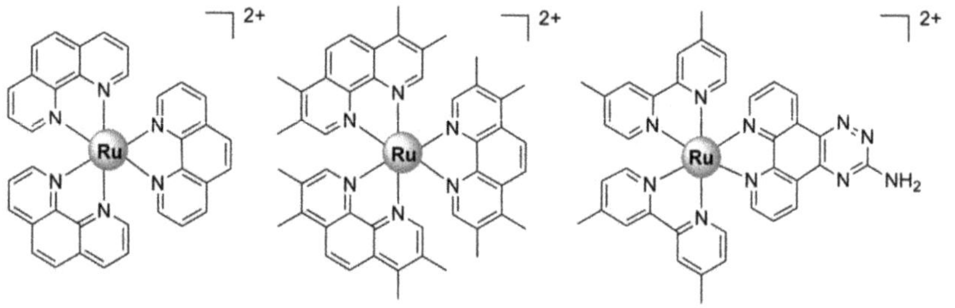

Figure 3. Examples of inert structural mononuclear polypyridylruthenium (II) complexes.

Following up on this remarkable work, various heteroleptic mononuclear polypyridyl Ru (II) complexes were tested for antibacterial activity. Their activities (MIC values) against various bacterial strains, as well as toxicity towards healthy eukaryotic cells and modes of action, where available, are listed in Table 1.

Table 1. Activities of selected ruthenium complexes against bacteria, toxicity to healthy mammalian cells, and mode of action.

Complex [Reference]	Activity Strain: MIC Values (µg/mL)		Toxicity to Healthy Mammalian Cells (IC_{50}, µg/mL, 24 h, unless Stated Otherwise)	Modes of Action
	Gram-Positive Strains	Gram-Negative Strains		
Polypyridylruthenium (II) complexes				
[Ru(2,9-Me$_2$phen)$_2$(dppz)]$^{2+}$ [40]	S. aureus MRSA252: 2, MRSA41: 4, MSSA160: 8, B. subtilis 168: 4	Not active on E. coli MC4100	-	bactericidal; DNA intercalation
R-825 [41]	S. pneumoniae D39 WT: 27.5 piuA mutant: 55	-	Not toxic to human alveolar epithelial A549 cells up to 480 µM	interference with iron acquisition systems in S. pneumoniae cells
X-03 [42]	S. pneumoniae D39: 25, Streptococcus suis 05ZYH33: 100, S. pyogenes MGAS5005: 25, Listeria monocytogenes 19,117: 25, S. aureus 29,213: 50	E. coli K12: > 200, Vibrio alginolyticus V12G01: > 200, Vibrio parahaemolyticus RIMD 2,210,633: > 200, A. baumanii 19,606: > 200	Not toxic to human alveolar A549 and bronchial HBE epithelial cells up to 100 µg/mL	interference with iron acquisition systems in S. pneumoniae cells; oxidative stress, membrane damage
[Ru(bpy)$_2$Cl(clbzpy)]$^+$ [43]	S. aureus ATCC 25,923: 500, S. epidermidis ATCC 12,228: 250	P. aeruginosa ATCC 10,145: not active	-	membrane damage
[Ru(bpy)$_2$(methionine)]$^{2+}$ [44]	upon blue LED irradiation S. aureus ATCC 25,923: 62.5, S. epidermidis ATCC 12,228: 125	P. aeruginosa ATCC 10,145: not active E. coli ATCC 11,303: 500	-	DNA photodamage
[Ru(dmb)$_2$(ETPIP)]$^{2+}$ [45]	S. aureus Newman: 50	-	-	-
[Ru(phen)$_2$(ETPIP)]$^{2+}$ [45]	S. aureus Newman: 25	-	-	inhibits biofilm formation; interacts with intracellular thiols
[Ru(bpy)$_2$(BTPIP)]$^{2+}$ [46]	S. aureus Newman: 16	-	-	inhibits biofilm formation

Table 1. Cont.

Complex [Reference]	Activity Strain: MIC Values (µg/mL)		Toxicity to Healthy Mammalian Cells (IC_{50}, µg/mL, 24 h, unless Stated Otherwise)	Modes of Action
	Gram-Positive Strains	Gram-Negative Strains		
[Ru(bpy)$_2$curcumin]$^+$ [47]	S. aureus ATCC 29,213: 1	A. baumanii BAA-1605: > 64, E. coli ATCC 25,922: > 64, K. pneumoniae BAA-1705: > 64, P. aeruginosa ATCC 27,853: > 64	Vero (African green monkey kidney epithelial) cells: > 80	bactericidal; inhibits biofilm formation
[Ru(phen)$_2$curcumin]$^+$ [47]	S. aureus ATCC 29,213: 1	A. baumanii BAA-1605: 8–16, E. coli ATCC 25,922: > 64, K. pneumoniae BAA-1705: > 64, P. aeruginosa ATCC 27,853: > 64	Vero (African green monkey kidney epithelial) cells: > 80	-
Mono-bb$_7$ [38]	S. aureus MSSA ATCC 25,923: 4 MRSA (JCU culture collection): 16	E. coli ATCC 25,922: 16 P. aeruginosa ATCC 27,853: > 128	-	bactericidal; membrane damage
Mono-bb$_{10}$ [37,38]	S. aureus MSSA ATCC 25,923: 4 MRSA (JCU culture collection): 16	E. coli ATCC 25,922: 16 P. aeruginosa ATCC 27,853: 32	-	bactericidal
Mono-bb$_{16}$ [37]	S. aureus MSSA ATCC 25,923: 16 MRSA (JCU culture collection): 16	E. coli ATCC 25,922: 64 P. aeruginosa ATCC 27,853: 64	-	-
cis-α-[Ru(phen)bb$_{12}$]$^{2+}$ [48]	S. aureus MSSA ATCC 25,923: 0.5 MRSA (JCU culture collection): 4	E. coli ATCC 25,922: 8 P. aeruginosa ATCC 27,853: 8	-	DNA binding
cis-β-[Ru(phen)(bb$_{12}$)]$^{2+}$ [48]	S. aureus MSSA ATCC 25,923: 0.5 MRSA (JCU culture collection): 4	E. coli ATCC 25,922: 16 P. aeruginosa ATCC 27,853: 32	-	DNA binding
[Ru(bb$_7$)(dppz)]$^{2+}$ [49]	S. aureus SH 1000: 2 MRSA USA 300 LAC JE2: 2	E. coli avian pathogenic: 8 uropathogenic: 8 E. coli MG1655: 8 P. aeruginosa PAO1: 16	human embryonic kidney HEK-293 cells: 27 (48 h), human fetal hepatocyte L02 cells: 64 (48 h)	bactericidal, DNA binding
[Ru(Me$_4$phen)$_2$(dppz)]$^{2+}$ [50]	S. aureus SH1000: 9.7, E. faecalis V583: 38.8	E. coli MG1655: 4.9, EC958: 4.9, P. aeruginosa PA2017: 9.7 A. baumannii AB184: 9.7	-	bactericidal, chromosomal DNA binding
SCAR4 [51]	M. tuberculosis H$_{37}$Rv ATCC 27,294 (neither G+, nor G-): 0.63	-	Mouse monocyte macrophage J774A.1 cell line: 19.5	covalent binding to DNA
SCAR5 [51]	M. tuberculosis H$_{37}$Rv ATCC 27,294 (neither G+, nor G-): 0.26	-	J774A.1: 3.9	covalent binding to DNA
SCAR6 [51]	M. tuberculosis H$_{37}$Rv ATCC 27,294 (neither G+, nor G-): 3.90	-	J774A.1: 78.2	covalent binding to DNA
RuNN [52]	S. aureus ATCC 25,923: 15.6, S. aureus ATCC 700,698 (MRSA): 62.5 S. epidermidis ATCC 12,228: 31.2, S. epidermidis ATCC 358,983: 62.5	-	no cytotoxic effect against human erythrocytes	bactericidal; inhibits biofilm formation
[Ru(hexpytri)$_3$](PF$_6$)$_2$ [53]	S. aureus MSSA ATCC 25,923: 8, S. aureus MSSA NZRM 9653: 1, S. aureus MRSA MR 9519: 4, S. pyogenes: 4	E. coli ATCC 25,922: non-active	Vero cells: IC_{50} > 128 (48h)	cell wall/cytoplasmic membrane damage

Table 1. Cont.

Complex [Reference]	Activity Strain: MIC Values (μg/mL)		Toxicity to Healthy Mammalian Cells (IC$_{50}$, μg/mL, 24 h, unless Stated Otherwise)	Modes of Action
	Gram-Positive Strains	Gram-Negative Strains		
[Ru(hexyltripy)(heptyltripy)]Cl$_2$ [54]	S. aureus ATCC 25,923: 2	E. coli ATCC 25,922: 8	HDFa (skin cells): 16.4	abnormal cellular division
ΔΔ-Rubb$_7$ [37,38]	S. aureus MSSA ATCC 25,923: 16 MRSA (JCU culture collection): 16	E. coli ATCC 25,922: 16 P. aeruginosa ATCC 27853: 128	Red blood cells: > 1024	bactericidal; membrane damage, interaction with ribosomal RNA
ΔΔ-Rubb$_{12}$ [55,56]	S. aureus MSSA ATCC 25,923: 1 MRSA (JCU culture collection): 1	E. coli ATCC 25,922: 2 P. aeruginosa ATCC 27,853: 16	Baby hamster kidney (BHK): 113.9, HEK-293: 82.2	bactericidal; membrane damage, interaction with ribosomal RNA
ΔΔ-Rubb$_{16}$ [56]	S. aureus MSSA ATCC 25,923: 1 MRSA (JCU culture collection): 1	E. coli ATCC 25,922: 4 P. aeruginosa ATCC 27,853: 8	Red blood cells: 22, BHK: 49.8, HEK-293: 35.1	bactericidal; membrane damage, interaction with ribosomal RNA
[Ru$_2$(Me$_4$phen)$_2$(tpphz)]$^{4+}$ [57–59]	S. aureus MSSA SH1000: 86, Enterococcus faecalis V583: 1	E. coli WT G1655: 2.5, EC958 ST131 (multi-drug-resistant, clinical isolate): 3.5, P. aeruginosa (clinical isolate): 4, K. pneumoniae (clinical isolate): 3.5, A. baumannii (clinical isolate): 3.5	HEK-293: 270	membrane and DNA damage
Cl-Rubb$_7$-Cl [55,60]	S. aureus MSSA ATCC 25,923: 8 MRSA (JCU culture collection): 8	E. coli ATCC 25,922: 8 P. aeruginosa ATCC 27,853: 32	-	bactericidal
Cl-Rubb$_{12}$-Cl [55,60]	S. aureus MSSA ATCC 25,923: 1 MRSA (JCU culture collection): 1	E. coli ATCC 25,922: 2 P. aeruginosa ATCC 27,853: 8	-	bactericidal
Cl-Rubb$_{16}$-Cl [55,60]	S. aureus MSSA ATCC 25,923: 8 MRSA (JCU culture collection): 8	E. coli ATCC 25,922: 8 P. aeruginosa ATCC 27,853: > 128	-	bactericidal
Rubb$_7$-Cl [56]	S. aureus MSSA ATCC 25,923: 8 MRSA (JCU culture collection): 16	E. coli ATCC 25,922: 1 P. aeruginosa ATCC 27,853: 16	BHK: 337.5, HEK-293: 98	interaction with chromosomal DNA and ribosomal RNA
Rubb$_{12}$-Cl [56]	S. aureus MSSA ATCC 25,923: 1 MRSA (JCU culture collection): 1	E. coli ATCC 25,922: 1 P. aeruginosa ATCC 27,853: 16	BHK: 70.6, HEK-293: 87.3	interaction with chromosomal DNA and ribosomal RNA
Rubb$_{16}$-Cl [56]	S. aureus MSSA ATCC 25,923: 1 MRSA (JCU culture collection): 2	E. coli ATCC 25,922: 4 P. aeruginosa ATCC 27,853: 64	BHK: 34.9, HEK-293: 63.5	interaction with chromosomal DNA and ribosomal RNA
Rubb$_7$-tri [37,61]	S. aureus MSSA ATCC 25,923: 4 MRSA (JCU culture collection): 4	E. coli ATCC 25,922: 16 P. aeruginosa ATCC 27,853: 2	-	interaction with DNA
Rubb$_7$-tetra (Rubb$_7$-TL) [62]	S. aureus MSSA ATCC 25,923: 8 MRSA (JCU culture collection): 16	E. coli avian pathogenic: 16 uropathogenic: 16 E. coli MG1655: 16 P. aeruginosa PAO1: 32	BHK: 176 (24 h) BHK: 36.4 (72 h)	interaction with proteins

Table 1. Cont.

Complex [Reference]	Activity Strain: MIC Values (μg/mL)		Toxicity to Healthy Mammalian Cells (IC$_{50}$, μg/mL, 24 h, unless Stated Otherwise)	Modes of Action
	Gram-Positive Strains	Gram-Negative Strains		
Rubb$_7$-TNL [62]	S. aureus MSSA ATCC 25,923: 4 MRSA (JCU culture collection): 8	E. coli avian pathogenic: 16 uropathogenic: 16 E. coli MG1655: 8 P. aeruginosa PAO1: 16	BHK: 276 (24 h) BHK: 81.6 (72 h)	interaction with proteins
Rubb$_{12}$-tri [37,55,61]	S. aureus: 1 MRSA (JCU culture collection): 1	E. coli: 4 P. aeruginosa: 32	BHK: 50.9 (72 h), HEK-293: 21.8 (72 h)	bactericidal, interaction with DNA
Rubb$_{12}$-tetra [37,55,61]	S. aureus: 2 MRSA (JCU culture collection): 2	E. coli: 2 P. aeruginosa: 16	BHK: 43.7 (72 h), HEK-293: 21.3 (72 h)	bactericidal, interaction with DNA
Rubb$_{16}$-tri [37,55,61]	S. aureus: 2 MRSA (JCU culture collection): 2	E. coli: 8 P. aeruginosa: 32	BHK: 25.1 (72 h), HEK-293: 20.2 (72 h)	bactericidal, interaction with DNA
Rubb$_{16}$-tetra [37,55,61]	S. aureus: 2 MRSA (JCU culture collection): 2	E. coli: 8 P. aeruginosa: 32	BHK: 19.8 (72 h), HEK-293: 15.8 (72 h)	bactericidal, interaction with DNA
Ruthenium-based CORMs				
CORM-2 [63–65]	Growth inhibitory effects on S. aureus (MIC value not reported)	E. coli avian pathogenic: 250, uropathogenic: 250, E. coli MG1655: 250, P. aeruginosa PAO1: 3.8 H. pylori strains (including antibiotic resistant): 100–200	Murine RAW264.7 monocyte macrophages: > 50 (DMEM culture medium)	Bactericidal, inhibition of aerobic respiration, inhibition of biofilm formation and disruption of mature biofilms, ROS generation, interaction with chromosomal DNA and intracellular proteins, interference with iron homeostasis
CORM-3 [64,66,67]	Growth inhibitory effects on S. aureus, Lactobacillus lactis (MIC value not reported)	E. coli MG1655: 4 (minimal GDMM medium) and > 512 (in rich MH-II medium) H. pylori 26,695: 420 (antibiotic resistant strains)	L929 murine fibroblast cells: 63 (RPMI culture medium), RAW264.7: > 30 (DMEM culture medium)	
Ruthenium complexes in Antimicrobial Photodynamic Therapy				
[Ru(dmob)$_3$]$^{2+}$ [68]	S. aureus NCTC 10788: 12.5	P. aeruginosa NCTC 8626: 50	-	Light activation
cis-[Ru(bpy)$_2$(INH)$_2$]$^{2+}$ [69]	Mycobacterium smegmatis: 4		human lung fibroblast MRC-5 cell line: > 200	465 nm blue light activation
[Ru(Ph$_2$phen)$_2$(dpp) PtCl$_2$]$^{2+}$ [70]	-	E. coli JM109: 8	-	visible light activation, binding to chromosomal DNA
[Ru(CO)$_2$Cl$_2$]$_n$ [71]	S. aureus CETC 240, coincident with ATCC 6538 P: 0.033	E. coli CET 516, coincident with ATCC 8739: 0.0066	human dermal fibroblasts hDF: > 3.33	365 nm UV light activation, ROS generation, biofilm inhibition

5.1.1. Mononuclear Polypyridyl Ru (II) Complexes

R-825 (Figure 3) was shown to interfere with the iron acquisition systems in *S. pneumoniae*, which led to a dramatic decrease in intracellular iron, correlated with a bactericidal effect. In addition, R-825 was essentially non-toxic to human A549 non-small-cell lung cancer cells in vitro [41]. Iron is an essential nutrient for the development and survival of bacteria, as well as a key factor in host infection. In order to scavenge iron from their surroundings, bacteria make use of highly effective iron acquisition systems. In *S. pneumoniae*, the ABC transporters PiaABC, PiuABC, and PitABC play a major role in the acquisition of heme, ferrichrome, and ferric irons, respectively [72]. The deletion of the *piuA* gene in a mutant strain of *S. pneumoniae* resulted in a significant decrease in ruthenium uptake, leading to an increased resistance of the mutant to R-825 treatment. These results suggest that the mechanism of uptake for R-825 appears to involve active transport via the PiuABC iron uptake pathway [41]. Note that this mechanism of uptake is different than those used by the currently approved antibiotics. Generally, due to the chemical similarity between iron and ruthenium, the ability of novel antibiotics to interfere with iron acquisition systems in bacteria (including ABC transporters) is considered to be a viable strategy for the discovery of new antibacterial drugs.

A variety of mononuclear heteroleptic polypyridyl ruthenium (II) chelates bearing bpy, phen, dmp (4,4′-dimethyl-2,2′-bipyridine), or hdpa (2,2′-dipyridylamine) and other mono/bidentate ligands were active in various degrees against Gram-positive and Gram-negative bacteria and fungi [73–81]. Although their mechanisms of action have not been determined, all complexes were shown to interact with DNA duplexes and several exerted photoactivated cleavage of plasmid DNA in vitro [75,77,79–81] with singlet oxygen ($^1O_2$) probably playing a significant role in the cleavage mechanism.

Mononuclear Ru(II) Heteroleptic Complexes Bearing 2,2′-Bipyridine (bpy) Ligands

Numerous octahedral heteroleptic Ru(II) complexes containing 2,2′-bipyridine (bpy), with the general formula [Ru(bpy)$_2$L]Y$_n$ (where L = a mono/bidentate ligand, note that when L is monodentate, the first coordination sphere of Ru(II) is saturated with chloride ions; Y = counterion) have been synthesized and tested against bacteria. Generally, these complexes showed moderate to high activity on Gram-positive bacteria, but were inactive against Gram-negative strains. X-03 (Figure 4), for instance, was active against several Gram-positive bacteria, *S. pneumoniae*, *Listeria monocytogenes*, and *S. aureus*, but showed no toxicity at the tested concentrations against Gram-negative microorganisms. X-03 appears to interfere with iron acquisition systems in *S. pneumoniae* cells, in a similar manner to R-825. Proteomic data revealed that X-03 caused the downregulation of several proteins involved in oxidative stress response and fatty acid biosynthesis, suggesting a mechanism of action based on increased susceptibility to oxidative stress and membrane damage. Additionally, X-03 displayed low toxicity even at a concentration 8 times higher than the MIC value to the A549 alveolar and HBE bronchial epithelial cell lines, indicating selective toxicity against bacteria [42].

Complexes with photolabile ligands, in which L is unidentately coordinated, L = 4-(4-chlorobenzoyl)pyridine (clbzpy), Y = PF$_6-$, n = 1 ([Ru(bpy)$_2$Cl(clbzpy)]$^+$, Figure 4), was moderately active against *S. aureus* and *S. epidermidis*. Additionally, the complex was shown to suffer blue light photolysis (453 nm) in aqueous solution and the resulting photoproduct, cis-[Ru(bpy)$_2$(H$_2$O)Cl]$^+$, displayed high binding affinity towards DNA in vitro. The antibacterial activity, however, was not influenced by blue light irradiation, which indicates that the antibacterial activity is not due to DNA damage, but might be the result of bacterial membrane disruption [43]. Blue LED irradiation, however, has been shown to enhance the activity of [Ru(bpy)$_2$(methionine)]$^{2+}$, albeit not drastically, against *S. aureus* and *S. epidermidis* [44]. Methionine release and subsequent exchange with water molecules via photolysis at 453 and 505 nm in aqueous solution lead to cis-[Ru(bpy)$_2$(H$_2$O)$_2$]$^{2+}$, which can bind covalently to double-stranded DNA [44,82] and promote photocleavage [44].

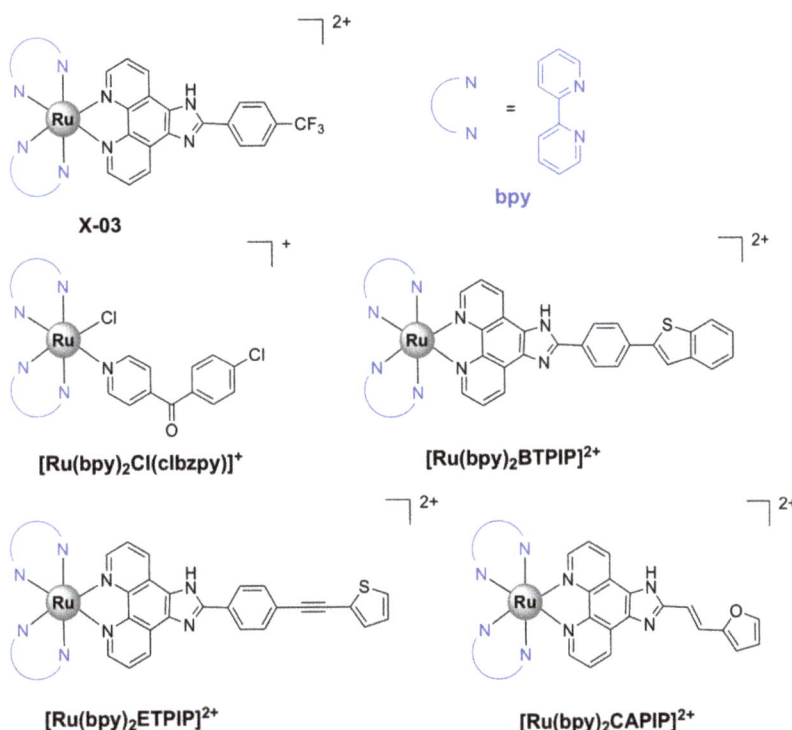

Figure 4. Chemical structures of heteroleptic Ru(II) complexes bearing 2,2′-bipyridine (bpy) ligands. BTPIP = (2-(4-(benzo[b]thiophen-2-yl)phenyl)-1H-imidazo [4,5-f][1,10]phenanthroline); ETPIP = 2-(4-(thiophen-2-ylethynyl)phenyl)-1H-imidazo[4,5-f][1,10]phenanthroline); CAPIP = (E)-2-(2-(furan-2-yl)vinyl)-1H-imidazo[4,5-f][1,10]phenanthroline; dmp = 4,4′-dimethyl-2,2′-bipyridine; bpy = 2,2′-bipyridine; phen = 1,10-phenanthroline.

[Ru(bpy)$_2$L]Y$_n$ complexes, where L = BTPIP, ETPIP, CAPIP, Y = ClO$_4-$, n = 2, [Ru(dmb)$_2$(ETPIP)]$^{2+}$, and [Ru(phen)$_2$(ETPIP)]$^{2+}$ (see Figure 4 for the chemical structures and the IUPAC names of the ligands) displayed good activities against drug-susceptible *S. aureus*. [Ru(bpy)$_2$(BTPIP)]$^{2+}$ was the most active compound of the series (MIC = 0.016 mg/mL) and was shown to inhibit biofilm formation and, thus, prevent bacteria from developing drug resistance. [Ru(bpy)$_2$(BTPIP)]$^{2+}$ [46] and [Ru(phen)$_2$(ETPIP)]$^{2+}$ [45] increased the susceptibility of *S. aureus* to certain aminoglycosidic antibiotics (kanamycin and gentamicin) [Ru(phen)$_2$(ETPIP)]$^{2+}$ was found to suppress the gene regulatory activity of the catabolite control protein A (CcpA) in *S. aureus*, which can explain the synergistic effects observed for this complex and kanamycin [45]. Studies conducted on a murine skin infection model for Ru(bpy)$_2$(BTPIP)]$^{2+}$ showed that Ru(bpy)$_2$(BTPIP)]$^{2+}$ ointments were effective as topical products against skin infection [46]. These complexes, however, have proven to be cytotoxic to A549 cancer cell lines, with IC$_{50}$ values lower than those required for the antibacterial activity [83–86], which might indicate poor selectivity towards bacteria. To the extent of our knowledge, no cytotoxic tests on normal cell lines have been performed.

The corresponding ruthenium(II) bipyridine complex in which L = curcumin and Y = PF$_6-$ (Figure 5) was tested against various ESKAPE pathogens. It displayed bactericidal activity against methicillin and vancomycin-resistant *S. aureus* strains (MIC = 1 µg/mL) and high selectivity towards bacteria as compared with eukaryotic Vero cells (SI > 80). Moreover, the complex strongly inhibited biofilm formation in *S. aureus* cells and displayed in vivo antibacterial activity against *S. aureus* comparable to that of vancomycin in a murine neutropenic thigh infection model. However, [Ru(bpy)$_2$curcumin]$^+$ was not toxic to the Gram-negative *E. coli*, *K. pneumoniae*, *A. baumanii*, and *P. aeruginosa* cells. In comparison, the corresponding Ru(II) complex, [Ru(phen)$_2$curcumin]$^+$, bearing 1,10-phenanthroline (Figure 5), was also active against the Gram-negative *A. baumanii* with a MIC value comparable to that of levofloxacin, in addition to its activity on the Gram-positive *S. aureus* bacteria and lack of toxicity against eukaryotic cells [47].

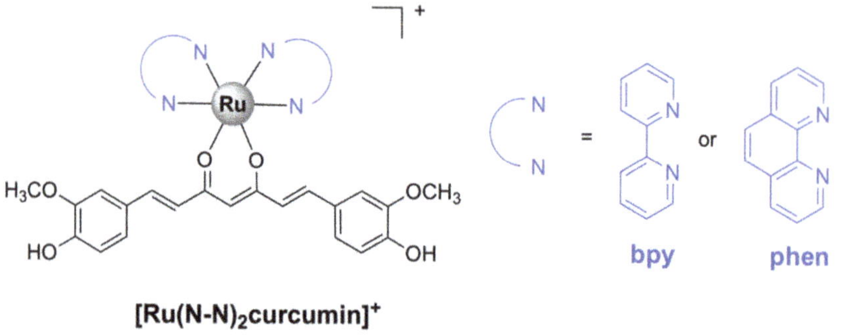

Figure 5. [Ru(N-N)$_2$curcumin]$^+$, where N-N is either 2,2′-bypiridine (bpy) or 1,10-phenanthroline (phen).

Mononuclear Ru(II) Heteroleptic Complexes Bearing 1,10-phenanthroline (phen)

Mononuclear Ru(II) complexes bearing phenanthroline ligands have also been investigated as potential antibacterial agents. Amongst these complexes, mono-bb$_n$ ([Ru(phen)$_2$bb$_n$]$^{2+}$) (Figure 6), where bb$_n$ is bis[4(4′-methyl-2,2′-bipyridyl)]-1,n-alkane and n stands for the number of methylene groups in the alkane chain of bb$_n$ (n = 7 or 10), have been extensively investigated. Although mono-bb$_{10}$ has a larger alkane chain and therefore is more lipophilic, it was less active than mono-bb$_7$ against drug-susceptible *S. aureus* [38,87,88]. The bactericidal activity of mono-bb$_7$ was linked to the extent of cellular accumulation, since its activity on Gram-negative strains is low and the uptake in *Staphylococcus* strains is much higher than in *E. coli* or *P. aeruginosa* [37,38]. Mono-bb$_7$ caused membrane depolarization in *S. aureus* cells and increased membrane permeability, which might suggest the membrane damage as part of its mode of action [88]. Morphological changes indicative of membrane damage have also been reported for a similar complex, [Ru(phen)$_2$(BPIP)]$^{2+}$, where BPIP = 2-(4′-biphenyl)imidazo[4,5-f][1,10]phenanthroline (Figure 6), in Gram-positive (*Micrococcus tetragenus* and *S. aureus*) bacteria [76]. Mono-bb$_7$ displayed selective activity against bacterial over healthy mammalian cells [38,89].

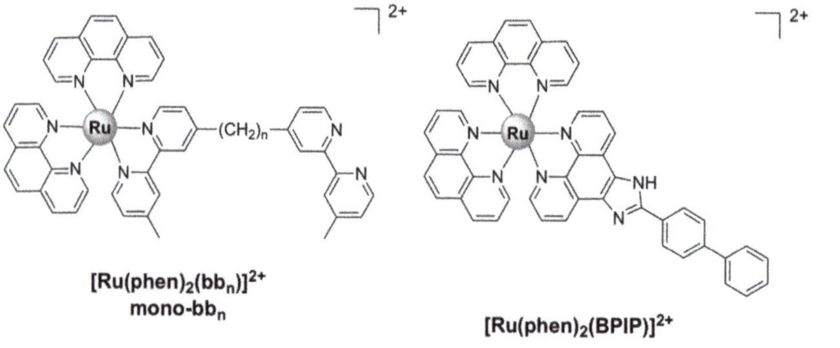

Figure 6. Chemical structures of heteroleptic Ru(II) complexes bearing 1,10-phenanthroline (phen) ligands.

A complex in which the bb_{12} ligand is tetradentately bound to Ru (II), cis-α-[Ru(phen)bb_{12}]$^{2+}$ (Figure 7a, see for comparison the other isomers of the compound, depicted in Figure 7b,c), was found to be more active against the Gram-negative *P. aeruginosa* than the more lipophilic mono-bb_7. The activity was found to be positively correlated with the uptake of the complex into the cells. Nonetheless, cis-α-[Ru(phen)bb_{12}]$^{2+}$ was still considerably more active against Gram-positive bacteria as compared with *P. aeruginosa*, the compound being more active against MRSA than ampicillin and gentamicin. Interestingly, cis-α-[Ru(phen)(bb_{12})]$^{2+}$ was found to be two to four times more active than its geometric isomer, cis-β-[Ru(phen)(bb_{12})]$^{2+}$, against the Gram-negative strains (*E. coli* and *P. aeruginosa*), while no difference in activity was found for the Gram-positive bacteria (*S. aureus* and MRSA). It is unclear why the cis-α isomer is more active, since no significant difference in cellular accumulation was observed for the two isomers. Moreover, both geometric isomers were shown to bind tightly and with similar potency to duplex DNA in vitro, but no correlation between the binding constants and activity was found [48]. It should be noted that DNA/RNA binding is a possible mechanism of action for these complexes, since several reports indicate that various inert Ru(II) polypyridyl complexes bearing phenanthroline ligands target DNA and RNA in bacterial and eukaryotic cells [76,90,91]. Notably, the similar complex cis-α-[Ru(Me$_4$phen)(bb_7)]$^{2+}$ displayed similar activity towards Gram-positive and Gram-negative bacteria as cis-α-[Ru(phen)(bb_{12})]$^{2+}$ and remarkably high DNA binding affinity ($\sim 10^7$) [92].

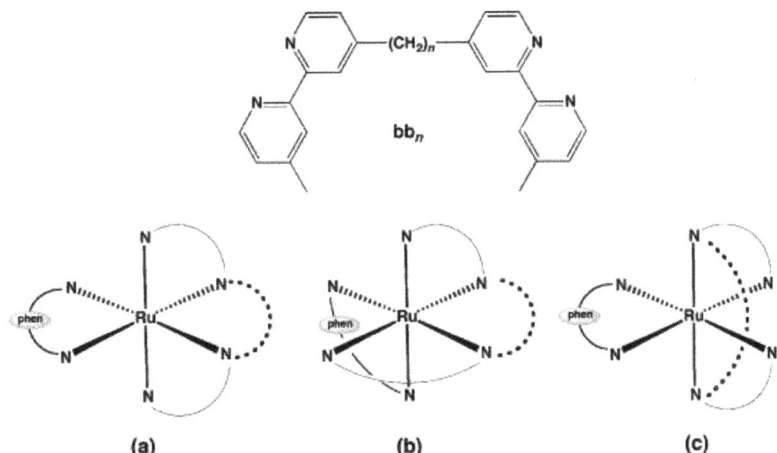

Figure 7. The ligand bb_n and the possible isomeric forms of the mononuclear complex [Ru(phen)(bb_n)]$^{2+}$ with bb_n as a tetradentate ligand: (**a**) cis-α isomer, (**b**) cis-β isomer, and (**c**) a form in which the central polymethylene chain spans the *trans*. Reproduced from [48] with permission. Copyright © 2015 WILEY-VCH Verlag GmbH & Co. KGaA, Weinheim.

Mononuclear Ru (II) Heteroleptic Complexes Bearing Pyridophenazine Ligands

[Ru(phen)$_2$(dppz)]$^{2+}$ (Figure 8), where dppz = dipyrido[3,2-a:2',3'-c]phenazine and phen = 1,10-phenanthroline, displayed good bactericidal activity against *M. smegmatis* (MIC = 2 µg/mL). Its mechanism of action was suggested to be linked to ROS generation and DNA intercalation [93]. A similar complex, [Ru(2,9-Me$_2$phen)$_2$(dppz)]$^{2+}$, was active against MRSA and *B. subtilis*, and displayed time–kill curves that were similar to those of currently used antibiotics, but displayed no activity against *E. coli*. The activity appeared to be correlated with the ability to intercalate into DNA double strands in vitro. In vivo antibacterial activity has been assessed using the nematode *Caenorhabditis elegans* infection model and [Ru(2,9-Me$_2$phen)$_2$(dppz)]$^{2+}$ proved to be non-toxic to the nematodes [40].

[Ru(bb$_7$)(dppz)]$^{2+}$ (Figure 8) (bb$_7$ = bis[4(4′-methyl-2,2′-bipyridyl)]-1,7-alkane) was 2–8 fold more active than its parent compound [Ru(phen)$_2$(dppz)]$^{2+}$ against both Gram-positive (*S. aureus*, MRSA) and Gram-negative bacteria (*E. coli*, *P. aeruginosa*). Although the two complexes have comparable lipophilicity, [Ru(bb$_7$)(dppz)]$^{2+}$ accumulated in *P. aeruginosa* to the same degree as in MRSA and was shown to permeabilize a model membrane system to a higher degree than [Ru(phen)$_2$(dppz)]$^{2+}$. Therefore, its higher cellular uptake might be responsible for the increase in activity. However, Ru(bb$_7$)(dppz)]$^{2+}$ was also ~3-fold more toxic to healthy eukaryotic cells than [Ru(phen)$_2$(dppz)]$^{2+}$, while still being more active against bacterial cells [49].

Complexes bearing tetrapyridophenazine (tpphz) are more lipophilic relative to their dppz analogues and generally more active. For instance, the luminescent, mononuclear ruthenium(II) complex bearing the tpphz ligand, [Ru(Me$_4$phen)$_2$(tpphz)]$^{2+}$ (Figure 8), displayed a comparable activity to that of ampicillin and oxacillin in drug-sensitive strains and the activity was retained in resistant strains. The complex was taken up by both Gram-positive (*E. faecalis*, *S. aureus*) and Gram-negative (*E. coli*, *A. baumannii*, *P. aeruginosa*) bacteria in a glucose-independent manner and was shown to target chromosomal DNA in both Gram-positive and Gram-negative strains. Moreover, model toxicity screens showed that the compound is non-toxic to *Galleria mellonella* larvae at concentrations that are 3–25 times higher than the MIC values [50]. This complex represents the starting point for the kinetically inert dinuclear polypyridylruthenium(II) complex [Ru$_2$(Me$_4$phen)$_2$(tpphz)]$^{4+}$ (see below), which displayed higher antibacterial activity (Table 1), except against *S. aureus*. Unlike the dinuclear derivative, [Ru(Me$_4$phen)$_2$(tpphz)]$^{2+}$ does not cause membrane damage.

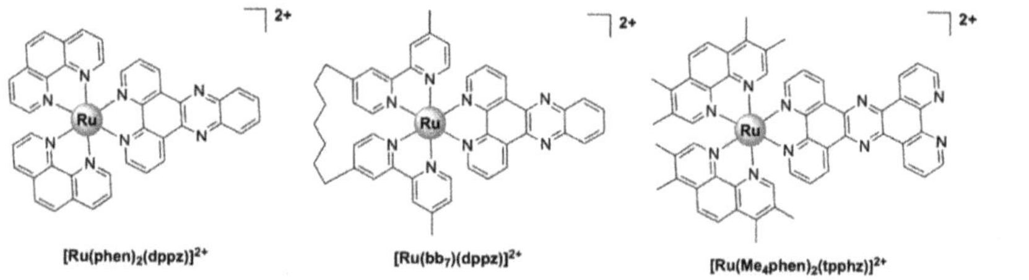

Figure 8. Chemical structures of heteroleptic Ru (II) complexes bearing pyridophenazine ligands.

5.1.2. Mononuclear Ru (II)–arene Complexes

Due to the promising anticancer activities of some representatives, the potential antibacterial properties of piano-stool Ru(II)-η^6–arene complexes, with the general structure shown in Figure 9, have also been considered for antimicrobial applications [94–103]. While some of them displayed modest activity [76,79,80], complexes of the general formulae [Ru(η^6-*p*-cymene)X$_2$(PTA)] (RAPTA-C complexes), where X = Cl, Br, I, NCS (labile) and PTA = 1, 3, 5-triaza-7-phosphaadamantane, were active in different degrees against bacteria (*E. coli*, *B. subtilis*, *P. aeruginosa*) and fungi (*Candida albicans*, *Cladosporium resinae*, and *Trichrophyton mentagrophytes*). The PTA ligand was suggested to play a role in facilitating the uptake of the complex into bacterial cells, while the antimicrobial activity was suggested to be mediated by the interaction of the Ru(II) ion with intracellular proteins. Although the complexes were found to cause DNA damage in vitro, their affinity towards DNA was not correlated with their antibacterial activities. Interestingly, extracts from *E. coli* cells treated with a PTA derivative show specific protein–ruthenium interactions, suggesting that the intracellular proteins are most likely targets of these complexes [94].

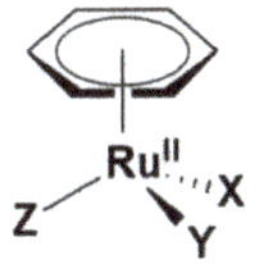

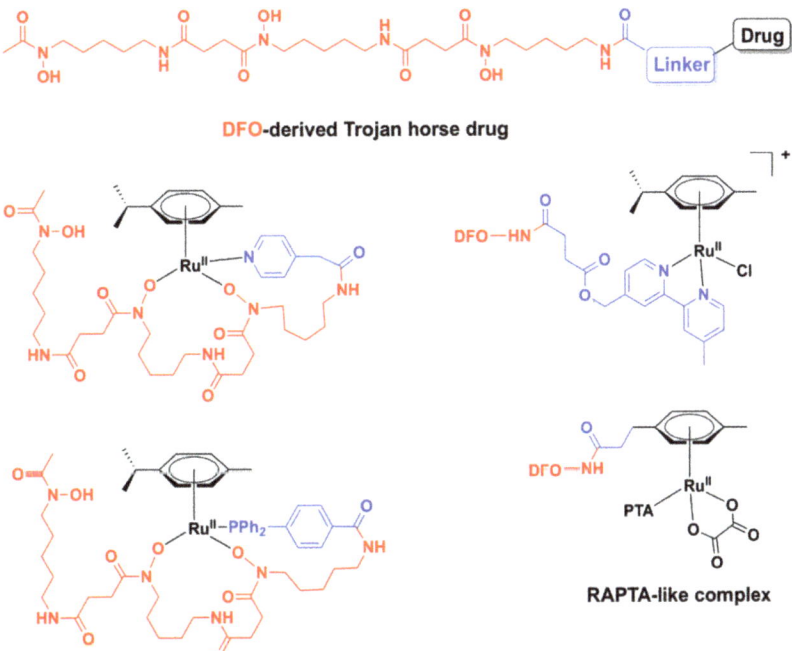

Figure 9. Representative 'piano stool' Ru^{II}-η^6-arene complex, where X, Y, and/or Z is a labile ligand.

Relying on potential interference with the iron-acquisition systems and in order to increase internalization of the complexes in bacteria, a Trojan Horse strategy was applied for three Ru (II)–arene complexes and one RAPTA-like complex bearing derivatives of deferoxamine B (DFO) (Figure 10) [104]. DFO is a commercially available siderophore, namely an iron chelator that is secreted by microorganisms to bind extracellular Fe (III) and aid in its transport across bacterial membranes inside the cells [105]. These compounds displayed only modest activity against three ESKAPE pathogens (*S. aureus*, *K. pneumoniae*, *A. baumannii*) and one fungal strain (*C. albicans*) when Fe (III) ions were present in the medium. Absence of iron in the media led to an increase in activity, particularly for *K. pneumoniae*. All Ru (II) complexes of this series, however, showed little to no activity against *P. aeruginosa*, *E. coli*, and *C. neoformans*, presumably because these bacterial and fungal strains are more susceptible to internalizing DFO. Antiproliferative studies on normal cells (HEK-293) showed that these complexes were essentially non-toxic towards normal eukaryotic cells in the presence of iron [104].

Figure 10. General structure of deferoxamine B (DFO)-derived Trojan Horse antibacterial drugs and some DFO-derived Ruthenium(II)–Arene Complexes [104].

Various Ru(II)–arene complexes with thiosemicarbazone ligands were more active against Gram-positive bacteria than Gram-negative bacteria and/or fungi, but were still less active than the antibiotics used as controls (ampicillin, streptomycin, or ciprofloxacin) [95,98,100,106]. As was seen for other ruthenium complexes, they were shown to bind DNA and human serum albumin with significant affinity in vitro, suggesting that DNA and/or proteins are potential targets of these complexes in bacterial cells. Several complexes were shown to exert low cytotoxicity towards healthy cell lines [95].

Ru(II)-η^6-p-cymene complexes bearing pyrazole derivatives containing *N,S* donor atoms exerted moderate antibacterial activity against Gram-positive strains, including *S. aureus*, *S. epidermidis*, and *E. faecalis*, while displaying very weak to no activity against Gram-negative bacteria (*P. vulgaris*, *P. aeruginosa*). Notably, the complexes were non-toxic against the healthy human fibroblast HFF-1 cells [107]. Other Ru(II)–arene complexes with various *N,N*- or *N,O*- bidendate ligands displayed moderate activity against various Gram-positive bacterial strains and, notably, were found to be more active against *P. aeruginosa* than various clinically used antibiotics used as controls [96,99].

While it is well known that Ru(II)–arene complexes have been widely investigated as potential anticancer agents, their clinical use as antibacterial drugs may be limited by their cytotoxic effects (and generally the poor selectivity for cancerous over healthy cells). Some of these complexes, however, exhibited dual antibacterial and anticancer activities [104]. This constitutes a desirable trait as current anticancer therapy weakens the immune system and often leaves patients susceptible to opportunistic infections. Conversely, patients suffering from a chronic infection are more prone to develop cancer due to certain defects in the immune response [108].

5.1.3. Other Mononuclear Ru Complexes

Various other Ru(II/III) complexes have been reported to possess antibacterial activity. However, microbiological studies for these complexes mainly involved disc diffusion assays or MIC testing, without any further research with regard to their modes of action [109–120]. These complexes were generally more active against Gram-positive strains, with little to no activity against Gram-negative or drug-resistant bacteria. However, a Ru(III) complex, [Ru(L)Cl$_2$]Cl, where L is a N,N,N,N- tetradentate macrocyclic ligand derived from 2,6-diaminopyridine and 3-ethyl-2,4-pentanedione, was moderately active against the Gram-negative bacteria *Xanthomonas campestris* and *P. aeruginosa* and displayed higher activity than the corresponding Pd(II), Pt(II), and Ir(III) complexes [114]. Three ruthenium half-sandwich complexes containing phenyl hydrazone Schiff base ligands also displayed good activity against the Gram-negative *P. aeruginosa*, comparable to that of the positive control, gentamicin, and generally higher than the corresponding Ir(III) and Rh(III) complexes [111].

There are few examples of Ru(II) complexes that display antimycobacterial activity. However, 'SCAR' compounds, consisting of a series of Ru(II) complexes containing phosphine/picolinate/diimine ligands (Figure 11), had low MIC values against multidrug-resistant strains of *M. tuberculosis* [51,121,122]. Moreover, the SCAR complexes exerted synergistic interactions with first-line antibiotics, with the best overall synergistic activity observed with isoniazid [122]. Although these complexes displayed some selectivity towards bacterial over healthy eukaryotic cells, an increase in the toxic effects against bacteria was correlated with higher toxicity against eukaryotic cells. *Cis*-[RuCl$_2$(dppb)(bpy)] (SCAR6), where dppb = 1,4-bis(diphenylphosphino)butane and bpy = 2,2′-bipyridine, the least active compound of the series, was found to be the least stable in aqueous solutions [121]. Upon dissolution in water, the chlorido ligands are released, and the resulting species was shown to bind covalently to DNA and induce DNA damage in a similar manner to cisplatin [51,121]. Moreover, the metabolic products of SCAR6 were responsible for the mutagenic effects of the compound observed in *Salmonella typhimurium*. In contrast, SCAR4 and SCAR5 did not display any mutagenic effect [51].

A biphosphinic ruthenium complex, *cis*-[Ru(dppb)(bqdi)Cl$_2$]$^{2+}$ (Figure 11, RuNN), where dppb = 1,4-bis(diphenylphosphino)butane and bqdi = o-benzoquinonediimine, displayed bacteriostatic and bactericidal activity against Gram-positive bacteria (*S. aureus*, including MRSA, and *S. epidermidis*). Time–kill kinetics studies indicated that RuNN displayed bactericidal activity in the first 1–5 h [52]. Note that this is a much shorter time than that reported for vancomycin or telavancin (24 h) [123]. Additionally, the combination treatment of RuNN and ampicillin (but not tetracycline) resulted in a dramatic increase in activity, highlighting the synergistic effect of the two drugs against *Staphylococcus* spp. For the drug-resistant *S. epidermidis* ATCC 35,984 strain, the MIC value for the RuNN + ampicillin treatment was 1/16 of that of ampicillin alone. Furthermore, RuNN inhibited the formation of *S. aureus* biofilms and reduced the total biomass of mature biofilms by ~50%. The complex displayed no hemolytic activity on erythrocytes [52].

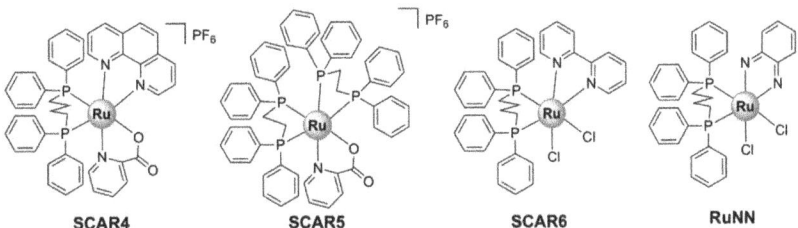

Figure 11. Chemical structures of selected SCAR complexes and RuNN.

Several ruthenium complexes with antibiotics have been reported. The activity of trimethoprim was, unfortunately, significantly decreased upon complexation with Ru(III) [124]. Complexes of the half-sandwich Ru(II)–arene complex [Ru(η^6-*p*-cymene)] with a ciprofloxacin derivative, CipA, exhibited higher activity against *E. coli* and *S. aureus* than CipA. These complexes are labile in aqueous solutions and, therefore, their activity is probably the result of additive or synergistic effects of the [Ru(η^6-*p*-cymene)] complex and CipA [125]. Ru(II) complexes with clotrimazole were active against mycobacteria, but were also found to be significantly toxic to mammalian cells [126]. Three Ru(III) complexes of ofloxacin, namely [Ru(OFL)$_2$(Cl)$_2$]Cl [Ru(OFL)(AA)(H$_2$O)$_2$]Cl$_2$, where OFL = ofloxacin and AA is either glycine or alanine, were active against Gram-negative bacteria (*E. coli* and *K. pneumoniae*), but showed little to no activity on Gram-positive bacteria (*S. epidermidis*, *S. aureus*) [127]. This is unsurprising, given that fluoroquinolones are particularly effective against Gram-negative microorganisms [128].

Homo- and hetero-leptic ruthenium(II) complexes with "click" pyridyl-1,2,3-triazole ligands with various aliphatic and aromatic substituents (generally denoted as Ru-pytri and Ru-tripy, Figure 12) have been reported to possess good antibacterial activity. Generally, the most active complexes displayed high activity against Gram-positive strains, including MRSA (MIC = 1–8 μg/mL), but were less effective against Gram-negative bacteria (MIC = 8–128 μg/mL) [53,54]. The Ru-tripy series was generally more effective against Gram-negative bacteria than the Ru-pytri compounds [54]. Notably, the water-soluble chloride salts of the most active Ru-pytri complexes ([Ru(hexpytri)$_3$]$^{2+}$ and Ru(octpytri)$_3$]$^{2+}$, Figure 12) displayed higher activity than the gentamicin control against two strains of MRSA (MR 4393 and MR 4549). Moreover, the Ru-pytri complexes exhibited only modest cytotoxic effects at concentrations higher than the MIC values on Vero (African green monkey kidney epithelial) and human dermal keratinocyte cell lines [53]. For the Ru-tripy series, the activity appears to be closely linked to the length of the alkyl chain, with hexyl or heptyl substituents on the "click" ligands resulting in the highest activity of the corresponding homo- and hetero- leptic Ru(II) complexes. The MIC values for the most active complex of the Ru-tripy series, [Ru(hexyltripy)(heptyltripy)]Cl$_2$, were 2 μg/mL and 8 μg/mL, respectively, against *S. aureus* and *E. coli*. Despite being generally more active than the Ru-pytri series, the Ru-tripy complexes demonstrated little to no selectivity for prokaryotic vs. eukaryotic cells (IC$_{50}$ = 2–25 μM on eukaryotic cells lines—cancer and skin). With regard to their mechanism of action, transmission electron microscopy (TEM) experiments and propidium iodide assays identified cell wall/cytoplasmic membrane disruption as the main mechanism for the Ru-pytri complexes [53], while [Ru(hexyltripy)(heptyltripy)]Cl$_2$ appears to cause abnormal cellular division [54].

Chitosan Schiff base derivatives conjugated to Ru(III) ions give polymers enhanced water solubility and antibacterial activity against Gram-positive (*B. subtilis* and *S. aureus*) and Gram-negative (*E. coli, K. pneumoniae,* and *P. aeruginosa*) bacteria [79].

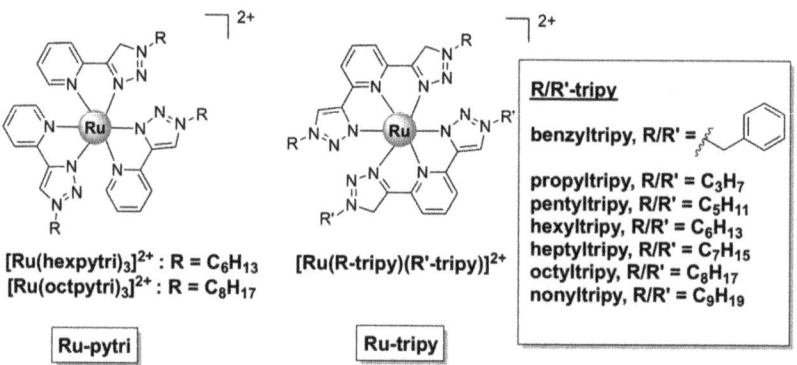

Figure 12. Chemical structures of ruthenium(II) complexes with "click" pyridyl-1,2,3-triazole ligands with various aliphatic and aromatic substituents (generally denoted as Ru-pytri [53] and Ru-tripy [54]). Adapted with permission from [53], Copyright © 2016, American Chemical Society and [54], © 2019 Wiley-VCH Verlag GmbH & Co. KGaA, Weinheim.

5.2. Polynuclear Ruthenium (II) Complexes

5.2.1. Kinetically Inert Dinuclear Polypyridylruthenium (II) Complexes

The ruthenium polynuclear complexes, commonly known as Rubb$_n$, are the most investigated ruthenium-based compounds with regard to their antimicrobial activities. Rubb$_n$ are kinetically inert dinuclear polypyridylruthenium (II) complexes with the general formula [(Ru(phen)$_2$)$_2$(μ-bb$_n$)]$^{4+}$ (Figure 13), where bb$_n$ = bis[4(4'-methyl-2-2'-bipyridyl)]-1, n-alkane. In the dinuclear Rubb$_n$ complexes, two mononuclear mono-bb$_n$ fragments (described above) are bridged by a flexible methylene linker, bb$_n$, where n represents the number of methylene groups in the alkyl chain. Rubb$_n$ are moderately active against Gram-negative bacteria (*E. coli, P. aeruginosa*) and exhibit excellent activity against Gram-positive strains (including MRSA—MIC Rubb$_{12/16}$ = 1 mg/L, while MIC gentamicin = 16 mg/L) [37,38]. The antibacterial activity appears to be closely linked to cellular uptake, which was, in turn, shown to be directly proportional to the length of the alkyl chain and therefore the lipophilicity of the compounds [38]. Of note, a follow-up study comparing the mononuclear [Ru(Me$_4$phen)$_3$]$^{2+}$ (Figure 3) with the dinuclear Rubb$_n$ complexes reported significant differences in the cellular uptake and mode of action. While Rubb$_n$ are taken up by *S. aureus* cells via a passive transport mechanism, the cellular uptake of [Ru(Me$_4$phen)$_3$]$^{2+}$ appears to be protein-mediated (active transport) [88]. In eukaryotic cells, however, Rubb$_n$ complexes are transported via either an active or a passive mechanism depending on the cell type and have been shown to localize to the mitochondria or the RNA-rich nucleolus [56,91,129].

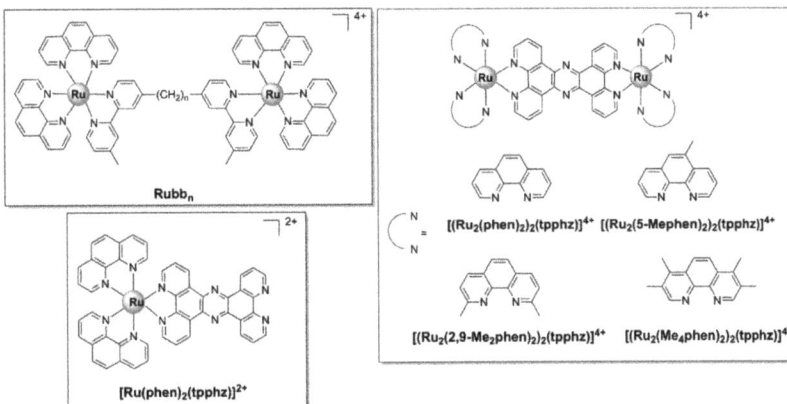

Figure 13. Chemical structures of the inert dinuclear Rubb$_n$ ([Ru$_2$(phen)$_2$(tpphz)]$^{4+}$, [Ru$_2$(5-Mephen)$_2$(tpphz)]$^{4+}$, [Ru$_2$(2,9-Me$_2$phen)$_2$(tpphz)]$^{4+}$, and [Ru$_2$(Me$_4$phen)$_2$(tpphz)]$^{4+}$) and mononuclear ([Ru(phen)$_2$(tpphz)]$^{2+}$) complexes.

The large positive charge (+4) and the hydrophobic alkyl chain are key structural features that contribute to the activity of the Rubb$_n$ complexes, allowing these compounds to pierce the bacterial cell walls and exert antibacterial activity. Based on the knowledge gained so far, two modes of action have been reported for dinuclear Rubb$_n$ complexes: membrane damage and/or interaction with nucleic acids, specifically ribosomal RNA.

Rubb$_n$ complexes were found to depolarize and permeabilize the membranes of *S. aureus* cells, while no membrane permeabilization was observed for [Ru(Me$_4$phen)$_3$]$^{2+}$, although it did cause depolarization [88]. Additionally, Rubb$_{12}$ was shown to embed via a pore-formation mechanism into negatively charged phospholipid multilamellar vesicles, an artificial model generally used to study drug–membrane interactions in vitro [130]. Interestingly, the corresponding Ir(III) complex, Irbb$_{12}$ (with a formal charge of +6), was not taken up by cells and was inactive [60]. Molecular dynamics (MD) simulations showed that the bulky, positively charged Rubb$_{12}$ spanned the bacterial membrane model at the negatively charged glycerol backbone and the bb$_{12}$ linker threaded the hydrophobic core. It is yet to be determined whether the interaction with bacterial membranes results in a change of state (fluidity, charge) of the membrane and if it plays a part in the activity of Rubb$_{12}$. It should be noted that the complex only interacted at the surface level with a neutrally charged eukaryotic membrane model, which could explain its lower toxicity towards healthy cells vs. bacteria (see below) [130]. This does not exclude the possibility of a protein-mediated transport of Rubb$_{12}$ inside eukaryotic cells.

The bactericidal mechanism of these complexes [38] was originally presumed to be linked to their ability to bind DNA [131,132]. Indeed, the dinuclear polypyridyl complex [(phen)$_2$Ru-(µ-tpphz)-Ru(phen)$_2$]$^{4+}$ [133] and Rubb$_7$ [132] were found to localize to *S. aureus* chromosomal DNA. However, despite binding with reasonably high affinity to double-stranded DNA in vitro, Rubb$_n$ complexes prefer non-duplex structures such as bulges and hairpins[132,134,135]. Live cell microscopy experiments on *E. coli* cells showed that Rubb$_{16}$ was found to localize at polysomes, with negligible binding to chromosomal DNA. Polysomes are formed when multiple ribosomes associate along the coding region of mRNA and therefore play an essential role in protein synthesis. The cationic charge of Rubb$_{16}$ is thought to promote its interaction with the highly negatively charged polysomes. Furthermore, Rubb$_{16}$ was found to induce condensation of the polysomes, an effect which is thought to hinder protein production and therefore inhibit bacterial growth [90]. Rubb$_n$ also displayed high affinity towards the serum transport proteins albumin and transferrin in vitro, which suggests that these complexes could potentially target intracellular proteins [88].

As was shown for $Rubb_{16}$, targeting ribosomal RNA (rRNA) in bacteria can be advantageous for the development of selective antibacterial agents, since there are significant differences between prokaryotic and eukaryotic rRNA [136]. Moreover, in vitro experiments and MD simulations have shown that $Rubb_{12}$ only interacts at a surface level with a neutral membrane bilayer mimic of a eukaryotic membrane [130]. Indeed, these inert Ru(II) complexes generally display selectivity for bacteria over normal eukaryotic cells. Although toxic to cancer cells, $Rubb_{12/16}$ were much less active (up to 100-fold) against healthy cell lines [89,90,129]. In spite of the fact that $Rubb_{16}$ is slightly more active against bacteria than $Rubb_{12}$, the higher in vitro toxicity of $Rubb_{16}$ to both healthy eukaryotic cells and red blood cells makes $Rubb_{12}$ a more promising drug candidate [37].

$Rubb_{12}$ injected intramuscularly was not toxic to mice at concentrations up to 64 mg/kg. Moreover, pharmacokinetic experiments have shown that 30 min post-administration, serum concentrations of $Rubb_{12}$ are higher than the MIC values for Gram-positive bacteria and were maintained for more than 3 h [55]. Encapsulation of $Rubb_{12}$ in cucurbit[10]uril ($Rubb_{12} \subset Q[10]$) resulted in a two-fold decrease in toxicity (free $Rubb_{12}$—1 mg/kg, $Rubb_{12} \subset Q[10]$—2 mg/kg) when administered intravenously to mice. Interestingly, while free $Rubb_{12}$ accumulated predominantly in the liver, $Rubb_{12} \subset Q[10]$ was found to be distributed in comparable amounts in both the liver and kidneys. A substantial reduction (~2-fold) in the ruthenium concentrations (quantified using Inductively Coupled Plasma Mass Spectrum, ICP-MS) found in the liver was reflected by an increase (~4-fold) in the kidneys. The significant increase in kidney accumulation is the result of the renal excretion of $Rubb_{12} \subset Q[10]$. The encapsulation in cucurbit[10]uril resulted in higher cellular accumulation, lower toxicity, and faster clearance of $Rubb_{12}$ [137].

As opposed to $Rubb_n$, which bear flexible linkers, systems bridged by a rigid, extended aromatic ligand possess a property that is rather unusual for this class of complexes, that is a generally higher activity against pathogenic Gram-negative as compared with Gram-positive bacteria. The more rigid structure of these complexes is thought to play an essential role in their activity against Gram-negative strains, as well as the presence of potentially ionizable nitrogen sites and the more complex 3D structure when compared with typical drug architectures [57,138]. Thus, a range of luminescent dinuclear Ru(II) complexes bearing tetrapyridophenazine (tpphz) (Figure 13) were found to be more active against Gram-negative (both a wild-type and a multidrug-resistant strain of *E. coli*) than Gram-positive (a vancomycin resistant strain of *E. faecalis*) bacteria. $[(Ru_2(5-Mephen)_2)_2(tpphz)]^{4+}$ was the least active compound of the series, most likely due to its low water solubility. For the other three complexes, a direct, positive relationship was observed between lipophilicity and activity. The lead compound of the series, $[Ru_2(Me_4phen)_2(tpphz)]^{4+}$, was also nontoxic to healthy eukaryotic cells (Table 1). Of note, all complexes showed appreciable activity against the ESKAPE pathogens and $[Ru_2(Me_4phen)_2(tpphz)]^{4+}$ even displayed higher activity than ampicillin against the wild-type strain of *E. coli* and against *E. faecalis*. Selectivity towards the Gram-negative strains has also been observed for the mononuclear parent compound, $[Ru(phen)_2(tpphz)]^{2+}$, even though it was found to be significantly less active than its dinuclear derivatives against all bacterial strains [57].

$[Ru_2(Me_4phen)_2(tpphz)]^{4+}$ was shown to be actively taken up into Gram-negative bacterial cells and to disrupt the bacterial membrane structure before internalization [57], results which were further substantiated by transcriptomic analysis. Thus, the complex caused a significant downregulation of genes involved in membrane transport and the tricarboxylic acid cycle and upregulation of the *spy* gene [58]. The *spy* gene, encoding a periplasmic chaperone, is involved in zinc homeostasis and in maintaining the homeostasis of protein folding under cellular stress [139]. Thus, overexpression of the *spy* gene in the $[Ru_2(Me_4phen)_2(tpphz)]^{4+}$-stressed cells indicates protein damage in the outer membrane. Moreover, multi-drug resistant *E. coli* cells developed resistance to $[Ru_2(Me_4phen)_2(tpphz)]^{4+}$ much slower, and only in low levels, in comparison with various clinically available antibiotics. Encouragingly, $[Ru_2(Me_4phen)_2(tpphz)]^{4+}$ was active at low micromolar concentrations against other Gram-negative ESKAPE pathogens, including *P. aeruginosa* and *A. baumannii* [58].

A similar mode of action involving membrane and DNA damage was reported in the less susceptible, Gram-positive *S. aureus* cells. However, [Ru$_2$(Me$_4$phen)$_2$(tpphz)]$^{4+}$ was found to accumulate to a lower extent in Gram-positive when compared with Gram-negative bacteria, which may account for the lower efficacy of these complexes against the former. This was shown to be related to a resistance mechanism developed by Gram-positive bacteria against cationic species, which involves upregulation of the *mprF* gene. Overexpression of this gene leads to the accumulation of positively charged phospholipids on the outer leaflet of the cytoplasmic membrane, which repel cationic molecules, such as metal complexes. Consequently, it was found that [Ru$_2$(Me$_4$phen)$_2$(tpphz)]$^{4+}$ was more active against a *mprF*-deficient *S. aureus* strain and in mutant *S. aureus* strains missing, or with altered, wall teichoic acids [59].

This class of compounds, particularly [Ru$_2$(Me$_4$phen)$_2$(tpphz)]$^{4+}$, shows remarkable promise for the treatment of infections caused by Gram-negative pathogens. In addition, the lead compound displays good kinetic solubility, which suggests good bioavailability and possible oral administration [58]. Clearly, animal experiments are needed to further assess the efficacy of this class of compounds as novel antibacterial agents in vivo.

5.2.2. Chlorido Dinuclear Polypyridylruthenium (II) Complexes

A range of symmetrical dinuclear polypyridylruthenium(II) complexes with the general formula [(Ru(terpy)Cl)$_2$(μ-bb$_n$)]$^{2+}$ (where terpy = 2,2′:6′,2″-terpyridine) have been reported [55,60]. These labile complexes are commonly denoted as Cl-Rubb$_n$-Cl (Figure 14). These complexes have a positive charge of +2; however, upon dissolution in water followed by the substitution of the chloride ions with solvent molecules, their charge increases to +4 [60]. The Cl-Rubb$_{7/12/16}$-Cl complexes exert bactericidal activity against Gram-positive strains (*S. aureus* and MRSA), *E. coli*, and *P. aeruginosa*, with Cl-Rubb$_{12}$-Cl being the lead compound of the series. Cl-Rubb$_{7/12}$-Cl are more active than their dinuclear inert analogues; however, the Cl-Rubb$_{16}$-Cl complex was significantly less active than Rubb$_{16}$ [60]. It is uncertain why this variation occurs, but a possible reason is speculated to be that the enhanced cellular uptake of the Cl-Rubb$_{7/12}$-Cl complexes can compensate for a reduction in activity. Since Rubb$_{16}$ readily accumulates into cells, the addition of chlorido groups only results in a lower activity.

Asymmetrical chloride-containinig dinuclear polypyridylruthenium(II) complexes, Rubb$_{7/12/16}$-Cl (Figure 14), have also been reported. The Rubb$_n$-Cl complexes contain two ruthenium centers bridged by a flexible methylene linker. One ruthenium center bears a labile chlorido ligand, while the second is kinetically inert. The MIC values calculated for these complexes are comparable with those reported for the previously described Cl-Rubb$_{7/12/16}$-Cl series. Furthermore, with the exception of Rubb$_{16}$-Cl, Rubb$_n$-Cl complexes exert superior antibacterial activities as compared with their inert dinuclear analogues, with Rubb$_{12}$-Cl being the most active against both Gram-positive and Gram-negative strains. Rubb$_{12}$-Cl was found to be 30- to 80-fold more toxic to the bacteria than to eukaryotic cell lines—two healthy cell lines (baby hamster BHK and embryonic HEK-293 kidney) and one cancerous cell line (liver carcinoma HepG2). Interestingly, large differences were found in the cytotoxic activity of Rubb$_7$-Cl as compared with Rubb$_{12/16}$-Cl. It was significantly more active towards the Gram-negative *E. coli* than against the Gram-positive *S. aureus* and MRSA, significantly more toxic to HepG2 (IC$_{50}$ = 3.7 μM), and far less toxic to BHK (IC$_{50}$ = 238 μM) cells than Rubb$_{12/16}$-Cl. Cellular localization studies in HepG2 cells suggest that all complexes of this series were shown to accumulate preferentially in the rRNA-rich nucleolus. In addition, the large differences in the toxicity profile of the Rubb$_n$-Cl complexes might be related to the fact that Rubb$_7$-Cl binds to chromosomal DNA to a greater extent than Rubb$_{12/16}$-Cl [56].

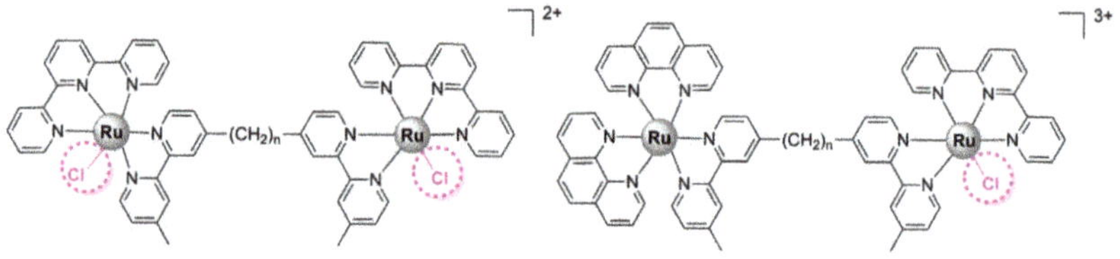

Figure 14. Chemical structures of labile dinuclear Cl-Rubb$_n$-Cl and Rubb$_n$-Cl complexes, where $n = 7, 12, 16$.

5.2.3. Tri-/Tetra-Nuclear Polypyridylruthenium(II) Complexes

Generally, the more lipohilic tri- and tetra- nuclear complexes, Rubb$_{7/10/12/16}$-tri and Rubb$_{7/10/12/16}$-tetra (Figure 15), displayed higher activities against Gram-positive and Gram-negative strains, as well as a range of bacterial clinical isolates, than the dinuclear Rubb$_n$ complexes [37,61]. The linear tetranuclear [Rubb$_n$-tetra]$^{8+}$ complexes were more active, with MIC values < 1 µM against Gram-positive bacteria, than their non-linear trinuclear [Rubb$_n$-tri]$^{6+}$ analogues. Time–kill curve experiments showed that Rubb$_{12}$-tri and Rubb$_{12}$-tetra exert bactericidal activity and kill bacteria within 3–8 h [55].

As opposed to the inert dinuclear Rubb$_n$ complexes, there is no apparent relationship between the antibacterial activities of the Rubb$_n$-tri and Rubb$_n$-tetra complexes and lipophilicity or cellular uptake. The more active tetranuclear [Rubb$_n$-tetra]$^{8+}$ complexes are less lipophilic than their trinuclear [Rubb$_n$-tri]$^{6+}$ analogues, despite the additional non-polar bb$_n$ ligand. This is unsurprising, considering the difference in the overall charge of the tri- and tetra- nuclear complexes. Moreover, even though Rubb$_n$-tri and Rubb$_n$-tetra complexes were more active against Gram-positive bacteria, they were shown to accumulate to a greater extent in Gram-negative bacteria [61]. Within eukaryotic Hep-G2 cells, Rubb$_{12}$-tri and Rubb$_{12}$-tetra have been shown to accumulate preferentially in the RNA-rich nucleolus, as was previously described for the dinuclear Rubb$_n$ complexes [91].

The mechanism of action of the Rubb$_n$-tri and Rubb$_n$-tetra complexes is yet to be determined, but it is thought to be related to their abilities to bind to nucleic acids and/or proteins [1,61]. The Rubb$_n$-tri and Rubb$_n$-tetra complexes have been shown to interact with single-stranded oligonucletides and proteins in vitro, with significantly higher affinities than their dinuclear analogues [87,88,91]. The mechanism underlying their interactions with the DNA backbone may differ for the linear tetranuclear and the three dimensional non-linear trinuclear species [87].

Two inert polypyridylruthenium(II) tetranuclear complexes, containing the bridging ligand bis[4(4'-methyl-2,2'-bipyridyl)]-1,7-heptane, with linear (Rubb$_7$-tetra or Rubb$_7$-TL) and non-linear (Rubb$_7$-TNL) (Figure 15) structures, displayed good antibacterial activity against both Gram-positive (S. aureus, MRSA) and Gram-negative (E. coli, P. aeruginosa) bacteria. The non-linear (branched) species displayed slightly higher activity than the corresponding linear analogue and accumulated in the nucleolus and cytoplasm but not in the mitochondria [62].

Rubb$_n$-tri and Rubb$_n$-tetra complexes were found to be more toxic than Rubb$_n$ to carcinoma and healthy mammalian cell lines in vitro, with IC$_{50}$ values lower than or comparable to that of cisplatin [55,89,91]. However, the tri- and tetra- nuclear complexes were still ~50-fold more toxic to Gram-positive bacteria and 25 times more toxic to the susceptible Gram-negative strains than to eukaryotic cells [55]. Rubb$_7$-TNL was slightly less toxic to healthy eukaryotic BHK cells than its linear analogue (Table 1), yet still more toxic than cisplatin [62]. In comparison, the dinuclear ΔΔ-Rubb$_{12}$ complex was ~100-fold more toxic to Gram-positive bacteria. The cytotoxic effects of the tri- and tetra- nuclear ruthenium complexes towards eukaryotic cells suggest that merely increasing the lipophilicity and charge is likely to result in decreased selectivity. Therefore, the general goal now is the development of new ruthenium complexes that are highly selective towards bacteria.

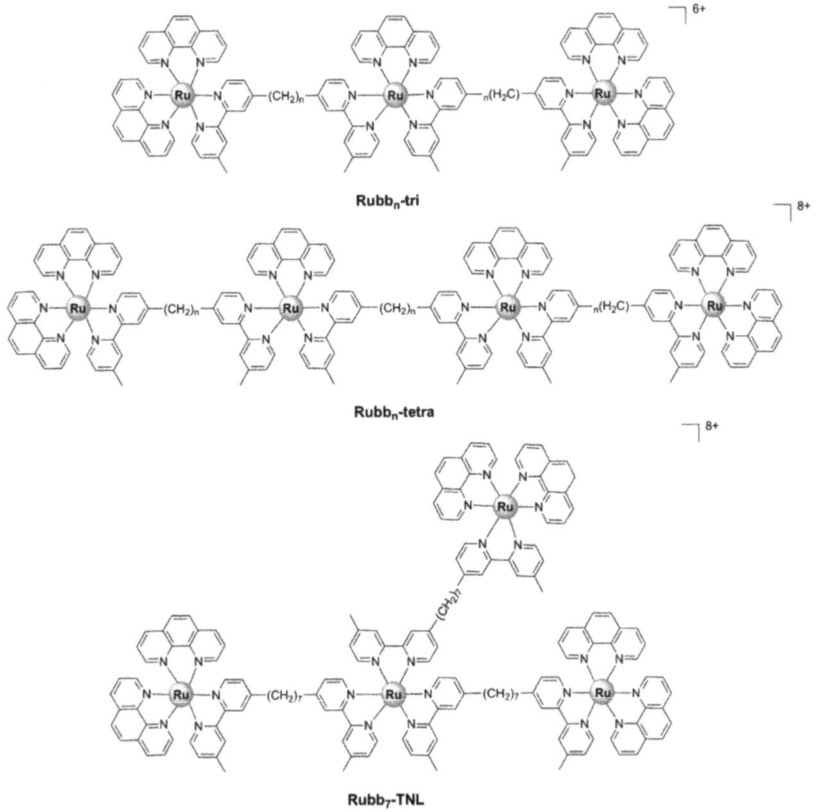

Figure 15. Chemical structures of inert tri- and tetra- nuclear ruthenium complexes, where $n = 7$, 10, 12 or 16.

5.2.4. Other Polynuclear Complexes

The dinuclear $[Ru_2L_3]^{4+}$ ruthenium(II) triply stranded helicate, bearing bidentate "click" pyridyl-1,2,3-triazole ligands, displayed modest antimicrobial activity (MIC > 256 µg/mL) [140] as compared with similar mononuclear Ru(II) complexes bearing "click" ligands [53,54]. However, in contrast to the similarly structured $[Fe_2L_3]^{4+}$ helicates, the more kinetically inert $[Ru_2L_3]^{4+}$ system proved stable over a period of at least 3 days in DMSO solutions [140].

The binuclear ruthenium (III) complexes $[RuX_3L]_2$ (X = Cl, X = Br), $[RuX_3L_{1.5}]_2$ (X = Br), and $[RuX_3L_2]_2$ (X = Br), where L stands for 2-substituted benzimidazole derivatives, were moderately active against Gram-negative bacteria (*E. coli* and *S. typhi*) as tested by the agar diffusion method. The activity on the Gram-positive bacteria *S. aureus* and *Bacillus aureus* was, however, low when compared with the standard antibiotics ampicillin and fluconazole [141].

5.3. *Hetero-bi/tri-Metallic Complexes*

The organometallic complex containing ruthenocene (Compound 1, Figure 16a) was moderately active against MRSA, admittedly less so than the ferrocene derivative (Compound 2, Figure 16a). The organometallic complex containing ferrocene (2) (Figure 16a) was found to generate ROS, in contrast to 1, as indicated by oxidative stress assays. Consequently, the difference in activity was suggested to result from their differing abilities to generate ROS [142].

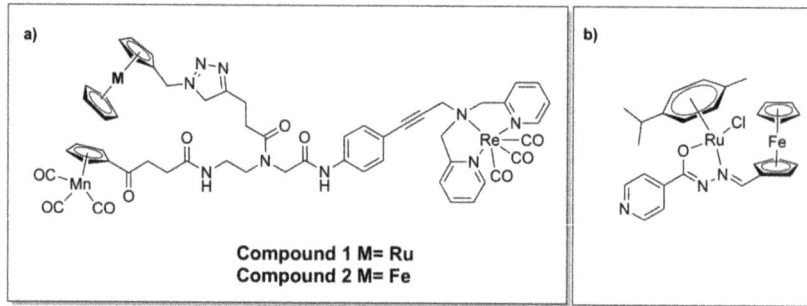

Figure 16. Chemical structures of hetero- (**a**) trimetallic complexes bearing ruthenocene or ferrocene moieties and (**b**) bimetallic complex bearing a ferrocenyl–salicylaldimine moiety.

Incorporation of ferrocene as well as ruthenium in a half-sandwich heterobimetallic complex bearing a ferrocenyl–salicylaldimine moiety (Figure 16b) showed promising activity against *Mycobacterium tuberculosis*. Due to the observed glycerol-dependent antimycobacterial activity, a possible mechanism of action involves disruption of glycerol metabolism and accumulation of toxic intermediate metabolites. The complex was found to possess relatively low cytotoxicity in vitro against normal microbial flora, which also suggests selectivity [143].

A Ru(II)–Pt(II) bimetallic complex, [RuCl(tpy)(dpp)PtCl$_2$](PF$_6$), where dpp = 2,3- bis(2-pyridyl)pyrazine and tpy = 2,2′:6′,2″-terpyridine, was reported to inhibit the growth of *E. coli* cells (albeit at a relatively high concentration of 400 µM). In contrast, its monometallic Ru(II) precursor, [RuCl(tpy)(dpp)](PF$_6$), was inactive against *E. coli*. The improved activity of the Ru(II)/Pt(II) heteronuclear complex was attributed to the *cis*-PtCl$_2$ moiety, although the heterobimetallic complex was still less effective than cisplatin alone [144]. Although [RuCl(tpy)(dpp)PtCl$_2$](PF$_6$) was reported in a follow-up study to induce DNA photocleavage, the effect of light irradiation on its antibacterial activity was not assessed [145].

5.4. Ruthenium-Based Carbon-Monoxide-Releasing Molecules (CORMs)

With a unique mode of action involving ligand exchange, carbon-monoxide-releasing molecules (CORMs) represent an emerging class of biologically active organometallic derivatives. Although their mechanism of action is fairly complex and not yet fully understood (Figure 17), CORMs release carbon monoxide (CO) to bind to intracellular targets, which is partially responsible for their activity. The chemistry and antimicrobial activity of ruthenium-based CORMs have already been reviewed in several excellent works [32,146–149]. The reader can find in the following pages a summary of what has already been reviewed, as well as references to more recent research.

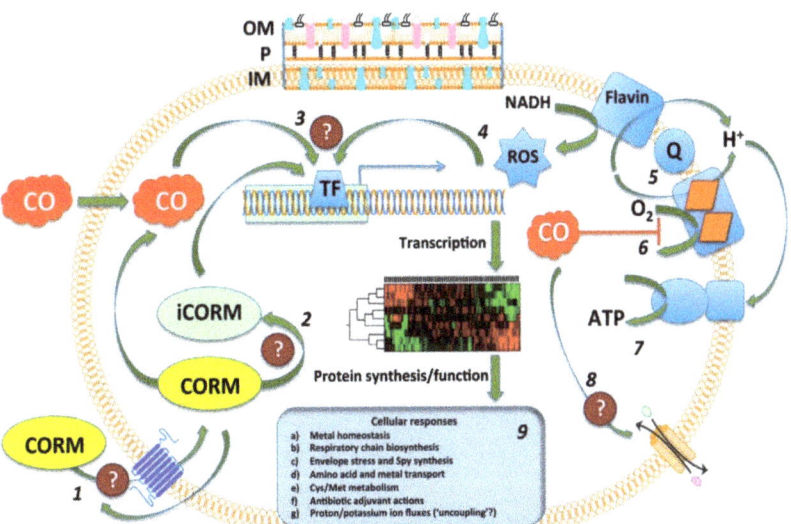

Figure 17. Modes of action and intracellular targets of CORMs. The bacterial membrane includes the inner membrane (IM), the outer membrane (OM), and periplasm (P), which are represented at the top. *1.* CORMs enter bacteria by unknown pathways and mechanisms; CO enters the cells by diffusion. *2.* After they enter the cell, CORMs release CO, forming inactivated CORM (iCORM). *3.* CO, CORM, and iCORM are detected by transcription factors (TFs), causing transcriptional changes. *4.* TFs are activated by ROS that may be generated directly by CORMs or can be generated as a result of the interaction of CORMs with the respiratory chain. *5.* A simplified aerobic respiratory chain of bacteria is represented, consisting of a flavin-containing NADH dehydrogenase, a ubiquinone (Q) pool, and a terminal heme-containing quinol oxidase. *6.* CO binds to the heme-containing quinol oxidase active site, competing with oxygen and impeding respiration. *7.* Impairment of ATP generation by ATP synthase. *8.* CO or CORM may directly or indirectly interact with IM transporters. *9.* Diverse cellular responses to CO and CORM. Question marks represent unknown targets, effects, or mechanisms: transport into (or out of) cells; intracellular mechanisms of CO release from CORMs; interaction with TFs and modification of gene expression by CORMs; effects of CORMs on membrane transporters. Figure reproduced from [146].

CORM-2, a highly lipophilic dinuclear ruthenium(II) complex with the formula $[Ru(CO)_3Cl_2]_2$ (Figure 18), and the water-soluble mononuclear CORM-3, $[Ru(CO)_3Cl(glycinate)]$ (Figure 18), have been intensely investigated over the last two decades. Various reports have shown that CORM 2 and CORM-3 exhibit broad-spectrum antibacterial activity against several strains and clinical isolates of Gram-positive (*S. aureus*, *Lactobacillus lactis*) and Gram-negative (*E. coli*, *H. pylori*, *Campylobacter jejuni*, *P. aeruginosa*, *Salmonella enterica* serovar Typhimurium) bacteria [63,64,66,67,150–153]. Notably, CORM-3 displays bactericidal activity against antibiotic-resistant *P. aeruginosa* [66], *H. pylori* [64], and *E. coli* [67] strains.

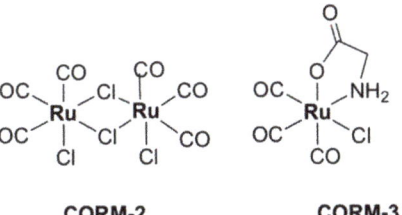

Figure 18. Chemical structures of CORM-2 and CORM-3.

Studies in various buffers indicated that significant ligand exchange is likely to occur in biological media. Both the Cl^- and glycinate ligands of CORM-3 are labile and undergo partial or full displacement by either water molecules or other counter-ions (e.g., phosphate) existing in the buffer or growth medium constituents [154].

5.4.1. Mechanisms of Action

The Role of CO

CO is an inorganic compound that can bind hemoglobin with highly toxic effects. CO is produced endogenously as a result of heme breakdown by heme oxygenase. It is generally known to interact with metalloproteins due to its affinity towards transition metals (for instance, the ferrous ions in hemoglobin). Despite its notorious toxic effects, CO acts as a signaling molecule with important therapeutical properties, which include anti-inflammatory, anti-apoptotic and anti-proliferative effects [146]. The possibility of limiting its intrinsic severe toxicity and enhancing the biological activity has been explored with pro-drugs acting as CO-releasing molecules (CORMs), including transition metal (Mn, Ru, Fe, Mo) carbonyl complexes.

Ru-carbonyl CORMs were initially thought to act merely as vectors designed to deliver the toxic CO gas inside bacterial cells and, hence, the respiratory chain was presumed to be the main target of these molecules. The antibacterial activity of Ru-based CORMs was attributed to their ability to release CO in certain microenvironments of the cell, effecting an increase in the ratio of CO relative to O_2, which eventually impedes the oxygen metabolism [35,142,150]. Indeed, there is substantial evidence in the literature that CORM-2 and CORM-3 impair aerobic respiration in *E. coli* [152,155,156], *P. aeruginosa* [66,157], *H. pylori* [64], *C. jejuni* [150], and *S. enterica* [152]. However, administration of BSA-Ru(II)(CO)$_2$, an adduct formed between BSA and the hydrolytic decomposition products of CORM-3 in vitro, was demonstrated to release CO in a controlled manner in tumor-bearing mice, but did not produce any significant effect on bacterial growth in *E. coli* cells [158]. Additionally, in physiological conditions CORM-3 was found to release low amounts of CO inside bacterial cells (for 100 μM CORM-3, the concentration of CO detected in cells was < 0.1 μM) [159]. Thus, the toxicity of CO alone appears to be insufficient to explain the antibacterial activity of these compounds.

ROS Generation

ROS-induced oxidative stress has also been assessed as a possible mechanism of action responsible for the antimicrobial activity of CORMs. This assumption was based on the positive correlation observed in *E. coli* between the bactericidal activity and the ROS levels generated upon treatment with CORMs [35,160]. In vitro studies performed in aqueous solutions indicated that CORM-2 and CORM-3 are able to generate OH• [160,161] and $O_2^{•-}$ [151,161] radicals. However, the amount of superoxide ions was measured to be only ~1% of the total CORM-3 concentration, which does not account for the bactericidal activity of the compound [151]. In airway smooth muscle cells, CORM-2 stimulated ROS production through inhibition of cytochromes on both NAD(P)H oxidase and the respiratory chain [162,163]. Furthermore, *E. coli* mutant strains in which genes encoding catalases and superoxide dismutases (SODs) have been deleted are more susceptible to CORM-2 treatment due to an increase in intracellular ROS content; this effect is alleviated upon supplementation of the culture medium with antioxidants (reduced glutathione or cysteine) [160]. For CORM-3, however, addition of catalase or SOD did not have any significant impact on its respiratory effects in *E. coli*, implying that peroxide or superoxide are not involved in the activity of CORM-3 in these cells [152,155]. In *C. jejuni*, however, CORM-3 was shown to inhibit respiration and generate hydrogen peroxide, although no effect on cell growth was observed even at concentrations as high as 500 μM [150]. Addition of various sulfur-containing antioxidants, namely cysteine, N-acetyl cysteine (NAC), or glutathione (GSH), abolished the respiratory and growth inhibitory effects of ruthenium–carbonyl CORMs in *E. coli* and *P. aeruginosa* [66,151,157,160,164]. However, this effect is presumed to be independent of the antioxidant activity of CORMs, based on two reports showing that NAC strongly inhibits the uptake of CORMs in *E. coli* cells [155] and a NAC–CORM-2 complex displays no activity against bacterial cells [165]. It is more likely that the Ru(II) species derived from CORMs in biological environments form adducts with exogenous compounds bearing thiol groups, which cannot be readily internalized into bacteria and are therefore less potent antibacterial agents. Non-thiol antioxidants do not alleviate the inhibitory effects of CORMs on respiration [155]. Moreover, CORM-3 was shown to impair the tricarboxylic acid (TCA) cycle, also known as the Krebs cycle, in *E. coli* cells treated under anaerobic conditions, suggesting that its activity extends beyond ROS generation [67]. Hence, it is unlikely that ROS-induced oxidative stress represents the main mechanism behind the CORMs' bactericidal activity, although ROS generation probably plays some part in inhibiting the growth and respiration of CORM-2 on *E. coli* cells.

Membrane Damage

The bactericidal activity of CORM-3 has also been linked to membrane damage in *E. coli* cells, as penetration of propidium iodide [156] and N-phenyl-1-napthylamine [166], fluorescent dyes that cannot pierce healthy membranes, is allowed after CORM-3 treatments. Clearly, loss of membrane integrity can occur in the aftermath of cell death; therefore, it is not necessarily part of the antibacterial mechanism.

The Role of the Ru(II) ion Interactions with Proteins and DNA

In ruthenium-based CORMs, the Ru ion was assumed to have more of a structural role. This paradigm was based on the assumption that ruthenium–carbonyl CORMs were stable enough to reach the intracellular environment, where reducing agents (e.g., sulfites) would trigger CO release [35]. However, more recent research suggests that CORM-2 and CORM-3 undergo ligand exchange and interact with serum proteins in vivo to form protein–Ru(CO)$_2$ adducts. CO release occurs following decomposition of these adducts [158,167–170]. Additionally, no CO release was detected in vitro upon addition of CORM-2 and CORM-3 in phosphate buffers and cell culture media in the absence of sulfur-containing reducing agents [159].

Therefore, CO release cannot be solely responsible for the cytotoxic effects of CORMs, which is further inferred by the fact that CORM-3 is toxic even for heme-deficient cells [166]. Moreover, Ru-carbonyl CORMs are considerably more active than other non-ruthenium-based CORMs [63,102,157] and inhibit aerobic respiration and bacterial growth more potently than CO gas alone [66,156]. Taking into account all of the above-mentioned arguments, it stands to reason that the ruthenium ion plays an essential role in the antimicrobial activity of these metal complexes.

The Ru(II) ion in CORM-3 was found to bind tightly to thiols. Addition of various compounds containing thiol groups in growth media protected both bacterial and mammalian cells against CORM-3. The binding affinities of CORM-3 for the compounds tested vary in the order cysteine ≈ GSH >> histidine > methionine. Moreover, a direct positive correlation was found between the protective effects of these compounds and the dissociation constants of the complexes formed between CORM-3 and the respective thiol compounds. Other amino acids (alanine and aspartate) did not exert significant protective effects. Southam et al. suggest a mechanism in which CORM-3 undergoes ligand displacement reactions in buffers or media to generate complex species in which the Ru(II) centers are readily available to bind to intracellular components such as glutathione. Another mode of action for CORMs is therefore presumed to involve Ru(II) binding to intracellular targets, impairment of glutathione-dependent systems, and disruption of redox homeostasis [159].

Indeed, CORMs have been shown to interact with various intracellular or membrane-bound proteins. CORM-3 has been shown to interact in vitro with the serum proteins myoglobin, hemoglobin, transferrin, and albumin, forming protein–Ru(II)(CO)$_2$ adducts [167,168]. As described above, CORM-3 possesses two labile ancillary ligands (Cl$^-$ and glycinate), which can be readily released in aqueous media, allowing further interaction with serum proteins to occur [168]. With BSA, CORM-3 forms in vitro a [BSA-(Ru(II)(CO)$_2$)$_{16}$] complex, in which the Ru(II)(CO)$_2$ adducts bind to histidine residues exposed on the surface of the protein. As stated above, the CO-releasing protein–Ru(II)(CO)$_2$ complex did not have any significant effect on bacterial growth in *E. coli* cells [158]. The reason is unknown. In addition, CORM-2 has also been shown to inhibit urease activity in *H. pylori* [64] and lactate dehydrogenase in primary rat cardiocytes [171]. *H. pylori* urease is essential to the survival of the bacterium in the acidic gastric milieu [172]; therefore, its inhibition can represent a viable strategy against *H. pylori* infections. The histidine-rich active site involved in coordination of Ni(II) ions is presumed to be the target of CORM-2. It is uncertain whether urease inhibition occurs via direct binding of the Ru(II) ion to the active site accompanied by Ni(II) displacement, or CO binding to the Ni(II) ion in the active site.

Soft and borderline transition metals have been shown to bind to Fe–S clusters, which are important cofactors of various enzymes including several pertaining to the Krebs (or TCA) cycle [173]. CO is also reported to bind to iron–sulfur clusters in a redox-dependent manner [174]. Therefore, Fe–S enzymes have been studied as potential targets for CORMs. Indeed, treatment of *E. coli* cells with CORM-2 resulted in an increase in intracellular iron, suggesting degradation of the Fe–S clusters. This assumption was further supported by the significant inhibition of two Fe–S proteins, aconitase B and glutamate synthase, following exposure of *E. coli* extracts to CORM-2. Although the presence of intracellular Fe–S clusters was shown to correlate with the antimicrobial activity of CORM-2, it was not clearly determined whether the Ru(II) ion of CORM-2 binds directly to Fe–S clusters, or if the degradation of the clusters occurs indirectly as a result of other processes [160]. However, a cell extract from *E. coli* overexpressing aconitase B displayed a 50% decrease in the activity of the enzyme after incubation with CORM-3, relative to untreated cells, suggesting that the protein–CORM-3 complex occurs at a post-translational level. Additionally, recent metabolomics studies in *E. coli* cells revealed that CORM-3 inhibits the activity of several Fe–S proteins, namely the glutamate synthase GOGAT and enzymes of the TCA cycle (aconitase B, isocitrate dehydrogenase, and fumarase). In response to the severe imbalance in the energy and redox homeostasis caused by the Ru-carbonyl complex, activation of the glycolysis pathway was detected in the CORM-3-stressed cells. Notably, other non-CO-releasing Ru(II) species, used as controls, were non-toxic to *E. coli* cells and had no effect on the Fe–S enzymes at the concentration used in this study (120 µM—a growth inhibitory but nonlethal concentration of CORM-3) [67].

Although numerous cytotoxic ruthenium complexes developed as anticancer agents have been shown to interact with DNA, no in vitro or in vivo studies clearly demonstrate whether Ru-based CORMs bind directly to DNA or not. However, CORM-2 has been shown to induce DNA damage and increase the expression of a double-strand break repair gene, *recA*, in *E. coli* [65,160]. DNA damage can be the result of CORM-2-induced generation of intracellular ROS, although this has not been clearly established [65].

Effects on Gene Expression

Transcriptome studies on *E. coli* revealed that CORM treatments under either aerobic or anaerobic conditions trigger complex transcriptional responses of gene expression [151,156,166,175,176] that exceed those induced by CO alone [177]. CORM-2 and CORM-3 downregulate genes involved in aerobic respiration, energy metabolism, and biosynthesis pathways and upregulate those involved in the SOS response and DNA damage and repair mechanisms. A recent gene profiling study analyzed the effects induced by CORM-2 exposure on a multidrug-resistant extended-spectrum beta-lactamase (ESBL)-producing uropathogenic *E. coli* clinical isolate [65]. Numerous genes encoding the NADH dehydrogenase complex were repressed by CORM-2 [65], as was previously shown for CORM-3 in the *E. coli* K12 strain [156]. Transcriptomics analysis of *E. coli* cells treated with CORM-3 indicated altered expression of the cytochrome genes *cyoABCDE* and *cydAB* [151,156]. However, CORM-2 had no effect on the expression of cytochrome genes, which could be attributed to the differences in the growth media [65].

Exposure to CORM-2 and CORM-3 increased the expression of genes coding for proteins with roles in stress response and adaptation, e.g., *ibBA, ibpA,* and *spy* [65,151,156, 166,176]. The *spy* gene appears to be one of the main non-heme targets for CORMs. Several genes coding for multidrug efflux pump proteins were also upregulated by CORM-2 [65] and CORM-3 [166]. Upregulation of multidrug efflux pump systems has been shown to lead to the development of resistant phenotypes over time [178]. However, the growth inhibitory activity of CORM-2 was not diminished by repeated exposure (20 times), neither in the multidrug-resistant ESBL-producing *E. coli* strain, nor in two other antibiotic-susceptible *E. coli* strains [65].

Significant upregulation has also been found for genes involved in metal homeostasis, such as iron or zinc [151,156,166], and genes involved in the uptake and/or metabolism of sulfur compounds (sulphate-thiosulphate, methionine, cysteine, glutathione) and the sulfur starvation response [67,151,166,176]. In agreement with the already-discussed inhibitory effects of CORMs on Fe–S enzymes [67,160], genes involved in Fe–S cluster biosynthesis and repair are also upregulated by CORM-2 and CORM-3 [151,166,176]. Transcriptomic data, therefore, correlate well with the in vitro observation that sulfur species represent intracellular targets of Ru(II)-based CORM [151].

5.4.2. Ruthenium-Based CORM Polymers

Encapsulation of drugs into polymers is a modern therapeutic strategy that makes use of building blocks with 3D structures that enable controlled ligand exchange [179]. Conjugation to lipophilic polymers reduces the access of water molecules to CORMs, causing the solvent-assisted ligand exchange reactions to occur at a slower, sustainable pace. A Ru-based CORM was conjugated to the side chain of polymeric fibers bearing different thiol moieties, yielding the three water-soluble CO-releasing macromolecules CORM-polymers 1–3 (Figure 19). The resulting polymers have been shown to exhibit bactericidal activity against *P. aeruginosa* and to prevent biofilm formation more efficiently than CORM-2, most likely due to their high CO-loading capacity, controlled release of CO, and prolonged half-lives. Notably, the antimicrobial activity was not directly proportional to the half-lives of the complexes, since CORM-polymer 2 was the most active compound of the series, while CORM-polymer 1 had the longest half-life [180].

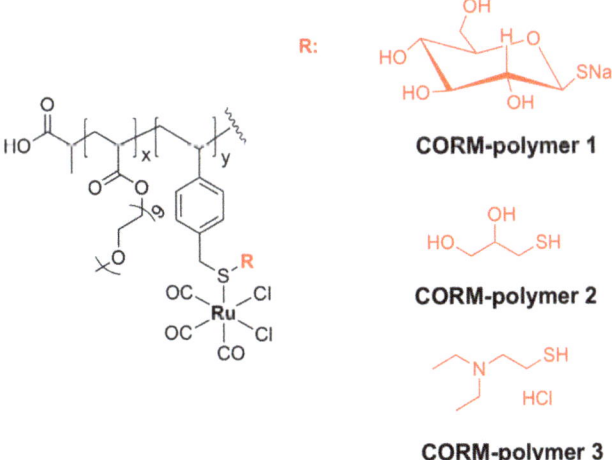

Figure 19. Chemical structures of ruthenium-based CORM-polymers 1–3.

5.4.3. Cellular Uptake

The mechanisms of uptake of CORM-2 and CORM-3 complexes are unknown. It is also unclear which are the Ru-CORM-derived species that pierce the bacterial membranes and it is likely that different species use different mechanisms of uptake. However, ruthenium species (quantified using ICP-MS) have been found to accumulate to high levels in *E. coli* cells treated with either CORM-2 or CORM-3 [155,156]. CORM-3 was found to be rapidly taken up by *E. coli* cells at an initial rate of 85 µM/min over the first 2.5 minutes after treatment, with intracellular Ru levels reaching a plateau after ~40 min [151]. CORM-3 accumulated to higher levels in *S. enterica* serovar Typhimurium than in *E. coli*, and at a faster initial uptake rate (>120 µM/min). This may explain, at least partially, why *Salmonella* strains are more susceptible to CORM-3 than *E. coli* [153]. Notably, simultaneous addition of NAC and CORM-2 or CORM-3 reduced the ruthenium accumulation inside bacterial cells, which is probably why exogenous thiols, such as NAC, are able to interfere with the antibacterial activity of both CORM-2 and CORM-3 [155]. These findings also suggest that the bactericidal effects of these compounds are dependent on the ruthenium uptake by the bacterial cells [151]. It has been suggested that Ru-based CORMs could be transported actively, or diffuse, inside the cells via an unidentified route against the concentration gradient and, due to the reactions that occur inside the cells, uptake can continue passively [153].

5.4.4. Toxicity and Pharmacokinetics

The more lipophilic, DMSO-soluble, CORM-2 is generally more toxic to mammalian cells than the water-soluble CORM-3. It has been suggested that the use of DMSO is at least partially accountable for the increased cytotoxicity [102,171,181]. Toxic concentrations reported for eukaryotic cells are considerably higher than the MIC values [66,102,153,164,169–171,181]. For instance, the bactericidal effects against *P. aeruginosa* occurred at concentrations of CORM-3 that are 50-fold lower than the toxic concentrations for macrophages [66]. However, survival of the mammalian cells was drastically increased by the presence of exogenous thiols in the growth media. For instance, treatment with 25 µM CORM-3 in phosphate-buffered saline (PBS) decreased survival relative to untreated human colon carcinoma RKO cells in PBS by 92%, compared with only 23% in RPMI-1640 growth medium, whilst in DMEM the survival rate was enhanced relative to untreated controls [159].

In vivo studies revealed that a two-week CORM-3 treatment (with increasing doses from 7.5 to 22.5 mg/kg) caused no mortality or any apparent side effects to healthy mice [66]. In contrast, consecutive administrations of 15–37 mg CORM-3/kg in rats caused severe liver and kidney damage after 21 days of treatment. Biodistribution studies in CORM-3-treated mice concluded that the ruthenium species derived from CORM-3 mostly accumulated in the blood for the first hour after the intravenous administration and then were slowly distributed to the kidneys, liver, lungs, and heart. Notably, only trace amounts of ruthenium were found in the brain, suggesting that the complex and its derived species did not cross the blood–brain barrier. Both ruthenium and elevated levels of protein were found in the urine of the CORM-3-treated mice, indicating kidney damage. Moreover, the Ru^{II} center was oxidized to Ru^{III} in vivo by enzymes such as cytochrome P450 [170].

5.4.5. In Vivo Studies Regarding the Antibacterial Activity of CORMs

Several studies have reported the in vivo antibacterial activity of Ru–carbonyl CORMs [66,157,182]. In a murine model of polymicrobial sepsis, treatment with 10 µM CORM-2/kg 12 and 2 h before the inoculation of bacteria resulted in a significant decrease in bacterial counts relative to the vehicle-treated mice. CORM-2 improved the survival rates of heme oxygenase (HO)-1 null mice, mutants that are more susceptible to polymicrobial infection, even when administered intraperitoneally after the onset of sepsis [182]. Administration of CORM-2 (12.8 mg/kg) was also shown to significantly increase the survival rates of BALB/c mice infected with *P. aeruginosa* [157].

Injections of CORM-3 (7.5–22.5 mg/kg) in the murine model of *P. aeruginosa* infection reduced bacterial counts in the spleen and increased the survival rates of the infected mice (from 20% in the vehicle-treated group to 100% in the CORM-3-treated mice). Moreover, treatment with CORM-3 reduced bacterial counts in the spleen of immunosuppressed mice to a similar degree to in immunocompetent mice, suggesting a direct, rather than host-mediated, antibacterial effect of CORM-3 [66].

The modes of action in vivo of these compounds are still unknown and require further assessment. The promising results of these studies, however, pave the way for a more extensive preclinical evaluation of the antibacterial efficacy of Ru-based CORMs.

5.5. Ruthenium Complexes in Antimicrobial Photodynamic Therapy

Photodynamic therapy (PDT) is a therapeutic strategy that makes use of a combination of photosensitive molecules, light, and molecular oxygen. PDT has been investigated against a range of medical conditions, including atherosclerosis, psoriasis, and malignant cancers [183,184]. Antimicrobial photodynamic therapy (aPDT) has been used against a variety of microbial pathogens (bacteria, fungi, and viruses). It relies on the ability of a compound, a photosensitizer, to generate singlet oxygen ($^1O_2$) and other ROS upon light irradiation, causing bacteria inactivation [185].

Ru(II) complexes, particularly Ru(II)–polypyridyl complexes, have been intensively investigated for PDT applications against malignant cancers due to their optical properties, such as the long luminescence lifetimes of the triplet metal-to-ligand charge transfer (MLCT) excited state [184,186]. The remarkable potential of Ru complexes as PDT agents has been confirmed by TLD-1433 [18], which is currently undergoing phase II clinical studies as a photosensitizer for PDT against bladder cancer.

Taking into account the remarkable success of Ru(II)-based PDT agents in the treatment of cancer, several Ru(II) complexes have been considered as potential photosensitizers for aPDT. For instance, $[Ru(dmob)_3]^{2+}$ (Figure 20), where dmob = 4,4'-dimethoxy-2,2'-bipyridine, was more active than the corresponding complexes bearing bpy and phen ligands against *S. aureus*, *P. aeruginosa*, and *C. albicans* strains. The enhanced activity was attributed to the increased lipophilicity of the complex due to the presence of methoxy groups in its structure, which can translate to enhanced uptake by the bacterial cells [68].

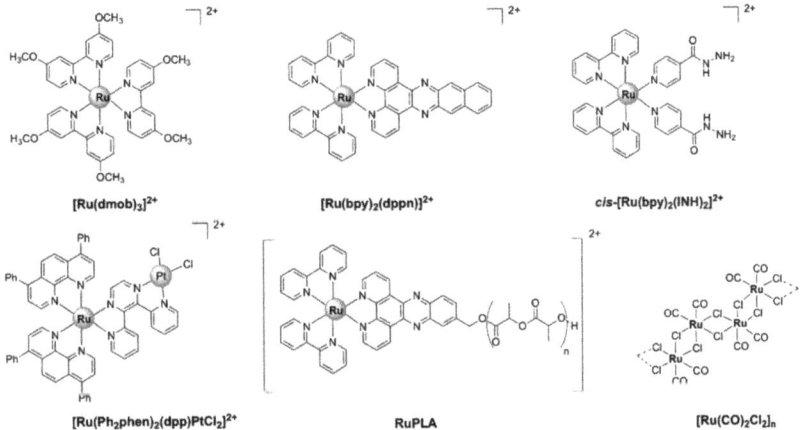

Figure 20. Chemical structures of ruthenium complexes developed for Antimicrobial Photodynamic Therapy.

$[Ru(bpy)_2(dppn)]^{2+}$ (Figure 20), where bpy = 2,2'-bipyridine and dppn = 4,5,9,16-tetraazadibenzo[*a,c*]-napthacene, was shown to cause potent photoinactivation of *E. coli* cells, while dark incubation with the compound had no effect on the viability of the microorganism. Treatment with [Ru(bpy)$_2$(dppn)]$^{2+}$ led to a 70% CFU decrease at 0.1 µM and complete inactivation at 0.5 µM following light activation [187].

The ruthenium(II) complex cis-[Ru(bpy)$_2$(INH)$_2$]$^{2+}$ (Figure 20), where INH = isoniazid, has been shown to undergo stepwise photoactivation in aqueous media after irradiation with 465 nm blue light. The resulting products of this process are two equivalents of the antituberculosis drug isoniazid and cis-[Ru(bpy)$_2$(H$_2$O)$_2$]$^{2+}$. cis-[Ru(bpy)$_2$(INH)$_2$]$^{2+}$ was inactive in the dark; however, upon photoactivation, it was 5.5-fold more efficient against *Mycobacterium smegmatis* in comparison with isoniazid. Notably, cis-[Ru(bpy)$_2$(INH)$_2$]$^{2+}$ displayed high selectivity towards mycobacteria over healthy MRC-5 human lung cells in vitro [69].

A heterobimetallic complex [Ru(Ph$_2$phen)$_2$(dpp)PtCl$_2$]$^{2+}$ (Figure 20), where Ph$_2$phen = 4,7-diphenyl-1,10-phenanthroline and dpp = 2,3-bis(2-pyridyl)pyrazine, has been reported to induce photocytotoxic effects in *E. coli* cells in the presence of oxygen and visible light. The dose required for complete cell growth inhibition under visible light irradiation was 5 µM, as opposed to 20 µM in the dark [70]. In comparison, cisplatin induced complete cell growth inhibition at 5 µM in the dark, but a similar complex, [RuCl(tpy)(dpp)PtCl$_2$]$^+$ (see above), had the same effect at 200 µM [145]. Inside the cells, photoactivated [Ru(Ph$_2$phen)$_2$(dpp)PtCl$_2$]$^{2+}$ was shown to bind to chromosomal DNA [70]. Further experiments are needed to assess the nature of the DNA binding, as well as what species are responsible for the activity.

Incorporation in or conjugation with biocompatible polymers has been used as an efficient strategy to increase the ability of ruthenium complexes to penetrate bacterial cell walls and therefore their antimicrobial activity. A Ru(II)–polypyridyl complex, [Ru(bpy)$_2$-dppz-7-hydroxymethyl][PF$_6$]$_2$ (RuOH), where bpy = 2,2′-bipyridine and dppz = dipyrido[3,2-a:2;2′,3′-c]phenazine, was found to be inactive against Gram-positive and Gram-negative bacteria. This lack of activity was thought to stem from its low uptake by bacterial cells. In order to solve this issue, RuOH was conjugated to the end-chain of a hydrophobic polylactide (PLA) polymer to form ruthenium–polylactide (RuPLA) nanoconjugates (Figure 20). Although RuPLA nanoconjugates displayed superior photophysical properties, including luminescence and enhanced ^{1}O$_2$ generation, they were only moderately active against Gram-positive (*S. aureus*, *S. epidermidis*) bacteria, with MIC values of 25 µM. The RuPLA nanoconjugates remained non-toxic to the Gram-negative (*E. coli* and *P. aeruginosa*) bacterial strains and displayed phototoxicity against human cervical carcinoma cells (IC$_{50}$ = 4.4 µM) [185].

In a recent study, the antibacterial activity of the purely inorganic polymer [Ru(CO)$_2$Cl$_2$]$_n$ (Figure 20), with repeating dicarbonyldichlororuthenium (II) monomers, was studied against *E. coli* and *S. aureus*. Significant inhibitory effects were observed on both strains at concentrations as low as 6.6 ng/mL after irradiation with 365 nm UV light. Interestingly, the polymer displayed stronger photobactericidal activity against the Gram-negative *E. coli* (MIC ~33 ng/mL) than the Gram-positive *S. aureus* (MIC ~166 ng/mL) bacteria. In addition, [Ru(CO)$_2$Cl$_2$]$_n$ remained non-toxic to human dermal fibroblasts and red blood cells at concentrations much higher than the MIC values. Although the complex was considerably toxic to both bacterial strains in the dark, the antibacterial activity of [Ru(CO)$_2$Cl$_2$]$_n$ was significantly increased upon photoirradiation, which can be attributed to the enhanced generation of ROS under UV light. SEM analysis revealed that its mode of action might involve disruption of bacterial membranes. Moreover, [Ru(CO)$_2$Cl$_2$]$_n$ was able to cause morphological changes to biofilm structures and to disassemble the biofilm matrix [71]. It should be noted that although the structure of [Ru(CO)$_2$Cl$_2$]$_n$ is similar to that of CORMs, there is no information available in the literature on the ability of the polymer to release CO or undergo ligand exchange in aqueous media.

The antibacterial photosensitizing activity towards a panel of bacterial strains has been assessed for seventeen homo- or heteroleptic polypyridyl Ru(II) complexes with the following formulae: [Ru(Phen)$_3$](PF$_6$)$_2$, [Ru(Phen)$_2$(Phen-X)](PF$_6$)$_2$, [Ru(Phen)(Phen-X)$_2$](PF$_6$)$_2$, [Ru(Phen-X)$_3$](PF$_6$)$_2$, [Ru(Phen-X)$_2$Cl$_2$], or [Ru(Phen)$_2$Cl$_2$] (Figure 21), varying due to the number and the nature of the substituents. With regard to the most active complexes, **2**, **5**, and **6** stood out, **5** was highly efficient against MRSA N315 even without light irradiation, and **2** demonstrated activity against four *S. aureus* strains, one *E. coli* strain, and three *P. aeruginosa* strains. However, **2** and **5** were more toxic towards eukaryotic cells upon light irradiation, with **6** being non-toxic. The counterion (PF_6^- vs. Cl^-) did not appear to have a significant effect on the antibacterial activity. In contrast, a dicationic charge was vital to the activity, taking into account that the two neutral Ru(II) complexes, **16** and **17**, were inactive. Surprisingly, the best photosensitizers for $^1O_2$ production (**8**, **9**, **10**, **15**) did not correspond to the most efficient aPDT agents (**2**, **5**, **6**). The ability of the complexes to interact efficiently with bacteria seems to be crucial for aPDT activity, considering the short half-life of ROS generated upon light irradiation. Thus, solely increasing $^1O_2$ production is not sufficient to yield more efficient aPDT agents. Parameters impacting the interactions with bacteria, such as lipophilicity and ability to form aggregates, should also be considered in the development of optimized future compounds for aPDT [184].

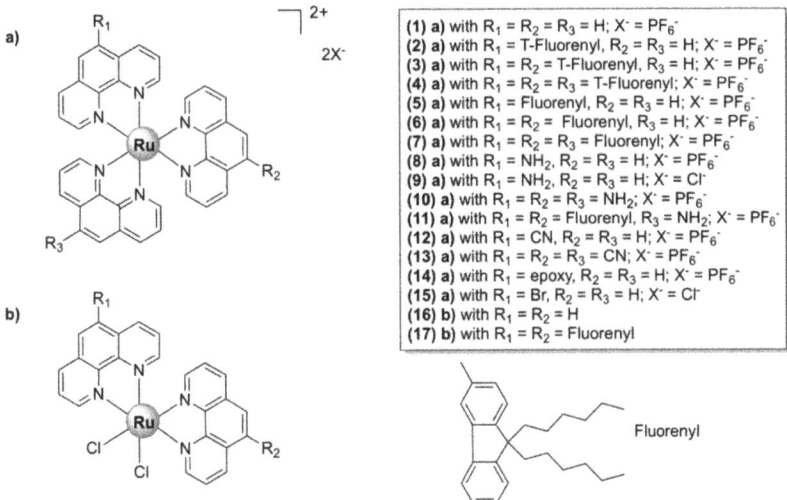

Figure 21. Chemical structures of the homo- or heteroleptic polypyridyl Ru(II) complexes (**1**)–(**17**) with the general formulae [Ru(Phen)$_3$](PF$_6$)$_2$, [Ru(Phen)$_2$(Phen-X)](PF$_6$)$_2$, [Ru(Phen)(Phen-X)$_2$](PF$_6$)$_2$, [Ru(Phen-X)$_3$](PF$_6$)$_2$, [Ru(Phen-X)$_2$Cl$_2$], or [Ru(Phen)$_2$Cl$_2$]. The core structures of the complexes (**1**)–(**17**) correspond to either (**a**) or (**b**), as denoted in the top right corner of the figure. The fluorene unit was bonded to the 1,10-phenanthroline moiety ligand either directly (Fluorenyl, bottom right corner) or via a triple bond (T-Fluorenyl).

6. Antiparasitic Activity of Ruthenium Complexes

Parasitic infections, including malaria (*Plasmodium* sp.), Chagas' disease (*Trypanosoma cruzi*), African trypanosomiasis (*Trypanosoma brucei*), and leishmaniasis (*Leishmania* sp.), mainly affect the tropical and subtropical regions of Africa and Asia and only a narrow spectrum of effective drugs is available for treatment. In this context, several ruthenium complexes have been reported as efficient antiparasitic agents active against malaria, leishmaniasis, trypanosomiasis, and Chagas' disease [188]. Generally, the enhanced antiplasmodial activity of these complexes when compared to the free ligands is thought to be related to their increased lipophilicity, which translates to increased uptake into the parasite's cells and/or increased ability to evade the parasite's drug efflux pumps.

6.1. Antiplasmodial Activity

Malaria is a highly infectious parasitic disease, with over 40% of the world's population living in an endemic region. Malaria parasites belong to the genus *Plasmodium*, the most virulent strain being *P. falciparum* [189,190]. Conventional treatment strategies use either quinoline-based drugs, such as chloroquine (CQ)) and its derivatives, or fixed-dose combination therapies containing a derivative of the Chinese natural product artemisinin. The increasing widespread resistance to these compounds requires urgent attention to the development of new therapeutic strategies [190,191].

An organometallic complex, [RuCl$_2$(CQ)]$_2$ (Figure 22a), where CQ = chloroquine, displayed 2–5-fold increased activity against *P. falciparum* compared with chloroquine diphosphate in vitro [192]. Moreover, the complex was significantly more active when compared with its organic derivative in mice infected with *Plasmodium berghei*, with no apparent signs of acute toxicity up to 30 days after treatment [193]. [RuCl$_2$(CQ)]$_2$ was shown to bind to hematin and inhibit aggregation of β-hematin (synthetic hemozoin—a target of the malaria parasite) in vitro, albeit to a slightly lower extent than chloroquine diphosphate. However, the heme aggregation inhibitory activity of the complex is significantly higher than that displayed by chloroquine, suggesting that the main target of the complex is the heme aggregation process. [RuCl$_2$(CQ)]$_2$ was shown to be significantly more lipophilic than chloroquine diphosphate, suggesting that the addition of Ru(II) induced drastic changes in the pharmacokinetic profile of the organometallic compound. One chlorido ligand from each of the two Ru(II) centers is displaced by water molecules upon addition to aqueous solutions. The resulting species, [RuCl(OH$_2$)$_3$(CQ)]$_2$[Cl]$_2$, is considered to be the active species in vitro and in vivo. The enhanced activity of the complex against CQ-resistant strains of *P. falciparum* was suggested to relate to its lipophilicity. This can be explained by the fact that the parasite efflux pump, usually involved in the resistance mechanism to chloroquine, has a lower ability to bind to highly lipophilic drugs [192].

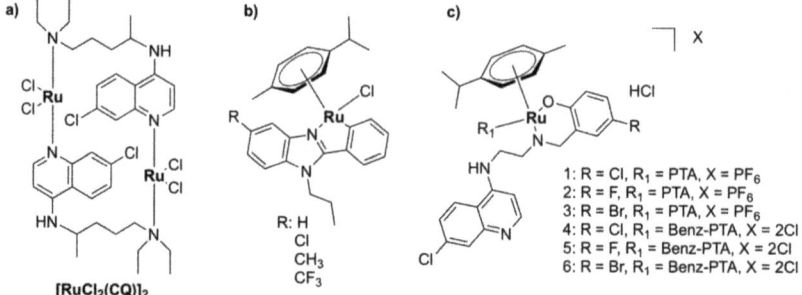

Figure 22. Chemical structures of ruthenium complexes with antiplasmodial activity. (a) [RuCl$_2$(CQ)]$_2$, (b) cyclometallated Ru(II) complexes of 2-phenylbenzimidazoles, and (c) PTA-derived ruthenium(II) quinoline complexes.

CQ has also been used as a chelating ligand in a series of organoruthenium complexes with the general formula [RuCQ(η^6-C$_{10}$H$_{14}$)(N–H)]$^{2+}$, where η^6-C$_{10}$H$_{14}$ is α-phellandrene and N–H is either 2′-bipyridine (BCQ), 5,5′-dimethyl-2,2′-bipyridine (MCQ), 1,10-phenanthroline (FCQ), or 4,7-diphenyl-1,10-phenanthroline (FFCQ). As was previously shown for [RuCl$_2$(CQ)]$_2$, the Ru–CQ bonds are stable, and CQ is not released upon aquation. The organoruthenium complexes displayed intraerythrocytic activity against CQ-sensitive and -resistant strains of *P. falciparum*. Unlike CQ, the complexes exerted moderate activity against the liver stage and potent activity against the sexual stage of the parasite, suggesting that they operate via a different mechanism than that of CQ. It has been shown that [RuCQ(η^6-C$_{10}$H$_{14}$)(N–H)]$^{2+}$ induces oxidative stress in the parasite, which might be linked to their mode of action. In addition, the organoruthenium complexes displayed low mammalian cytotoxicity and inhibited parasitemia in mice infected with *P. berghei* [194].

A range of Ru(II)–arene complexes were developed in the knowledge that increasing the lipophilic properties of a drug is likely to increase passive diffusion through membranes and hence the antiplasmodial activity. For instance, a series of half-sandwich Ru(II) complexes with aryl-functionalized organosilane thiosemicarbazone ligands were more active against *P. falciparum* at low micromolar concentrations (2.29–6.66 μM) and less cytotoxic to the Chinese Hamster Ovarian (CHO) cell line in comparison with the corresponding free ligands. It should be stated that the activity of the complexes was still much lower than that of both CQ and artesunate, which were used as controls. However, the complexes also displayed much lower resistance index values relative to the control drugs, which suggests that the parasites are less likely to develop cross-resistance to the metal complexes [195].

An enhancement of the antiplasmodial activity has also been observed for cyclometallated Ru(II) complexes of 2-phenylbenzimidazoles (Figure 22b), when compared with the free ligands. These complexes were found to be active against CQ-sensitive and multidrug-resistant *P. falciparum* strains, with IC_{50} values in the low to submicromolar range (0.12–3.02 μM). The nature of the substituent on the η^6-*p*-cymene moiety does not seem to influence the activity to a great extent. Although CQ was still more active than the cyclometallated complexes against both strains, the latter displayed lower resistance index values relative to CQ. In addition, the metal complexes displayed relatively low cytotoxicity against the mammalian CHO cells. Notably, the Ru(II) complexes were found to be more active than the Ir(III) analogues on the resistant strain [196], which was also reported for other Ru(II)–arene complexes [197]. PTA-derived ruthenium(II) quinoline complexes (Figure 22c) were, however, generally less effective against CQ-sensitive and resistant strains of *P. falciparum* than their Ir(III) correspondents, but were also much less toxic to the CHO cells. In addition, these RAPTA-like complexes inhibited β-hematin formation, suggesting that their mechanism of action is similar to that of CQ [198].

Di- and tri- nuclear Ru(II)-η^6-*p*-cymene complexes (Figure 23a), in which the ruthenium centers are bridged by pyridyl aromatic ether ligands, were evaluated against CQ-sensitive and -resistant *P. falciparum* strains. While the dinuclear derivative displayed only moderate activity, the trinuclear complex proved to be highly active in both strains, displaying activities in the nanomolar range (IC_{50} = 240 nM and 670 nM for the CQ-sensitive and -resistant *P. falciparum* strains, respectively). The trinuclear complex was also able to inhibit more efficiently β-hematin formation in vitro, in comparison with the dinuclear derivative, which suggests that hemozoin might be a target of the complexes in vivo. Notably, the trinuclear Ru(II) complex was only slightly more toxic than the corresponding tripyridyl ether ligand, indicating that it was the incorporation of a triazine moiety that had a more significant impact on activity [197]. This was confirmed by the fact that trinuclear Ru(II)-η^6-*p*-cymene complexes, in which the ruthenium centers are bridged by pyridyl aromatic ester ligands lacking the triazine moiety (Figure 23b), are much less efficient antiparasitic agents [199].

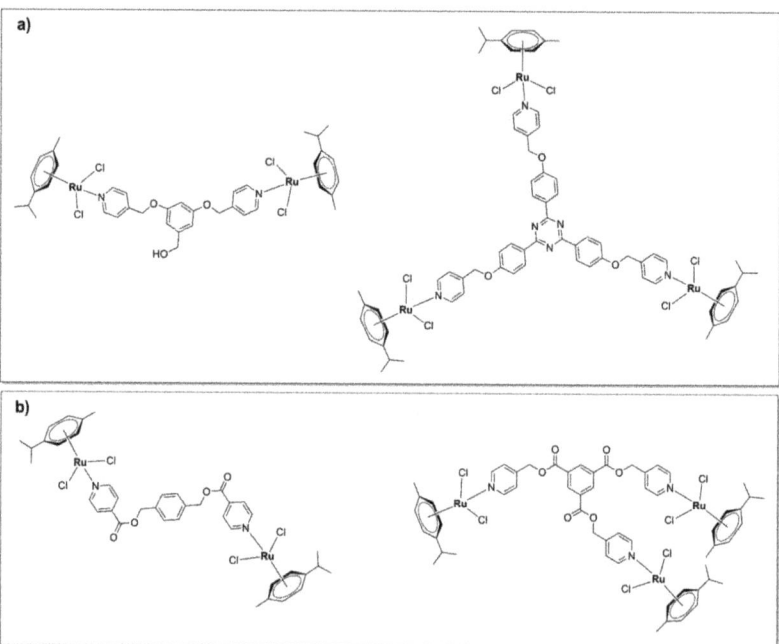

Figure 23. Di- and tri- nuclear Ru(II)-η^6-p-cymene complexes in which the ruthenium centers are bridged by (**a**) pyridyl aromatic ether ligands and (**b**) pyridyl aromatic ester ligands.

Using 'old' drugs to assist in the search for new agents that are more efficient for either common or rare diseases is the scope of a relatively new therapeutic strategy called drug repositioning/repurposing. For instance, a series of ferrocenyl and ruthenocenyl derivatives incorporating tamoxifen-based compounds were tested against CQ-resistant *P. falciparum* blood forms. Tamoxifen (Figure 24) is an anticancer agent used in current treatment plans to prevent and treat breast cancer. The results within this series indicated that the ruthenocenyl-containing complexes (Figure 24) were more active than their ferrocenyl analogues, but still only displayed moderate activity (IC$_{50}$ = 4.7–16.5 mM) against *P. falciparum*. The ruthenocenyl complexes were considered nontoxic to HepG2 cells [200].

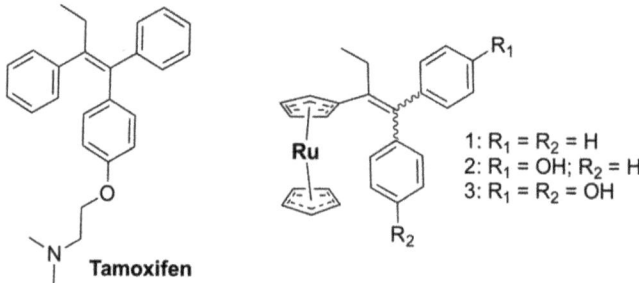

Figure 24. Chemical structures of tamoxifen and the ruthenocenyl complexes incorporating tamoxifen-based ligands.

6.2. Antitrypanosomal Activity

Chagas' disease (American trypanosomiasis) affects millions of people worldwide, mainly in Central and South America, where the disease is endemic. It is a life-threatening disease caused by the parasite *Trypanosoma cruzi*. No vaccines are currently available, and treatment options are limited to only two drugs, benznidazole and nirfurtimox [201]. Sleeping sickness (African trypanosomiasis) predominantly affects people living in sub-Saharan Africa and is transmitted by the bite of the tsetse fly. The disease is caused by the insect-borne *T. brucei* parasite [202].

Two Ru(II)–NO donor compounds, namely *trans*-[Ru(NO)(NH$_3$)$_4$(isn)](BF$_4$)$_3$ (Figure 25) where isn = isonicotinamide and *trans*-[Ru(NO)(NH$_3$)$_4$(imN)](BF$_4$)$_3$ (Figure 25) where imN = imidazole, displayed significant activity against *T. cruzi* both in vitro and in vivo. NO release upon reduction of the ruthenium nitrosyls in culture cells and animal models is thought to play an essential role in the antiproliferative and trypanocidal activities. Notably, *trans*-[Ru(NO)(NH$_3$)$_4$(imN)](BF$_4$)$_3$ allowed for survival of up to 80% of infected mice at a much lower dose (100 nmol/kg/day) than that required for benznidazole (385 µmol/kg/day) [203,204]. Ru(II) complexes with the formulae *cis*-[Ru(NO)(bpy)$_2$(imN)](PF$_6$)$_3$ and *cis*-[Ru(NO)(bpy)$_2$SO$_3$]PF$_6$ displayed inhibitory effects on the *T. cruzi* glyceraldehyde 3-phosphate dehydrogenase (GAPDH) (IC$_{50}$ = 89 and 153 µM, respectively), which is a potential molecular target. These compounds exhibited in vitro and in vivo trypanocidal activities at doses up to 1000-fold lower than the clinical dose for benznidazole [205]. Furthermore, in a series of nitro/nitrosyl-Ru(II) complexes, *cis*, *trans*-[RuCl(NO)(dppb)(5,5'-mebipy)](PF$_6$)$_2$, where 5,5'-mebipy = 5,5'-dimethyl-2,2'-bipyridine and dppb = 1,4-*bis*(diphenylphosphino)butane, was the most active compound. The complex displayed an IC$_{50}$ of 2.1 µM against trypomastigotes (the form of the parasite during the acute stage of the disease) and an IC$_{50}$ of 1.3 µM against amastigotes (the form of the parasite during the chronic stage of the disease), while it was less toxic to macrophages. Moreover, the complex exerted synergistic activity with benznidazole in vitro against trypomastigotes and in vivo in infected mice [206].

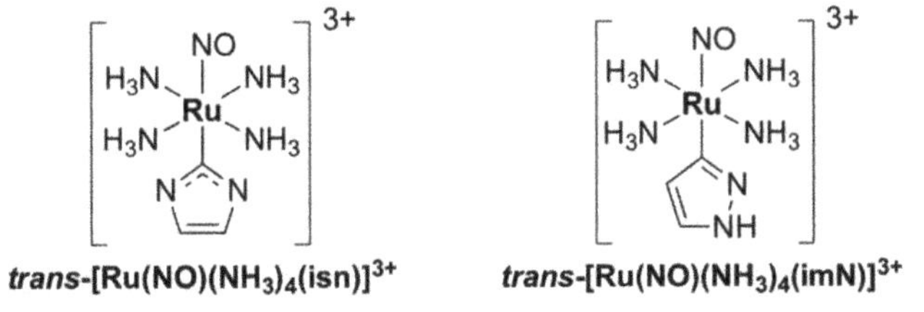

Figure 25. Chemical structures of the ruthenium NO-donor complexes *trans*-[Ru(NO)(NH$_3$)$_4$(isn)]$^{3+}$ and *trans*-[Ru(NO)(NH$_3$)$_4$(imN)]$^{3+}$.

A series of symmetric trinuclear ruthenium complexes bearing azanaphthalene ligands with the general formula [Ru$_3$O(CH$_3$COO)$_6$(L)$_3$]PF$_6$ (Figure 26), where L = (1) quinazoline (qui), (2) 5-nitroisoquinoline (5-nitroiq), (3) 5-bromoisoquinoline (5-briq), (4) isoquinoline (iq), (5) 5-aminoisoquinoline (5-amiq), and (6) 5,6,7,8-tetrahydroisoquinoline (thiq), were developed. All complexes presented in vitro trypanocidal activity, complex 6 being the lead compound of the series, with IC$_{50}$ values of 1.39 µM against trypomastigotes and 1.06 µM against amastigotes. Complex 6 was up to 10 times more effective than benznidazole, while being essentially non-toxic to healthy mammalian cells (SI trypomastigote: 160, SI amastigote: 209) [207].

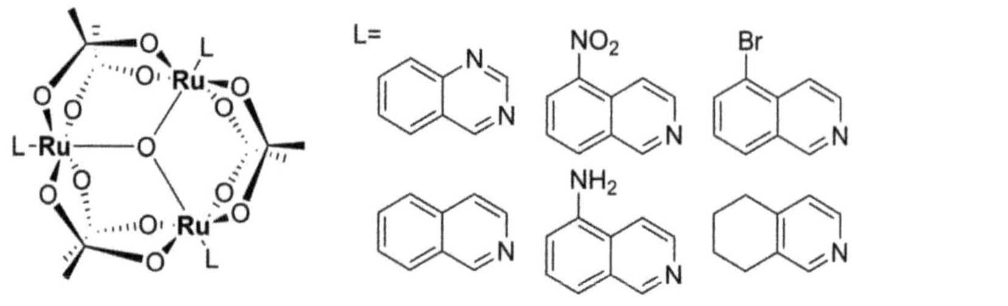

Figure 26. Chemical structures of symmetric trinuclear ruthenium complexes bearing azanaphthalene ligands with the general formula [Ru$_3$O(CH$_3$COO)$_6$(L)$_3$]PF$_6$.

A range of Ru (II)–cyclopentadienyl thiosemicarbazone complexes displayed sub- or micromolar IC$_{50}$ values against *T. cruzi* and *T. brucei*. Notably, [RuCp(PPh$_3$)L] (Figure 27), where HL is the *N*-methyl derivative of 5-nitrofuryl containing thiosemicarbazone and Cp is cyclopentadienyl, exhibited high (IC$_{50}$ *T. cruzi* = 0.41 µM; IC$_{50}$ *T. brucei* = 3.5 µM) and selective activity (SI *T. cruzi* > 49 and SI *T. brucei* SI > 6). These complexes had the ability to interact with DNA in vitro, but no correlation with the biological activity was observed [208]. A Ru(II)–cyclopentadienyl clotrimazole complex, [RuCp(PPh$_3$)$_2$(CTZ)](CF$_3$SO$_3$) (Figure 27), where Cp = cyclopentadienyl and CTZ = clotrimazole, was more cytotoxic on *T. cruzi* than nifurtimox. With regard to its mechanism of action, the complex was shown to impair the sterol biosynthetic pathway in *T. cruzi* [209]. In another series of Ru(II)–cyclopentadienyl clotrimazole complexes, [Ru^{II}(*p*-cymene)(bpy)(CTZ)][BF$_4$]$_2$ (Figure 27) was found to be the most active compound, increasing the activity of CTZ by a factor of 58 against *T. cruzi* (IC$_{50}$ = 0.1 µM), with no appreciable toxicity to human osteoblasts [210].

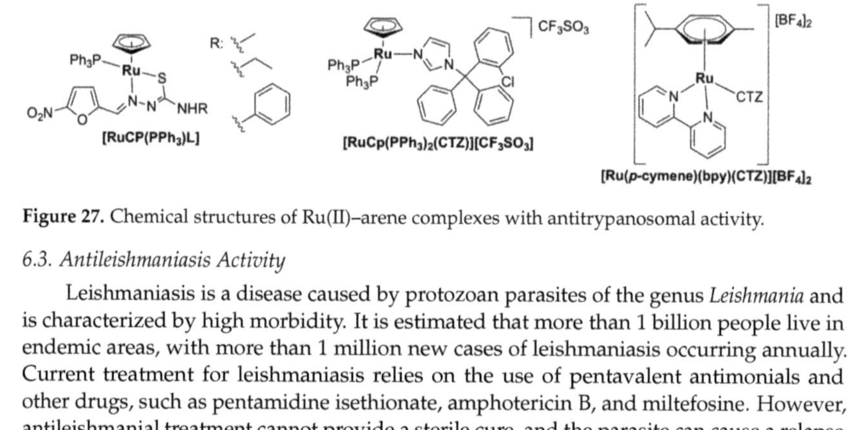

Figure 27. Chemical structures of Ru(II)–arene complexes with antitrypanosomal activity.

6.3. Antileishmaniasis Activity

Leishmaniasis is a disease caused by protozoan parasites of the genus *Leishmania* and is characterized by high morbidity. It is estimated that more than 1 billion people live in endemic areas, with more than 1 million new cases of leishmaniasis occurring annually. Current treatment for leishmaniasis relies on the use of pentavalent antimonials and other drugs, such as pentamidine isethionate, amphotericin B, and miltefosine. However, antileishmanial treatment cannot provide a sterile cure, and the parasite can cause a relapse when the human body is immunosuppressed [211,212].

An improved antiplasmodial activity in comparison with that of the free ligand has been reported for Ru(II)–lapachol complexes. [RuCl$_2$(Lap)(dppb)] was active against *L. amazonensis* promastigotes and infected macrophages, with submicromolar IC$_{50}$ values comparable with that of the reference drug, amphotericin B. In addition, the complex was not toxic to macrophages at concentrations much higher than the IC$_{50}$ values [212].

[Ru^{II}(*p*-cymene)(bpy)(CTZ)][BF$_4$]$_2$ (Figure 27) was found to be active against promastigotes of *L. major* at nanomolar concentrations (IC$_{50}$ = 15 nM) and displayed no appreciable toxicity against human osteoblasts (SI > 500). Moreover, in *L. major*-infected mice macrophages, the complex caused a significant inhibition of the proliferation of intracellular amastigotes (IC$_{70}$ = 29 nM) [210].

7. Antiviral Activity of Ruthenium Complexes

7.1. Anti-HIV Activity

The mixed-valent tetranuclear ruthenium–oxo oxalato cluster $Na_7[Ru_4(\mu_3\text{-}O)_4(C_2O_4)_6]$ exerted promising anti-HIV-1 activity with over 98% inhibition of viral replication toward the R5-tropic HIV-1 strain at a 5 µM concentration and similar inhibitory activity toward X4-tropic viral replication. Moreover, the ruthenium–oxo oxalato cluster displayed selective anti-viral activity, with over 90% survival of the host cells registered at concentrations up to 50 µM. Notably, $Na_7[Ru_4(\mu_3\text{-}O)_4(C_2O_4)_6]$ was 10-fold more effective against HIV-1 reverse transcriptase (IC_{50} = 1.9 nM) than the commonly used HIV-1 RT inhibitor 3'-azido-3'-deoxythmidine-5'-triphosphate (IC_{50} = 68 nM) [213].

Another ruthenium cluster, $[H_4Ru_4(\eta^6\text{-}p\text{-benzene})_4]^{2+}$, displayed selective activity against Polio virus, without inhibiting the growth of healthy human cells. It has been suggested that the complex might only be cytotoxic in Polio-infected cells, as the virus alters cell membrane permeability, facilitating passage for the cluster [94].

$[Ru(bpy)_2eilatin]^{2+}$ (Figure 28), where eilatin = dibenzotetraazaperylene, inhibited HIV-1 replication in CD4+ HeLa cells and in human peripheral blood monocytes (IC_{50} values ~1 µM). Eilatin is a fused, heptacyclic aromatic alkaloid that was isolated from the sea squirts belonging to *Eudistoma* sp., reported to possess cytotoxic and antiproliferative activities. $[Ru(bpy)_2eilatin]^{2+}$ is a kinetically inert complex and in vitro studies suggest that its mechanism of action relies upon inhibition of key protein–RNA interactions. The planar structure of the bidentate ligand, eilatin, was found to be essential for the activity of the complex [214].

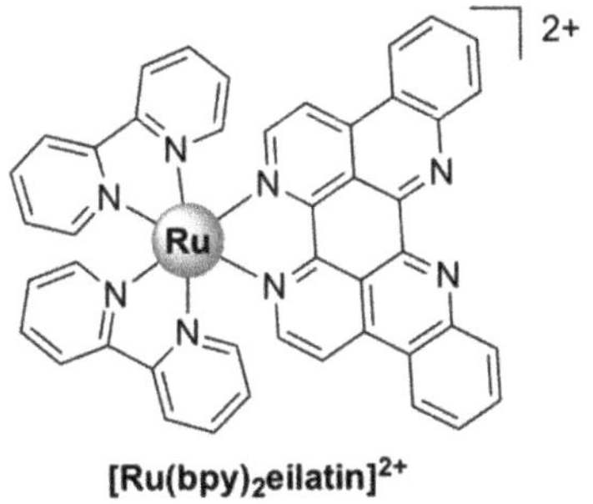

Figure 28. Chemical structure of $[Ru(bpy)_2eilatin]^{2+}$.

7.2. Anti-SARS-Cov-2 Activity

In spite of the extensive vaccination campaigns that are currently ongoing, the severe acute respiratory syndrome coronavirus 2 (SARS-CoV-2) is spreading at an alarming pace across the world. The large number of mutations rendered several new variants less susceptible to treatment options, and possibly to vaccines. Thus, there is still an urgent need for the development of new drugs with a broader spectrum of activity [215,216].

BOLD-100 (sodium trans-[tetrachlorobis(1H-indazole)ruthenate(III)], KP1339, Figure 29), developed as an anticancer agent, was shown to selectively inhibit stress-induced upregulation of 78-kDa glucose-regulated protein (GRP78) [217–219], which is a master chaperone protein serving critical functions in the endoplasmic reticulum of normal cells [220,221]. The interaction of SARS-CoV-2 spike protein with the GRP78 protein located on the cell membrane can mediate viral entry. Therefore, disruption of this interaction may be used to develop novel therapeutic strategies against coronavirus [222]. Indeed, BOLD-100 was reported to reduce viral loads in various COVID-19 variants, including the more virulent B.1.1.7, originally identified in the United Kingdom. Unlike vaccines, which are more effective against certain viral variants, BOLD-100, with a broad antiviral mechanism of action, appears to remain active on all mutant strains [223]. In vivo studies are currently in progress.

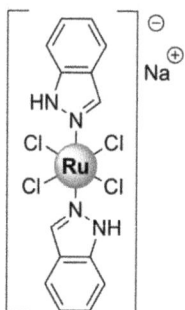

Figure 29. Chemical structure of BOLD-100 (sodium trans-[tetrachlorobis(1H-indazole)ruthenate(III)], KP1339).

BOLD-100 has a tolerable safety profile (minimal neurological or hematological effects), as was shown in a recently completed phase I clinical study involving 41 patients with advanced cancer. Moreover, it is currently undergoing clinical trials in combination with FOLFOX chemotherapy (which includes folinic acid, 5-fluorouracil, and oxaliplatin) for gastrointestinal solid tumors [224]. Therefore, BOLD-100 has already been successfully developed as a clinical-stage product, which suggests its potential for rapid further clinical development against COVID-19.

Additionally, [Ru(bpy)$_3$]$^{2+}$ is used in the Elecsys® Anti-SARS-CoV-2, a chemiluminescence immunoassay intended for qualitative detection of antibodies to SARS-CoV-2 in human serum and plasma, which has been approved worldwide. In this assay, the SARS-CoV-2-specific recombinant antigen is labeled with the ruthenium complex [225,226]. Other metal complexes identified as potential anti-SARS-Cov-2 agents include auranofin [227,228] and Re(I) tricarbonyl complexes [229].

8. Conclusions

Ruthenium-based antimicrobial agents have a fairly complex mode of action involving multiple mechanisms acting in synergy. The knowledge gained so far in this area suggests that the activity of ruthenium compounds against microbial cells is based upon their ability to induce oxidative stress, interact with the genetic material, proteins, or other intracellular targets, and/or damage the cell membranes. The complex interplay between these modes of action is likely responsible for the activity of some ruthenium-based compounds against drug-resistant strains.

Generally, ruthenium complexes exert excellent activity against Gram-positive bacteria (e.g., *S. aureus* and MRSA) and, with some exceptions (see, for instance, the dinuclear polypyridylruthenium(II) complexes and ruthenium-based CORMs), display lower activity towards Gram-negative strains (e.g., *E. coli* and *P. aeruginosa*). With regard to their activity against Gram-negative bacteria, one can notice a trend towards higher efficacy against *E. coli* when compared with *P. aeruginosa* and *K. pneumoniae*. For most classes of compounds, activity towards both Gram-negative and Gram-positive strains has been correlated to the uptake of the complex into the cells.

Additionally, this work highlights recent advances in ruthenium-based compounds that are active against neglected tropical diseases caused by parasites, such as malaria, Chagas' disease, and leishmaniasis. Notably, several complexes possess excellent activity, at submicromolar concentrations, results that raise awareness about the potential use of ruthenium compounds as effective antiparasitic agents. Moreover, the antiviral activity of ruthenium complexes, particularly the anti-HIV and anti-SARS-Cov-2 activities, has been reviewed herein. It is worth noting that BOLD-100 (formerly denoted KP1339) displays a broad antiviral mechanism of action and appears to remain active on all mutant strains of the SARS-Cov-2 virus.

In general terms, ruthenium complexes have been shown to display low levels of toxicity towards healthy eukaryotic cells in vitro and in vivo. This finding underlines the potential of these compounds for future clinical development, since selective toxicity against microbial over host cells in vitro and in vivo is imperative for a potential drug to advance in clinical trials. More in vivo studies are clearly needed in order to provide proof beyond a reasonable doubt that ruthenium complexes are strong candidates in the field of antimicrobial drug discovery.

In conclusion, this work aimed to highlight the potential of ruthenium-based compounds as novel antimicrobial agents due to the diverse range of complex 3D structures and modes of action they provide. Given that the pipeline of new antibiotics is running dry, the ruthenium species with high activity and selectivity presented herein may represent the starting point for a much-needed new class of antimicrobial agents. Therefore, we hope that this review will succeed in raising awareness about the potential of ruthenium complexes for antimicrobial applications and spur further research into their development.

Author Contributions: A.-C.M. performed a literature search, conceptualized the manuscript, and contributed to the writing of, corrections to, and the final shape of the manuscript. V.U. performed a literature search and contributed to the writing of and corrections to the manuscript. All authors have read and agreed to the published version of the manuscript.

Funding: This research was funded by The Executive Unit for the Financing of Higher Education, Research, Development, and Innovation (UEFISCDI), Project No. 383PED/2020 and Project No. PD 219/2020.

Acknowledgments: We thank Joseph Cowell for proofreading the manuscript and improving the use of English throughout the paper.

Conflicts of Interest: The authors declare no conflicts of interest. The funders had no role in the design of the study; in the collection, analyses, or interpretation of data; in the writing of the manuscript; or in the decision to publish the results.

References

1. Li, F.; Collins, J.G.; Keene, F.R. Ruthenium complexes as antimicrobial agents. *Chem. Soc. Rev.* **2015**, *44*, 2529–2542. [CrossRef]
2. Frei, A.; Zuegg, J.; Elliott, A.G.; Baker, M.; Braese, S.; Brown, C.; Chen, F.G.; Dowson, C.; Dujardin, G.; Jung, N.; et al. Metal complexes as a promising source for new antibiotics. *Chem. Sci.* **2020**, *11*, 2627–2639. [CrossRef]
3. Keogan, D.M.; Griffith, D.M. Current and potential applications of bismuth-based drugs. *Molecules* **2014**, *19*, 15258–15297. [CrossRef]
4. Silver, S. Bacterial silver resistance: Molecular biology and uses and misuses of silver compounds. *FEMS Microbiol. Rev.* **2003**, *27*, 341–353. [CrossRef]
5. Sánchez-López, E.; Gomes, D.; Esteruelas, G.; Bonilla, L.; Lopez-Machado, A.L.; Galindo, R.; Cano, A.; Espina, M.; Ettcheto, M.; Camins, A.; et al. Metal-based nanoparticles as antimicrobial agents: An overview. *Nanomaterials* **2020**, *10*, 292. [CrossRef] [PubMed]
6. Morrison, C.N.; Prosser, K.E.; Stokes, R.W.; Cordes, A.; Metzler-Nolte, N.; Cohen, S.M. Expanding medicinal chemistry into 3D space: Metallofragments as 3D scaffolds for fragment-based drug discovery. *Chem. Sci.* **2020**, *11*, 1216–1225. [CrossRef]
7. Hung, A.W.; Ramek, A.; Wang, Y.; Kaya, T.; Wilson, J.A.; Clemons, P.A.; Young, D.W. Route to three-dimensional fragments using diversity-oriented synthesis. *Proc. Natl. Acad. Sci. USA* **2011**, *108*, 6799–6804. [CrossRef] [PubMed]
8. Galloway, W.R.J.D.; Isidro-Llobet, A.; Spring, D.R. Diversity-oriented synthesis as a tool for the discovery of novel biologically active small molecules. *Nat. Commun.* **2010**, *1*, 80. [CrossRef]
9. Frei, A. Metal complexes, an untapped source of antibiotic potential? *Antibiotics* **2020**, *9*, 90. [CrossRef]
10. Anthony, E.J.; Bolitho, E.M.; Bridgewater, H.E.; Carter, O.W.L.; Donnelly, J.M.; Imberti, C.; Lant, E.C.; Lermyte, F.; Needham, R.J.; Palau, M.; et al. Metallodrugs are unique: Opportunities and challenges of discovery and development. *Chem. Sci.* **2020**, *11*, 12888–12917. [CrossRef]
11. Claudel, M.; Schwarte, J.V.; Fromm, K.M. New Antimicrobial Strategies Based on Metal Complexes. *Chemistry* **2020**, *2*, 849–899.
12. Munteanu, A.-C.; Notaro, A.; Jakubaszek, M.; Cowell, J.; Tharaud, M.; Goud, B.; Uivarosi, V.; Gasser, G. Synthesis, Characterization, Cytotoxic Activity, and Metabolic Studies of Ruthenium(II) Polypyridyl Complexes Containing Flavonoid Ligands. *Inorg. Chem.* **2020**, *59*, 4424–4434. [CrossRef]
13. Rademaker-Lakhai, J.M.; van den Bongard, D.; Pluim, D.; Beijnen, J.H.; Schellens, J.H.M. A Phase I and Pharmacological Study with Imidazolium-trans-DMSO-imidazole-tetrachlororuthenate, a Novel Ruthenium Anticancer Agent. *Clin. Cancer Res.* **2004**, *10*, 3717–3727. [CrossRef]

14. Leijen, S.; Burgers, S.A.; Baas, P.; Pluim, D.; Tibben, M.; Van Werkhoven, E.; Alessio, E.; Sava, G.; Beijnen, J.H.; Schellens, J.H.M. Phase I/II study with ruthenium compound NAMI-A and gemcitabine in patients with non-small cell lung cancer after first line therapy. *Invest. New Drugs* **2015**, *33*, 201–214. [CrossRef] [PubMed]
15. Hartinger, C.G.; Jakupec, M.A.; Zorbas-Seifried, S.; Groessl, M.; Egger, A.; Berger, W.; Zorbas, H.; Dyson, P.J.; Keppler, B.K. KP1019, A New Redox-Active Anticancer Agent – Preclinical Development and Results of a Clinical Phase I Study in Tumor Patients. *Chem. Biodivers.* **2008**, *5*, 2140–2155. [CrossRef] [PubMed]
16. Lentz, F.; Drescher, A.; Lindauer, A.; Henke, M.; Hilger, R.A.; Hartinger, C.G.; Scheulen, M.E.; Dittrich, C.; Keppler, B.K.; Jaehde, U. Pharmacokinetics of a novel anticancer ruthenium complex (KP1019, FFC14A) in a phase I dose-escalation study. *Anticancer. Drugs* **2009**, *20*, 97–103. [CrossRef]
17. Trondl, R.; Heffeter, P.; Kowol, C.R.; Jakupec, M.A.; Berger, W.; Keppler, B.K. NKP-1339, the first ruthenium-based anticancer drug on the edge to clinical application. *Chem. Sci.* **2014**, *5*, 2925–2932. [CrossRef]
18. Monro, S.; Colón, K.L.; Yin, H.; Roque, J.; Konda, P.; Gujar, S.; Thummel, R.P.; Lilge, L.; Cameron, C.G.; McFarland, S.A. Transition Metal Complexes and Photodynamic Therapy from a Tumor-Centered Approach: Challenges, Opportunities, and Highlights from the Development of TLD1433. *Chem. Rev.* **2019**, *119*, 797–828. [CrossRef]
19. Antibiotic Resistance. Available online: https://www.who.int/news-room/fact-sheets/detail/antibiotic-resistance (accessed on 20 April 2021).
20. Silhavy, T.J.; Kahne, D.; Walker, S. The bacterial cell envelope. *Cold Spring Harb. Perspect. Biol.* **2010**, *2*, a000414. [CrossRef] [PubMed]
21. Pizarro-Cerdá, J.; Cossart, P. Bacterial Adhesion and Entry into Host Cells. *Cell* **2006**, *124*, 715–727. [CrossRef] [PubMed]
22. Huan, Y.; Kong, Q.; Mou, H.; Yi, H. Antimicrobial Peptides: Classification, Design, Application and Research Progress in Multiple Fields. *Front. Microbiol.* **2020**, *11*, 582779. [CrossRef] [PubMed]
23. Uivarosi, V.; Munteanu, A.-C.; Nițulescu, G.M. Chapter 2—An Overview of Synthetic and Semisynthetic Flavonoid Derivatives and Analogues: Perspectives in Drug Discovery. In *Studies in Natural Products Chemistry*; Atta-ur-Rahman, Ed.; Elsevier: Amsterdam, The Netherlands, 2019; Volume 60, pp. 29–84. ISBN 1572-5995.
24. Provenzani, A.; Hospodar, A.R.; Meyer, A.L.; Leonardi Vinci, D.; Hwang, E.Y.; Butrus, C.M.; Polidori, P. Multidrug-resistant gram-negative organisms: A review of recently approved antibiotics and novel pipeline agents. *Int. J. Clin. Pharm.* **2020**, *42*, 1016–1025. [CrossRef] [PubMed]
25. Kim, B.; Kim, E.S.; Yoo, Y.-J.; Bae, H.-W.; Chung, I.-Y.; Cho, Y.-H. Phage-Derived Antibacterials: Harnessing the Simplicity, Plasticity, and Diversity of Phages. *Viruses* **2019**, *11*, 268. [CrossRef] [PubMed]
26. Alfei, S.; Schito, A.M. Positively charged polymers as promising devices against multidrug resistant gram-negative bacteria: A Review. *Polymers* **2020**, *12*, 1195. [CrossRef]
27. Guo, C.; Mandalapu, D.; Ji, X.; Gao, J.; Zhang, Q. Chemistry and Biology of Teixobactin. *Chem. – A Eur. J.* **2018**, *24*, 5406–5422. [CrossRef]
28. Reygaert, W.C. An overview of the antimicrobial resistance mechanisms of bacteria. *AIMS Microbiol.* **2018**, *4*, 482–501. [CrossRef]
29. Raafat, D.; Otto, M.; Reppschläger, K.; Iqbal, J.; Holtfreter, S. Fighting *Staphylococcus aureus* Biofilms with Monoclonal Antibodies. *Trends Microbiol.* **2019**, *27*, 303–322. [CrossRef]
30. Stewart, P.S. Mechanisms of antibiotic resistance in bacterial biofilms. *Int. J. Med. Microbiol.* **2002**, *292*, 107–113. [CrossRef]
31. Gholizadeh, P.; Köse, Ş.; Dao, S.; Ganbarov, K.; Tanomand, A.; Dal, T.; Aghazadeh, M.; Ghotaslou, R.; Ahangarzadeh Rezaee, M.; Yousefi, B.; et al. How CRISPR-Cas System Could Be Used to Combat Antimicrobial Resistance. *Infect. Drug Resist.* **2020**, *13*, 1111–1121. [CrossRef]
32. Southam, H.M.; Butler, J.A.; Chapman, J.A.; Poole, R.K. The Microbiology of Ruthenium Complexes. In *Advances in Microbial Physiology*; Poole, R.K., Ed.; Elsevier: London, UK, 2017; Volume 71, pp. 1–96. ISBN 0065-2911.
33. Dwyer, F.P.; Gyarfas, E.C.; Rogers, W.P.; Koch, J.H. Biological Activity of Complex Ions. *Nature* **1952**, *170*, 190–191. [CrossRef]
34. Dwyer, F.P.; Mayhew, E.; Roe, E.M.F.; Shulman, A. Inhibition of Landschütz Ascites Tumour Growth by Metal Chelates Derived from 3,4,7,8-Tetramethyl-1,10-phenanthroline. *Br. J. Cancer* **1965**, *19*, 195–199. [CrossRef]
35. Abd-El-Aziz, A.S.; Agatemor, C.; Etkin, N. Antimicrobial resistance challenged with metal-based antimicrobial macromolecules. *Biomaterials* **2017**, *118*, 27–50. [CrossRef]
36. Shulman, A.; Dwyer, F.P. Metal Chelates in Biological Systems. In *Chelating Agents and Metal Chelates*; Dwyer, F.P., Mellor, D.P., Eds.; Academic Press: Cambridge, MA, USA, 1964; ISBN 978-0-12-395499-2.
37. Li, F.; Mulyana, Y.; Feterl, M.; Warner, J.M.; Collins, J.G.; Keene, F.R. The antimicrobial activity of inert oligonuclear polypyridyl-ruthenium(II) complexes against pathogenic bacteria, including MRSA. *Dalt. Trans.* **2011**, *40*, 5032–5038. [CrossRef] [PubMed]
38. Li, F.; Feterl, M.; Mulyana, Y.; Warner, J.M.; Collins, J.G.; Keene, F.R. *In vitro* susceptibility and cellular uptake for a new class of antimicrobial agents: Dinuclear ruthenium(II) complexes. *J. Antimicrob. Chemother.* **2012**, *67*, 2686–2695. [CrossRef]
39. Dwyer, F.P.; Gyarfas, E.C.; Wright, R.D.; Shulman, A. Effect of Inorganic Complex Ions on Transmission at a Neuromuscular Junction. *Nature* **1957**, *179*, 425–426. [CrossRef]
40. Bolhuis, A.; Hand, L.; Marshall, J.E.; Richards, A.D.; Rodger, A.; Aldrich-Wright, J. Antimicrobial activity of ruthenium-based intercalators. *Eur. J. Pharm. Sci.* **2011**, *42*, 313–317. [CrossRef]
41. Yang, X.-Y.; Sun, B.; Zhang, L.; Li, N.; Han, J.; Zhang, J.; Sun, X.; He, Q.-Y. Chemical Interference with Iron Transport Systems to Suppress Bacterial Growth of *Streptococcus pneumoniae*. *PLoS One* **2014**, *9*, e105953. [CrossRef] [PubMed]

42. Yang, X.-Y.; Zhang, L.; Liu, J.; Li, N.; Yu, G.; Cao, K.; Han, J.; Zeng, G.; Pan, Y.; Sun, X.; et al. Proteomic analysis on the antibacterial activity of a Ru(II) complex against Streptococcus pneumoniae. *J. Proteomics* **2015**, *115*, 107–116. [CrossRef]
43. de Sousa, A.P.; Ellena, J.; Gondim, A.C.S.; Lopes, L.G.F.; Sousa, E.H.S.; de Vasconcelos, M.A.; Teixeira, E.H.; Ford, P.C.; Holanda, A.K.M. Antimicrobial activity of cis-[Ru(bpy)2(L)(L′)]n+ complexes, where L = 4-(4-chlorobenzoyl)pyridine or 4-(benzoyl)pyridine and L′ = Cl− or CO. *Polyhedron* **2018**, *144*, 88–94. [CrossRef]
44. De Sousa, A.P.; Gondim, A.C.S.; Sousa, E.H.S.; de Vasconcelos, M.A.; Teixeira, E.H.; Bezerra, B.P.; Ayala, A.P.; Martins, P.H.R.; Lopes, L.G.d.F.; Holanda, A.K.M. An unusual bidentate methionine ruthenium(II) complex: Photo-uncaging and antimicrobial activity. *J. Biol. Inorg. Chem.* **2020**, *25*, 419–428. [CrossRef] [PubMed]
45. Liao, X.; Jiang, G.; Wang, J.; Duan, X.; Liao, Z.; Lin, X.; Shen, J.; Xiong, Y.; Jiang, G. Two ruthenium polypyridyl complexes functionalized with thiophen: Synthesis and antibacterial activity against *Staphylococcus aureus*. *New J. Chem.* **2020**, *44*, 17215–17221. [CrossRef]
46. Bu, S.; Jiang, G.; Jiang, G.; Liu, J.; Lin, X.; Shen, J.; Xiong, Y.; Duan, X.; Wang, J.; Liao, X. Antibacterial activity of ruthenium polypyridyl complexes against *Staphylococcus aureus* and biofilms. *J. Biol. Inorg. Chem.* **2020**, *25*, 747–757. [CrossRef] [PubMed]
47. Srivastava, P.; Shukla, M.; Kaul, G.; Chopra, S.; Patra, A.K. Rationally designed curcumin based ruthenium(ii) antimicrobials effective against drug-resistant Staphylococcus aureus. *Dalt. Trans.* **2019**, *48*, 11822–11828. [CrossRef] [PubMed]
48. Gorle, A.K.; Feterl, M.; Warner, J.M.; Primrose, S.; Constantinoiu, C.C.; Keene, F.R.; Collins, J.G. Mononuclear Polypyridylruthenium(II) Complexes with High Membrane Permeability in Gram-Negative Bacteria—in particular Pseudomonas aeruginosa. *Chem. - A Eur. J.* **2015**, *21*, 10472–10481. [CrossRef] [PubMed]
49. Liu, X.; Sun, B.; Kell, R.E.M.; Southam, H.M.; Butler, J.A.; Li, X.; Poole, R.K.; Keene, F.R.; Collins, J.G. The Antimicrobial Activity of Mononuclear Ruthenium(II) Complexes Containing the dppz Ligand. *Chempluschem* **2018**, *83*, 643–650. [CrossRef] [PubMed]
50. Smitten, K.L.; Thick, E.J.; Southam, H.M.; Bernardino de la Serna, J.; Foster, S.J.; Thomas, J.A. Mononuclear ruthenium(ii) theranostic complexes that function as broad-spectrum antimicrobials in therapeutically resistant pathogens through interaction with DNA. *Chem. Sci.* **2020**, *11*, 8828–8838. [CrossRef]
51. De Grandis, R.A.; Resende, F.A.; da Silva, M.M.; Pavan, F.R.; Batista, A.A.; Varanda, E.A. In vitro evaluation of the cyto-genotoxic potential of Ruthenium(II) SCAR complexes: a promising class of antituberculosis agents. *Mutat. Res. Genet. Toxicol. Environ. Mutagen.* **2016**, *798–799*, 11–18. [CrossRef]
52. Andrade, A.L.; de Vasconcelos, M.A.; Arruda, F.V.d.F.; do Nascimento Neto, L.G.; Carvalho, J.M.d.S.; Gondim, A.C.S.; Lopes, L.G.d.F.; Sousa, E.H.S.; Teixeira, E.H. Antimicrobial activity and antibiotic synergy of a biphosphinic ruthenium complex against clinically relevant bacteria. *Biofouling* **2020**, *36*, 442–454. [CrossRef]
53. Kumar, S.V.; Scottwell, S.O.; Waugh, E.; McAdam, C.J.; Hanton, L.R.; Brooks, H.J.L.; Crowley, J.D. Antimicrobial Properties of Tris(homoleptic) Ruthenium(II) 2-Pyridyl-1,2,3-triazole "click" Complexes against Pathogenic Bacteria, Including Methicillin-Resistant Staphylococcus aureus (MRSA). *Inorg. Chem.* **2016**, *55*, 9767–9777. [CrossRef]
54. van Hilst, Q.V.C.; Vasdev, R.A.S.; Preston, D.; Findlay, J.A.; Scottwell, S.; Giles, G.I.; Brooks, H.J.L.; Crowley, J.D. Synthesis, Characterisation and Antimicrobial Studies of some 2,6-bis(1,2,3-Triazol-4-yl)Pyridine Ruthenium(II) "Click" Complexes. *Asian J. Org. Chem.* **2019**, *8*, 496–505. [CrossRef]
55. Gorle, A.K.; Li, X.; Primrose, S.; Li, F.; Feterl, M.; Kinobe, R.T.; Heimann, K.; Warner, J.M.; Keene, F.R.; Collins, J.G. Oligonuclear polypyridylruthenium(II) complexes: Selectivity between bacteria and eukaryotic cells. *J. Antimicrob. Chemother.* **2016**, *71*, 1547–1555. [CrossRef] [PubMed]
56. Li, X.; Heimann, K.; Li, F.; Warner, J.M.; Richard Keene, F.; Grant Collins, J. Dinuclear ruthenium(II) complexes containing one inert metal centre and one coordinatively-labile metal centre: Syntheses and biological activities. *Dalt. Trans.* **2016**, *45*, 4017–4029. [CrossRef]
57. Smitten, K.L.; Southam, H.M.; de la Serna, J.B.; Gill, M.R.; Jarman, P.J.; Smythe, C.G.W.; Poole, R.K.; Thomas, J.A. Using Nanoscopy To Probe the Biological Activity of Antimicrobial Leads That Display Potent Activity against Pathogenic, Multidrug Resistant, Gram-Negative Bacteria. *ACS Nano* **2019**, *13*, 5133–5146. [CrossRef] [PubMed]
58. Varney, A.M.; Smitten, K.L.; Thomas, J.A.; McLean, S. Transcriptomic Analysis of the Activity and Mechanism of Action of a Ruthenium(II)-Based Antimicrobial That Induces Minimal Evolution of Pathogen Resistance. *ACS Pharmacol. Transl. Sci.* **2021**, *4*, 168–178. [CrossRef]
59. Smitten, K.L.; Fairbanks, S.D.; Robertson, C.C.; Bernardino de la Serna, J.; Foster, S.J.; Thomas, J.A. Ruthenium based antimicrobial theranostics – using nanoscopy to identify therapeutic targets and resistance mechanisms in Staphylococcus aureus. *Chem. Sci.* **2020**, *11*, 70–79. [CrossRef] [PubMed]
60. Pandrala, M.; Li, F.; Feterl, M.; Mulyana, Y.; Warner, J.M.; Wallace, L.; Keene, F.R.; Collins, J.G. Chlorido-containing ruthenium(II) and iridium(III) complexes as antimicrobial agents. *Dalt. Trans.* **2013**, *42*, 4686–4694. [CrossRef]
61. Gorle, A.K.; Feterl, M.; Warner, J.M.; Wallace, L.; Keene, F.R.; Collins, J.G. Tri- and tetra-nuclear polypyridyl ruthenium(II) complexes as antimicrobial agents. *Dalt. Trans.* **2014**, *43*, 16713–16725. [CrossRef]
62. Sun, B.; Sundaraneedi, M.K.; Southam, H.M.; Poole, R.K.; Musgrave, I.F.; Keene, F.R.; Collins, J.G. Synthesis and biological properties of tetranuclear ruthenium complexes containing the bis[4(4′-methyl-2,2′-bipyridyl)]-1,7-heptane ligand. *Dalt. Trans.* **2019**, *48*, 14505–14515. [CrossRef]
63. Nobre, L.S.; Seixas, J.D.; Romão, C.C.; Saraiva, L.M. Antimicrobial Action of Carbon Monoxide-Releasing Compounds. *Antimicrob. Agents Chemother.* **2007**, *51*, 4303–4307. [CrossRef]

64. Tavares, A.F.; Parente, M.R.; Justino, M.C.; Oleastro, M.; Nobre, L.S.; Saraiva, L.M. The bactericidal activity of carbon monoxide-releasing molecules against *Helicobacter pylori*. *PLoS One* **2013**, *8*, e83157. [CrossRef]
65. Sahlberg Bang, C.; Demirel, I.; Kruse, R.; Persson, K. Global gene expression profiling and antibiotic susceptibility after repeated exposure to the carbon monoxide-releasing molecule-2 (CORM-2) in multidrug-resistant ESBL-producing uropathogenic *Escherichia coli*. *PLoS One* **2017**, *12*, e0178541. [CrossRef] [PubMed]
66. Desmard, M.; Davidge, K.S.; Bouvet, O.; Morin, D.; Roux, D.; Foresti, R.; Ricard, J.D.; Denamur, E.; Poole, R.K.; Montravers, P.; et al. A carbon monoxide-releasing molecule (CORM-3) exerts bactericidal activity against Pseudomonas aeruginosa and improves survival in an animal model of bacteraemia. *FASEB J.* **2009**, *23*, 1023–1031. [CrossRef] [PubMed]
67. Carvalho, S.M.; Marques, J.; Romão, C.C.; Saraiva, L.M. Metabolomics of Escherichia coli Treated with the Antimicrobial Carbon Monoxide-Releasing Molecule CORM-3 Reveals Tricarboxylic Acid Cycle as Major Target. *Antimicrob. Agents Chemother.* **2019**, *63*, e00643–e00719. [CrossRef]
68. Donnelly, R.F.; Fletcher, N.C.; McCague, P.J.; Donnelly, J.; McCarron, P.A.; Tunney, M.M. Design, Synthesis and Photodynamic Antimicrobial Activity of Ruthenium Trischelate Diimine Complexes. *Lett. Drug Des. Discov.* **2007**, *4*, 175–179. [CrossRef]
69. Smith, N.A.; Zhang, P.; Greenough, S.E.; Horbury, M.D.; Clarkson, G.J.; McFeely, D.; Habtemariam, A.; Salassa, L.; Stavros, V.G.; Dowson, C.G.; et al. Combatting AMR: Photoactivatable ruthenium(II)-isoniazid complex exhibits rapid selective antimycobacterial activity. *Chem. Sci.* **2017**, *8*, 395–404. [CrossRef]
70. Hopkins, S.L.; Stepanyan, L.; Vahidi, N.; Jain, A.; Winkel, B.S.J.; Brewer, K.J. Visible light induced antibacterial properties of a Ru(II)–Pt(II) bimetallic complex. *Inorganica Chim. Acta* **2017**, *454*, 229–233. [CrossRef]
71. Ghosh, S.; Amariei, G.; Mosquera, M.E.G.; Rosal, R. Polymeric ruthenium precursor as a photoactivated antimicrobial agent. *J. Hazard. Mater.* **2021**, *402*, 123788. [CrossRef]
72. Yang, X.-Y.; He, K.; Du, G.; Wu, X.; Yu, G.; Pan, Y.; Zhang, G.; Sun, X.; He, Q.-Y. Integrated Translatomics with Proteomics to Identify Novel Iron–Transporting Proteins in *Streptococcus pneumoniae*. *Front. Microbiol.* **2016**, *7*, 78. [CrossRef] [PubMed]
73. Srishailam, A.; Gabra, N.M.; Kumar, Y.P.; Reddy, K.L.; Devi, C.S.; Anil Kumar, D.; Singh, S.S.; Satyanarayana, S. Synthesis, characterization; DNA binding and antitumor activity of ruthenium(II) polypyridyl complexes. *J. Photochem. Photobiol. B Biol.* **2014**, *141*, 47–58. [CrossRef] [PubMed]
74. Reddy, M.R.; Reddy, P.V.; Kumar, Y.P.; Srishailam, A.; Nambigari, N.; Satyanarayana, S. Synthesis, Characterization, DNA Binding, Light Switch "On and Off", Docking Studies and Cytotoxicity, of Ruthenium(II) and Cobalt(III) Polypyridyl Complexes. *J. Fluoresc.* **2014**, *24*, 803–817. [CrossRef]
75. Mallepally, R.R.; Putta, V.R.; Chintakuntla, N.; Vuradi, R.K.; Kotha, L.R.; Sirasani, S. DNA Binding Behavior, Sensor Studies, Antimicrobial, Photocleavage and In vitro Cytotoxicity of Synthesized Ru(II) Complexes with Assorted Intercalating Polypyridyl Ligands. *J. Fluoresc.* **2016**, *26*, 1101–1113. [CrossRef] [PubMed]
76. Sun, D.; Zhang, W.; Lv, M.; Yang, E.; Zhao, Q.; Wang, W. Antibacterial activity of ruthenium(II) polypyridyl complex manipulated by membrane permeability and cell morphology. *Bioorg. Med. Chem. Lett.* **2015**, *25*, 2068–2073. [CrossRef] [PubMed]
77. Putta, V.R.; Chintakuntla, N.; Mallepally, R.R.; Avudoddi, S.; K, N.; Nancherla, D.; V V N, Y.; R S, P.; Surya, S.S.; Sirasani, S. Synthesis and Evaluation of In Vitro DNA/Protein Binding Affinity, Antimicrobial, Antioxidant and Antitumor Activity of Mononuclear Ru(II) Mixed Polypyridyl Complexes. *J. Fluoresc.* **2016**, *26*, 225–240. [CrossRef]
78. Ravi Kumar, V.; Nagababu, P.; Srinivas, G.; Rajender Reddy, M.; Vinoda Rani, M.; Ravi, M.; Satyanarayana, S. Investigation of DNA/BSA binding of three Ru(II) complexes by various spectroscopic methods, molecular docking and their antimicrobial activity. *J. Coord. Chem.* **2017**, *70*, 3790–3809. [CrossRef]
79. Vadivel, T.; Dhamodaran, M. Synthesis, characterization and antibacterial studies of ruthenium(III) complexes derived from chitosan schiff base. *Int. J. Biol. Macromol.* **2016**, *90*, 44–52. [CrossRef]
80. Ashwini Kumar, K.; Laxma Reddy, K.; Satyanarayana, S. Study of the interaction between ruthenium(II) complexes and CT-DNA: synthesis, characterisation, photocleavage and antimicrobial activity studies. *Supramol. Chem.* **2010**, *22*, 629–643. [CrossRef]
81. Ashwini Kumar, K.; Reddy, K.L.; Vidhisha, S.; Satyanarayana, S. Synthesis, characterization and DNA binding and photocleavage studies of [Ru(bpy)2BDPPZ]2+, [Ru(dmb)2BDPPZ]2+ and [Ru(phen)2BDPPZ]2+ complexes and their antimicrobial activity. *Appl. Organomet. Chem.* **2009**, *23*, 409–420. [CrossRef]
82. Garner, R.N.; Gallucci, J.C.; Dunbar, K.R.; Turro, C. [Ru(bpy)2(5-cyanouracil)2]2+ as a Potential Light-Activated Dual-Action Therapeutic Agent. *Inorg. Chem.* **2011**, *50*, 9213–9215. [CrossRef]
83. Jiang, G.-B.; Zhang, W.-Y.; He, M.; Gu, Y.-Y.; Bai, L.; Wang, Y.-J.; Yi, Q.-Y.; Du, F. New ruthenium polypyridyl complexes functionalized with fluorine atom or furan: Synthesis, DNA-binding, cytotoxicity and antitumor mechanism studies. *Spectrochim. Acta. A. Mol. Biomol. Spectrosc.* **2020**, *227*, 117534. [CrossRef]
84. Jiang, G.-B.; Zhang, W.-Y.; He, M.; Gu, Y.-Y.; Bai, L.; Wang, Y.-J.; Yi, Q.-Y.; Du, F. Design and synthesis of new ruthenium polypyridyl complexes with potent antitumor activity in vitro. *Spectrochim. Acta. A. Mol. Biomol. Spectrosc.* **2019**, *220*, 117132. [CrossRef]
85. Jiang, G.-B.; Zhang, W.-Y.; He, M.; Gu, Y.-Y.; Bai, L.; Wang, Y.-J.; Yi, Q.-Y.; Du, F. Development of four ruthenium polypyridyl complexes as antitumor agents: Design, biological evaluation and mechanism investigation. *J. Inorg. Biochem.* **2020**, *208*, 111104. [CrossRef]
86. Jiang, G.-B.; Zhang, W.-Y.; He, M.; Gu, Y.-Y.; Bai, L.; Wang, Y.-J.; Yi, Q.-Y.; Du, F. Anticancer activity of two ruthenium(II) polypyridyl complexes toward Hepatocellular carcinoma HepG-2 cells. *Polyhedron* **2019**, *169*, 209–218. [CrossRef]

87. Mulyana, Y.; Weber, D.K.; Buck, D.P.; Motti, C.A.; Collins, J.G.; Keene, F.R. Oligonuclear polypyridylruthenium(II) complexes incorporating flexible polar and non-polar bridges: synthesis, DNA-binding and cytotoxicity. *Dalt. Trans.* **2011**, *40*, 1510–1523. [CrossRef] [PubMed]
88. Li, F.; Feterl, M.; Warner, J.M.; Keene, F.R.; Collins, J.G. Dinuclear polypyridylruthenium(II) complexes: Flow cytometry studies of their accumulation in bacteria and the effect on the bacterial membrane. *J. Antimicrob. Chemother.* **2013**, *68*, 2825–2833. [CrossRef]
89. Pisani, M.J.; Fromm, P.D.; Mulyana, Y.; Clarke, R.J.; Körner, H.; Heimann, K.; Collins, J.G.; Keene, F.R. Mechanism of cytotoxicity and cellular uptake of lipophilic inert dinuclear polypyridylruthenium(II) complexes. *ChemMedChem* **2011**, *6*, 848–858. [CrossRef] [PubMed]
90. Li, F.; Harry, E.J.; Bottomley, A.L.; Edstein, M.D.; Birrell, G.W.; Woodward, C.E.; Keene, F.R.; Collins, J.G. Dinuclear ruthenium(II) antimicrobial agents that selectively target polysomes in vivo. *Chem. Sci.* **2014**, *5*, 685–693. [CrossRef]
91. Li, X.; Gorle, A.K.; Ainsworth, T.D.; Heimann, K.; Woodward, C.E.; Collins, J.G.; Keene, F.R. RNA and DNA binding of inert oligonuclear ruthenium(II) complexes in live eukaryotic cells. *Dalt. Trans.* **2015**, *44*, 3594–3603. [CrossRef]
92. Sun, B.; Southam, H.M.; Butler, J.A.; Poole, R.K.; Burgun, A.; Tarzia, A.; Keene, F.R.; Collins, J.G. Synthesis, isomerisation and biological properties of mononuclear ruthenium complexes containing the bis[4(4′-methyl-2,2′-bipyridyl)]-1,7-heptane ligand. *Dalt. Trans.* **2018**, *47*, 2422–2434. [CrossRef]
93. Liao, G.; Ye, Z.; Liu, Y.; Fu, B.; Fu, C. Octahedral ruthenium (II) polypyridyl complexes as antimicrobial agents against mycobacterium. *PeerJ* **2017**, *5*, e3252. [CrossRef]
94. Allardyce, C.S.; Dyson, P.J.; Ellis, D.J.; Salter, P.A.; Scopelliti, R. Synthesis and characterisation of some water soluble ruthenium(II)–arene complexes and an investigation of their antibiotic and antiviral properties. *J. Organomet. Chem.* **2003**, *668*, 35–42. [CrossRef]
95. Beckford, F.A.; Stott, A.; Gonzalez-Sarrías, A.; Seeram, N.P. Novel microwave synthesis of half-sandwich [(η6-C6H6)Ru] complexes and an evaluation of the biological activity and biochemical reactivity. *Appl. Organomet. Chem.* **2013**, *27*, 425–434. [CrossRef]
96. Gichumbi, J.M.; Friedrich, H.B.; Omondi, B.; Singh, M.; Naicker, K.; Chenia, H.Y. Synthesis, characterization, and cytotoxic and antimicrobial activities of ruthenium(II) arene complexes with N,N-bidentate ligands. *J. Coord. Chem.* **2016**, *69*, 3531–3544. [CrossRef]
97. Singh, K.S.; Devi, P.; Sawant, S.G.; Kaminsky, W. Arene ruthenium(II) complexes with 2-acetamidothiazole derived ligands: Synthesis, structural studies, antifouling and antibacterial properties. *Polyhedron* **2015**, *100*, 321–325. [CrossRef]
98. Obradović, D.; Nikolić, S.; Milenković, I.; Milenković, M.; Jovanović, P.; Savić, V.; Roller, A.; Đorđić Crnogorac, M.; Stanojković, T.; Grgurić-Šipka, S. Synthesis, characterization, antimicrobial and cytotoxic activity of novel half-sandwich Ru(II) arene complexes with benzoylthiourea derivatives. *J. Inorg. Biochem.* **2020**, *210*, 111164. [CrossRef] [PubMed]
99. Turan, N.; Buldurun, K.; Alan, Y.; Savci, A.; Çolak, N.; Mantarcı, A. Synthesis, characterization, antioxidant, antimicrobial and DNA binding properties of ruthenium(II), cobalt(II) and nickel(II) complexes of Schiff base containing o-vanillin. *Res. Chem. Intermed.* **2019**, *45*, 3525–3540. [CrossRef]
100. Shadap, L.; Banothu, V.; Adepally, U.; Adhikari, S.; Kollipara, M.R. Variable structural bonding modes and antibacterial studies of thiosemicarbazone ligands of ruthenium, rhodium, and iridium metal complexes. *J. Coord. Chem.* **2020**, *73*, 175–187. [CrossRef]
101. Lapasam, A.; Banothu, V.; Addepally, U.; Kollipara, M.R. Synthesis, structural and antimicrobial studies of half-sandwich ruthenium, rhodium and iridium complexes containing nitrogen donor Schiff-base ligands. *J. Mol. Struct.* **2019**, *1191*, 314–322. [CrossRef]
102. Nobre, L.S.; Jeremias, H.; Romão, C.C.; Saraiva, L.M. Examining the antimicrobial activity and toxicity to animal cells of different types of CO-releasing molecules. *Dalt. Trans.* **2016**, *45*, 1455–1466. [CrossRef]
103. Dkhar, L.; Banothu, V.; Kaminsky, W.; Kollipara, M.R. Synthesis of half sandwich platinum group metal complexes containing pyridyl benzothiazole hydrazones: Study of bonding modes and antimicrobial activity. *J. Organomet. Chem.* **2020**, *914*, 121225. [CrossRef]
104. Laurent, Q.; Batchelor, L.K.; Dyson, P.J. Applying a Trojan Horse Strategy to Ruthenium Complexes in the Pursuit of Novel Antibacterial Agents. *Organometallics* **2018**, *37*, 915–923. [CrossRef]
105. Chhabra, R.; Saha, A.; Chamani, A.; Schneider, N.; Shah, R.; Nanjundan, M. Iron Pathways and Iron Chelation Approaches in Viral, Microbial, and Fungal Infections. *Pharmaceuticals* **2020**, *13*, 275. [CrossRef] [PubMed]
106. Yildirim, H.; Guler, E.; Yavuz, M.; Ozturk, N.; Kose Yaman, P.; Subasi, E.; Sahin, E.; Timur, S. Ruthenium (II) complexes of thiosemicarbazone: Synthesis, biosensor applications and evaluation as antimicrobial agents. *Mater. Sci. Eng. C* **2014**, *44*, 1–8. [CrossRef] [PubMed]
107. Namiecińska, E.; Sadowska, B.; Więckowska-Szakiel, M.; Dolęga, A.; Pasternak, B.; Grazul, M.; Budzisz, E. Anticancer and antimicrobial properties of novel η6-p-cymene ruthenium(ii) complexes containing a N,S-type ligand, their structural and theoretical characterization. *RSC Adv.* **2019**, *9*, 38629–38645. [CrossRef]
108. Felício, M.R.; Silva, O.N.; Gonçalves, S.; Santos, N.C.; Franco, O.L. Peptides with Dual Antimicrobial and Anticancer Activities. *Front. Chem.* **2017**, *5*, 5. [CrossRef] [PubMed]
109. Appelt, P.; Fagundes, F.D.; Facchin, G.; Gabriela Kramer, M.; Back, D.F.; Cunha, M.A.A.; Sandrino, B.; Wohnrath, K.; de Araujo, M.P. Ruthenium (II) complexes containing 2-mercaptothiazolinates as ligands and evaluation of their antimicrobial activity. *Inorganica Chim. Acta* **2015**, *436*, 152–158. [CrossRef]

110. Beloglazkina, E.K.; Manzheliy, E.A.; Moiseeva, A.A.; Maloshitskaya, O.A.; Zyk, N.V.; Skvortsov, D.A.; Osterman, I.A.; Sergiev, P.V.; Dontsova, O.A.; Ivanenkov, Y.A.; et al. Synthesis, characterisation, cytotoxicity and antibacterial activity of ruthenium(II) and rhodium(III) complexes with sulfur-containing terpyridines. *Polyhedron* **2016**, *107*, 27–37. [CrossRef]
111. Lapasam, A.; Dkhar, L.; Joshi, N.; Poluri, K.M.; Kollipara, M.R. Antimicrobial selectivity of ruthenium, rhodium, and iridium half sandwich complexes containing phenyl hydrazone Schiff base ligands towards B. thuringiensis and P. aeruginosa bacteria. *Inorganica Chim. Acta* **2019**, *484*, 255–263. [CrossRef]
112. Elnagar, M.M.; Samir, S.; Shaker, Y.M.; Abdel-Shafi, A.A.; Sharmoukh, W.; Abdel-Aziz, M.S.; Abou-El-Sherbini, K.S. Synthesis, characterization, and evaluation of biological activities of new 4′-substituted ruthenium (II) terpyridine complexes: Prospective anti-inflammatory properties. *Appl. Organomet. Chem.* **2021**, *35*, 1–16. [CrossRef]
113. Nyawade, E.A.; Friedrich, H.B.; Omondi, B.; Chenia, H.Y.; Singh, M.; Gorle, S. Synthesis and characterization of new α,α′-diaminoalkane-bridged dicarbonyl(η5-cyclopentadienyl)ruthenium(II) complex salts: Antibacterial activity tests of η5-cyclopentadienyl dicarbonyl ruthenium(II) amine complexes. *J. Organomet. Chem.* **2015**, *799–800*, 138–146. [CrossRef]
114. Rani, S.; Kumar, S.; Chandra, S. Synthesis, structural, spectral, thermal and antimicrobial studies of palladium(II), platinum(II), ruthenium(III) and iridium(III) complexes derived from N,N,N,N-tetradentate macrocyclic ligand. *Spectrochim. Acta Part A Mol. Biomol. Spectrosc.* **2011**, *78*, 1507–1514. [CrossRef]
115. Balasubramian, K.P.; Raju, V.V.; Chinnusamy, V. Synthesis, characteristic, catalytic and antimicrobial activities of imidazolo substituted benzylidene imines with ruthenium(II) complexes. *J. Indian Chem. Soc.* **2009**, *86*, 570–576.
116. Thilagavathi, N.; Manimaran, A.; Priya, N.P.; Sathya, N.; Jayabalakrishnan, C. Synthesis, characterization, electrochemical, catalytic and antimicrobial activity studies of hydrazone Schiff base ruthenium(II) complexes. *Appl. Organomet. Chem.* **2010**, *24*, 301–307. [CrossRef]
117. Thilagavathi, N.; Manimaran, A.; Padma Priya, N.; Sathya, N.; Jayabalakrishnan, C. Synthesis, spectroscopic, redox, catalytic and antimicrobial properties of some ruthenium(II) Schiff base complexes. *Transit. Met. Chem.* **2009**, *34*, 725–732. [CrossRef]
118. Thilagavathi, N.; Jayabalakrishnan, C. Synthesis, characterization, catalytic and antimicrobial studies of ruthenium(III) complexes. *Cent. Eur. J. Chem.* **2010**, *8*, 842–851. [CrossRef]
119. Thangadurai, T.D.; Ihm, S.-K. Ruthenium(II) Complexes Derived from Substituted Cyclobutane and Substituted Thiazole Schiff Base Ligands: Synthetic, Spectral, Catalytic and Antimicrobial Studies. *Synth. React. Inorganic, Met. Nano-Metal Chem.* **2005**, *35*, 499–507. [CrossRef]
120. Matshwele, J.T.P.; Nareetsile, F.; Mapolelo, D.; Matshameko, P.; Leteane, M.; Nkwe, D.O.; Odisitse, S. Synthesis of Mixed Ligand Ruthenium (II/III) Complexes and Their Antibacterial Evaluation on Drug-Resistant Bacterial Organisms. *J. Chem.* **2020**, *2020*, 2150419. [CrossRef]
121. Pavan, F.R.; Poelhsitz, G.V.; Barbosa, M.I.F.; Leite, S.R.A.; Batista, A.A.; Ellena, J.; Sato, L.S.; Franzblau, S.G.; Moreno, V.; Gambino, D.; et al. Ruthenium(II) phosphine/diimine/picolinate complexes: Inorganic compounds as agents against tuberculosis. *Eur. J. Med. Chem.* **2011**, *46*, 5099–5107. [CrossRef] [PubMed]
122. Pavan, F.R.; Poelhsitz, G.V.; da Cunha, L.V.P.; Barbosa, M.I.F.; Leite, S.R.A.; Batista, A.A.; Cho, S.H.; Franzblau, S.G.; de Camargo, M.S.; Resende, F.A.; et al. In Vitro and In Vivo Activities of Ruthenium(II) Phosphine/Diimine/Picolinate Complexes (SCAR) against Mycobacterium tuberculosis. *PLoS One* **2013**, *8*, e64242.
123. Rolston, K.V.; Wang, W.; Nesher, L.; Smith, J.R.; Rybak, M.J.; Prince, R.A. Time-kill determination of the bactericidal activity of telavancin and vancomycin against clinical methicillin-resistant *Staphylococcus aureus* isolates from cancer patients. *Diagn. Microbiol. Infect. Dis.* **2017**, *87*, 338–342. [CrossRef]
124. Demirezen, N.; Tarınç, D.; Polat, D.; Çeşme, M.; Gölcü, A.; Tümer, M. Synthesis of trimethoprim metal complexes: Spectral, electrochemical, thermal, DNA-binding and surface morphology studies. *Spectrochim. Acta Part A Mol. Biomol. Spectrosc.* **2012**, *94*, 243–255. [CrossRef]
125. Ude, Z.; Romero-Canelón, I.; Twamley, B.; Fitzgerald Hughes, D.; Sadler, P.J.; Marmion, C.J. A novel dual-functioning ruthenium(II)–arene complex of an anti-microbial ciprofloxacin derivative — Anti-proliferative and anti-microbial activity. *J. Inorg. Biochem.* **2016**, *160*, 210–217. [CrossRef] [PubMed]
126. Colina-Vegas, L.; Dutra, J.L.; Villarreal, W.; Neto, J.H.d.A.; Cominetti, M.R.; Pavan, F.; Navarro, M.; Batista, A.A. Ru(II)/clotrimazole/diphenylphosphine/bipyridine complexes: Interaction with DNA, BSA and biological potential against tumor cell lines and Mycobacterium tuberculosis. *J. Inorg. Biochem.* **2016**, *162*, 135–145. [CrossRef]
127. Naglah, A.M.; Al-Omar, M.A.; Almehizia, A.A.; Obaidullah, A.J.; Bhat, M.A.; Al-Shakliah, N.S.; Belgacem, K.; Majrashi, B.M.; Refat, M.S.; Adam, A.M.A. Synthesis, Spectroscopic, and Antimicrobial Study of Binary and Ternary Ruthenium(III) Complexes of Ofloxacin Drug and Amino Acids as Secondary Ligands. *Crystals* **2020**, *10*, 225. [CrossRef]
128. Măciucă, A.-M.; Munteanu, A.-C.; Uivarosi, V. Quinolone Complexes with Lanthanide Ions: An Insight into their Analytical Applications and Biological Activity. *Molecules* **2020**, *25*, 1347. [CrossRef]
129. Pisani, M.J.; Weber, D.K.; Heimann, K.; Collins, J.G.; Keene, F.R. Selective mitochondrial accumulation of cytotoxic dinuclear polypyridyl ruthenium(II) complexes. *Metallomics* **2010**, *2*, 393–396. [CrossRef] [PubMed]
130. Weber, D.K.; Sani, M.-A.; Downton, M.T.; Separovic, F.; Keene, F.R.; Collins, J.G. Membrane Insertion of a Dinuclear Polypyridyl-ruthenium(II) Complex Revealed by Solid-State NMR and Molecular Dynamics Simulation: Implications for Selective Antibacterial Activity. *J. Am. Chem. Soc.* **2016**, *138*, 15267–15277. [CrossRef] [PubMed]

131. Morgan, J.L.; Spillane, C.B.; Smith, J.A.; Buck, D.P.; Collins, J.G.; Keene, F.R. Dinuclear ruthenium(II) complexes with flexible bridges as non-duplex DNA binding agents. *Dalt. Trans.* **2007**, 4333–4342. [CrossRef]
132. Li, F.; Weber, D.K.; Morgan, J.L.; Collins, J.G.; Keene, F.R. An approach to therapeutic agents through selective targeting of destabilised nucleic acid duplex sequences. *Dalt. Trans.* **2012**, *41*, 6528–6535. [CrossRef]
133. Gill, M.R.; Garcia-Lara, J.; Foster, S.J.; Smythe, C.; Battaglia, G.; Thomas, J.A. A ruthenium(II) polypyridyl complex for direct imaging of DNA structure in living cells. *Nat. Chem.* **2009**, *1*, 662–667. [CrossRef] [PubMed]
134. Millimouno, F.M.; Dong, J.; Yang, L.; Li, J.; Li, X. Targeting Apoptosis Pathways in Cancer and Perspectives with Natural Compounds from Mother Nature. *Cancer Prev. Res.* **2014**, *7*, 1081. [CrossRef] [PubMed]
135. Buck, D.P.; Paul, J.A.; Pisani, M.J.; Collins, J.G.; Keene, F.R. Binding of a Flexibly-linked Dinuclear Ruthenium(II) Complex to Adenine-bulged DNA Duplexes. *Aust. J. Chem.* **2010**, *63*, 1365–1375. [CrossRef]
136. Recht, M.I.; Douthwaite, S.; Puglisi, J.D. Basis for prokaryotic specificity of action of aminoglycoside antibiotics. *EMBO J.* **1999**, *18*, 3133–3138. [CrossRef] [PubMed]
137. Li, F.; Gorle, A.K.; Ranson, M.; Vine, K.L.; Kinobe, R.; Feterl, M.; Warner, J.M.; Keene, F.R.; Collins, J.G.; Day, A.I. Probing the pharmacokinetics of cucurbit[7, 8 and 10]uril: And a dinuclear ruthenium antimicrobial complex encapsulated in cucurbit[10]uril. *Org. Biomol. Chem.* **2017**, *15*, 4172–4179. [CrossRef]
138. Brown, D.G.; May-Dracka, T.L.; Gagnon, M.M.; Tommasi, R. Trends and exceptions of physical properties on antibacterial activity for Gram-positive and Gram-negative pathogens. *J. Med. Chem.* **2014**, *57*, 10144–10161. [CrossRef]
139. Kitamura, Y.; Ihara, T.; Tsujimura, Y.; Osawa, Y.; Sasahara, D.; Yamamoto, M.; Okada, K.; Tazaki, M.; Jyo, A. Template-directed formation of luminescent lanthanide complexes: Versatile tools for colorimetric identification of single nucleotide polymorphism. *J. Inorg. Biochem.* **2008**, *102*, 1921–1931. [CrossRef] [PubMed]
140. Kumar, S.V.; Lo, W.K.C.; Brooks, H.J.L.; Crowley, J.D. Synthesis, structure, stability and antimicrobial activity of a ruthenium(II) helicate derived from a bis-bidentate "click" pyridyl-1,2,3-triazole ligand. *Inorganica Chim. Acta* **2015**, *425*, 1–6. [CrossRef]
141. Roopashree, B.; Gayathri, V.; Gopi, A.; Devaraju, K.S. Syntheses, characterizations, and antimicrobial activities of binuclear ruthenium(III) complexes containing 2-substituted benzimidazole derivatives. *J. Coord. Chem.* **2012**, *65*, 4023–4040. [CrossRef]
142. Wenzel, M.; Patra, M.; Senges, C.H.R.; Ott, I.; Stepanek, J.J.; Pinto, A.; Prochnow, P.; Vuong, C.; Langklotz, S.; Metzler-Nolte, N.; et al. Analysis of the mechanism of action of potent antibacterial hetero-tri-organometallic compounds: a structurally new class of antibiotics. *ACS Chem. Biol.* **2013**, *8*, 1442–1450. [CrossRef]
143. Stringer, T.; Seldon, R.; Liu, N.; Warner, D.F.; Tam, C.; Cheng, L.W.; Land, K.M.; Smith, P.J.; Chibale, K.; Smith, G.S. Antimicrobial activity of organometallic isonicotinyl and pyrazinyl ferrocenyl-derived complexes. *Dalt. Trans.* **2017**, *46*, 9875–9885. [CrossRef] [PubMed]
144. Jain, A.; Winkel, B.S.J.; Brewer, K.J. In vivo inhibition of E. coli growth by a Ru(II)/Pt(II) supramolecule [(tpy)RuCl(dpp)PtCl2](PF6). *J. Inorg. Biochem.* **2007**, *101*, 1525–1528. [CrossRef]
145. Jain, A.; Wang, J.; Mashack, E.R.; Winkel, B.S.J.; Brewer, K.J. Multifunctional DNA Interactions of Ru–Pt Mixed Metal Supramolecular Complexes with Substituted Terpyridine Ligands. *Inorg. Chem.* **2009**, *48*, 9077–9084. [CrossRef]
146. Wareham, L.K.; Poole, R.K.; Tinajero-Trejo, M. CO-releasing Metal Carbonyl Compounds as Antimicrobial Agents in the Post-antibiotic Era. *J. Biol. Chem.* **2015**, *290*, 18999–19007. [CrossRef]
147. Ling, K.; Men, F.; Wang, W.-C.; Zhou, Y.-Q.; Zhang, H.-W.; Ye, D.-W. Carbon Monoxide and Its Controlled Release: Therapeutic Application, Detection, and Development of Carbon Monoxide Releasing Molecules (CORMs). *J. Med. Chem.* **2018**, *61*, 2611–2635. [CrossRef]
148. Adach, W.; Błaszczyk, M.; Olas, B. Carbon monoxide and its donors - Chemical and biological properties. *Chem. Biol. Interact.* **2020**, *318*, 108973. [CrossRef]
149. Yan, H.; Du, J.; Zhu, S.; Nie, G.; Zhang, H.; Gu, Z.; Zhao, Y. Emerging Delivery Strategies of Carbon Monoxide for Therapeutic Applications: From CO Gas to CO Releasing Nanomaterials. *Small* **2019**, *15*, 1904382. [CrossRef] [PubMed]
150. Smith, H.; Mann, B.E.; Motterlini, R.; Poole, R.K. The carbon monoxide-releasing molecule, CORM-3 (Ru(CO)$_3$Cl(glycinate)), targets respiration and oxidases in *Campylobacter jejuni*, generating hydrogen peroxide. *IUBMB Life* **2011**, *63*, 363–371. [CrossRef] [PubMed]
151. McLean, S.; Begg, R.; Jesse, H.E.; Mann, B.E.; Sanguinetti, G.; Poole, R.K. Analysis of the bacterial response to Ru(CO)$_3$Cl(Glycinate) (CORM-3) and the inactivated compound identifies the role played by the ruthenium compound and reveals sulfur-containing species as a major target of CORM-3 action. *Antioxid. Redox Signal.* **2013**, *19*, 1999–2012. [CrossRef] [PubMed]
152. Wilson, J.L.; Jesse, H.E.; Hughes, B.; Lund, V.; Naylor, K.; Davidge, K.S.; Cook, G.M.; Mann, B.E.; Poole, R.K. Ru(CO)$_3$Cl(Glycinate) (CORM-3): A carbon monoxide-releasing molecule with broad-spectrum antimicrobial and photosensitive activities against respiration and cation transport in *Escherichia coli*. *Antioxidants Redox Signal.* **2013**, *19*, 497–509. [CrossRef]
153. Rana, N.; McLean, S.; Mann, B.E.; Poole, R.K. Interaction of the carbon monoxide-releasing molecule Ru(CO)$_3$Cl(glycinate) (CORM-3) with Salmonella enterica serovar Typhimurium: In situ measurements of carbon monoxide binding by integrating cavity dual-beam spectrophotometry. *Microbiology* **2014**, *160*, 2771–2779. [CrossRef]
154. Johnson, T.R.; Mann, B.E.; Teasdale, I.P.; Adams, H.; Foresti, R.; Green, C.J.; Motterlini, R. Metal carbonyls as pharmaceuticals? [Ru(CO)$_3$Cl(glycinate)], a CO-releasing molecule with an extensive aqueous solution chemistry. *Dalt. Trans.* **2007**, 1500–1508. [CrossRef]

155. Jesse, H.E.; Nye, T.L.; McLean, S.; Green, J.; Mann, B.E.; Poole, R.K. Cytochrome bd-I in *Escherichia coli* is less sensitive than cytochromes bd-II or bo' to inhibition by the carbon monoxide-releasing molecule, CORM-3: N-acetylcysteine reduces CO-RM uptake and inhibition of respiration. *Biochim. Biophys. Acta - Proteins Proteomics* **2013**, *1834*, 1693–1703. [CrossRef]
156. Davidge, K.S.; Sanguinetti, G.; Yee, C.H.; Cox, A.G.; McLeod, C.W.; Monk, C.E.; Mann, B.E.; Motterlini, R.; Poole, R.K. Carbon monoxide-releasing antibacterial molecules target respiration and global transcriptional regulators. *J. Biol. Chem.* **2009**, *284*, 4516–4524. [CrossRef]
157. Desmard, M.; Foresti, R.; Morin, D.; Dagouassat, M.; Berdeaux, A.; Denamur, E.; Crook, S.H.; Mann, B.E.; Scapens, D.; Montravers, P.; et al. Differential antibacterial activity against Pseudomonas aeruginosa by carbon monoxide-releasing molecules. *Antioxid. Redox Signal.* **2012**, *16*, 153–163. [CrossRef] [PubMed]
158. Chaves-Ferreira, M.; Albuquerque, I.S.; Matak-Vinkovic, D.; Coelho, A.C.; Carvalho, S.M.; Saraiva, L.M.; Romão, C.C.; Bernardes, G.J.L. Spontaneous CO Release from RuII(CO)2–Protein Complexes in Aqueous Solution, Cells, and Mice. *Angew. Chemie Int. Ed.* **2015**, *54*, 1172–1175. [CrossRef]
159. Southam, H.M.; Smith, T.W.; Lyon, R.L.; Liao, C.; Trevitt, C.R.; Middlemiss, L.A.; Cox, F.L.; Chapman, J.A.; El-Khamisy, S.F.; Hippler, M.; et al. A thiol-reactive Ru(II) ion, not CO release, underlies the potent antimicrobial and cytotoxic properties of CO-releasing molecule-3. *Redox Biol.* **2018**, *18*, 114–123. [CrossRef]
160. Tavares, A.F.N.; Teixeira, M.; Romão, C.C.; Seixas, J.D.; Nobre, L.S.; Saraiva, L.M. Reactive oxygen species mediate bactericidal killing elicited by carbon monoxide-releasing molecules. *J. Biol. Chem.* **2011**, *286*, 26708–26717. [CrossRef]
161. Marazioti, A.; Bucci, M.; Coletta, C.; Vellecco, V.; Baskaran, P.; Szabó, C.; Cirino, G.; Marques, A.R.; Guerreiro, B.; Gonçalves, A.M.L.; et al. Inhibition of nitric oxide-stimulated vasorelaxation by carbon monoxide-releasing molecules. *Arterioscler. Thromb. Vasc. Biol.* **2011**, *31*, 2570–2576. [CrossRef] [PubMed]
162. Taillé, C.; El-Benna, J.; Lanone, S.; Boczkowski, J.; Motterlini, R. Mitochondrial respiratory chain and NAD(P)H oxidase are targets for the antiproliferative effect of carbon monoxide in human airway smooth muscle. *J. Biol. Chem.* **2005**, *280*, 25350–25360. [CrossRef] [PubMed]
163. Zuckerbraun, B.S.; Chin, B.Y.; Bilban, M.; D'Avila, J.d.C.; Rao, J.; Billiar, T.R.; Otterbein, L.E. Carbon monoxide signals via inhibition of cytochrome c oxidase and generation of mitochondrial reactive oxygen species. *FASEB J.* **2007**, *21*, 1099–1106. [CrossRef]
164. Murray, T.S.; Okegbe, C.; Gao, Y.; Kazmierczak, B.I.; Motterlini, R.; Dietrich, L.E.P.; Bruscia, E.M. The Carbon Monoxide Releasing Molecule CORM-2 Attenuates Pseudomonas aeruginosa Biofilm Formation. *PLoS One* **2012**, *7*, e35499. [CrossRef]
165. Seixas, J.D.; Chaves-Ferreira, M.; Montes-Grajales, D.; Gonçalves, A.M.; Marques, A.R.; Saraiva, L.M.; Olivero-Verbel, J.; Romão, C.C.; Bernardes, G.J.L. An N-Acetyl Cysteine Ruthenium Tricarbonyl Conjugate Enables Simultaneous Release of CO and Ablation of Reactive Oxygen Species. *Chem. Eur. J.* **2015**, *21*, 14708–14712. [CrossRef]
166. Wilson, J.L.; Wareham, L.K.; McLean, S.; Begg, R.; Greaves, S.; Mann, B.E.; Sanguinetti, G.; Poole, R.K. CO-Releasing Molecules Have Nonheme Targets in Bacteria: Transcriptomic, Mathematical Modeling and Biochemical Analyses of CORM-3 [Ru(CO)3Cl(glycinate)] Actions on a Heme-Deficient Mutant of Escherichia coli. *Antioxid. Redox Signal.* **2015**, *23*, 148–162. [CrossRef]
167. Santos-Silva, T.; Mukhopadhyay, A.; Seixas, J.D.; Bernardes, G.J.L.; Romão, C.C.; Romão, M.J. CORM-3 Reactivity toward Proteins: The Crystal Structure of a Ru(II) Dicarbonyl–Lysozyme Complex. *J. Am. Chem. Soc.* **2011**, *133*, 1192–1195. [CrossRef] [PubMed]
168. Santos-Silva, T.; Mukhopadhyay, A.; Seixas, J.D.; Bernardes, G.J.L.; Romão, C.C.; Romão, M.J. Towards improved therapeutic CORMs: Understanding the reactivity of CORM-3 with proteins. *Curr. Med. Chem.* **2011**, *18*, 3361–3366. [CrossRef] [PubMed]
169. Seixas, J.D.; Santos, M.F.A.; Mukhopadhyay, A.; Coelho, A.C.; Reis, P.M.; Veiros, L.F.; Marques, A.R.; Penacho, N.; Gonçalves, A.M.L.; Romão, M.J.; et al. A contribution to the rational design of Ru(CO)3Cl2L complexes for in vivo delivery of CO. *Dalt. Trans.* **2015**, *44*, 5058–5075. [CrossRef] [PubMed]
170. Wang, P.; Liu, H.; Zhao, Q.; Chen, Y.; Liu, B.; Zhang, B.; Zheng, Q. Syntheses and evaluation of drug-like properties of CO-releasing molecules containing ruthenium and group 6 metal. *Eur. J. Med. Chem.* **2014**, *74*, 199–215. [CrossRef]
171. Winburn, I.C.; Gunatunga, K.; McKernan, R.D.; Walker, R.J.; Sammut, I.A.; Harrison, J.C. Cell damage following carbon monoxide releasing molecule exposure: Implications for therapeutic applications. *Basic Clin. Pharmacol. Toxicol.* **2012**, *111*, 31–41. [CrossRef]
172. Stingl, K.; De Reuse, H. Staying alive overdosed: How does Helicobacter pylori control urease activity? *Int. J. Med. Microbiol.* **2005**, *295*, 307–315. [CrossRef]
173. Lemire, J.A.; Harrison, J.J.; Turner, R.J. Antimicrobial activity of metals: Mechanisms, molecular targets and applications. *Nat. Rev. Microbiol.* **2013**, *11*, 371–384. [CrossRef]
174. Arnett, C.H.; Chalkley, M.J.; Agapie, T. A Thermodynamic Model for Redox-Dependent Binding of Carbon Monoxide at Site-Differentiated, High Spin Iron Clusters. *J. Am. Chem. Soc.* **2018**, *140*, 5569–5578. [CrossRef]
175. Wilson, J.L.; McLean, S.; Begg, R.; Sanguinetti, G.; Poole, R.K. Analysis of transcript changes in a heme-deficient mutant of Escherichia coli in response to CORM-3 [Ru(CO)$_3$Cl(glycinate)]. *Genomics Data* **2015**, *5*, 231–234. [CrossRef] [PubMed]
176. Nobre, L.S.; Al-Shahrour, F.; Dopazo, J.; Saraiva, L.M. Exploring the antimicrobial action of a carbon monoxide-releasing compound through whole-genome transcription profiling of Escherichia coli. *Microbiology* **2009**, *155*, 813–824. [CrossRef] [PubMed]
177. Wareham, L.K.; Begg, R.; Jesse, H.E.; Van Beilen, J.W.A.; Ali, S.; Svistunenko, D.; McLean, S.; Hellingwerf, K.J.; Sanguinetti, G.; Poole, R.K. Carbon Monoxide Gas Is Not Inert, but Global, in Its Consequences for Bacterial Gene Expression, Iron Acquisition, and Antibiotic Resistance. *Antioxid. Redox Signal.* **2016**, *24*, 1013–1028. [CrossRef]

178. Li, X.-Z.; Nikaido, H. Efflux-mediated drug resistance in bacteria: An update. *Drugs* **2009**, *69*, 1555–1623. [CrossRef]
179. Villemin, E.; Ong, Y.C.; Thomas, C.M.; Gasser, G. Polymer encapsulation of ruthenium complexes for biological and medicinal applications. *Nat. Rev. Chem.* **2019**, *3*, 261–282. [CrossRef]
180. Nguyen, D.; Nguyen, T.-K.; Rice, S.A.; Boyer, C. CO-Releasing Polymers Exert Antimicrobial Activity. *Biomacromolecules* **2015**, *16*, 2776–2786. [CrossRef]
181. Bang, C.S.; Kruse, R.; Demirel, I.; Önnberg, A.; Söderquist, B.; Persson, K. Multiresistant uropathogenic extended-spectrum β-lactamase (ESBL)-producing Escherichia coli are susceptible to the carbon monoxide releasing molecule-2 (CORM-2). *Microb. Pathog.* **2014**, *66*, 29–35. [CrossRef]
182. Chung, S.W.; Liu, X.; Macias, A.A.; Baron, R.M.; Perrella, M.A. Heme oxygenase-1-derived carbon monoxide enhances the host defense response to microbial sepsis in mice. *J. Clin. Invest.* **2008**, *118*, 239–247. [CrossRef] [PubMed]
183. Josefsen, L.B.; Boyle, R.W. Photodynamic Therapy and the Development of Metal-Based Photosensitisers. *Met. Based. Drugs* **2008**, *2008*, 276109. [CrossRef]
184. Le Gall, T.; Lemercier, G.; Chevreux, S.; Tücking, K.-S.; Ravel, J.; Thétiot, F.; Jonas, U.; Schönherr, H.; Montier, T. Ruthenium(II) Polypyridyl Complexes as Photosensitizers for Antibacterial Photodynamic Therapy: A Structure-Activity Study on Clinical Bacterial Strains. *ChemMedChem* **2018**, *13*, 2229–2239. [CrossRef]
185. Soliman, N.; Sol, V.; Ouk, T.-S.; Thomas, C.M.; Gasser, G. Encapsulation of a Ru(II) Polypyridyl Complex into Polylactide Nanoparticles for Antimicrobial Photodynamic Therapy. *Pharmaceutics* **2020**, *12*, 961. [CrossRef]
186. Rensmo, H.; Lunell, S.; Siegbahn, H. Absorption and electrochemical properties of ruthenium(II) dyes, studied by semiempirical quantum chemical calculations. *J. Photochem. Photobiol. A Chem.* **1998**, *114*, 117–124. [CrossRef]
187. Lei, W.; Zhou, Q.; Jiang, G.; Zhang, B.; Wang, X. Photodynamic inactivation of Escherichia coli by Ru(II) complexes. *Photochem. Photobiol. Sci.* **2011**, *10*, 887–890. [CrossRef] [PubMed]
188. Allardyce, C.; Dyson, P. Ruthenium in Medicine: Current Clinical Uses and Future Prospects. *Platin. Met. Rev.* **2001**, *45*, 62–69.
189. Wassmer, S.C.; Grau, G.E.R. Severe malaria: What's new on the pathogenesis front? *Int. J. Parasitol.* **2017**, *47*, 145–152. [CrossRef] [PubMed]
190. Baartzes, N.; Stringer, T.; Smith, G.S. Targeting Sensitive-Strain and Resistant-Strain Malaria Parasites Through a Metal-Based Approach. In *Advances in Bioorganometallic Chemistry*; Hirao, T., Moriuchi, T., Eds.; Elsevier: Amsterdam, The Netherlands, 2019; pp. 193–213, ISBN 978-0-12-814197-7.
191. Miotto, O.; Almagro-Garcia, J.; Manske, M.; Macinnis, B.; Campino, S.; Rockett, K.A.; Amaratunga, C.; Lim, P.; Suon, S.; Sreng, S.; et al. Multiple populations of artemisinin-resistant Plasmodium falciparum in Cambodia. *Nat. Genet.* **2013**, *45*, 648–655. [CrossRef]
192. Martínez, A.; Rajapakse, C.S.K.; Naoulou, B.; Kopkalli, Y.; Davenport, L.; Sánchez-Delgado, R.A. The mechanism of antimalarial action of the ruthenium(II)-chloroquine complex [RuCl(2)(CQ)] (2). *J. Biol. Inorg. Chem.* **2008**, *13*, 703–712. [CrossRef] [PubMed]
193. Sánchez-Delgado, R.A.; Navarro, M.; Pérez, H.; Urbina, J.A. Toward a Novel Metal-Based Chemotherapy against Tropical Diseases. 2. Synthesis and Antimalarial Activity in Vitro and in Vivo of New Ruthenium— and Rhodium—Chloroquine Complexes. *J. Med. Chem.* **1996**, *39*, 1095–1099. [CrossRef]
194. Macedo, T.S.; Colina-Vegas, L.; DA Paixão, M.; Navarro, M.; Barreto, B.C.; Oliveira, P.C.M.; Macambira, S.G.; Machado, M.; Prudêncio, M.; D'Alessandro, S.; et al. Chloroquine-containing organoruthenium complexes are fast-acting multistage antimalarial agents. *Parasitology* **2016**, *143*, 1543–1556. [CrossRef]
195. Adams, M.; de Kock, C.; Smith, P.J.; Land, K.M.; Liu, N.; Hopper, M.; Hsiao, A.; Burgoyne, A.R.; Stringer, T.; Meyer, M.; et al. Improved antiparasitic activity by incorporation of organosilane entities into half-sandwich ruthenium(II) and rhodium(III) thiosemicarbazone complexes. *Dalt. Trans.* **2015**, *44*, 2456–2468. [CrossRef]
196. Rylands, L.-I.; Welsh, A.; Maepa, K.; Stringer, T.; Taylor, D.; Chibale, K.; Smith, G.S. Structure-activity relationship studies of antiplasmodial cyclometallated ruthenium(II), rhodium(III) and iridium(III) complexes of 2-phenylbenzimidazoles. *Eur. J. Med. Chem.* **2019**, *161*, 11–21. [CrossRef]
197. Chellan, P.; Land, K.M.; Shokar, A.; Au, A.; An, S.H.; Taylor, D.; Smith, P.J.; Chibale, K.; Smith, G.S. Di- and Trinuclear Ruthenium-, Rhodium-, and Iridium-Functionalized Pyridyl Aromatic Ethers: A New Class of Antiparasitic Agents. *Organometallics* **2013**, *32*, 4793–4804. [CrossRef]
198. Stringer, T.; Quintero, M.A.S.; Wiesner, L.; Smith, G.S.; Nordlander, E. Evaluation of PTA-derived ruthenium(II) and iridium(III) quinoline complexes against chloroquine-sensitive and resistant strains of the Plasmodium falciparum malaria parasite. *J. Inorg. Biochem.* **2019**, *191*, 164–173. [CrossRef] [PubMed]
199. Chellan, P.; Land, K.M.; Shokar, A.; Au, A.; An, S.H.; Taylor, D.; Smith, P.J.; Riedel, T.; Dyson, P.J.; Chibale, K.; et al. Synthesis and evaluation of new polynuclear organometallic Ru(ii), Rh(iii) and Ir(iii) pyridyl ester complexes as in vitro antiparasitic and antitumor agents. *Dalt. Trans.* **2014**, *43*, 513–526. [CrossRef]
200. De Souza, N.B.; Aguiar, A.C.C.; de Oliveira, A.C.; Top, S.; Pigeon, P.; Jaouen, G.; Goulart, M.O.F.; Krettli, A.U. Antiplasmodial activity of iron(II) and ruthenium(II) organometallic complexes against Plasmodium falciparum blood parasites. *Mem. Inst. Oswaldo Cruz* **2015**, *110*, 981–988. [CrossRef]
201. Lidani, K.C.F.; Andrade, F.A.; Bavia, L.; Damasceno, F.S.; Beltrame, M.H.; Messias-Reason, I.J.; Sandri, T.L. Chagas Disease: From Discovery to a Worldwide Health Problem. *Front. public Heal.* **2019**, *7*, 166. [CrossRef] [PubMed]

202. Kennedy, P.G.E. Update on human African trypanosomiasis (sleeping sickness). *J. Neurol.* **2019**, *266*, 2334–2337. [CrossRef] [PubMed]
203. Silva, J.J.N.; Osakabe, A.L.; Pavanelli, W.R.; Silva, J.S.; Franco, D.W. In vitro and in vivo antiproliferative and trypanocidal activities of ruthenium NO donors. *Br. J. Pharmacol.* **2007**, *152*, 112–121. [CrossRef]
204. Silva, J.J.N.; Pavanelli, W.R.; Pereira, J.C.M.; Silva, J.S.; Franco, D.W. Experimental chemotherapy against Trypanosoma cruzi infection using ruthenium nitric oxide donors. *Antimicrob. Agents Chemother.* **2009**, *53*, 4414–4421. [CrossRef]
205. Silva, J.J.N.; Guedes, P.M.M.; Zottis, A.; Balliano, T.L.; Nascimento Silva, F.O.; França Lopes, L.G.; Ellena, J.; Oliva, G.; Andricopulo, A.D.; Franco, D.W.; et al. Novel ruthenium complexes as potential drugs for Chagas's disease: Enzyme inhibition and in vitro/in vivo trypanocidal activity. *Br. J. Pharmacol.* **2010**, *160*, 260–269. [CrossRef]
206. Bastos, T.M.; Barbosa, M.I.F.; da Silva, M.M.; Júnior, J.W.d.c.; Meira, C.S.; Guimaraes, E.T.; Ellena, J.; Moreira, D.R.M.; Batista, A.A.; Soares, M.B.P. Nitro/nitrosyl-ruthenium complexes are potent and selective anti-Trypanosoma cruzi agents causing autophagy and necrotic parasite death. *Antimicrob. Agents Chemother.* **2014**, *58*, 6044–6055. [CrossRef]
207. Possato, B.; Carneiro, Z.A.; de Albuquerque, S.; Nikolaou, S. New uses for old complexes: The very first report on the trypanocidal activity of symmetric trinuclear ruthenium complexes. *J. Inorg. Biochem.* **2017**, *176*, 156–158. [CrossRef] [PubMed]
208. Fernández, M.; Arce, E.R.; Sarniguet, C.; Morais, T.S.; Tomaz, A.I.; Azar, C.O.; Figueroa, R.; Diego Maya, J.; Medeiros, A.; Comini, M.; et al. Novel ruthenium(II) cyclopentadienyl thiosemicarbazone compounds with antiproliferative activity on pathogenic trypanosomatid parasites. *J. Inorg. Biochem.* **2015**, *153*, 306–314. [CrossRef]
209. Rodríguez Arce, E.; Sarniguet, C.; Moraes, T.S.; Vieites, M.; Tomaz, A.I.; Medeiros, A.; Comini, M.A.; Varela, J.; Cerecetto, H.; González, M.; et al. A new ruthenium cyclopentadienyl azole compound with activity on tumor cell lines and trypanosomatid parasites. *J. Coord. Chem.* **2015**, *68*, 2923–2937. [CrossRef]
210. Martínez, A.; Carreon, T.; Iniguez, E.; Anzellotti, A.; Sánchez, A.; Tyan, M.; Sattler, A.; Herrera, L.; Maldonado, R.A.; Sánchez-Delgado, R.A. Searching for new chemotherapies for tropical diseases: Ruthenium-clotrimazole complexes display high in vitro activity against Leishmania major and Trypanosoma cruzi and low toxicity toward normal mammalian cells. *J. Med. Chem.* **2012**, *55*, 3867–3877. [CrossRef]
211. Sundar, S.; Chakravarty, J. Leishmaniasis: an update of current pharmacotherapy. *Expert Opin. Pharmacother.* **2013**, *14*, 53–63. [CrossRef] [PubMed]
212. Barbosa, M.I.F.; Corrêa, R.S.; de Oliveira, K.M.; Rodrigues, C.; Ellena, J.; Nascimento, O.R.; Rocha, V.P.C.; Nonato, F.R.; Macedo, T.S.; Barbosa-Filho, J.M.; et al. Antiparasitic activities of novel ruthenium/lapachol complexes. *J. Inorg. Biochem.* **2014**, *136*, 33–39. [CrossRef]
213. Wong, E.L.-M.; Sun, R.W.-Y.; Chung, N.P.-Y.; Lin, C.-L.S.; Zhu, N.; Che, C.-M. A Mixed-Valent Ruthenium−Oxo Oxalato Cluster Na7[Ru4(μ3-O)4(C2O4)6] with Potent Anti-HIV Activities. *J. Am. Chem. Soc.* **2006**, *128*, 4938–4939. [CrossRef]
214. Luedtke, N.W.; Hwang, J.S.; Glazer, E.C.; Gut, D.; Kol, M.; Tor, Y. Eilatin Ru(II) complexes display anti-HIV activity and enantiomeric diversity in the binding of RNA. *Chembiochem* **2002**, *3*, 766–771. [CrossRef]
215. van Oosterhout, C.; Hall, N.; Ly, H.; Tyler, K.M. COVID-19 evolution during the pandemic – Implications of new SARS-CoV-2 variants on disease control and public health policies. *Virulence* **2021**, *12*, 507–508. [CrossRef]
216. Mahase, E. Covid-19: What new variants are emerging and how are they being investigated? *BMJ* **2021**, *372*, n158. [CrossRef] [PubMed]
217. Neuditschko, B.; Legin, A.A.; Baier, D.; Schintlmeister, A.; Reipert, S.; Wagner, M.; Keppler, B.K.; Berger, W.; Meier-Menches, S.M.; Gerner, C. Interaction with Ribosomal Proteins Accompanies Stress Induction of the Anticancer Metallodrug BOLD-100/KP1339 in the Endoplasmic Reticulum. *Angew. Chem. Int. Ed. Engl.* **2021**, *60*, 5063–5068. [CrossRef] [PubMed]
218. Guo, S.; Xiao, Y.; Li, D.; Jiang, Q.; Zhu, L.; Lin, D.; Jiang, H.; Chen, W.; Wang, L.; Liu, C.; et al. PGK1 and GRP78 overexpression correlates with clinical significance and poor prognosis in Chinese endometrial cancer patients. *Oncotarget* **2017**, *9*, 680–690. [CrossRef] [PubMed]
219. Bakewell, S.J.; Rangel, D.F.; Ha, D.P.; Sethuraman, J.; Crouse, R.; Hadley, E.; Costich, T.L.; Zhou, X.; Nichols, P.; Lee, A.S. Suppression of stress induction of the 78-kilodalton glucose regulated protein (GRP78) in cancer by IT-139, an anti-tumor ruthenium small molecule inhibitor. *Oncotarget* **2018**, *9*, 29698–29714. [CrossRef]
220. Ibrahim, I.M.; Abdelmalek, D.H.; Elfiky, A.A. GRP78: A cell's response to stress. *Life Sci.* **2019**, *226*, 156–163. [CrossRef]
221. Ha, D.P.; Van Krieken, R.; Carlos, A.J.; Lee, A.S. The stress-inducible molecular chaperone GRP78 as potential therapeutic target for coronavirus infection. *J. Infect.* **2020**, *81*, 452–482. [CrossRef]
222. Ibrahim, I.M.; Abdelmalek, D.H.; Elshahat, M.E.; Elfiky, A.A. COVID-19 spike-host cell receptor GRP78 binding site prediction. *J. Infect.* **2020**, *80*, 554–562. [CrossRef]
223. Bold Therapeutics Potential to Fight COVID-19. Available online: https://www.bold-therapeutics.com/COVID-19 (accessed on 18 April 2021).
224. O'Kane, G.M.; Spratlin, J.L.; Kavan, P.; Goodwin, R.A.; McWhirter, E.; Thompson, D.; Jones, M.; McAllister, E.R.; Machado, A.; Lemmerick, Y.; et al. BOLD-100-001 (TRIO039): A phase Ib dose-escalation study of BOLD-100 in combination with FOLFOX chemotherapy in patients with advanced gastrointestinal solid tumors. *J. Clin. Oncol.* **2021**, *39*, TPS145. [CrossRef]
225. Lippi, G.; Salvagno, G.L.; Pegoraro, M.; Militello, V.; Caloi, C.; Peretti, A.; De Nitto, S.; Bovo, C.; Lo Cascio, G. Preliminary evaluation of Roche Cobas Elecsys Anti-SARS-CoV-2 chemiluminescence immunoassay. *Clin. Chem. Lab. Med.* **2020**, *58*, e251–e253. [CrossRef]

226. Riester, E.; Findeisen, P.; Hegel, J.K.; Kabesch, M.; Ambrosch, A.; Rank, C.M.; Langen, F.; Laengin, T.; Niederhauser, C. Performance evaluation of the Roche Elecsys Anti-SARS-CoV-2 S immunoassay. *medRxiv* **2021**. [CrossRef]
227. Rothan, H.A.; Stone, S.; Natekar, J.; Kumari, P.; Arora, K.; Kumar, M. The FDA-approved gold drug auranofin inhibits novel coronavirus (SARS-COV-2) replication and attenuates inflammation in human cells. *Virology* **2020**, *547*, 7–11. [CrossRef] [PubMed]
228. Marzo, T.; Messori, L. A Role for Metal-Based Drugs in Fighting COVID-19 Infection? The Case of Auranofin. *ACS Med. Chem. Lett.* **2020**, *11*, 1067–1068. [CrossRef] [PubMed]
229. Karges, J.; Kalaj, M.; Gembicky, M.; Cohen, S.M. ReI Tricarbonyl Complexes as Coordinate Covalent Inhibitors for the SARS-CoV-2 Main Cysteine Protease. *Angew. Chemie Int. Ed.* **2021**, *60*, 10716. [CrossRef] [PubMed]

Article

Antibacterial Activity of Co(III) Complexes with Diamine Chelate Ligands against a Broad Spectrum of Bacteria with a DNA Interaction Mechanism

Katarzyna Turecka [1,*], Agnieszka Chylewska [2], Michał Rychłowski [3], Joanna Zakrzewska [4] and Krzysztof Waleron [1]

1. Department of Pharmaceutical Microbiology, Faculty of Pharmacy, Medical University of Gdańsk, gen. Hallera 107, 80-416 Gdańsk, Poland; krzysztof.waleron@gumed.edu.pl
2. Department of Bioinorganic Chemistry, Faculty of Chemistry, University of Gdańsk, Wita Stwosza 63, 80-308 Gdańsk, Poland; agnieszka.chylewska@ug.edu.pl
3. Laboratory of Virus Molecular Biology, Intercollegiate Faculty of Biotechnology, University of Gdańsk and Medical University of Gdańsk, Abrahama 58, 80-307 Gdańsk, Poland; michal.rychlowski@biotech.ug.edu.pl
4. Centre of Molecular and Macromolecular Studies, Polish Academy of Sciences, Henryka Sienkiewicza 112, 90-001 Łódź, Poland; jzakrzew@cbmm.lodz.pl
* Correspondence: katarzyna.turecka@gumed.edu.pl; Tel.: +48-58-349-19-72

Abstract: Cobalt coordination complexes are very attractive compounds for their therapeutic uses as antiviral, antibacterial, antifungal, antiparasitic, or antitumor agents. Two Co(III) complexes with diamine chelate ligands ([CoCl$_2$(dap)$_2$]Cl (**1**) and [CoCl$_2$(en)$_2$]Cl (**2**)) (where dap = 1,3-diaminopropane, en = ethylenediamine) were synthesized and characterized by elemental analysis, an ATR technique, and a scan method and sequentially tested against Gram-positive and Gram-negative bacteria. The minimum inhibitory concentration results revealed that anaerobic and microaerophilic bacteria were found to be the most sensitive; the serial passages assay presented insignificant increases in bacterial resistance to both compounds after 20 passages. The synergy assay showed a significant reduction in the MIC values of nalidixic acid when combined with Compounds (**1**) or (**2**). The assessment of cell damage by the complexes was performed using scanning electron microscopy, transmission electron microscopy, and confocal microscopy, which indicated cell membrane permeability, deformation, and altered cell morphology. DNA interaction studies of the Co(III) complexes with plasmid pBR322 using spectrophotometric titration methods revealed that the interaction between Complex (**1**) or (**2**) and DNA suggested an electrostatic and intercalative mode of binding, respectively. Furthermore, the DNA cleavage ability of compounds by agarose gel electrophoresis showed nuclease activity for both complexes. The results suggest that the effect of the tested compounds against bacteria can be complex.

Keywords: Co(III) coordination complexes; antibacterial activity; microbroth dilution method; minimum inhibitory concentration; minimum bactericidal concentration; synergy assay; serial passages assay; DNA interactions

1. Introduction

Increased antimicrobial resistance to the current antibiotics among bacteria is a serious problem globally. To overcome this problem, new and effective antibacterial compounds with low toxicity are needed. A promising group of antimicrobial compounds seem to be metallopharmaceuticals due to their abundance and structural diversity. The most remarkable achievements in the research on this type of compound refer to d-block metal-based drugs. D-block metal ion complexes encounter a large number of biomolecules in biological systems (amino acids, proteins, oligonucleotides, or DNA) and can interact with them. Comprehensive in vitro studies (evaluations of the structure of the complex, including detailed knowledge of bond length, the angles between them, their energy, the acid–base nature, and behaviour in the aquatic and non-aqueous environment) are necessary to design a metal drug or metal pro-drug useful for treatment. The kinetic and thermodynamic stability of metal-based pharmaceuticals against pH changes, temperature, chemical agents, the resistance of compounds to metabolism, the hydrophilic–lipophilic nature or ionization, and particle size is very important in drug development as well [1]. The growing interest of researchers in this type of compound is due to ligand complexes of transition metals resulting in antibacterial, antifungal, antiviral, antitumor, and anti-inflammatory properties [2–8]. There have been many reports on the use of metal-containing drugs. Complexes of platinum (cisplatin), gold (auranofin used in therapy of rheumatoid arthritis), rhenium (radiopharmaceutical used in imaging and radiotherapy), ruthenium (anticancer drugs) or cobalt, lithium, bismuth, iron, calcium, copper, and zinc have been used in medicine [9–14]. Recently, the interest in cobalt coordination complexes, especially Co(III) complexes, due to their antimicrobial and antitumor properties has grown [15–24].

The main feature allowing the use of cobalt(III) complexes as components of chemotherapeutic agents is the presence of stable Co(III) and labile Co(II). Complexes of Co(II) are stable in solid form but present a remarkable ease of oxidation under biological conditions. The antibacterial properties of Co(III) complexes have been frequently reported, and the increased effectiveness of cobalt ion coordination to the appropriate ligand when compared to the free ligand itself has been emphasized. It was confirmed that the values of the electrochemical redox potential of the complex and the structure of the ligand have a significant impact on the effectiveness and the stability of compounds used [25,26]. Optical isomers of Co(III) with ethylenediamine as N,N-bidentate ligand [Co(en)$_3$](NO$_3$)$_3$ have been studied and have exhibited high antimicrobial activity, irrespective of the isomer used [27]. Coordination compounds of cobalt(III) with pyridine-amide tri- or bidentate ligands have also been studied [28] and presented strong antibacterial properties for *Escherichia coli*, *Shigella flexneri*, and *Klebsiella planticola*. These complexes were also tested for the cytotoxic activity on the HEK cell lines and showed less cytotoxicity compared with the commercial antibiotic (gentamycin) at all tested concentrations.

There is a large number of cobalt(III) complex compounds that also exhibit potent antiviral activity, such as the CTC-96 (CTC series is a class of Co(III) complexes containing N, O-donor ligands), a potent agent against herpes simplex virus type 1 (HSV-1) [29]. This compound is present in the medication to prevent conjunctivitis, and it prevents epithelial corneal inflammation.

In the scientific literature, the anticancer activity of Co(III) complexes has also been described. Although the mechanism of this action has not been resolved yet, it is known that the important role in the antitumor activity is played by ligand activity, redox potential, and the different durability of Co^{2+} (unstable) ions and Co^{3+} (neutral and stable) ions. The active ligand is deactivated when combined with the cobalt atom. The cytotoxic agent is released due to the reduction of Co(III) to Co(II) under hypoxic conditions. Compounds investigated for this effect are cobalt (III) complexes with Schiff's four-coarse bases, nitrogen mustards, other DNA alkylating agents, and MMP (extracellular matrix metalloproteinase) inhibitors. Measurements involving substances used in anticancer therapies consist of finding cytostatic factors that strongly interact with cancer cells and very weakly influence the body's health cells [30,31].

The Co(III)-based antimicrobial and anticancer compounds can target DNA [32], block metal binding sites in enzymes [33], and interact with cytoplasmic proteins or other biomolecules [34].

In the search for new antibacterial agents, due to the growing resistance to antibiotics, the metallopharmaceuticals is a promising alternative. In the presented study, we determined the antibacterial activity of Co(III) complexes with simple bidentate inorganic ligands (en = ethylenediamine; dap = 1,3-diaminopropane) (Figure 1) on a broad spectrum of bacteria cultured in both aerobic and anaerobic conditions. The influence of the tested compounds on the bacterial DNA was also evaluated.

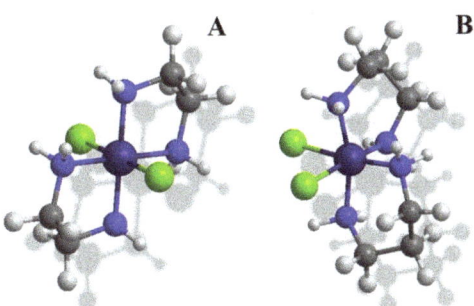

Figure 1. The structures of Co(III) coordination cations adopted from Ref. [5], Front. Microbiol. 2018 presented (**A**) trans-configuration of $[CoCl_2(en)_2]^+$ (for solid state) and (**B**) cis-configuration of $[CoCl_2(dap)_2]^+$ (for solution).

2. Materials and Methods

2.1. Materials and Growth Conditions

The reference and clinical strains of bacteria used in the study are listed in Table 1. The reference strains originated from the LGC standards. The clinical strains of bacteria from the Department of Pharmaceutical Microbiology collection were used. Strains were stored as glycerol stocks at −70 °C. For research purposes, cultures were conducted at 37 °C for 24 h in Mueller-Hinton (MH) broth, with 5% sheep blood (*S. pneumoniae* and *S. pyogenes*) and thioglycolate broth (*P. acnes* and *Clostridium* spp.) (Merck, Warsaw, Poland).

2.2. Synthesis of $[CoCl_2(N,N)_2]Cl$

All starting materials were commercially available (Sigma-Aldrich): cobalt(III) chloride hexahydrate, hydrochloride acid, hydrogen peroxide (30%), ethylenediammine, 1,3-diamminepropane, and methanol. All the solutions under study were prepared with twice-distilled water (Hydrolab-Reference purified) with conductivity not exceeding 0.09 µS/cm. The synthesis and physicochemical characterization of $[CoCl_2(dap)_2]Cl$ (**1**) and $[CoCl_2(en)_2]Cl$ (**2**) were performed according to the procedure described previously [35].

2.3. Synthesis of $[Co(dap)_2FLU]Cl_2$

A mixture of $[CoCl_2(dap)_2]Cl \cdot 2H_2O$ (1.05 g, 3 mmol) and fluorescein sodium salt (FLU) (1.51 g; 4 mmol) was dissolved in ethanol (6 mL), and NaBr (0.30 g; 3 mmol) in H_2O was added (5 mL). The mixture was heated in a water bath until the final volume was reduced to half of its initial volume. It was then cooled on ice, and a dark violet solid was formed. The complex $[Co(dap)_2FLU]Cl_2$ was collected and recrystallized from H_2O (20 mL). The yield through this method was ca. 60%. UV–vis: maxima at 231, 444, and 479 nm; ATR (cm^{-1}): (NH amine) 3418 and 3191; (C=O) 1583; (C=C) 1470; (Co-N(dap)) 610; (Co-O (FLU)) 734; see Figures S1 and S2 of SI. Anal. calc. for C, 54.32; H, 5.61; N, 9.74; found C, 54.35; H, 5.57; N, 9.79.

2.4. Physicochemical Measurements

The structural analyses of Co(III) synthesized complexes were prepared by using three independent analytical techniques. To determine percentage compositions of the elements (C, H, N, S) of the synthesized compounds an element analyzer Carlo Erba EA 1108 CHNS (Elementar, Langenselbold, Germany) was used. The oscillatory spectra were recorded in the wavenumber range 4000–400 cm^{-1} on a Spectrum Two FT-IR instrument (Perkin Elmer, Waltham, MA, USA) using the ATR technique. ^1H NMR spectra were recorded with a Brüker AVANCE 700 MHz spectrometer (Brüker, Billerica, MA, USA) at the NMR Laboratory at the Faculty of Chemistry (University of Gdańsk). Chemical shifts of proton NMR spectra were obtained by using two samples, FLU and $[Co(dap)_2FLU]Cl_2$, in the d^6-DMSO as solvent. The XRD powder diffractograms of three Co(III) complexes were recorded by using a diffractometer to prove the synthetic products differences in their structures. The D2 Physier X-ray powder diffractometer (D2 Phaser model by Brüker) was used to collect the XRD patterns for the solid samples using CuKα1 radiation (measurement parameters: 2 Theta between 5–60. The scan method used a double beam mode with a zero/baseline correction. A jacketed titration cell connected to a constant temperature water bath set to 25.0 ± 0.1 °C was used to all mentioned spectroscopic measurements.

2.5. Determination of the Minimum Inhibitory Concentration (MIC) and Minimum Bactericidal Concentration (MBC)

The MIC and MBC of tested compounds were performed according to the procedure described by Turecka et al. [5], except that MH broth was used. Anaerobic bacteria were cultured using Genbaganaer (bioMerieux, Marcy l'Etoile, France).

2.6. Serial Passages Assay

Four strains of bacteria (*S. aureus* ATCC 6538, *S. aureus* MRSA/h-VISA 6347, *P. aeruginosa* ATCC 9027, and *P. aeruginosa* 12274) were selected for the passages studies. Assay was performed according to the procedure described by Turecka et al. [5], except that MH broth was used.

2.7. Synergy Assay

To determine the fractional inhibitory concentrations (FICs) of antibiotics (ampicillin, gentamicin, polymyxin B, and nalidixic acid) (Merck, Warsaw, Poland) in combination with Co(III) complexes, a checkerboard assay (CLSI) was used in 96-well microtiter plates. The concentration ranges for antibiotics were from 4096 to 0.125 µg/mL, and those for the Co(III) complexes were from 8000 to 125 µg/mL. All steps of the assay were performed according to the procedure described by Turecka et al. [5], except that MH broth was used. The results were interpreted as described in Meletiadis et al. (2005) and Odds (2003) [36,37].

2.8. Microscopic Analysis

2.8.1. Transmission Electron Microscopy (TEM)

The suspension of *S. aureus* ATCC 6538 and *P. aeruginosa* ATCC 9027, cultured overnight in the MH broth, were diluted to 0.5 McFarland (with the same broth). The tested compounds in a concentration equivalent to MIC were introduced to 5 mL of the bacteria suspension and then incubated at 37 °C for 24 h. Following the incubation period and centrifugation, probes were fixed for 18 h in 2.5% glutaraldehyde (Polysciences, Warrington, PA, United States) in PBS (phosphate-buffered saline, pH 7.4), washed three times in the same buffer, and postfixed overnight in 1% osmium tetroxide (Polyscience, Warrington, PA, United States). Next, ethanol was dehydrated, and probes were embedded in Epon resin (Merck, Warsaw, Poland) and cut on the ultramicrotome Leica UC7 (Leica Microsystems, Wetzlar, Germany). Finally, probes were contrasted in uranyl acetate and lead citrate. A Philips CM100 transmission electron microscope (Philips, Amsterdam, the Netherlaands) was used [38].

2.8.2. Scanning Electron Microscopy (SEM)

The potential effect of Co(III) complexes on the bacterial cell morphology using SEM was determined according to the procedure described by Khan et al. [39] for reference strains of *S. aureus* and *P. aeruginosa* cells. Scanning Electron Microscope JSM-6010LA by JEOL (Akishima, Tokyo, Japan), equipped with energy-dispersive X-ray spectrometer EDX, was used.

2.8.3. Confocal Microscopy Assay

The cultures of *S. aureus* and *P. aeruginosa* were grown in LB broth until mid-log phase and then centrifuged. The bacterial pellets were washed three times using PBS buffer, pH 7.4, and resuspended in the same buffer to achieve the optical density corresponding to 10^6 CFU/mL. Bacterial cells were incubated with FITC-labelled [Co(dap)$_2$]Cl$_2$ at MIC concentration and with fluorescein alone for 1 h at 37 °C. After incubation, the cells were centrifuged, washed three times with PBS buffer, and fixed on a glass slide. After that, the cells were evaluated using Confocal microscopes from Leica Microsystems (Wetzlar, Germany) and the images were produced. The same studies were performed for fluorescein alone.

2.9. Interactions of Compounds (1) and (2) with Bacterial DNA

2.9.1. DNA Binding Studies of Diamine Co(III) Complexes

The electronic spectra were recorded on an Evolution 300 spectrophotometer (Thermo Fischer Scientific, Waltham, MA, USA) in the range of 200–700 nm in the case of UV detection of intermolecular interactions with biomolecules together with a spectral band with a 2 nm width. The binding ability of Co(III) complexes with diamines to DNA (plasmid pBR322) was investigated by spectrophotometric titration. The tris-(hydroxymethyl)-amino methane (Tris-HCl) buffer, pH 7.39, was used to prepare a solution of DNA. The concentration of freshly prepared DNA was calculated using an absorbance value at 258 nm according to the buffer solvent used (Figures S1 and S2, Supplementary Materials) and the calibration curve, which indicates the DNA molar absorption coefficient (ε_{DNA} 6600 M^{-1} cm^{-1}) [40,41]. The spectrophotometric titrations were performed at room temperature by gradually increasing the DNA concentration and constant concentrations of the complexes studied. Additionally, a second type of spectrophotometric titration, where a constant concentration of DNA and a gradual increase of [CoCl$_2$(dap)$_2$]Cl were maintained, was prepared to check the possibility of interaction between this coordination compound and DNA (Figure S3). After each addition of a different amount of DNA solution, electronic absorption spectra were recorded (Figures S11 and S12). The calculations were always made from the experimental titration data measured in the absence of any precipitate in the solution.

2.9.2. DNA Cleavage Study

Agarose gel electrophoresis was used to evaluate the Co(III) complexes' DNA cleavage ability. We used plasmid pBR322 isolated from *E. coli* DH5α by Plasmid Midi AX (A&A Biotechnology, Gdańsk, Poland). The concentration of freshly prepared DNA was measured with a spectrophotometer (Infinite M200 PRO by Tecan, Männedorf, Switzerland) using an absorbance at a 260 and 280 nm value according to the solvent buffer (Tris-HCl/NaCl 5 mM/50 mM). Dilution in the geometric progression of the tested compounds were prepared in the final concentration ranged from 1000 to 15.6 µg/mL and were mixed with the DNA at a constant concentration (62.5 µg/mL). The mixtures of DNA and Co(III) complexes were incubated at 37 °C for 2 h. To enhance the DNA cleaving ability by the complexes, H$_2$O$_2$ (100 µM) was added to each sample (two concentrations were examined, 500 and 62.5 µg/mL of complexes) and incubated for 5, 10, 15, 30, 60, and 120 min in 37 °C. Controls with DNA and H$_2$O$_2$ (100 µM) without compounds were also performed. After incubation, the samples were analysed by 0.8% agarose gel electrophoresis in 0.5% TAE buffer for 3 h at 50 V and then detected by a UV illuminator (ChemiDoc^{TM} Touch Imaging System Bio-Rad, Hercules, California, United States).

2.10. Statistical Analysis

All experiments were carried out in triplicates, in three independent experimental sets. The means ± SD were used in the statistical analysis of the data and the graphics.

3. Results

3.1. The Minimum Inhibitory Concentration (MIC) and Minimum Bactericidal Concentration (MBC)

The synthetized and characterized complexes ([CoCl$_2$(dap)$_2$]Cl (1) and [CoCl$_2$(en)$_2$]Cl (2) were screened in vitro for their antimicrobial activity against a broad spectrum of Gram-positive and Gram-negative bacteria (the reference and clinical strains) using a microbroth dilution method (Table 1). No significant differences in the sensitivity of Gram-positive and

Gram-negative bacteria to the tested compounds were observed. The MICs of compounds (**1**) and (**2**) were within the range from 167 to 9333 µg/mL (MBC from 208 to >9333 µg/mL) and were much higher than they were for commercial antibiotics (ampicillin and ciprofloxacin). The most sensitive proved to be S. pyogenes and S. pneumoniae (MIC/MBC for compound (**1**): 229/521 and 208/208 µg/mL; for (**2**): 208/229 and 229/292 µg/mL, respectively), S. aureus MSSA 56/AS, P. acnes (MIC/MBC for Compound (**1**): 333/458 and 208/208 µg/mL; for (**2**): 583/583 and 229/229 µg/mL, respectively), C. sporogenes (MIC/MBC for (**1**): 208/1667 µg/mL; for (**2**): 115/1833 µg/mL), and H. pylori (MIC/MBC for (**1**): 167/1833 µg/mL; for (**2**): 208/3000 µg/mL). The most resistant proved to be the strain of E. faecium 3844825 (MIC for (**1**): 6833; for (**2**): 9333 µg/mL; MBC: 7333 and >9333 µg/mL, respectively).

In order to examine whether the availability of oxygen affects the activity of cobalt compounds, several bacteria (S. aureus ATCC 6538, S. aureus MRSA 12673, E. coli ATCC 8739, and E. coli 12519) were also tested in anaerobic conditions by culturing in GENbaganaer. There were no differences in the activity of the compounds under both conditions.

Table 1. MIC and MBC values in µg/mL of $[CoCl_2(dap)_2]Cl$ (**1**), $[CoCl_2(en)_2]Cl$ (**2**), ampicillin, and ciprofloxacin against selected bacteria strains.

Strains	$[CoCl_2(dap)_2]Cl$ (1)		$[CoCl_2(en)_2]Cl$ (2)		Ampicillin		Ciprofloxacin	
	MIC	MBC	MIC	MBC	MIC	MBC	MIC	MBC
P. aeruginosa ATCC 9027	1667 ± 516	2333 ± 817	1500 ± 548	2333 ± 817	>2333	>2333	0.67 ± 0.3	0.83 ± 0.3
P. aeruginosa 12274	667 ± 258	1500 ± 548	1333 ± 516	1500 ± 548	>2333	>2333	107 ± 33	341 ± 132
P. mirabilis	750 ± 246	833 ± 258	1167 ± 408	1333 ± 204	>2333	>2333	21 ± 8.3	19 ± 6.5
P. mirabilis 1268	667 ± 258	917 ± 204	1333 ± 516	1333 ± 516	>2333	>2333	17 ± 6.5	21 ± 8.3
E. hirae ATCC 1052	2167 ± 983	2333 ± 817	2333 ± 817	2333 ± 817	117 ± 26	192 ± 70	107 ± 33	149 ± 52
E. faecium 38344825	6833 ± 2858	7333 ± 1633	9333 ± 3266	>9333	>2333	>2333	85 ± 33	171 ± 66
E. faecalis ATCC 51299	2333 ± 817	4667 ± 1633	2667 ± 1033	7333 ± 1633	171 ± 66	171 ± 52	1.33 ± 0.5	1.5 ± 0.6
E. faecalis 3937158	1333 ± 516	1733 ± 653	1333 ± 516	2667 ± 1033	>2333	>2333	53 ± 17	171 ± 66
E. faecalis 16274	458 ± 102	833 ± 258	1200 ± 408	1600 ± 516	235 ± 52	1195 ± 418	149 ± 52	234 ± 52
S. aureus ATCC 6538	375 ± 137	750 ± 433	667 ± 258	1333 ± 516	27 ± 8.3	27 ± 8.3	0.38 ± 0.1	0.58 ± 0.3
S. aureus MSSA 56/AS	333 ± 129	458 ± 102	583 ± 204	583 ± 204	1365 ± 529	>2333	0.67 ± 0.3	0.67 ± 0.3
S. aureus MRSA 12673	667 ± 258	750 ± 418	833 ± 258	916 ± 204	>2333	>2333	149 ± 52	149 ± 52
S. aureus MRSA (hetero-VISA) 6347	458 ± 102	667 ± 258	667 ± 516	667 ± 204	>2333	>2333	0.42 ± 0.1	0.67 ± 0.3
S. aureus MRSA N315 (ref.)	667 ± 258	750 ± 204	583 ± 204	583 ± 204	>2333	>2333	1.33 ± 0.5	1.33 ± 0.5
S. aureus MRSA 13251	542 ± 225	583 ± 204	833 ± 258	833 ± 258	>2333	>2333	107 ± 33	213 ± 66
S. aureus MRSA 15732	458 ± 102	833 ± 258	917 ± 204	917 ± 204	>2333	>2333	171 ± 66	171 ± 52
S. aureus MRSA 13318	667 ± 258	833 ± 258	458 ± 102	833 ± 258	>2333	>2333	149 ± 52	149 ± 33
K. pneumoniae ATCC 700603	1333 ± 516	1667 ± 516	1667 ± 516	3000 ± 1095	853 ± 264	1365 ± 529	43 ± 16	107 ± 66
K. pneumoniae 16205	750 ± 274	667 ± 258	750 ± 274	833 ± 258	1877 ± 418	>2333	85 ± 33	149 ± 52
K. pneumoniae 12828	667 ± 274	1167 ± 408	1333 ± 516	1333 ± 204	1877 ± 418	>2333	43 ± 17	171 ± 66
E. coli ATCC 8739	833 ± 258	1083 ± 491	1500 ± 548	1833 ± 408	107 ± 33	384 ± 140	0.23 ± 0.08	0.84 ± 0.3
E. coli 12519	667 ± 258	833 ± 258	1167 ± 408	1333 ± 516	>2333	>2333	13 ± 4.1	171 ± 66
E. coli 12293	833 ± 258	1667 ± 516	1667 ± 516	2333 ± 817	>2333	>2333	21 ± 8.3	107 ± 33
S. marcescens 12795	583 ± 333	1333 ± 516	917 ± 258	917 ± 204	149 ± 52	213 ± 66	0.19 ± 0.07	0.21 ± 0.07
S. marcescens 13148/2	667 ± 258	1833 ± 408	917 ± 204	1333 ± 516	341 ± 132	427 ± 132	0.33 ± 0.1	0.33 ± 01
C. sporogenes	208 ± 65	1667 ± 516	115 ± 25	1833 ± 408	0.833 ± 0.3	1.17 ± 0.4	0.83 ± 0.3	1.17 ± 0.4
Propionibacterium acnes	208 ± 65	208 ± 65	229 ± 51	229 ± 51	171 ± 66	171 ± 66	0.75 ± 0.3	1.13 ± 0.5
S. epidermidis ATCC 1499	667 ± 258	1083 ± 492	1667 ± 516	1667 ± 516	21 ± 8.3	21 ± 6.5	0.21 ± 0.06	0.42 ± 0.1
S. epidermidis MRSE 13199	917 ± 204	1833 ± 1602	1833 ± 408	1833 ± 408	683 ± 264	>2333	0.19 ± 0.07	0.19 ± 0.07
Salmonella enterica	1333 ± 516	1667 ± 516	1833 ± 408	2333 ± 817	341 ± 132	>2333	48 ± 18	170 ± 66.1
Helicobacter pylori	167 ± 65	1833 ± 408	208 ± 65	3000 ± 1095	3.33 ± 1.03	5.3 ± 2.1	0.67 ± 0.3	1.17 ± 0.4
S. pyogenes	229 ± 51	521 ± 26	208 ± 65	229 ± 51	1.7 ± 0.52	4.7 ± 1.6	6 ± 1.9	24 ± 8.8
S. pneumoniae	208 ± 65	208 ± 65	229 ± 51	292 ± 102	1.8 ± 0.41	1.8 ± 0.5	11 ± 4.1	-

3.2. Serial Passages Assay

In order to assess the increase in bacterial resistance to tested compounds, a serial passages assay was performed using four strains of bacteria (S. aureus ATCC 6538, S. aureus MRSA 6347, P. aeruginosa ATCC 9027, and P. aeruginosa 12274) in a medium supplemented with (**1**) and (**2**) below their active concentrations (Table 2 and Figure 2). Each MIC value of Compounds (**1**) and (**2**) was determined by the microbroth dilution method. There was no significant increase in MIC values after 20 passages, both for Compounds (**1**) and (**2**). After 5 passages, there was no increase in the MIC value in any case (the MIC value was the same as the initial value), and after 10 passages, the MIC value doubled only in the case of *S. aureus* MRSA 6347 for Compound (**2**). The following reduction (two times) of susceptibility was observed for *S. aureus* MRSA 6347 and *P. aeruginosa* 12274 after 15 passages for Compound (**1**); the same results were found in the case of *P. aeruginosa* ATCC 9027 for Compound (**2**). After 20 passages, an approximately two-fold reduction in sensitivity was obtained for *S. aureus* ATCC 6538 (Compounds (**1**) and (**2**)) and for *P. aeruginosa* 12274 in the case of Compound (**2**). The MIC value for *S. aureus* MRSA 6347 increased by about three times in comparison to the initial MIC. The presented increases in bacterial resistance to the test compounds were insignificant.

Table 2. MIC (μg/mL) values in the presence of [CoCl$_2$(dap)$_2$]Cl (**1**) and [CoCl$_2$(en)$_2$]Cl (**2**) passaging results for selected bacterial strains.

Strains	Compound	Initial MIC (μg/mL)	MIC after 20 Passages (μg/mL)
S. aureus ATCC 6538	[CoCl$_2$(dap)$_2$]Cl (**1**)	375 ± 137	667 ± 258
	[CoCl$_2$(en)$_2$]Cl (**2**)	667 ± 258	1333 ± 516
S. aureus MRSA 6347	[CoCl$_2$(dap)$_2$]Cl (**1**)	458 ± 102	1333 ± 516
	[CoCl$_2$(en)$_2$]Cl (**2**)	667 ± 516	2333 ± 817
P. aeruginosa ATCC 9027	[CoCl$_2$(dap)$_2$]Cl (**1**)	1667 ± 516	2333 ± 817
	[CoCl$_2$(en)$_2$]Cl (**2**)	1500 ± 548	2333 ± 817
P. aeruginosa 12274	[CoCl$_2$(dap)$_2$]Cl (**1**)	667 ± 258	1500 ± 548
	[CoCl$_2$(en)$_2$]Cl (**2**)	1333 ± 516	1500 ± 548

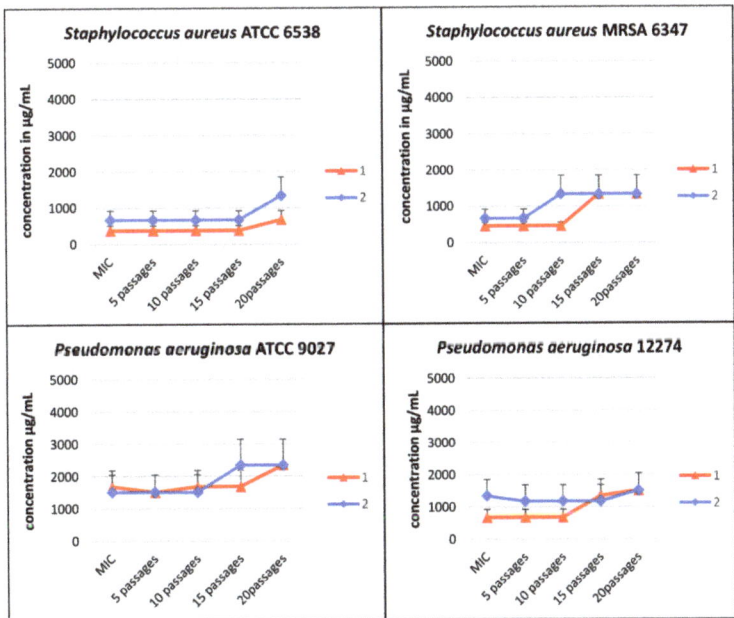

Figure 2. Serial passages assay results for the [CoCl$_2$(dap)$_2$]Cl (**1**) and [CoCl$_2$(en)$_2$]Cl (**2**) after 20 subsequent passages of reference and clinical strains of *S. aureus* and *P. aeruginosa*. The compounds below MIC (0.5 × MIC) were used. Data shown are mean ± SD.

3.3. Synergy Assay

The antimicrobial activity of selected antibiotics (ampicillin, gentamicin, ciprofloxacin, polymyxin B, and nalidixic acid) in combination with compounds (**1**) and (**2**) was also determined against both Gram-positive (*S. aureus* ATCC 6538 and *S. aureus* MRSA 6347) and Gram-negative (*P. coli* ATCC 8739 and *E. coli* 12519) bacterial strains by the checkerboard titration method (CSLI) using MH broth in 96-well microtiter plates. Results are shown in Table 3. The significant reductions in MIC values are noted in the case of the combination of compounds (**1**) and (**2**) with nalidixic acid. The mixture of nalidixic acid and compound (**1**) against *S. aureus* MRSA 12673 showed a reduction of MIC values by 8 times (from 448 to 56 µg/mL), and that against *E. coli* 12519 reduced by 4 times (from 1792 to 448 µg/mL), compared to nalidixic acid alone. An eight-fold reduction in MICs was also observed for the combination of the aforementioned antibiotic and Compound (**2**) against *S. aureus* ATCC 6530 and an almost 6-fold reduction in the case of *E. coli* 12519 (from 56 to 7.0 and from 1792 to 320 µg/mL, respectively). On the other hand, there was no reduction in MIC values when nalidixic acid + (**1**) and nalidixic acid + (**2**) mixtures were used against *E. coli* ATCC 8739.

Fractional inhibitory concentration index (FICi) values were also calculated and were in the range of 0.5–4.0 in most cases. These values indicate that there is no interaction in the mixture between the components of antibiotics and either (**1**) or (**2**) (FICi values of >0.5 and ≤4 reflect indifference), even though fold reductions in MIC values for both antimicrobials were observed in some cases (Table 3). The exception is the combination of polymyxin and (**1**) for *E. coli* 12519, where the FIC is 5.0, which would indicate an antagonistic effect.

3.4. Microscopic Analysis

3.4.1. Transmission Electron Microscopy

Tested bacterial strains treated for 18 h with MIC concentrations of compounds (**1**) and (**2**) were subjected to transmission electron microscopy, observed in solution and paraffin-embedded bacteria, to visualize their effect on bacterial cell morphology. After incubation in the presence of compounds (**1**) and (**2**) at the MIC level, the shape and morphology of the bacterial cells were distorted. The regular shape of the control cells was clearly visible (Figure 3A,B, control). The images of the bacterial cells treated with the tested compounds, prepared for observation in solution, showed disordered and structural disorganization within the cytoplasm (Figure 3A, +(**1**) and +(**2**)). Some cells turned from the normal round shape into irregular shapes presenting broken and lysed cells. Moreover, the cells coated probably with tested compounds were also seen (black arrows) (Figure 3A, +(**1**)). In the case of paraffin-embedded control bacteria, a regular shape and a cytoplasm of appropriate density inside the cells were observed (Figure 3B, control), whereas an alternation of the intracellular masses and obvious cytoplasmic clear zones were found in the bacterial cells after treatment with compounds (**1**) and (**2**) (Figure 3B, +(**1**), +(**2**)). Visible changes in bacterial cell morphology can indicate that cell membrane permeability was disrupted.

3.4.2. Scanning Electron Microscopy

To visualize the effect of compounds (**1**) and (**2**) on bacterial cell morphology, scanning electron microscopy was carried out. *S. aureus* ATCC 6538 and *P. aeruginosa* ATCC 9027 cells were treated for 24 h with tested compounds at an MIC concentration. The SEM images of untreated cells of bacteria show a well-defined shape free of visible distortions (Figure 4, control). Treatment with both compounds induced remarkable changes in the morphology of the cells in comparison to the control probe (Figure 4, +(**1**) and +(**2**)). Deformation and altered cell morphology were observed in both cases. Cells of different sizes for the *S. aureus* strain and collapsing cells for the *P. aeruginosa* strain were observed. The surfaces of *P. aeruginosa* cells treated with the MIC level of both compounds were wrinkled and irregular. In the case of the microphotograph of *S. aureus*, malformed cells were observed. Moreover, most of the bacterium were ruptured to different degrees.

Table 3. (a) Fractional inhibitory concentration index (FICi) values of [CoCl₂(dap)₂]Cl (1), ampicillin, gentamicin, nalidixic acid, and polymyxin B. (b) Fractional inhibitory concentration index (FICi) values of [CoCl₂(en)₂]Cl (2), ampicillin, gentamicin, nalidixic acid, and polymyxin B.

(a)

The Bacterial Strain	Antibiotic	MIC of Antibiotics (μg/mL)		MIC of (1) (μg/mL)		Fold Reduction of MIC of Antibiotic	Fold Reduction of MIC of (1)	FIC	Interpretation
		Alone	Com.	Alone	Com.				
S. aureus ATCC 6530	Ampicillin	27 ± 8.3	27 ± 8.3	458 ± 102	417 ± 144	-	0.9	2.1	indifference
	Gentamicin	0.438 ± 0.13	0.438 ± 0.13	375 ± 137	375 ± 137	-	-	2	indifference
	Ciprofloxacin	0.38 ± 0.1	0.38 ± 0.1	375 ± 137	375 ± 137	-	-	2	indifference
	Nalidixic acid	53.3 ± 18.5	53.3 ± 18.5	375 ± 137	375 ± 137	-	-	2	indifference
	Polymyxin B	85.3 ± 37	85.3 ± 37	417 ± 144	208 ± 72	-	2	1.5	indifference
S. aureus MRSA 12673	Ampicillin	>4096	>4096	667 ± 258	667 ± 258	-	-	-	-
	Gentamicin	0.23 ± 0.08	0.12 ± 0.03	667 ± 258	667 ± 258	1.9	-	1.5	indifference
	Ciprofloxacin	149 ± 52	85.3 ± 37	4116.7 ± 144	208 ± 72	1.8	2	1	indifference
	Nalidixic acid	448 ± 128	56 ± 16	667 ± 258	667 ± 258	8	-	1.1	indifference
	Polymyxin B	224 ± 64	224 ± 64	667 ± 258	667 ± 258	-	-	2	indifference
E. coli ATCC 8739	Ampicillin	107 ± 37	53.5 ± 28.5	833 ± 258	417 ± 144	2	2	0.7	indifference
	Gentamicin	0.42 ± 0.14	0.22 ± 0.06	437 ± 125	219 ± 63	2	2	1	indifference
	Ciprofloxacin	0.23 ± 0.08	0.12 ± 0.03	900 ± 223	313 ± 125	1.9	4	0.7	indifference
	Nalidixic acid	7.0 ± 2.0	3.6 ± 0.9	900 ± 223	437 ± 125	1.9	2	1	indifference
	Polymyxin B	0.438 ± 0.13	0.89 ± 0.25	875 ± 250	875 ± 250	-	-	3	indifference
E. coli 12519	Ampicillin	3584 ± 1024	3584 ± 1024	667 ± 258	667 ± 258	-	-	2	indifference
	Gentamicin	112 ± 32	56 ± 16	667 ± 258	667 ± 258	2	-	1.5	indifference
	Ciprofloxacin	13 ± 4.1	13 ± 4.1	667 ± 258	667 ± 258	-	-	2	indifference
	Nalidixic acid	1792 ± 512	448 ± 128	667 ± 258	219 ± 63	4	3	0.6	indifference
	Polymyxin B	0.112 ± 0.03	0.438 ± 0.13	667 ± 258	667 ± 258	-	-	5	antagonistic

129

Table 3. Cont.

(b)

The Bacterial Strain	Antibiotic	MIC of Antibiotics (µg/mL)		MIC of (2) (µg/mL)		Fold Reduction of MIC of Antibiotic	Fold Reduction of MIC of (2)	FIC	Interpretation
		Alone	Com.	Alone	Com.				
S. aureus ATCC 6530	Ampicillin	27 ± 8.3	27 ± 8.3	667 ± 258	667 ± 258	-	-	2	indifference
	Gentamicin	0.438 ± 0.13	0.23 ± 0.08	667 ± 258	667 ± 258	2	-	1.5	indifference
	Ciprofloxacin	0.38 ± 0.1	0.17 ± 0.06	667 ± 258	667 ± 258	2.2	-	1.5	indifference
	Nalidixic acid	56 ± 16	7.0 ± 2.0	667 ± 258	667 ± 258	8	-	1.1	indifference
	Polymyxin B	80 ± 32	80 ± 32	667 ± 258	333 ± 63	-	2	1	indifference
S. aureus MRSA 12673	Ampicillin	>4096	>4096	883 ± 258	883 ± 258	-	-	1.2	indifference
	Gentamicin	0.23 ± 0.08	0.12 ± 0.03	438 ± 125	438 ± 125	2	-	1.5	indifference
	Ciprofloxacin	149 ± 52	74.5 ± 29	438 ± 125	225 ± 56	2	1.9	1	indifference
	Nalidixic acid	461 ± 114	115 ± 33	438 ± 125	225 ± 56	4	1.9	0.7	indifference
	Polymyxin B	224 ± 64	224 ± 64	438 ± 125	438 ± 125	-	-	2	indifference
E. coli ATCC 8739	Ampicillin	107 ± 33	53.5 ± 19	1500 ± 548	750 ± 274	2	2	1	indifference
	Gentamicin	0.438 ± 0.13	0.12 ± 0.03	1750 ± 500	875 ± 250	4	2	0.7	indifference
	Ciprofloxacin	0.23 ± 0.08	0.23 ± 0.08	1750 ± 500	875 ± 250	-	2	1.5	indifference
	Nalidixic acid	7.2 ± 1.8	7.2 ± 1.8	1750 ± 500	875 ± 250	-	2	1.5	indifference
	Polymyxin B	0.438 ± 0.13	0.22 ± 0.06	1750 ± 500	875 ± 250	2	2	1	indifference
E. coli 12519	Ampicillin	3584 ± 1024	3584 ± 1024	1167 ± 408	1167 ± 408	-	-	2	indifference
	Gentamicin	115 ± 29	115 ± 29	1200 ± 447	1200 ± 447	-	-	2	indifference
	Ciprofloxacin	13 ± 4.1	13 ± 4.1	1167 ± 408	600 ± 224	-	1.9	1.5	indifference
	Nalidixic acid	1792 ± 512	320 ± 128	1200 ± 447	1200 ± 447	5.6	-	1.1	indifference
	Polymyxin B	0.109 ± 0.03	0.22 ± 0.06	1167 ± 408	1167 ± 408	-	-	3	indifference

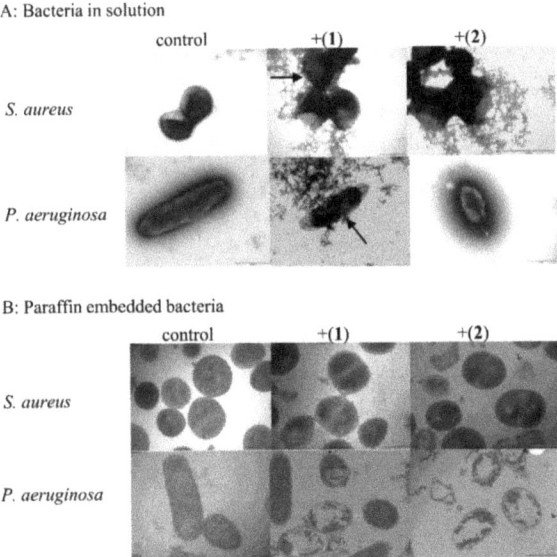

Figure 3. Changes in the cell morphology of *S. aureus* and *P. aeruginosa* cells treated with [CoCl$_2$(dap)$_2$]Cl- (**1**) and [CoCl$_2$(en)$_2$]Cl- (**2**). Microscopic preparations prepared in solution and as paraffin-embedded bacteria. Transmission electron microscopy images of *S. aureus* ATCC 6538 and *P. aeruginosa* ATCC 9077 in the absence (control) and presence of Compounds (**1**) (+(**1**)) and (**2**) (+(**2**)). Magnification 20,000×.

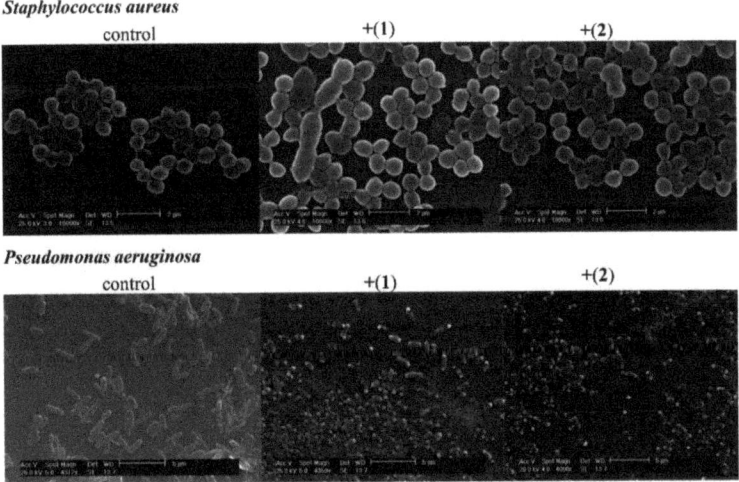

Figure 4. Changes in the cell morphology of *Staphylococcus aureus* and *Pseudomonas aeruginosa* cells treated with [CoCl2(dap)2]Cl- (**1**) and [CoCl2(en)2]Cl- (**2**). Scanning electron microscopy images of *S. aureus* ATCC 6538 (magnification 10000x) and *Pseudomonas aeruginosa* ATCC 9027 (magnification 4000×) in the absence (control) and presence of compound (**1**) (+(**1**)) and compound (**2**) (+(**2**)).

3.4.3. Fluorescent Microscopy Assay

To evaluate whether Co(III) complexes are able to penetrate bacterial cells, a fluorescent microscopy assay was performed. For these tests, [CoCl$_2$(dap)$_2$]Cl was selected as a more reactive compound. *P. aeruginosa* ATCC 9077 and *S. aureus* ATCC 6538 were incubated with FITC-labelled [Co(dap)$_2$]Cl$_2$ for 1 h at 37 °C. Localization of the fluorescence complex in the bacterial cell was visualized using a confocal microscope from Leica Microsystems. Fluorescein conjugated with compound (**1**) ([Co(dap)$_2$FLU]Cl$_2$) in subinhibitory concentrations (subMIC) penetrated the bacterial cell membrane and has been found to be evenly distributed inside bacterial cells (Figure 5) in the case of both bacteria. Cells of both bacteria in the presence of fluorescein alone did not show any fluorescence.

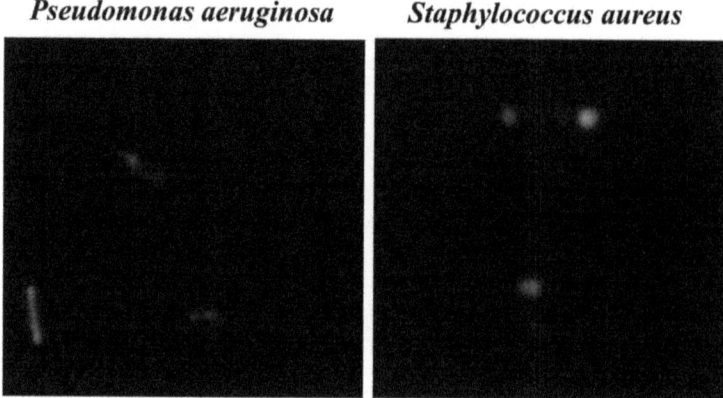

Figure 5. *Pseudomonas aeruginosa* ATCC 9077 and *Staphylococcus aureus* ATCC 6538 with FITC-labeled [CoCl$_2$(dap)$_2$]Cl. Magnification 2000×.

*3.5. Interactions of Compounds (**1**) and (**2**) with DNA*

3.5.1. Binding Studies in the Presence of *E. coli* DNA

The binding properties of the diamine complexes of Co(III) with DNA (pBR322) were studied using electronic absorption spectroscopy. To compare quantitatively the binding strength of the two complexes, the intrinsic binding constants, K_b, of the complexes studied with DNA extracted from bacteria were obtained by monitoring the changes in absorbance at 520 nm for complex (**1**) and 510 nm for complex (**2**). The absorption spectra of the free cobalt(III) complexes, treated also as precursors and of their adducts with DNA (at a constant concentration of the compounds) are given in Figure 6 for complexes (**1**) and (**2**), respectively. The UV–vis spectra of Co(III) complexes (**1**) and (**2**) at different contents of DNA show that, in the visible region, the absorption peaks of these solutions showed moderate shifts towards longer wavelengths, which indicates that complexes (**1**) and (**2**) interact with plasmid pBR322 DNA. However, the detailed analysis and comparison of results received for both titrations suggest that Co(III) complex (**2**) with ethylenediamine ligands interacts much more strongly than the analogical Co(III) complex (**1**) with 1,3-diamminepropane ligands inside.

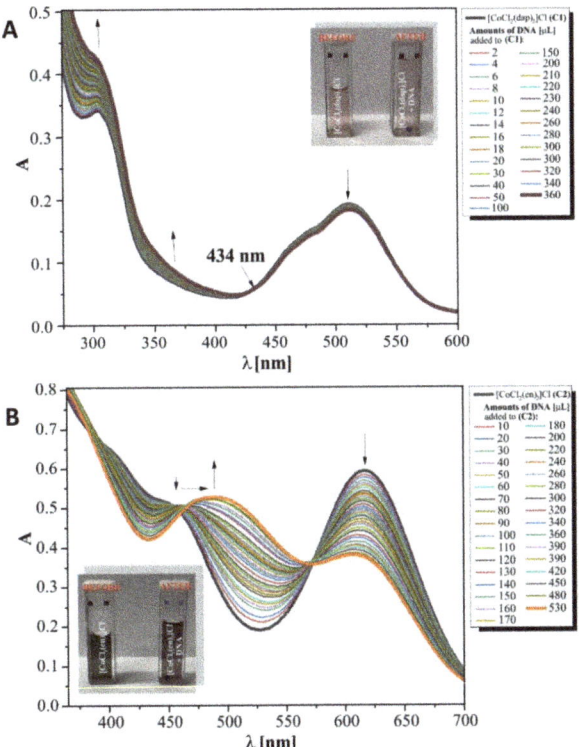

Figure 6. Electronic spectral titration of complex (**1**) and (**2**) with DNA (pBR322) in Tris–HCl buffer, pH 7.39; (**A**): (C1) = 25 mM of compound (**1**), [DNA] = 0.27 mM; (**B**): (C2) = 12 mM of compound (**2**); [DNA] = 0.12 mM. The arrows denote the absorbance changes during the gradual increase of DNA concentration. The photos inside present the colour change of complex (**1**) and (**2**) solutions studied.

In order to quantitatively compare the ability and strength binding of both complexes with DNA independently, the binding constant (K_b) was determined by calculation based on the changes in the absorbance of the $\pi \rightarrow \pi^*$ (261 nm) peaks for (**1**) and of d-d transitions (616 nm) for complex (**2**) after the subsequent addition of amounts of DNA in Tris-HCl solutions. The linear relationships received for both complexes studied are presented in Figure 7 and are according to the Wolfe–Shimer equation [42] below:

$$\frac{[DNA]}{\varepsilon_a - \varepsilon_f} = \frac{[DNA]}{\varepsilon_b - \varepsilon_f} + \frac{1}{K_b(\varepsilon_b - \varepsilon_f)}$$

where:
  [DNA] is the concentration of DNA (*E. coli*),
  ε is the appropriate extinction coefficients:
  $\varepsilon_a = A_{obsd}/[complex]$
  ε_f = for the free complexes (**1**) or (**2**)
  ε_b = for compounds (**1**) or (**2**) in the fully bound with DNA form, respectively.

The results obtained for complex (**1**), [CoCl$_2$(dap)$_2$]Cl, from UV–vis titrations suggest that a weak binding mode of interactions between the studied molecules resulted in low hypochromicity with a red shift. Admittedly, we observed wavelengths at 434 nm, whose light absorption by the test mixed solution remained constant. The aforementioned regions discovered suggest that there could be a balance between the components in the solution, but interactions between (**1**) and DNA are rather due to the electrostatic binging mode.

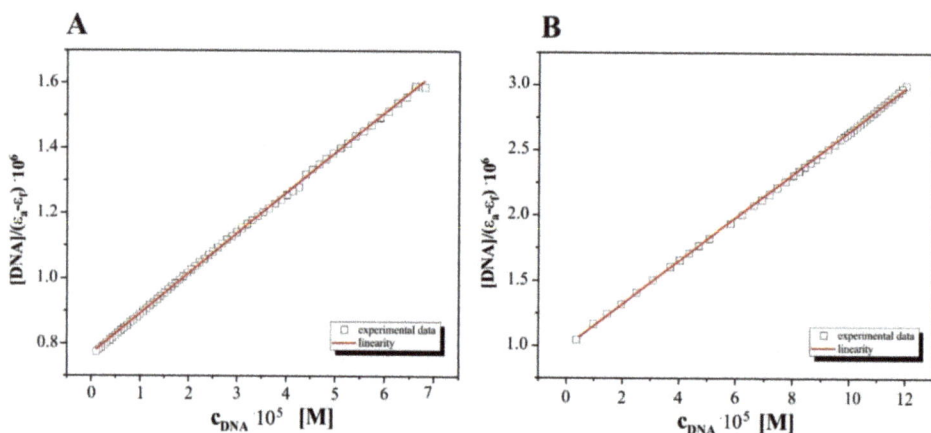

Figure 7. Individual plots of [DNA]/($\varepsilon_a - \varepsilon_f$) vs. [DNA] for the absorption titration of DNA (*E.coli*) with complexes: (**A**). [CoCl$_2$(dap)$_2$]Cl (**1**) and (**B**). [CoCl$_2$(en)$_2$]Cl (**2**) studied in Tris–HCl buffer; association constant K_b: $0.75 \cdot 10^3$ M^{-1} (R = 0.99950, n = 70 experimental points) for (**1**); K_b: $8.0 \cdot 10^5$ M^{-1} (R = 0.99987, n = 46 experimental points) for (**2**).

In our opinion, the results for the interactions of complex (**2**), [CoCl$_2$(en)$_2$]Cl, with DNA of bacteria suggest that it can be assigned as an intercalation type of process. This mode of action is presented by a decrease in absorbance (hypochromism), registered here at 600 nm together with an isosbestic point (575 nm), indicating the equilibria in the medium studied. The value of the binding constants equal to $8.0 \cdot 10^5$ M^{-1} for the studied Complex (**2**)–DNA system suggests that this intercalation mode is quantitatively more competitive with groove binding.

3.5.2. DNA Cleavage Study

Agarose gel electrophoresis was used to evaluate the DNA cleavage ability of compounds (**1**) and (**2**). Different amounts of (**1**) and (**2**) complexes were mixed with a fixed amount of supercoiled pBR322 DNA in the medium of 5 mM Tris-HCl, 50 mM NaCl buffer, pH 7.4, in the presence and absence of H$_2$O$_2$ and incubated for 5, 10, 15, 30, 60, and 120 min at 37 °C. The cleavage patterns of the Co(III) complexes are shown in Figure 8. Control line (DNA in buffer, c) showed a non-cleaved plasmid. The addition of hydrogen peroxide contributed to the active cleavage of the DNA molecule and the appearance of a linear conformation (Form III) of DNA (Figure 8B,C). Compound (**1**) (Figure 8A) did not contribute to a visible change in DNA conformation, and a slight strengthening of the band corresponding to the linear form of DNA (Form III) was observed (Figure 8A). Complex (**2**) (Figure 8A) actively cleaved the plasmid DNA at higher concentrations (1000 and 500 µg/mL). Additionally, DNA retention in the gel well was also observed (Figure 8A, 1000 µg/mL). Furthermore, both complexes cleaved DNA more efficiently in the presence of an oxidant, H$_2$O$_2$, as compared to the control DNA. After 5 min, at a higher concentration of the tested compounds (500 µg/mL), the bands corresponding to the supercoiled form (Form I) of DNA were invisible, and after 2 h, only smears were observed (Figure 8B). The addition of compound (**1**) at a lower concentration (62.5 µg/mL) resulted in the cleavage of DNA into nicked (Form II) and linear forms after 5 min (Figure 8C), while compound (**2**) cleaved DNA into Forms II and III after 10 min (Figure 8C). After 2 h, the DNA completely disappeared from the gel for both Co(III) complexes (Figure 8C). This means that the DNA was damaged.

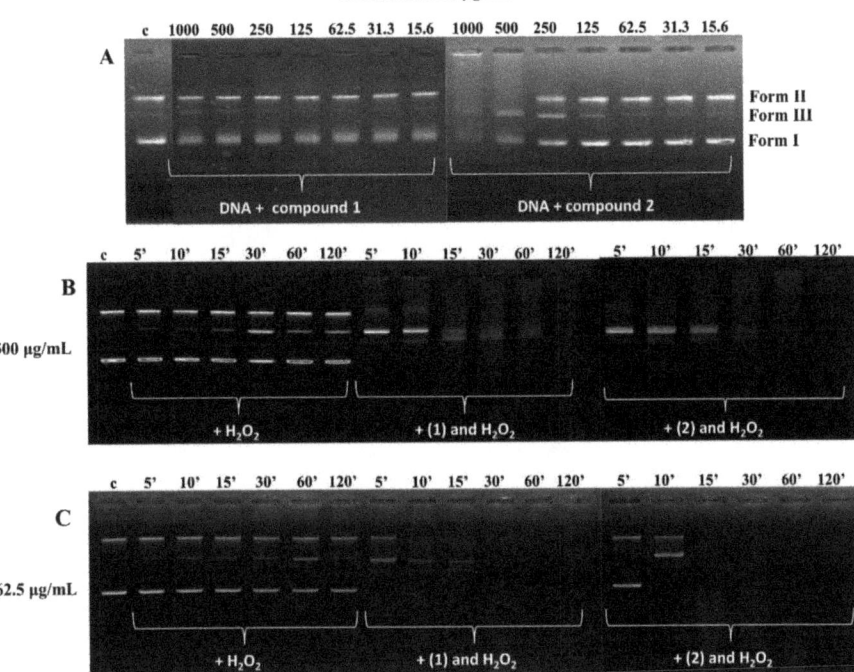

Figure 8. The cleavage of supercoiled pBR322 DNA (62.5 µg/mL) by the complexes at 37 °C in 5 mM Tris HCl, 50 mM NaCl buffer. (**A**)—DNA incubated with compounds (**1**) and (**2**), respectively; c, control line—DNA in buffer (5 mM Tris HCl, 50 mM NaCl) (1:1), 1000–15.6 µg/mL, decreasing concentration of compounds (**1**) and (**2**). (**B**)—DNA incubated with H_2O_2 (100 µM), compound (**1**) (500 µg/mL) + H_2O_2 (100 µM), and (**2**) (500 µg/mL) + H_2O_2 (100 µM), respectively; c, control line—DNA in buffer (5 mM Tris HCl, 50 mM NaCl) (1:1), 5–120 min, time of incubation. (**C**)—DNA incubated with H_2O_2 (100 µM), compound (**1**) (62.5 µg/mL) + H_2O_2 (100 µM) and (**2**) (62.5 µg/mL) + H_2O_2 (100 µM), respectively; c, control line—DNA in buffer (5 mM Tris HCl, 50 mM NaCl) (1:1), 5–120 min, time of incubation.

4. Discussion

4.1. The Minimum Inhibitory Concentration (MIC) and Minimum Bactericidal Concentration (MBC)

In the presented study, two Co(III) complexes with a diamine chelate ligands (en—ethylenediamine; dap—1,3-diaminopropane) were synthesized, and the complete physicochemical as well as biological profiles of both compounds were established. A previous report using a broad spectrum of reference and clinical strains of *Candida* spp. showed strong antifungal activity, especially against *C. glabrata* (MIC 16 µg/mL) [5]. The similar results presented Dias et al. (2020) against *Candida glabrata* strains treated with Co(II) complexes with thiocabamoyl–pyrazoline ligands with an MIC from 3.9 to 15.62 µg/mL [24]. In this research, tested compounds were shown to present anti-bacterial activity against a broad spectrum of bacteria, and no significant differences in the sensitivity of the Gram-positive and Gram-negative bacteria to the test compounds were observed. The bacterial strains *S. pyogenes*, *S. pneumoniae*, *P. acnes*, *C. sporogenes*, and *H. pylori* were assessed as the most sensitive. The most resistant proved to be the strain of *E. faecium* 3844825 (Table 1). Studies performed by Dwyer and Sargeson (1959) concerning an evaluation of the antimicrobial activity of the optical isomers of Co(III) with ethylenediamine as N,N-bidentate ligand [Co(en)$_3$](NO$_3$)$_3$ compared with other metal ion complexes revealed that they exhibit high antimicrobial activity, irrespective of the isomer used [27]. Mishra et al. (2008) also showed strong antibacterial properties of the coordination compounds of cobalt(III) with pyridine-amide tri- or bidentate ligands for *P. aeruginosa*, *E. coli*, *S. flexneri*, and *K. planticola* [28].

In our work, the MIC values for Co(III) complexes against bacteria (*Streptococcus* spp., *H. pylori*, *C. sporogenes*, or *P. acnes*) grown under anaerobic and microaerophilic conditions were the lowest. To evaluate whether the respiration conditions affect the MIC values of tested complexes, several relatively anaerobic bacterial species, reference and clinical strains of *S. aureus* and *E. coli*, were examined under anaerobic conditions. The obtained results illustrated the lack of influence of the oxygen accessibility in the culture on the anti-bacterial activity of the Co(III) compounds, as compared to studies under aerobic conditions, as MIC results have not changed. However, more tests need to be carried out on a broader spectrum of bacteria strains. Suller and Lloyd (2001) showed in their work that MIC values of vancomycin against *S. aureus* were similar whether tested aerobically or anaerobically [43]. In turn, Oliveira et al. (2019) showed that the Schiff-base ligands and their silver(I) and bismuth(III) complexes were inactive against Gram-positive and Gram-negative aerobic bacteria but were highly active against anaerobic strains. The authors suggested that the mode of action of the tested compounds probably involves the anaerobic reduction of the nitro group by the microorganisms, with a formation of metabolites that are toxic to the tested microorganisms [44].

4.2. Serial Passages Assay

We also accessed multi-step resistance studies to evaluate antimicrobial resistance development. Multi-step resistance studies allow for the determination of the effect of the selective pressure of antimicrobials on bacteria, causing the acquisition of mutations at the genetic level [45,46]. These studies involve exposing the bacteria to the sub-inhibitory concentration of antimicrobial agents over many passages, allowing for the formation of resistance mutation over time [47]. In this study, 20 consecutive passages were performed with four strains of bacteria, *S. aureus* ATCC 6538, *S. aureus* MRSA 6347, *P. aeruginosa* ATCC 9027, and *P. aeruginosa* 12274, cultured in a medium supplemented with Compounds (1) and (2) below their MIC values. No significant reduction in the tested bacterial susceptibility to Co(III) compounds was observed. For these compounds, the active concentration after 20 passages was two (*S. aureus* ATCC 6538) or four (*S. aureus* MRSA 6347) times as high as the initial MIC. Only in the case of *P. aeruginosa* for Compound (1) did the MIC value remain at the same level as the initial MIC. The studies assessing bacterial resistance by Mohammad et al. (2017) showed that MIC values for ciprofloxacin against *S. aureus* MRSA increased sevenfold after 14 passages [48]. The study by D'Lima et al. [49] showed that MIC values for reference strains of *S. aureus* ATCC 29213 and *P. aeruginosa* PAO1 for ciprofloxacin after 25 passages increased by about 32 times and for *E. coli* ATCC 25922 by 256 times.

4.3. Synergy Assay

The synergy assay was performed for the combination of compounds (1) and (2) with selected antibiotics (ampicillin, gentamicin, ciprofloxacin, nalidixic acid, and polymyxin B) and showed significant reductions in MIC values only in the case of the mixture of the tested complexes with nalidixic acid. Co(III) complexes with diamine chelate ligands enhance the activity of the aforementioned antibiotic. Nalidixic acid (1-ethyl-1,4-dihydro-7-methyl-4-oxo-1,8-naphthiridin-3-carboxylic acid) is a first-generation quinolone antibiotic used for the treatment of urinary tract infections. This antibiotic selectively and reversibly blocks DNA replication in bacteria by inhibiting a subunit of DNA gyrase and topoisomerase IV. The enzyme is inhibited by trapping the cleavage complex (drug–enzyme–DNA complexes) in which the DNA is broken [50]. It is not clear why the addition of compounds (1) and (2) increases the activity of nalidixic acid. It is possible that the tested compounds attach to the cleavage complexes or affect the DNA, thus enhancing the effects of the drug.

4.4. Microscopic Analysis

The effect of Co(III) complexes with diamine chelate ligands on the bacterial cell were also studied by confocal, scanning electron, and transmission electron microscopes. Using the scanning electron microscope, we observed deformations in the morphology of both tested bacteria, *S. aureus* and *P. aeruginosa*, in the presence of compounds (**1**) and (**2**), while the untreated cells were seen intact. Similarly, in the transmission electron microscope analysis, the bacterial cells showed a distorted shape and morphology. Moreover, we observed irregular shapes of the cells, broken cells, and structural disorganization within the cytoplasm. The described changes in bacterial cells may indicate that cell membrane permeability was disrupted. This was confirmed by analysis using a confocal microscope with the newly synthetized photosensitive complex of the type [Co(dap)$_2$FLU]Cl$_2$, where the luminescence of the cells was observed, suggesting cell membrane permeability.

*4.5. Interactions of Compounds (**1**) and (**2**) with DNA*

In this research, we explored the biomolecule affinity of Co(III) diamine complexes by UV–vis titrations. Small molecules, as in our case, can interact selectively with DNA by intercalation and/or groove binding, but the interaction preferences depend on the structure of the DNA-interacting molecules and the nature of the DNA. Small differences in the structure of Co(III) homological complexes may affect the binding types and stability of the complex/DNA adducts. Co(III) complex (**2**), containing a shorter hydrocarbon chain than in the case of complex (**1**), is more favourable for intercalation, in which the moiety can slide between the adjacent base pairs and facilitate the intercalation. The intercalation mode was interpreted in the literature as enhanced π→π* stacking interactions between the aromatic ring of the chromophores and the DNA-base pair's red shift of the peak to a longer wavelength (bathochromism) [51], which we observed during our spectral intermolecular detection between the complex [CoCl$_2$(en)$_2$]Cl (**2**) and the DNA. The value of the binding constants equal to $8.0 \cdot 10^5$ M^{-1} for the studied complex (**2**)–DNA system suggests that this intercalation mode is quantitatively more competitive with groove binding. It can be certainly related to the ionization form of (**2**) formed as a result of the aquatation process, a form that exists at pH 7.4 to interact with the biomolecule [35]. The value of K_b obtained for interactions of the (**1**) complex with DNA is definitely much lower than those above (0.75×10^3 M^{-1}), according to the other interaction mechanism promoted by the Co(III)—dap complex. Liu et al., Zhang et al. and Carter et al. [25,52–54] showed that Co(III) complexes with a surfactant can bind to the DNA in different binding modes on the basis of their structure, charge, and type of ligands. For example, complexes of the surfactant contain several methyl groups that bind to the DNA by van der Waals interactions and hydrophobic interactions. Moreover, Kumar and Arunachalam (2008) exhibited that surfactant-Co(III) complexes, containing ligands ethylenediamine, triethylenetetramine, 2,2′-bipyridyl, or 1,10-phenantroline, have electrostatic interactions, van der Waals interactions, and/or partial intercalative binding [32]. According to our results, the bacterial DNA can be considered as a cellular target for both complexes studied, susceptible to the formation of adducts with the small Co(III)-diamine complexes (**1**) and (**2**).

The cleaving ability (metallonuclease activity) of complexes (**1**) and (**2**) with supercoiled pBR322 DNA by gel electrophoresis was also performed. The experiment was carried out in the presence and absence of hydrogen peroxide as an oxidant. Supercoiled DNA cleavage is controlled by the relaxation of supercoiled circular conformation of pBR322 DNA in nicked, circular, and/or linear conformations. In our study, complex (**2**) effectively cleaved the DNA in a higher concentration. The same effect was obtained by Thamilarasan et al. (2016) with a higher concentration of the complexes ([Co(acac)(bpy)(N$_3$)$_2$·H$_2$O, ([Co(acac)(en)(N$_3$)$_2$ and ([Co(acac)(2-pic)(N$_3$)$_2$, where acac = acetylacetone, bpy = 2,2′-bipyridine, en = ethylenediamine, 2-pic = picolylamine, and NaN$_3$ = sodium azide), and the cleavage was found to be much more efficient [55]. This suggested that the cleavage of pBR322 DNA depends on the concentration of the complexes. The different DNA cleavage efficiency of complexes (**1**) and (**2**), but especially (**2**), may be due to the different binding affinity of the complexes to DNA [56,57], as it has been demonstrated by UV–vis titrations experiments. Moreover, the addition of hydrogen peroxide to the DNA + complex (**1**)/(**2**) mixture contributed to the active cleavage of the DNA molecule after 5 min and caused its degradation after 2 h. This may be attributed to the formation of hydroxyl free radicals. Mahalakshmi and Raman (2013) also proposed the occurrence of this phenomenon in their work [58]. They presented that N-(4-aminophenyl)acetamide-derived Schiff-base mixed ligand complexes with Mn(II), Co(II), Ni(II), Cu(II), and Zn(II) show nuclease activity in the presence of oxidant H_2O_2, which may be due to the increased production of hydroxyl radicals. The scientific literature indicates that the cleavage of double-stranded DNA by small metal complexes involves two mechanisms: oxidative cleavage and hydrolytic cleavage. The first one to initiate the cleavage requires light and oxidative (leads to the formation of reactive oxygen species, such as $^1O_2$, O_2^-, and OH·) and/or reductive agents [59–67], whereas the hydrolytic mechanism requires a *cis*-nucleophile activation to the cleavage of phosphodiester bonds in DNA [68–73]. The results of our studies suggested an oxidative mechanism of cleavage with the formation of hydroxyl free radicals.

The studies aiming to explain the metallo-pharmaceutical action mechanisms are still intensively developing [74–76]. Interestingly, a significant number of reports about metallo-drugs concern the structure–activity relationship (SAR) determination together with the molecular target(s) assignation. The complexes studied in our work contained short *N,N*-donor organic ligands and simple monodentate inorganic ligands (en—ethylenediamine; dap—1,3-diaminopropane) in their composition. The exact mode of action of these compounds is still unexplained. In our previous work on *Candida* species, we suggested that tested complexes can change membrane permeability and damage the mitochondrial membrane or the membrane of the endoplasmic reticulum [5]. In the presented study we observed, using TEM and SEM, visible changes in bacterial cell morphology, and the confocal microscope showed the luminescence of cells as well. These results may indicate a disruption of cell membrane permeability. Tümer et al. (1999) suggested that complexes containing ligands with the N and O donor system might be responsible for the inhibition of enzyme production, since enzymes requiring a free hydroxy group for their activity seem to be particularly sensitive to deactivation by the ions of the complexes [77]. The partial sharing of the central ion positive charge with the donor groups and the possible p-electron delocalization within the whole chelate ring decreases the polarity of the molecule, which in turn causes an increase in the lipophilicity of the complex, which enhances the penetration of the complexes into lipid membranes [19] and the blocking of the metal binding sites in the enzymes of the microorganism. Notably, both Co(III) complexes studied in this work are hydrophilic, low-molecular mass compounds. Indeed, they are polar with high water solubility, and their molar mass does not exceed 300 $g \cdot mol^{-1}$. In our opinion, these properties contribute to the lower antibacterial activity. We also hypothesize that the lower antibacterial activity observed for both diamine-chelate Co(III) compounds are due to the active transport out (efflux pumps) of the bacteria cells. Researchers suggest that efflux pumps may be used by the cell as a first-line defense mechanism, avoiding the drug to reach lethal concentrations [78,79].

In summary, special attention was paid to the characterization of coordination compound action modes and to the interactions' strength. According to the issues discussed above, the possibilities of interactions between complexes (**1**) or (**2**) and the bacterial DNA were planned and examined, and are discussed in detail herein. Studies assessing the interaction of the Co(III) complexes with pBR322 showed a strong mode of interaction in the case of complex (**2**), suggesting an intercalation mode of process, whereas in the case of complex (**1**), these interactions were much weaker and instead indicated an electrostatic binging mode. Kumar and Arunachalam (2008) also proposed the binding of Co(III) complexes with surfactants to DNA as a mode of action of these kind of compounds [29]. Thus, the mode of action of Co(III) complexes with diamine chelate ligands against bacterial cells can be complex, and more studies are necessary to understand the effect of these compounds on bacteria.

5. Conclusions

In this study, we evaluated the antibacterial activity of Co(III) complexes with a simple bidentate inorganic ligands (en = ethylenediamine; dap = 1,3-diaminopropane) on a broad spectrum of Gram-positive and Gram-negative bacteria. The analyzed compounds revealed lower activity against bacteria than tested earlier fungi, and no significant differences in the sensitivity of the Gram-positive and Gram-negative bacteria to the test compounds were observed. We hypothesized that the lower activity of compounds against bacteria from the difficulties of overcoming the barrier created by the lipid membranes of bacterial cells, which hinders possible reactions with the target(s) inside the bacterial cell. We also hypothesize that the lower antibacterial activity observed for both diamine-chelate Co(III) compounds, especially for *Pseudomonas aeruginosa* or *Enterococcus* spp., are due to the active transport out (efflux pumps) of the bacteria cells. It was shown that the bacteria grown under anaerobic and microaerophilic conditions (*Streptococcus* spp., *H. pylori*, *C. sporogenes*, or *P. acnes*) turned out to be the most sensitive. We proved, by conducting experiments using relatively anaerobic bacteria in anaerobic conditions, that oxygen is not a factor affecting the antibacterial activity of the tested complexes. To evaluate the antimicrobial resistance development, the multi-step resistance studies were performed, and they showed no significant reduction in tested bacterial susceptibility to Co(III) compounds, whereas the synergy assay results revealed significant reductions in MIC values in the case of the mixture of the tested complexes with nalidixic acid. We hypothesized that the aforementioned compounds attach to the cleavage complexes or affect the DNA, thus enhancing the effects of the antibiotic. Indeed, the experiments included the DNA interaction of the Co(III) complexes with plasmid DNA (pBR322) using spectrophotometric titration and DNA cleavage ability of compounds by agarose gel electrophoresis methods revealed that complex (**2**) showed a strong interaction with DNA and indicated an intercalative mode of binding to pBR322. Results for complex (**1**) indicated a much weaker binding mode of interaction between molecules and suggested an electrostatic binding mode. Furthermore, the DNA cleavage ability of the compounds showed, by agarose gel electrophoresis methods, nuclease activity, especially in the presence of oxidant H_2O_2 for both complexes. We concluded that this phenomenon may be attributed to the formation of hydroxyl free radicals, but we did not rule out the hydrolytic mechanism of cleavage, highlighting that more tests are needed. Studies using microscopic analysis suggested cell membrane permeability, as evidenced by deformations in the morphology of both tested bacteria.

Finally, we concluded that the mode of action of Co(III) complexes with diamine chelate ligands against bacterial cells can be complex, and a wider spectrum of tests are necessary to understand their antimicrobial effect against bacteria.

Supplementary Materials: The following are available online at https://www.mdpi.com/article/10.3390/pharmaceutics13070946/s1, Figure S1: The Lambert-Beer law presentation used as a calibration curve for determining DNA concentration in Tris-HCl solutions studied, Figure S2: The procedure of selection the optimal concentration of DNA used further as a titrant during spectrophotometric titrations with complex (**2**), Figure S3: The spectrophotometric titration of DNA (*E. coli*) by using the complex (**1**) solution as a titrant, Figure s4: ^1H NMR spectra comparison together with signals assignments requested to confirm the [Co(dap)$_2$FLU]Cl$_2$ structure, Figure S5: ATR spectra of Co(III) complex with neutral dap form (blue spectrum) and anionic form of FLU (fluoresceine) and free fluoresceine sodium salt (black spectrum), Figure S6: The comparison of electronic spectra obtained for buffer solutions: [Co^{III}(dap)$_2$FLU]Cl$_2$ sensor (black), fluoresceine sodium salt FLU (blue) and [Co^{III}Cl$_2$(dap)$_2$]Cl (red); note the similarities and differences between absorption maxima positions in the compounds spectra above 400 nm, Figure S7: The analysis effect as a confirmation of the Co ions presence in the indicator formula: [CoCl$_2$(en)$_2$]Cl (**1**); [CoCl$_2$(dap)$_2$]Cl (**2**); FLU (**3**); [Co(dap)$_2$FLU]Cl$_2$ (**4**), Figure S8: The effect of the qualitative analysis to confirm the Co(III) presence in the formula [Co(dap)$_2$FLU]Cl$_2$, Figure S9: The XRD structural analysis prepared for solid states FLU and *trans*-[CoCl$_2$(dap)$_2$]Cl solid states together with [Co(dap)$_2$FLU]Cl$_2$ designed intentionally as sensor to investigate cell penetration by the motif Co(III) coordinated by two 1,3-diaminepropane ligands as well as it localization inside the fungus cell. Figure S10: The proposed enantiomer structures of the coordination cation formula [Co(dap)$_2$FLU]$^{2+}$, Figure S11: Absorption spectra of complex (**2**) in the presence of DNA (*E. coli*): $c_{(1)}$ = 0.025 M; c_{DNA} = 2.68 × 10^{-4} M; the last spectrum of titration system presented the adduct formed between complex (**2**) and DNA, Figure S12: Absorption spectra of complex (**1**) in the presence of DNA (*E. coli*): $c_{(1)}$ = 12 mM; c_{DNA} = 0.12 mM; the last spectrum of titration system presented the adduct formed between complex (**1**) and DNA.

Author Contributions: Conceptualization, methodology, and investigation, K.T. and A.C.; the biological component, K.T.; the chemical component, A.C.; preparing slides and taking pictures, J.Z. and M.R.; formal analysis, K.T.; writing—original draft preparation, K.T.; writing—review, A.C. and K.W.; editing, K.T. and A.C. All authors have read and agreed to the published version of the manuscript.

Funding: This work was financially supported by the Ministry of Science and Higher Education Republic of Poland from the quality-promoting subsidy under the Leading National Research Centre (KNOW) programme 2012–2017 Faculty of Pharmacy with Subfaculty of Laboratory Medicine [dec. MNiSW-DS-6002-4693-23/WA/12]. The presented project was also maintained by DS/531-T120-D601-20 (University of Gdańsk).

Institutional Review Board Statement: Not applicable.

Informed Consent Statement: Not applicable.

Data Availability Statement: Not applicable.

Acknowledgments: The authors would like to thank Magdalena Płotka (Department of Microbiology, Faculty of Biology, University of Gdańsk, Poland) for the valuable comments.

Conflicts of Interest: The authors declare no conflict of interest.

References

1. Patrick, G.L. *An introduction to Medicinal Chemistry*; Oxford University Press: Oxford, UK, 2001; p. 264.
2. Giordano, T.J.; Palenik, G.J.; Palenik, R.C.; Sullivan, D.A. Preparation and x-ray crystal structure of a seven-coordinate cobalt(II) complex with 2,6-diacetylpyridine bis(2-picolinoylhydrazone. *Inorg. Chem.* **1979**, *18*, 2445. [CrossRef]
3. Rekha, T.H.; Ibrahim, K.M.; Abdallah, A.M.; Hassanian, M.M. Synthesis, spectral and antimicrobial activity studies of *o*-aminoacetophenone *o*-hydroxybenzoylhydrazone complexes. *Synth. React. Inorg. Met. Org. Chem.* **1996**, *26*, 1113.
4. Nawar, N.; Hosny, N.M. Mono- and Bi-nuclerar Schiff base complexes derived from glycine, 3-acetylpyridine and transition metal ions. *Transit. Met. Chem.* **2000**, *25*, 1–8. [CrossRef]
5. Turecka, K.; Chylewska, A.; Kawiak, A.; Waleron, K. Antifungal activity and mechanism of action of the Co(III) coordination complexes with diamine chelate ligands against reference and clinical strains of *Candida* spp. *Front. Microbiol.* **2018**, *9*, 1594. [CrossRef]
6. Da Silva Dantas, F.G.; de Almeida-Apolonio, A.A.; de Araújo, R.P.; Favarin, L.R.V.; de Castilho, P.F.; de Oliveira Galvão, F.; Svidzinski, T.I.E.; Casagrande, G.A.; de Oliveira, K.M.P. A promising copper(II) complex as antifungal and anibiofilm drug against yeast infection. *Molecules* **2018**, *23*, 1856. [CrossRef] [PubMed]
7. Favarin, L.R.V.; Oliveira, L.B.; Silva, H.; Micheletti, A.C.; Pizzuti, L.; Machulek-Júnior, A.; Caires, A.R.L.; Back, D.F.; Lima, S.M.; Andrade, L.H.C.; et al. Sonochemical synthesis of highly luminescent silver complexes: Photophysical properties and preliminary in vitro antitumor and antibacterial assays. *Inorg. Chim. Acta* **2018**, *492*, 235–242. [CrossRef]
8. Favarin, L.R.V.; Laranjeira, G.B.; Teixeira, C.F.A.; Silva, H.; Micheletti, A.C.; Pizzuti, L.; Machulek-Júnior, A.; Caires, A.R.L.; Deflon, V.M.; Pesci, R.R.B.P.; et al. Harvesting greenish blue luminescence in gold(I) complexes and their application as promising bioactive molecules and cellular bioimaging agents. *New J. Chem.* **2020**, *44*, 6862–6871. [CrossRef]
9. Rosenberg, B. Platinum complexes for the treatment of cancer. *Interdiscipl. Sci. Rev.* **1978**, *3*, 134–147. [CrossRef]
10. Sadler, P.J. The biological chemistry of gold. *Struct. Bond.* **1984**, *29*, 171–214. [CrossRef]
11. Clark, M.J.E. *Ruthenium and Other Metal Complexes in Cancer Chemotherapy*; Springer: Heidelberg, Germany, 1989.
12. Cowan, J.A. *Inorganic Biochemistry*, 2nd ed.; Wiley-VCH: New York, NY, USA, 1997.
13. Merchant, B. Gold, the noble metal and the paradoxes of its toxicology. *Biologicals* **1998**, *26*, 49–59. [CrossRef]
14. Bertini, L.; Gray, H.B.; Stiefel, E.I.; Valentine, J.S. *Biological Inorganic Chemistry: Structure and Rectivity*; University Science Books: Sausalito, CA, USA, 2007.
15. Walker, G.W.; Gene, R.J.; Sargeson, A.M.; Behm, C.A. Surface-active cobalt cage complexes: Synthesis, surface chemistry, biological activity, and redox properties. *Dalton Trans.* **2003**, 2992–3001. [CrossRef]
16. Yilmaz, I.; Cukurovali, A. Characterization and Antimicrobial Activity of the Schiff Bases Derived from 2,4-Disubstituted Thiazole and 3-Methoxy Salicylaldehyde and Their Cobalt(II), Copper(II), Nickel(II) and Zinc(II) Complexes. *Trans Met. Chem.* **2003**, *28*, 399–404. [CrossRef]

17. Liang, F.; Wang, P.; Zhou, X.; Li, T.; Li, Z.; Lin, H.; Gao, D.; Zheng, C.; Wu, C. Nickle(II) and cobalt(II) complexes of hydroxyl-substituted triazamacrocyclic ligand as potential antitumor agents. *Bioorg Med. Chem Lett.* **2004**, *14*, 1901–1904. [CrossRef] [PubMed]
18. Belicchi-Ferrari, M.; Bisceglie, F.; Casoli, C.; Durot, S.; Morgerstern-Badarau, I.; Pelosi, G.; Pilloti, E.; Pinelli, S.; Tarasconi, P. Copper(II) and Cobalt(III) Pyridoxal Thiosemicarbazone Complexes with Nitroprusside as Counterion: Syntheses, Electronic Properties, and Antileukemic Activity. *J. Med. Chem.* **2005**, *48*, 1671–1679. [CrossRef] [PubMed]
19. Lv, J.; Liu, T.; Cai, S.; Wang, X.; Liu, L.; Wang, Y. Synthesis, structure and biological activity of cobalt(II) and copper(II) complexes of valine-derived schiff bases. *J. Inorg. Biochem.* **2006**, *100*, 1888–1896. [CrossRef]
20. Zhong, X.; Yi, J.; Sun, J.; Wei, H.L.; Liu, W.S.; Yu, K.B. Synthesis and crystal structure of some transition metal complexes with a novel bis-Schiff base ligand and their antitumor activities. *Eur. J. Med. Chem.* **2006**, *41*, 1090–1092. [CrossRef] [PubMed]
21. Bisceglie, F.; Baldini, M.; Belicchi-Ferrari, M.; Buluggiu, E.; Careri, M.; Pelosi, G.; Pinelli, S.; Tarasconi, P. Metal complexes of retinoid derivatives with antiproliferative activity: Synthesis, characterization and DNA interaction studies. *Eur. J. Med. Chem.* **2007**, *42*, 627–634. [CrossRef]
22. Penumaka, N.; Satyanarayana, S. DNA Binding and Photocleavage Studies of Cobalt(III) Polypyridine Complexes: [Co(en)2PIP]3+, [Co(en)2IP]3+, and [Co(en)2phen-dione]3+. *Bioinorg. Chem. Appl.* **2007**, *8*, 1–8. [CrossRef]
23. Konidaris, K.F.; Raptopoulou, C.P.; Psycharis, V.; Perlepes, S.P.; Manessi-Zoupa, E.; Stamatatos, T.C. Use of the 2-Pyridinealdoxime/N,N′-Donor Ligand Combination in Cobalt (III) Chemistry: Synthesis and Characterization of Two Cationic Mononuclear Cobalt (III) Complexes. *Bioinorg. Chem. Appl.* **2010**, *7*, 1–7. [CrossRef] [PubMed]
24. Dias, B.B.; da Silva Dantas, F.G.; Galvão, F.; Cupozk-Pinheiro, W.J.; Wender, H.; Pizzuti, L.; Rosa, P.P.; Tenório, K.V.; Gatto, C.C.; Negri, M.; et al. Synthesis, structural characteryzation, and prospects for new cobalt (II) complexes with tiocarbamoyl-pyrazoline ligands as promising antifungal agents. *J. Ion. Bioch.* **2020**, *213*, 111277. [CrossRef] [PubMed]
25. Carter, M.T.; Rodriguez, M.; Bard, A.J. Voltammetric studies of the interaction of metal chelates with DNA. 2. Tris-chelated complexes of co(III) and iron(III) with 1,10-phenanthroline and 2,2′-bipyridine. *J. Am. Chem. Soc.* **1989**, *111*, 8901–8911. [CrossRef]
26. Jungwirth, U.; Kowol, C.R.; Keppler, B.K.; Hartinger, C.G.; Berger, W.; Heffeter, P. Anticancer Activity of Metal Complexes: Involvement of Redox Processes. Europe PubMed Central. *Antioxid Redox Signal.* **2011**, *15*, 1085–1127. [CrossRef] [PubMed]
27. Dwyer, F.P.; Sargeson, A.M. Stereospecific Influences in Metal Complexes Containing Optically Active Ligands. III. The Reaction of Dichlorobis-(ethylenediamine)-cobalt(III) Chloride with levoprophylenediamine. *J. Am. Chem. Soc.* **1959**, *81*, 5269–5272. [CrossRef]
28. Mishra, A.; Kaushik, N.K.; Verma, A.K.; Gupta, R. Synthesis, characterization and antibacterial activity of cobalt(III) complexes with pyridine–amide ligands. *Eur. J. Med. Chem.* **2008**, *43*, 2189–2196. [CrossRef] [PubMed]
29. Asbell, P.A.; Epstein, S.P.; Wallace, J.A.; Epstein, D.; Stewart, C.C.; Burger, R.M. Efficacy of kobalt chelates in the Rabbit eye model for epithelial herpetic keratitis. *Cornea* **1998**, *17*, 550–557. [PubMed]
30. Brown, J.M. The Hypoxic Cell: A Target for Selective Cancer Theraphy—Eighteenth Bruce F. Cain Memorial Award Lecture. *Cancer Res.* **1999**, *59*, 5863–5870. [PubMed]
31. Dachs, G.U.; Tozer, G.M. Hypoxia modulated gene expression: Angiogenesis, metatesis and therapeutic exploitation. *Eur. J. Cancer* **2000**, *36*, 1649–1660. [CrossRef]
32. Kumar, R.S.; Arunachalam, S. Synthesis, micellar properties, DNA binding and antimicrobial studies of some surfactant-cobalt(III) complexes. *Biophys. Chem.* **2008**, *136*, 136–144. [CrossRef]
33. El-Ayaan, U.; Abdel-Aziz, A.A.M. Synthesis, antimicrobial activity and molecular modeling of cobalt and nickel complexes containing the bulky ligand: Bis[N-(2,6-diisopropylphenyl)imino]acenaphthene. *Eur. J. Med. Chem.* **2005**, *40*, 1214–1221. [CrossRef]
34. Chylewska, A.; Biedulsak, M.; Sumczyński, P.; Makowski, M. Metallopharmaceuticals in therapy—A new horizon for scientific research. *Cur. Med. Chem.* **2018**, *25*, 1729–1791. [CrossRef]
35. Chylewska, A.; Turecka, K.; Dąbrowska, A.; Werel, W.; Chmurzyński, L. Synthesis, physicochemical characterization and antimicrobial activity of Co (III) complexes with diamine chelate ligands. *IJAPBC* **2013**, *2*, 454–464.
36. Meletiadis, J.; Verweji, P.E.; TeDorsthorst, T.A.; Meis, J.F.G.M.; Mouton, J.W. Assessing in vitro combinations of antifungal drugs against yeasts and filamentous fungi: Comparison of different drug interaction models. *Med. Mycol.* **2005**, *43*, 133–152. [CrossRef] [PubMed]
37. Odds, F.C. Synergy, antagonism, and what the chequerboard puts between them. *J Ant. Chem.* **2003**, *52*, 1. [CrossRef]
38. Banasiuk, R.; Frackowiak, J.E.; Krychowiak, M.; Matuszewska, M.; Kawiak, A.; Ziabka, M.; Lendzion-Bielun, Z.; Narajczyk, M.; Królicka, A. Synthesis of antimicrobial silver nanoparticles through a photomediated reaction in an aqueous environment. *Inter. J. Nanomed.* **2016**, *11*, 315–324. [CrossRef]
39. Khan, I.; Bahuguna, A.; Kumar, P.; Bajpal, V.K.; Kang, S.C. Antimicrobial Potential of Carvacrol against Uropathogenic Escherichia coli via Membrane Disruption, Depolarization, and Reactive Oxygen Species Generation. *Front. Microbiol.* **2017**, *8*, 2421. [CrossRef]
40. Reichmann, M.E.; Rice, S.A.; Thomas, C.A.; Doty, P.A. Further Examination of the Molecular Weight and Size of Desoxypentose Nucleic Acid. *J. Am. Chem. Soc.* **1954**, *76*, 3047–3053. [CrossRef]

41. Bouwman, E.; Day, R.; Driessen, W.L.; Tremel, W.; Krebs, B.; Wood, J.S.; Reedijk, J. Two different copper(II) coordination geometries imposed by two closely related chelating imidazole-thioether (N2S2) ligands. Crystal structures of (1,6-bis(4-imidazolyl)-2,5-dithiahexane)chlorocopper(II) tetrafluoroborate, (1,6-bis(5-methyl-4-imidazolyl)-2,5-dithiahexane)chloro (tetrafluoroborato)copper(II), and (1,6-bis(5-methyl-4-imidazolyl)-2,5-dithiahexane)nitrato(thiocyanato-N)copper(II). *Inorg. Chem.* **1988**, *27*, 4614–4618. [CrossRef]
42. Vijayalakshmi, R.; Kanthimathi, M.; Subramanian, V.; Nair, B.U. Interaction of DNA with [Cr(Schiff base)(H$_2$O)$_2$]ClO$_4$. *Biochim. Biophys. Acta* **2000**, *1475*, 157–162. [CrossRef]
43. Suller, M.T.E.; Lloyd, D. The antibacterial activity of vancomycin towards *Staphylococcus aureus* under aerobic and anaerobic conditions. *J Appl. Microbiol.* **2001**, *92*, 866–872. [CrossRef]
44. Oliveira, A.P.A.; Ferreira, J.F.G.; Farias, L.M.; Magalhães, P.P.; Teixeira, L. l R.; Beraldo, H. Antimicrobial Effects of Silver(I) and Bismuth(III) Complexes with Secnidazole-Derived Schiff Base Ligands: The Role of the Nitro Group Reduction. *J. Braz. Chem. Soc.* **2019**, *30*, 2299–2307. [CrossRef]
45. Martinez, J.L.; Baquero, F.; Andersson, D.I. Beyond serial passages: New methods for predicting the emergence of resistance to novel antibiotics. *Curr. Opin. Pharmacol.* **2011**, *11*, 439–445. [CrossRef] [PubMed]
46. Davies, T.A.; Pankuch, G.A.; Dewasse, B.E.; Jacobs, M.R.; Appelbaum, P.C. In vitro development of resistance to five quinolones and amoxicillin-claulanate in *Streptococcus pneumoniae*. *Antimicrob. Agents Chemother.* **1999**, *42*, 1177–1182. [CrossRef] [PubMed]
47. Clark, C.; McGhee, P.; Appelbaum, P.C.; Kosowska-Shick, K. Multistep resistance development studies of ceftaroline in gram-positive and -negative bacteria. *Antimicrob. Agents Chemother.* **2011**, *55*, 2344–2351. [CrossRef]
48. Mohammad, H.; Younis, W.; Ezzat, H.G.; Peters, C.E.; Abdel-Khalek, A.; Cooper, B.; Pogliano, K.; Pogliano, J.; Mayhoub, A.S.; Seleem, M.N. Bacteriological profiling of diphenylureas as a novel class of antibiotics against methicillin-resistant *Staphylococcus aureus*. *PLoS ONE* **2017**, *12*, 6. [CrossRef]
49. D'Lima, L.; Friedman, L.; Wang, L.; Xu, P.; Anderson, M.; Debabov, D. No Decrease in Susceptibility to NVC-422 in Multiple-Passage Studies with Methicillin-Resistant *Staphylococcus aureus*, *S. aureus*, *Pseudomonas aeruginosa*, and *Escherichia coli*. *Antimicrob Agents Chemother.* **2012**, *56*, 2753–2755. [CrossRef]
50. Pommier, Y.; Leo, E.; Zhang, H.; Marchand, C. DNA topoisomerases and their poisoning by anticancer and antibacterial drugs. *Chem. Biol.* **2010**, *17*, 421–433. [CrossRef]
51. Shahabadi, N.; Kashanian, S.; Purfoulad, M. DNA interaction studies of a platinum(II) complex, PtCl$_2$(NN) (NN = 4,7-dimethyl-1,10-phenanthroline), using different instrumental methods. *Spectrochim. Acta Part A* **2009**, *72*, 757–761. [CrossRef] [PubMed]
52. Liu, J.; Zhang, T.; Lu, T.; Qu, L.; Zhou, H.; Zhang, Q.; Ji, L. DNA-binding and cleavage studies of macrocyclic copper(II) complexes. *J. Inorg. Biochem.* **2002**, *91*, 269–276. [CrossRef]
53. Liu, J.; Zhang, C.; Chen, H.; Deng, T.; Lu, T.; Ji, L. Interaction of macrocyclic copper(II) complexes with calf thymus DNA: Effects of the side chains of the ligands on the DNA-binding behaviors. *Dalton Trans.* **2003**, 114–119. [CrossRef]
54. Zhang, S.; Zhu, Y.; Tu, C.; Wei, H.; Yang, Z.; Lin, L.; Ding, J.; Zhang, Z.; Guo, A. A novel cytotoxic ternary copper(II) complex of 1,10-phenantroline and L-threonine with DNA nuclease activity. *J. Inorg Biochem.* **2004**, *98*, 2099–2106. [CrossRef]
55. Thamilarasan, V.; Sengottuvelan, N.; Sudha, A.; Srinivasan, P.; Chakkaravarthi, G. Cobalt(III) complexes as potential anticancer agents: Physicochemical, structural, cytotoxic activity and DNA/protein interactions. *J. Photochem. Photobiol. B Biol.* **2016**, *162*, 558–569. [CrossRef]
56. Haribabu, J.; Jeyallakshmi, K.; Arun, Y.; Bhuvanesh, N.S.P.; Perumal, P.T.; Karvembu, R. Synthesis, DNA/protein binding, molecular docking, DNA cleavage and in vitro anticancer activity of nickel(II) bis(thiosemicarbazone) complexes. *RSC Adv.* **2015**, *5*, 46031–46049. [CrossRef]
57. Kumar, M.P.; Tejaswi, S.; Rambabu, A.; Kalalbandi, V.K.A. Synthesis, crystal structure, DNA binding and cleavage studies of cooper(II) complexes with isoxazole Schiff bases. *Polyhedron* **2015**, *102*, 111–120. [CrossRef]
58. Mahalakshmi, R.; Raman, N. Enthused research on DNA-binding and DNA-cleavage aptitude of mixed ligand metal complexes. *Spectrochim. Acta A Mol. Biomol. Spectrosc.* **2013**, *112*, 198–205. [CrossRef] [PubMed]
59. Van Eldik, R.; Reedijk, J. *Advances in Inorganic Chemistry: Homogeneous Biomimetic Oxidation Catalysis*; Elsevier: Amsterdam, The Netherlands, 2006.
60. Qian, L.; Browne, W.R.; Roelfes, G. DNA cleavage activity of Fe(II)N4Py under photo irradiation in the presence of 1,8-naphthalimide and 9-aminocridine: Unexpected effects of reactive oxygen species scavengers. *Inorg. Chem.* **2011**, *50*, 8318–8325. [CrossRef]
61. Qian, L.; Browne, W.R.; Roelfes, G. Photoenhanced oxidative DNA cleavage with non-heme iron(II) complexes. *Inorg. Chem.* **2010**, *49*, 11009–11017. [CrossRef]
62. Zhao, Y.; Zhu, J.; He, W.; Yang, Z.; Zhu, Z.; Li, Y.; Zhang, J.; Guo, Z. Oxidative DNA cleavage promoted by multinuclear copper complexes: Activity dependence on the complex structure. *Chem.-Eur. J.* **2006**, *12*, 6621–6629. [CrossRef]
63. Uma, V.; Kanthimathi, M.; Nair, B.U. Oxidative DNA cleavage mediated by a new cooper(II) terpyridine complex: Crystal structure and DNA binding studies. *J. Inorg. Biochem.* **2005**, *99*, 2299–2307. [CrossRef]
64. Li, D.D.; Tian, J.L.; Gu, W.; Liu, X.; Zeng, H.H.; Yan, S.P. DNA binding, oxidative DNA cleavage, cytotoxicity and apoptosis-inducing activity of cooper(II) complexes with 1,4-Tpbd(N,N,N'N'-tetrakis(2-yridylme- thyl)benzene-1,4-diamine) ligand. *J. Inorg. Bioch.* **2011**, *105*, 894–901. [CrossRef]

65. Li, D.D.; Huang, F.P.; Chen, G.J.; Gao, C.Y.; Tian, J.L.; Gu, W.; Liu, X.; Yan, S.P. Four new copper(II) complexes with 1,3-tpbd ligand: Synthesis, crystal structures, magnetism, oxidative and hydrolytic cleavage of pBR322 DNA. *J. Inorg. Bioch.* **2009**, *104*, 431–441. [CrossRef] [PubMed]
66. Prakash, H.; Shodai, A.; Yasui, H.; Sakurai, H.; Hirota, S. Photocontrol of Spatial Orientation and DNA Cleavage Activity of Copper(II)-Bound Dipeptides Linked by an Azobenzene Derivative. *Inorg. Chem.* **2008**, *47*, 5045–5047. [CrossRef]
67. Li, H.; Le, X.Y.; Pang, D.W.; Deng, H.; Xu, Z.H.; Lin, Z.H. DNA-binding and cleavage studies of novel copper(II) complex with L-phenylalaninate and 1,4,8,9-tetra-aza-triphenylene ligands. *J. Inorg. Biochem.* **2005**, *99*, 2240–2247. [CrossRef]
68. Xu, W.; Louka, F.; Doulain, P.E.; Landry, C.A.; Mautner, F.A.; Massoud, S.S. Hydrolytic cleavage of DNA promoted by cobalt(III)–tetraamine complexes: Synthesis and characterization of carbonatobis [2-(2-pyridylethyl)]-(2-pyridylmethyl)aminecobalt(III) perchlorate. *Polyhedron* **2009**, *28*, 1221–1228. [CrossRef]
69. Massoud, S.S.; Perkins, R.S.; Louka, F.R.; Xu, W.; LeRoux, A.; Dutercq, Q.; Fischer, R.C.; Mautner, F.A.; Handa, M.; Hiraoka, Y.; et al. Efficient hydrolytic cleavage of plasmid DNA by chloro-cobalt(II) complexes based on sterically hindered pyridyl tripod tetraamine ligands: Synthesis, crystal structure and DNA cleavage. *Dalton. Trans.* **2014**, *43*, 10086–10103. [CrossRef]
70. Molenveld, P.; Engbersen, J.F.J.; Reinhoudt, D.N. Dinuclear metallo-phosphodiesterase models: Application of calix [4]arenes as molecular scaffolds. *Chem. Soc. Rev.* **2000**, *29*, 75–86. [CrossRef]
71. Jin, Y.; Lewis, M.A.; Gokhale, N.H.; Long, E.C.; Cowan, J.A. Influence of Stereochemistry and Redox Potentials on the Single- and Double-Strand DNA Cleavage Efficiency of Cu(II)· and Ni(II)·Lys-Gly-His-Derived ATCUN Metallopeptides. *J. Am. Chem. Soc.* **2007**, *129*, 8353–8361. [CrossRef] [PubMed]
72. Jin, Y.; Cowan, A. DNA Cleavage by Copper—ATCUN Complexes. Factors Influencing Cleavage Mechanism and Linearization of dsDNA. *J. Am. Chem. Soc.* **2005**, *127*, 8408–8415. [CrossRef]
73. Jiang, Q.; Xiao, N.; Shi, P.; Zhu, Y.; Guo, Z. Design of artificial metallonucleases with oxidative mechanism. *Coord. Chem. Rev.* **2007**, *251*, 1951–1972. [CrossRef]
74. Turel, I.; Kljun, J. Interactions of Metal Ions with DNA, Its Constituents and Derivatives, which may be Relevant for Anticancer Research. *Curr. Top. Med. Chem.* **2011**, *11*, 2661–2687. [CrossRef]
75. Ahmadi, R.A.; Amani, S.S. Synthesis, Spectroscopy, Thermal Analysis, Magnetic Properties and Biological Activity Studies of Cu(II) and Co(II) Complexes with Schiff Base Dye Ligands. *Molecules* **2012**, *17*, 6434–6448. [CrossRef]
76. Muhammad, N.; Guo, Z. Metal-based anticancer chemotherapeutic agents. *Curr. Opin. Chem. Biol.* **2014**, *19*, 144–153. [CrossRef]
77. Tümer, M.; Köksal, H.; Serin, S.; Dig, M. Antimicrobial activity studies of mononuclear and binuclear mixed-ligand copper (II) complexes derived from Schiff base ligands and 1,10-phenantroline. *Transit. Met. Chem.* **1999**, *24*, 13–17. [CrossRef]
78. Costa, S.S.; Viveiros, M.; Amaral, L.; Couto, I. Multidrug efflux pumps in *Staphylococcus aureus*: An uptade. *Open Microbiol. J.* **2013**, *7* (Suppl. 1-M5), 59–71. [CrossRef] [PubMed]
79. Anes, J.; McCusker, M.P.; Fanning, S.; Martins, M. The ins and outs of RND efflux pumps in *Escherichia coli*. *Front. Microbiol.* **2015**, *6*, 587. [CrossRef] [PubMed]

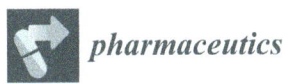

Article

Ceftriaxone Mediated Synthesized Gold Nanoparticles: A Nano-Therapeutic Tool to Target Bacterial Resistance

Farhan Alshammari [1], Bushra Alshammari [2], Afrasim Moin [1], Abdulwahab Alamri [3], Turki Al Hagbani [1], Ahmed Alobaida [1], Abu Baker [4], Salman Khan [4] and Syed Mohd Danish Rizvi [1,*]

1. Department of Pharmaceutics, College of Pharmacy, University of Ha'il, Ha'il 81442, Saudi Arabia; frh.alshammari@uoh.edu.sa (F.A.); afrasimmoin@yahoo.co.in (A.M.); t.alhagbani@uoh.edu.sa (T.A.H.); a.alobaida@uoh.edu.sa (A.A.)
2. Department of Medical Surgical Nursing, College of Nursing, University of Ha'il, Ha'il 81442, Saudi Arabia; bu.alshammari@uoh.edu.sa
3. Department of Pharmacology and Toxicology, College of Pharmacy, University of Ha'il, Ha'il 81442, Saudi Arabia; a.alamry@uoh.edu.sa
4. Nanomedicine and Nanotechnology Lab, Department of Biosciences, Integral University, Lucknow 226026, India; karimabubaker@gmail.com (A.B.); salmank@iul.ac.in (S.K.)
* Correspondence: syeddanishpharmacy@gmail.com

Abstract: Ceftriaxone has been a part of therapeutic regime for combating some of the most aggressive bacterial infections in the last few decades. However, increasing bacterial resistance towards ceftriaxone and other third generation cephalosporin antibiotics has raised serious clinical concerns especially due to their misuse in the COVID-19 era. Advancement in nanotechnology has converted nano-therapeutic vision into a plausible reality with better targeting and reduced drug consumption. Thus, in the present study, gold nanoparticles (GNPs) were synthesized by using ceftriaxone antibiotic that acts as a reducing as well as capping agent. Ceftriaxone-loaded GNPs (CGNPs) were initially characterized by UV-visible spectroscopy, DLS, Zeta potential, Electron microscopy and FT-IR. However, a TEM micrograph showed a uniform size of 21 ± 1 nm for the synthesized CGNPs. Further, both (CGNPs) and pure ceftriaxone were examined for their efficacy against *Escherichia coli*, *Staphylococcus aureus*, *Salmonella abony* and *Klebsiella pneumoniae*. CGNPs showed MIC_{50} as 1.39, 1.6, 1.1 and 0.9 µg/mL against *E. coli*, *S. aureus*, *S. abony* and *K. pneumoniae*, respectively. Interestingly, CGNPs showed two times better efficacy when compared with pure ceftriaxone against the tested bacterial strains. Restoring the potential of unresponsive or less efficient ceftriaxone via gold nanoformulations is the most alluring concept of the whole study. Moreover, applicability of the findings from bench to bedside needs further validation.

Keywords: antibiotics; antibacterial resistance; ceftriaxone; gold nanoparticles; MIC_{50}

Citation: Alshammari, F.; Alshammari, B.; Moin, A.; Alamri, A.; Al Hagbani, T.; Alobaida, A.; Baker, A.; Khan, S.; Rizvi, S.M.D. Ceftriaxone Mediated Synthesized Gold Nanoparticles: A Nano-Therapeutic Tool to Target Bacterial Resistance. *Pharmaceutics* **2021**, *13*, 1896. https://doi.org/10.3390/pharmaceutics13111896

Academic Editors: Corneliu Tanase, Valentina Uivarosi and Aura Rusu

Received: 5 October 2021
Accepted: 5 November 2021
Published: 8 November 2021

Publisher's Note: MDPI stays neutral with regard to jurisdictional claims in published maps and institutional affiliations.

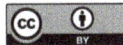

Copyright: © 2021 by the authors. Licensee MDPI, Basel, Switzerland. This article is an open access article distributed under the terms and conditions of the Creative Commons Attribution (CC BY) license (https://creativecommons.org/licenses/by/4.0/).

1. Introduction

According to Centers for Disease Control and Prevention (CDC) threat report on antibiotic resistance (2019) [1], every year around 2.8 million cases of resistant bacterial infection occur in the United States alone with 35 K mortality. However, COVID-19 co-infection with antibiotic-resistant bacterial pathogens has raised a serious clinical issue now-adays. The situation has worsened due to the increasing trend of self-medication of antibiotics in the COVID-19 era [2]. One such antibiotic is ceftriaxone, and scientists have grave concerns over the cautious use of antibiotics in COVID-19 management [3]. In fact, ceftriaxone is often prescribed to treat a wide range of bacterial infections, such as meningitis, bone infections, joints, middle ear, intra-abdominal, skin, and pelvic inflammatory diseases [4]. On the other hand, ceftriaxone resistance has also increased many fold in the recent past [5–7]. Thus, alternative novel approaches to tackle the current scenario are urgently needed, and nanotechnology appears to deliver a plausible solution to these resistant issues.

Application of nanoparticles in different fields of medicine has gained worldwide acceptance because of their unique physical and bio-chemical features, and controlled drug release ability [8]. In the past few years, several inorganic nanoparticles with antibacterial potential have been developed, such as gold nanoparticles, silver nanoparticles, zinc oxide nanoparticles, and titanium dioxide nanoparticles [9–15]. These inorganic nanoparticles can inhibit bacterial growth by various mechanisms such as hindering replication and transcription process, DNA damage via direct interaction, increasing reactive oxygen species, destroying the cell wall, etc. [13]. Importantly, they have shown effectiveness against resistant bacterial strains [14,15].

Among the different inorganic nanoparticles, gold nanoparticles (GNPs) are of major interest in diverse research fields such as therapeutics, antimicrobials, catalysis, and biomolecular detection [16–18]. A two-fold increase in antibiotic activity was observed when ampicillin was conjugated with chitosan-capped GNPs, compared to free ampicillin [9]. GNPs capped with Human Serum Albumin (HSA) have been used for the successful delivery of antibiotics of the amino-glycosidic group, such as sulfates of streptomycin, neomycin, gentamicin, and kanamycin [19]. Similarly, sericin-capped silver and GNPs have shown marked activity against both Gram-negative and Gram-positive bacteria [20]. In addition, silver and GNPs have shown the ability to overcome ampicillin and cefaclor resistance [21], although, GNPs are considered more biocompatible and safe than silver nanoparticles [22,23].

All these findings incited us to explore solution(s) for expanding ceftriaxone resistance via applying GNPs as a nano-carrier. The thought behind the current study is to increase ceftriaxone strength by loading them onto GNPs. The study involved synthesis of GNPs by employing ceftriaxone as a reducing and capping agent, and to boost ceftriaxone antibacterial potential in a coordinated manner against *Escherichia coli, Staphylococcus aureus, Salmonella abony* and *Klebsiella pneumoniae*.

2. Materials and Methods

2.1. Materials

All the chemicals, microbiological media and reagents, such as, Mueller–Hinton agar, ceftriaxone sodium and tetra chloroauric [III] acid (HAHuCl$_4$) were procured from Sigma–Aldrich (St. Louis, MO, USA).

2.2. Ceftriaxone-Mediated Synthesis of GNPs (CGNPs)

The reaction for the synthesis of CGNPs was performed at temperatures of 30 °C, 40 °C, 50 °C and 60 °C by adding ceftriaxone at concentrations of 50, 100, 150, 200, and 250 µg/mL to a 1 mL reaction mixture and incubating for 48 h. However, the reaction mixture consisted of 1 mM HAuCl$_4$ in 50 mM phosphate buffer at pH 7.4.

An autonomous reaction was performed for the control without ceftriaxone. At ten distinct time points, the mixture was removed and analyzed by UV-visible spectroscopy. The CGNPs were collected by centrifugation at 30,000× g for 30 min after the completion of the reaction. The CGNPs were then washed twice by Milli Q water followed by a final wash with 50% v/v ethanol to remove unbounded materials. For further analysis, the resultant CGNPs were used. For comparative analysis, the Khan et al. [24] method was applied to synthesize GNPs by bromelain (where bromelain acts as a reducing as well as stabilizing agent) to keep them as control naked GNPs (without ceftriaxone).

2.3. Characterization of CGNPs

2.3.1. UV/Vis Spectroscopy

The GNPs (control) and CGNPs were characterized via UV-vis spectrophotometry using a Shimadzu dual-beam spectrophotometer (UV-1601 PC, Shimadzu, Tokyo, Japan) at a resolution of 1 nm.

2.3.2. Dynamic Light Scattering (DLS)

The mean particle size of GNPs and CGNPs was measured with a DLS particle size analyzer (Zetasizer Nano-ZS, Malvern Instrument Ltd., Malvern, UK). The sample was taken in a DTS0112-low volume disposable sizing cuvette of 1.5 mL. The sample was sonicated for 1 min and filtered through syringe membrane filters with pores less than 0.45 µm before measurement. The mean particle size was determined by calculating the average of the measurements of a single sample in triplicate. Zeta potential was also measured to observe the nature of charge present on the surface of each sample by using Zetasizer Nano-ZS, Malvern Instrument Ltd., Malvern, UK. For zeta potential, DTS1070 disposable cuvette was used.

2.3.3. Scanning Electron Microscopy (SEM)

A drop from each sample, GNPs and CGNPs solutions, was deposited onto a conductive silicon substrate and dried on a hotplate at 60 °C for 20 min. The morphology of deposited GNPs and CGNPs on Si substrates were then imaged using FEI quanta 250 SEM (FEI Company, Hillsboro, OR, USA) with an accelerating voltage of 30 KV and a spot size of 3 nm.

2.3.4. Transmission Electron Microscopy (TEM)

TEM was performed using a Tecnai™ G2 Spirit Bio-TWIN equipped with a CCD camera (GatanDigital, Hillsboro, OR, USA). CGNPs sample was prepared using a carbon-coated TEM copper grid.

2.3.5. Fourier Transform Infrared Spectroscopy (FTIR)

FTIR (Shimadzu FTIR-8201 PC, PerkinElmer Inc., Waltham, MA, USA) was used to analyze the binding conformation and changes in secondary structures on the ceftriaxone present on the surface of CGNPs. The instrument was operated in diffuse reflectance mode at a resolution of 4 cm^{-1} to obtain good signal-to-noise ratios, 256 scans of CGNP films were obtained at a range of 400–4000 cm^{-1}.

2.4. Ceftriaxone Loading Efficiency on GNPs

2.4.1. Calculation by UV-Vis Spectrophotometry

The ceftriaxone loading efficacy onto GNPs was evaluated by using the methodology of Gomes et al. [25] as applied in Shaikh et al. [26]. Once the CGNPs were synthesized (without washing), the samples were centrifuged at 30,000× g for 30 min. Ceftriaxone in the supernatant was quantified by using UV-Visible spectrophotometer (λmax 241) after scanning [27,28]. However, the 5–70 µg/mL concentration range was used to plot calibration curve of ceftriaxone. For evaluating ceftriaxone loading efficacy, free ceftriaxone present in the supernatant was subtracted from the initial amount added for the CGNPs synthesis. The following equation was used to evaluate the % of loading efficacy.

$$\text{Percentage of loading efficacy} = \frac{[\text{Amt. of ceftriaxone used (Total)} - \text{Free ceftriaxone in supernatant}]}{\text{Amt. of ceftriaxone used (Total)}} \times 100$$

2.4.2. Calculation by High Performance Liquid Chromatography (HPLC)

The loading efficacy of ceftriaxone onto GNPs was also estimated by using the modified methodology of Pal et al. [29]. Shimadzu HPLC model fitted with UV/VIS detector (SPD-20A), AT pump (LC-20) and rheodyne injector with a 20-µL loop were used. Samples were analyzed on a reverse phase C-18 (Luna -5 µm, 250 × 4.6 mm inner diameter) column at 25 °C by applying a mobile phase (0.01 M KH2PO4:ACN buffer in 85:15 ratio) with 1 mL/min flow rate and UV-detection at 241 nm. Spinchrom software was used to record and evaluate the data. Before analyzing, a 0.22 µm filter was used to filter the mobile phase. Each sample was run in triplicate, and a calibration curve was plotted by using 5–70 µg/mL concentration of ceftriaxone. The amount of unbound ceftriaxone was calculated by using the calibration curve, and the amount of capped ceftriaxone onto GNPs was calculated by subtracting the unbound ceftriaxone from the total amount of ceftriaxone added. The exact amount of capped ceftriaxone was calculated using the following equation:

$$\text{Percentage of drug capping} = \frac{[\text{Amt. of ceftriaxone capped}]}{\text{Amt. of ceftriaxone used (Total)}} \times 100$$

2.5. Antibacterial Activity Evaluation

2.5.1. Bacteria and Growth Conditions

Escherichia coli (ATCC 25922), *Klebsiella pneumoniae* (ATCC 13883), *Salmonella abony* (NCIM 2257) and *Staphylococcus aureus* (ATCC 25923) were obtained from National Chemical Laboratory, India. Luria–Bertani (LB) broth was used to prepare fresh inoculum for each bacterial strain and incubated at 37 °C for 18 h. Prior to antibacterial activity, LB broth was used to adjust the turbidity of culture to 0.5 McFarland standard i.e., 1.5×10^8 CFU/mL.

2.5.2. Qualitative Assessment of Antibacterial Activity

Before performing the antibacterial assay, solutions were prepared by dispersing the synthesized CGNPs, GNPs (control) and ceftriaxone in PBS (phosphate saline buffer at pH 7.4). The agar well diffusion method was applied to assess the potency of synthesized CGNPs [30]. Fresh bacterial culture for each strain was spread on Mueller–Hinton agar and 6 mm wells were cut on 1 mg/mL) and GNPs (control) were dispensed in the wells. All the experiments were performed in triplicate, and the agar plates were placed in an incubator at a temperature of 37 °C overnight. The diameter of the zone of inhibition was measured.

2.5.3. Determination of the MIC

The synthesized CGNPs and ceftriaxone were tested against bacterial strains to determine their minimum inhibitory concentrations (MICs) by employing the broth microdilution method of Eloff [31]. To achieve the concentrations ranging from 0.025–32 µg/mL, aliquots of CGNPs and ceftriaxone were serially diluted in 96-well microtiter plates containing LB broth medium. The tested strains were cultured overnight in LB broth, and their turbidity was adjusted to 0.5 McFarland standard (1.5×10^8 CFU/mL), following these plates. A total of 50 µL of CGNPs (200 µg/mL ceftriaxone), ceftriaxone (which, 10 µL of the standard suspensions was placed in the aliquots. MICs are the lowest concentrations of synthesized CGNPs that completely inhibit bacterial growth after being incubated at 37 °C for 20 h.

3. Results and Discussion

3.1. CGNPs Synthesis

Several biomolecules and chemicals have been utilized as capping and reducing agents in the synthesis of multi-purpose inorganic nanoparticles [32]. Generally, conjugation of antibiotic/drug is performed on pre-formed GNPs by using different strategies. GNPs are synthesized either by chemicals (such as sodium borohydrate and trisodium citrate) or by herbal extracts and natural enzymes before conjugating antibiotics onto them [26,33–35]. In both the cases, residual contamination might create a doubt on the actual antibacterial results.

Typically, gold salt reduction followed by nucleation and nuclei growth leads to the synthesis of GNPs, and synthesized GNPs need a capping agent to be stabilized [36–38]. The highlight of the present study is that ceftriaxone acted as both reducing and capping/stabilizing agents for the synthesis of (ceftriaxone loaded gold nanoparticles) CGNPs (Figure 1). It is a fact that by changing the concentration of reducing agent (especially when it acts as a reducing as well as capping agent) and experimental conditions, the size of GNPs can be controlled [36–38]. Here, the different concentrations of ceftriaxone along with different temperature conditions were applied to synthesize CGNPs. Finally, the 250 µg/mL ceftriaxone concentration was selected to reduce HAuCl$_4$ to GNPs to obtain the desired size at a temperature of 40 °C and pH of 7.4. Khan et al. [24] and Khan et al. [39] have also applied the same strategy to synthesize GNPs of various sizes using bromelain and trypsin as reducing and capping agents. Similarly, the properties such as size, shape, mono-dispersity and stability of CGNPs in the present study basically relied on ceftriaxone concentration and temperature used for the reaction (data not shown for brevity). The synthesized GNPs and CGNPs showed visible characteristic color changes from yellow to ruby red (Figure S1).

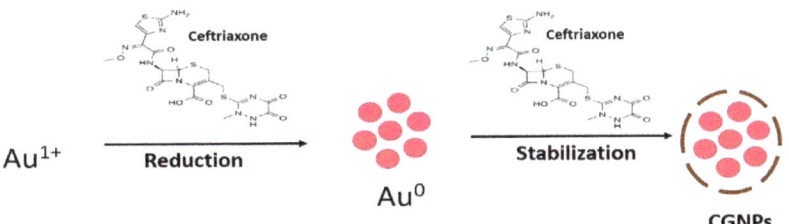

Figure 1. Scheme of ceftriaxone-mediated synthesis of gold nanoparticles. Here, CGNPs are the ceftriaxone-stabilized gold nanoparticles.

3.2. Characterization of CGNPs

3.2.1. Spectrophotometric

Typical 'Surface Plasma Resonance' band patterns for synthesized gold nanoformulations were characterized using UV-Visible spectroscopy. GNPs (control/without ceftriaxone showed absorption λmax at 520 nm, while CGNPs showed maximum absorption at 536 nm (Figure 2). The red shift of absorption from 520 to 536 nm can be correlated with the changes in size that might have occurred due to attachment of ceftriaxone to the CGNPs [40,41]. In a 2017 study, Shaikh et al. [26] also observed the same red shift after the attachment of cefotaxime antibiotic to the GNPs. However, they conjugated the antibiotic on preformed GNPs instead of synthesizing them by the one-pot synthesis method that has been developed during the present study. During CGNP spectrophotometric analysis, an additional peak at 241 nm was also detected that corresponds to ceftriaxone attached to CGNPs [27]. Similarly, other studies have also shown two peaks when antibiotics (secnidazole-320 nm and cefotaxime-298 nm) were conjugated to GNPs along with characteristic peaks of 525 [42] and 542 nm [26]. In fact, it has been observed that the capping agent has a major influence on the electrocatalytic activity of GNPs [43].

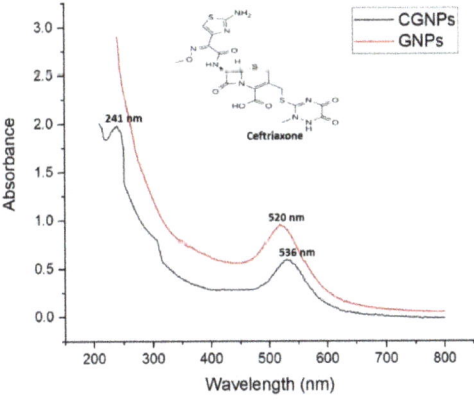

Figure 2. UV-Visible spectrophotometric characterization of GNPs and CGNPs.

3.2.2. Dynamic Light Scattering (DLS) and Electron Microscopy

Z-average size by DLS for GNPs and CGNPs was estimated as 51.59 and 95.07 nm, respectively (Figure 3). The size by DLS is based on the details of inner inorganic core of nanoparticles along with the solvent layer that has adhered to the nanoparticles once they are disseminated in the liquid medium. Thus, relying only on DLS is not enough to know the actual size of inorganic core. Zeta potential of GNPs and CGNPs was found to be −16.6 and −25.7 mV, respectively, which is an indicator of good stability of both the nanoparticles [44]. Usually, larger zeta potential either −ve or +ve implicates much more stable dispersion, that means nanoparticles will not get aggregated due to repulsion between each other [45,46]. However, emulsion and colloid stability are not always predicted by zeta-potential, as only repulsive electrostatic forces are measured, and the forces of attraction such as Van der Waals forces are not considered [47]. Thus, the stability was also checked by keeping the colloidal CGNPs at room temperature for months and no aggregation was found even after 5 months.

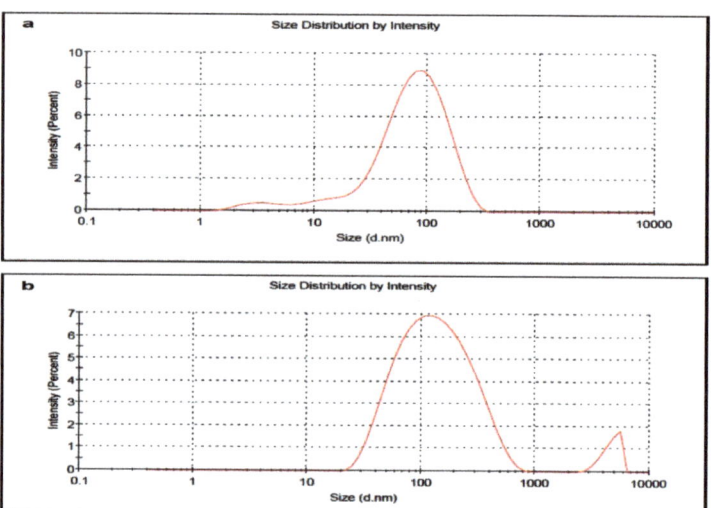

Figure 3. Z-average particle size of (**a**) GNPs and (**b**) CGNPs measured by DLS.

Scanning Electron Microscopy (SEM) results showed that both GNPs and CGNPs were spherical in shape and monodispersed (Figure 4). Ceftriaxone attachment/capping has not caused any changes in the shape of GNPs. In accordance, several other reports have also suggested the similar spherical pattern of GNPs after antibiotic conjugation [26,42].

Transmission Electron Microscopy (TEM) has been performed for GNPs and CGNPs to estimate the size of the inorganic core. Using the TEM analysis by Gatan Digital Micrograph (Figure 5), the size of the GNPs and CGNPs were confirmed to be 10.2 ± 1 and 21 ± 1 nm, respectively. The optical properties of GNPs were accredited to the 5 d (valence) and 6 sp (conduction) electrons. Well-defined monodispersed nanoparticles of equal size were revealed by the TEM micrograph. Estimating size by TEM and DLS covers two different aspects. DLS provide size distribution and polydispersity index results based on the quantification of several million particles present in the colloidal form, while TEM results are considered more biased in terms of selective imaging, where only a few hundred particles could be quantified at one time. Thus, correlating both the approaches has become an important strategy worldwide.

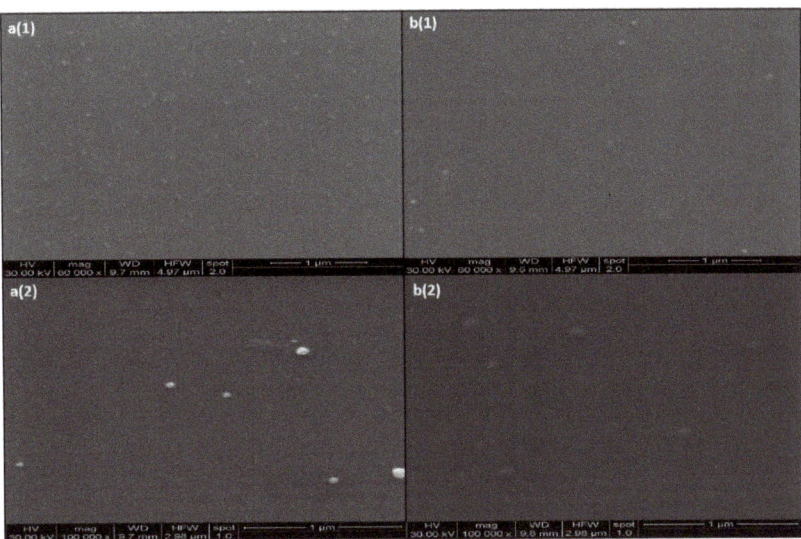

Figure 4. Scanning electron images of (**a1,a2**) GNPs at different magnifications and (**b1,b2**) CGNPs at different magnifications.

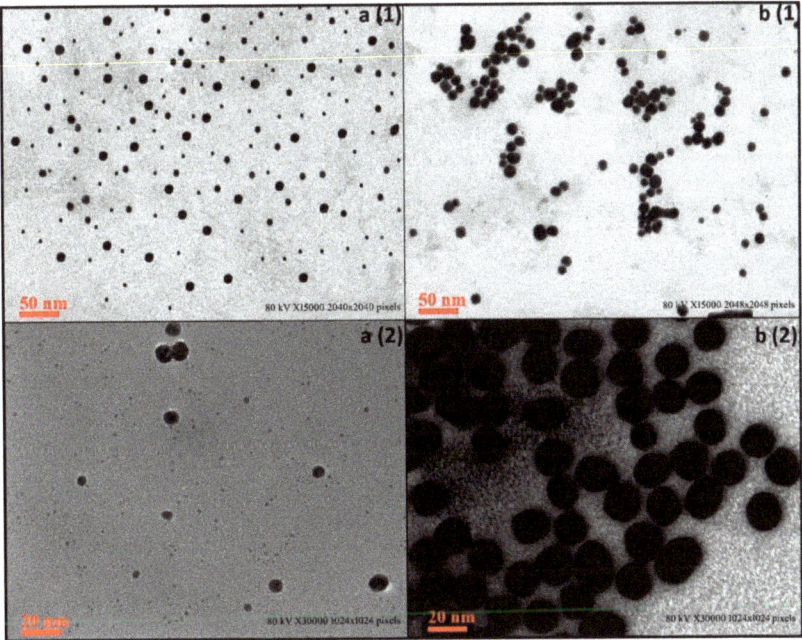

Figure 5. TEM Micrograph images of GNPs (**a1,a2**) and CGNPs (**b1,b2**).

3.3. FTIR Spectra of CGNPs and Ceftriaxone

Confirmation of the interactions between the surface of gold nanoparticles and ceftriaxone was done by FTIR spectroscopy (Figure 6a,b). The FTIR spectrum of ceftriaxone shows chief absorption bands at 3426 and 3265 cm^{-1}. The emergence of the aforementioned absorption bands indicates the stretching vibrations in the N–H and O–H groups, respectively. The absorption band at 2935 cm^{-1} indicates stretching band vibrations of C–H groups, range between 1741 and 1650 cm^{-1} is designated for the stretching vibrations of the carbonyl group (C=O), and the absorption band corresponding to 1538 cm^{-1} indicates torsional vibrations of the aromatic ring.

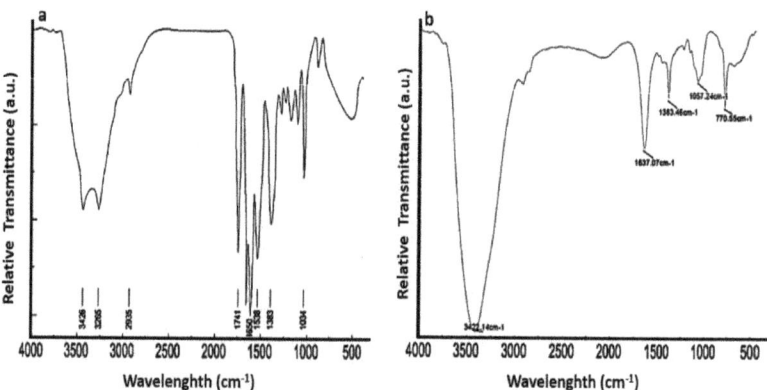

Figure 6. FTIR spectra of (**a**) pure ceftriaxone and (**b**) CGNPs.

Absorption bands corresponding to 1383 and 1034 cm^{-1} indicate the stretching vibration values of the C–N and C–O bonds. However, the interaction of ceftriaxone with the surface of gold nanoparticles causes the merging of the absorption bands and reduces the absorption intensities in C=O, N-H, and O-H groups. The absorption intensities of C=O, N-H, and O-H are 1798–1637, 3422, and 3265 cm^{-1}, respectively.

3.4. Calculation of Loading Efficiency

Prior to antibacterial assessment, loading efficiency of ceftriaxone on GNPs was calculated by UV-Visible spectrophotometric and HPLC method. Here, 199.8 µg of ceftriaxone (by UV-Visible spectrophotometry) and 199.5 µg of ceftriaxone (by HPLC) was found to be loaded to the GNPs, out of 250 µg of the ceftriaxone initially used for the synthesis. Thus, the loading efficiency percentage was estimated as 79.92% and 79.80%, respectively, for the methods used. Furthermore, the retention time for pure ceftriaxone and capped ceftriaxone is estimated as 3.512 min (Figure 7a) and 3.59 min (Figure 7b), respectively. The observable slight change in retention time was might be due to variation of pH in the mobile phase to the medium of the drug. The retention time for CGNPs is 2.61 min (Figure 7b). Similarly, in a 2015 study, secnidazole was estimated by HPLC, and found to have 70% loading efficacy onto GNPs [42]. In another study, cefotaxime loading efficacy on GNPs was found as 77.59% when estimated by UV-Visible spectrophotometry [26]. It is a fact that higher loading efficiency correlates inversely with unwanted loss of antibiotic/drug and shows better therapeutic application [25]. Therefore, the methodology applied in the present study was effective in loading a good amount of ceftriaxone onto gold nanoparticles. However, 200 µg ceftriaxone was considered as the final loaded amount on GNPs as an approximation for further antibacterial assay to avoid difficulties in calculations.

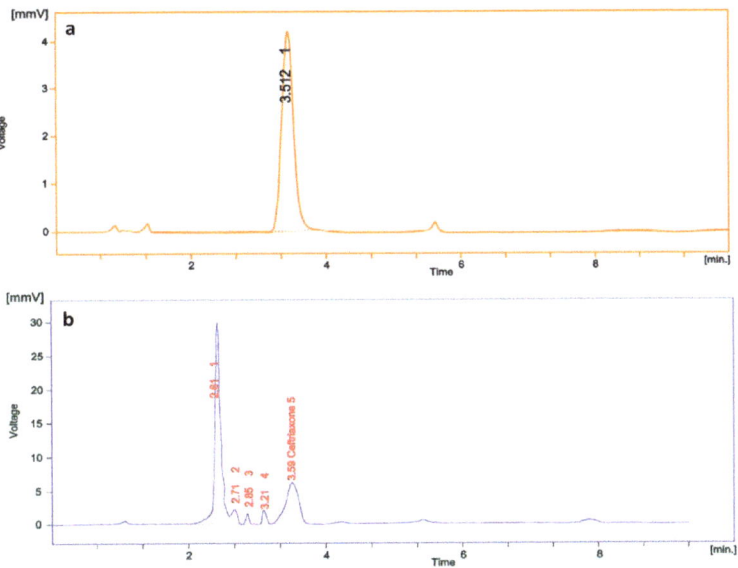

Figure 7. RP-HPLC chromatogram of (**a**) pure ceftriaxone and (**b**) CGNPs.

3.5. Antibacterial Activity of CGNPs

The antibacterial activities of GNPs (Control), CGNPs and ceftriaxone were evaluated by testing them against three gGram-negative strains, i.e., *Escherichia coli*, *Salmonella abony* and *Klebsiella pneumoniae* and one Gram-positive *Staphylococcus aureus*. These tested strains were chosen to represent different bacterial types of machinery nurturing several potent virulent factors other than their observable pathogenicity and their prevalence in day-to-day life. The promising detection revealed that CGNPs and ceftriaxone could inhibit the growth of bacteria after diffusion into the agar (Figure S2). Also, it was observed that both CGNPs and pure ceftriaxone had similar zones of inhibition. However, the total concentration of ceftriaxone in 50 µL CGNPs was equivalent to only 10 µg/well, whereas, the concentration of pure ceftriaxone was 50 µg/well. Thus, our primary findings confirmed that effectiveness of CGNPs was higher than pure ceftriaxone.

The MIC_{50} of CGNPs and pure ceftriaxone against all the tested bacterial strains was recorded (Figure 8). The MIC_{50} values for GNPs and pure ceftriaxone were 1.39 and 3.1 µg/mL against *E. coli* (Figure 8a), 1.60 and 2.9 µg/mL against *S. aureus* (Figure 8b), 1.1 and 2.07 µg/mL against *S. abony* (Figure 8c), 0.9 and 2.4 µg/mL against *K. pneumoniae* (Figure 8d), respectively.

Based on the antibacterial results, it can be suggested that ceftriaxone attachment to gold nanoparticles has enhanced its potency twice than the pure ceftriaxone. GNPs without ceftriaxone were used as a control and they did not show any activity against any tested strain. Similar results were observed when Shaikh et al. [26] and Brown et al. [48] tested naked GNPs while studying the cefotaxime- and ampicillin-conjugated GNPs against resistant bacterial strains, respectively. Thus, it can be inferred that the activity was due to ceftriaxone, and GNPs just aided in augmenting the potency. Due to biocompatibility, non-cytotoxicity and exceptional physiochemical properties, gold nanoformulations have always been the first choice among inorganic nanoparticles for drug delivery [22,23]. Importantly, it was observed that the reactive portion of antibiotic (ciprofloxacin) was surface exposed when it was attached to GNPs and activity is retained [49]. Our results were in harmony with the findings of Shaikh et al. [26] and Brown et al. [48], where cefotaxime and ampicillin also retained their potency after conjugation to GNPs.

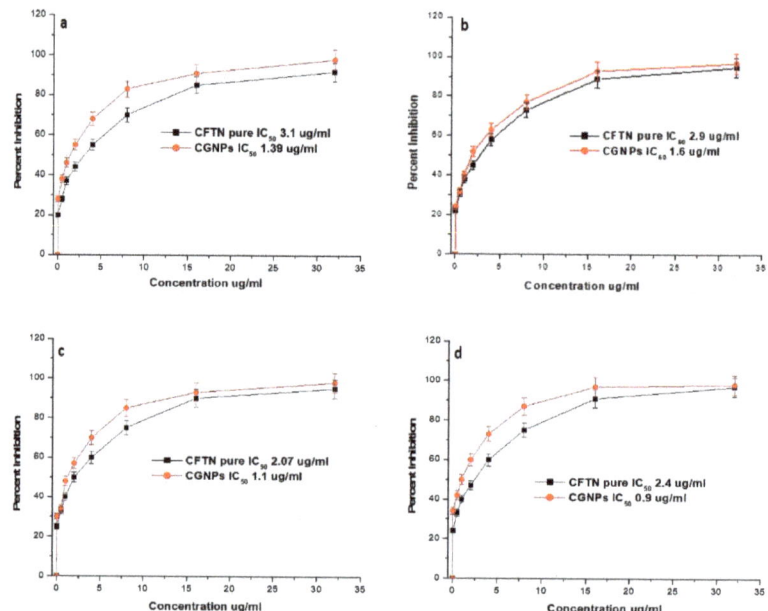

Figure 8. Determination of Minimum Inhibitory Concentration (MIC) of CGNPs and ceftriaxone (CFTN) against (**a**) *Escherichia coli*, (**b**) *Staphylococcus aureus*, (**c**) *Salmonella abony*, and (**d**) *Klebsiella pneumoniae*.

The hypothesis on the mechanistic aspect of CGNP antibacterial action is based on the earlier reports of Rai et al. [21] and Shaikh et al. [26]. Firstly, the effective delivered ceftriaxone concentration was increased due to its attachment to GNPs. It might be due to the typical properties of GNPs, i.e., high surface-to-volume ratio, high concentration of (ceftriaxone) molecules loaded onto it due to large surface area, increased permeability towards the biological membrane and higher uptake by the bacterial cell [50]. Secondly, GNPs might have increased the porosity of the targeted bacterial strains and ceftriaxone molecules have gained easy access to the bacterial cell for their action. In fact, increased delivered concentration of antibiotic could saturate the resistant enzymes such as beta-lactamses, and plausibly inhibit the growth of the beta-lactamase-containing resistant bacterial strains as well [26]. However, when we discuss human cellular uptake of the nanoparticles (within the nanometers size range), pinocytosis is considered as a major uptake mechanism [51]. In fact, pinocytosis is a continual process occurring in all the cells that could be subdivided as clathrin-mediated endocytosis, micropinocytosis, clathrin- and caveolae-independent endocytosis, and caveolae-mediated endocytosis [52,53]. It has been observed that if the size is below 100 nm, the pinocytosis uptake mechanism is preferred, whereas, if the size is large (250 nm), phagocytosis occurs [54,55]. In our study, the size of both GNPs and CGNPs (as observed by TEM) are appropriate for pinocytosis. Although, further studies are needed to pinpoint the exact pinocytosis mechanism followed by CGNPs for the cellar uptake.

The most persistent global public health issue after COVID-19 is antimicrobial resistance due to the resultant restriction in therapeutic options against infections, and misuse/self-medication of antibiotics in the COVID-19 era [2]. Recently, novel strategies have been designed to enhance the properties (distribution, penetration, specificity, and pharmacokinetics) of antimicrobial drugs. The formulation of antimicrobial nanoparticles or antimicrobial-conjugated nanoparticles is one such strategy. Impressive increases in drug specificity and enhanced pharmacokinetics were observed when GNPs are utilized for antimicrobial delivery. In this study, a similar approach has been used to enhance the potency of ceftriaxone. Ceftriaxone resistance was globally accepted before the arrival of COVID-19, but it is speculated to increase with time as suggested by several reports. Thus, the solutions are warranted urgently. In our study, it has been found GNPs can markedly enhance the potency of ceftriaxone. Moreover, its fate in the human body and toxicity aspects still needed to be deciphered. Currently, our team is working on exploring the exact mechanism of action, toxicity and lethal dose of CGNPs using in-vivo and in-vitro experimental designs. On the basis of preliminary findings on toxicity (data not shown), we found no toxicity on normal cell lines. Our team hopes that we can come up with fresh nanoformulations to tackle bacterial resistance issues in the near future.

4. Conclusions

The present study delivered an approach to synthesize gold nanoparticles by applying ceftriaxone as reducing as well as stabilizing agent. In addition, synthesized ceftriaxone-loaded gold nanoparticles (CGNPs) acted as an effective tool to deliver ceftriaxone to the tested bacterial strains and markedly enhanced the ceftriaxone potency. Comparative analysis of pure ceftriaxone and CGNPs revealed that ceftriaxone after loading onto GNPs could become two times more potent. This strategy has opened a path to synthesize and deliver different antibiotics through GNPs in a one-step process to resolve the issue of increasing resistance. However, in-vivo studies to evaluate the fate and toxicity of CGNPs are warranted before jumping into the conclusive statement on the applicability of synthesized nanoformulations. Moreover, the preliminary findings of the present study could be used as a base to develop applicable nanoformulations.

Supplementary Materials: The following are available online at https://www.mdpi.com/article/10.3390/pharmaceutics13111896/s1, Figure S1: Synthesized gold nanoparticles (a) Bromelain mediated synthesized (GNPs) (b) Ceftriaxone mediated synthesized (CGNPs); Figure S2: Qualitative assessment of the antibacterial activity of CGNPs and ceftriaxone (CFTN). Müeller-Hinton (MH) agar plates were seeded with standardized suspensions (equivalent to 0.5 McFarland) of (A) *Escherichia coli* (B) *Staphylococcus aureus*, (C) *Salmonella abony*, and (D) *Klebsiella pneumonia*. The dilutions of CGNPs 50 µL (200 µg/mL CFTN), CFTN 50 µL (1 mg/mL CFTN), and GNPs 50 µL (negative control) were poured in the wells made in MH plates. After overnight incubation at 37 °C, zones of inhibition around wells of CGNPs and CFTN against all tested bacterial species, in comparison to control, were observed.

Author Contributions: Conceptualization, F.A., A.M. and S.M.D.R.; methodology, B.A. and A.B.; validation, A.M., A.A. (Abdulwahab Alamri) and S.K.; formal analysis, T.A.H. and A.A. (Abdulwahab Alamri); resources, F.A. and S.M.D.R.; writing—original draft preparation, B.A., T.A.H. and A.B.; writing—review and editing, A.M. and A.A. (Ahmed Alobaida); supervision, F.A., S.K. and S.M.D.R.; project administration, F.A.; funding acquisition, F.A. and S.M.D.R. All authors have read and agreed to the published version of the manuscript.

Funding: This research work has been funded by Scientific Research Deanship at University of Ha'il-Saudi Arabia through project number BA-2026.

Institutional Review Board Statement: Not applicable.

Informed Consent Statement: Not applicable.

Data Availability Statement: Not applicable.

Acknowledgments: The authors are thankful to Scientific Research Deanship at University of Ha'il-Saudi Arabia for funding the project (BA-2026).

Conflicts of Interest: The authors declare no conflict of interest.

References

1. CDC's Antibiotic Resistance Threats Report 2019. Available online: https://www.cdc.gov/drugresistance/biggest-threats.html (accessed on 10 September 2021).
2. Ghosh, S.; Bornman, C.; Zafer, M.M. Antimicrobial Resistance Threats in the emerging COVID-19 pandemic: Where do we stand? *J. Infect. Public Health* **2021**, *14*, 555–560. [CrossRef]

3. Adebisi, Y.A.; Jimoh, N.D.; Ogunkola, I.O.; Uwizeyimana, T.; Olayemi, A.H.; Ukor, N.A.; Lucero-Prisno, D.E. The use of antibiotics in COVID-19 management: A rapid review of national treatment guidelines in 10 African countries. *Trop. Med. Health* **2021**, *49*, 51. [CrossRef] [PubMed]
4. Kumar, S.; Bhanjana, G.; Kumar, A.; Taneja, K.; Dilbaghi, N.; Kim, K.-H. Synthesis and optimization of ceftriaxone-loaded solid lipid nanocarriers. *Chem. Phys. Lipids* **2016**, *200*, 126–132. [CrossRef]
5. Chua, K.Y.L.; Stewardson, A.J. Individual and community predictors of urinary ceftriaxone-resistant *Escherichia coli* isolates, Victoria, Australia. *Antimicrob. Resist. Infect. Control.* **2019**, *8*, 36. [CrossRef] [PubMed]
6. Goldstein, F.W.; Péan, Y.; Gertner, J. Resistance to ceftriaxone and other beta-lactams in bacteria isolated in the community. The Vigil'Roc Study Group. *Antimicrob. Agents Chemother.* **1995**, *39*, 2516–2519. [CrossRef]
7. Al kraiem, A.A.; Yang, G.; Al kraiem, F.; Chen, T. Challenges associated with ceftriaxone resistance in *Salmonella*. *Front. Life Sci.* **2018**, *11*, 26–34. [CrossRef]
8. Núñez-Lozano, R.; Cano, M.; Pimentel, B.; de la Cueva-Méndez, G. 'Smartening' anticancer therapeutic nanosystems using biomolecules. *Curr. Opin. Biotechnol.* **2015**, *35*, 135–140. [CrossRef] [PubMed]
9. Chamundeeswari, M.; Sobhana, S.S.L.; Jacob, J.; Kumar, M.G.; Devi, M.P.; Sastry, T.P.; Mandal, A.B. Preparation, characterization and evaluation of a biopolymeric gold nanocomposite with antimicrobial activity. *Biotechnol. Appl. Biochem.* **2010**, *55*, 29–35. [CrossRef] [PubMed]
10. Pal, S.; Tak, Y.K.; Song, J.M. Does the antibacterial activity of silver nanoparticles depend on the shape of the nanoparticle? A study of the gram-negative bacterium Escherichia coli. *Appl. Environ. Microbiol.* **2007**, *73*, 1712–1720. [CrossRef]
11. Huang, X.; Jain, P.; El-Sayed, I.H.; El-Sayed, M.A. Plasmonic photothermal therapy (PPTT) using gold nanoparticles. *Lasers Med. Sci.* **2008**, *23*, 217. [CrossRef] [PubMed]
12. Maness, P.-C.; Smolinski, S.; Blake, D.M.; Huang, Z.; Wolfrum, E.J.; Jacoby, W.A. Bactericidal Activity of Photocatalytic TiO_2 Reaction: Toward an Understanding of Its Killing Mechanism. *Appl. Environ. Microbiol.* **1999**, *65*, 4094–4098. [CrossRef]
13. Rudramurthy, G.R.; Swamy, M.K.; Sinniah, U.R.; Ghasemzadeh, A. Nanoparticles: Alternatives against Drug-Resistant Pathogenic Microbes. *Molecules* **2016**, *21*, 836. [CrossRef] [PubMed]
14. Morones, J.R.; Elechiguerra, J.L.; Camacho, A.; Holt, K.; Kouri, J.B.; Tapia, J.; Yacaman, M.J. The bactericidal effect of silver nanoparticles. *Nanotechnology* **2005**, *16*, 2346–2353. [CrossRef]
15. Franci, G.; Falanga, A.; Galdiero, S.; Palomba, L.; Rai, M.; Morelli, G.; Galdiero, M. Silver nanoparticles as potential antibacterial agents. *Molecules* **2015**, *20*, 8856–8874. [CrossRef]
16. Dreaden, E.; Mwakwari, S.C.; Sodji, Q.H.; Oyelere, A.K.; El-Sayed, M.A. Tamoxifen−Poly(ethylene glycol)−Thiol Gold Nanoparticle Conjugates: Enhanced Potency and Selective Delivery for Breast Cancer Treatment. *Bioconjugate Chem.* **2009**, *20*, 2247–2253. [CrossRef] [PubMed]
17. Alba-Molina, D.; Giner-Casares, J.J.; Cano, M. Bioconjugated Plasmonic Nanoparticles for Enhanced Skin Penetration. *Top. Curr. Chem.* **2020**, *378*, 8. [CrossRef] [PubMed]
18. Fuster, M.G.; Montalbán, M.G.; Carissimi, G.; Lima, B.; Feresin, G.E.; Cano, M.; Giner-Casares, J.J.; López-Cascales, J.J.; Enriz, R.D.; Víllora, G. Antibacterial Effect of Chitosan–Gold Nanoparticles and Computational Modeling of the Interaction between Chitosan and a Lipid Bilayer Model. *Nanomaterials* **2020**, *10*, 2340. [CrossRef]
19. Rastogi, L.; Kora, A.J.; Arunachalam, J. Highly stable, protein capped gold nanoparticles as effective drug delivery vehicles for amino-glycosidic antibiotics. *Mater. Sci. Eng. C* **2012**, *32*, 1571–1577. [CrossRef] [PubMed]
20. Aramwit, P.; Bang, N.; Ratanavaraporn, J.; Ekgasit, S. Green synthesis of silk sericin-capped silver nanoparticles and their potent anti-bacterial activity. *Nanoscale Res. Lett.* **2014**, *9*, 79. [CrossRef]
21. Rai, A.; Prabhune, A.; Perry, C.C. Antibiotic mediated synthesis of gold nanoparticles with potent antimicrobial activity and their application in antimicrobial coatings. *J. Mater. Chem.* **2010**, *20*, 6789–6798. [CrossRef]
22. Fako, V.E.; Furgeson, D.Y. Zebrafish as a correlative and predictive model for assessing biomaterial nanotoxicity. *Adv. Drug Deliv. Rev.* **2009**, *61*, 478–486. [CrossRef] [PubMed]
23. Cobley, C.M.; Chen, J.; Cho, E.C.; Wang, L.V.; Xia, Y. Gold nanostructures: A class of multifunctional materials for biomedical applications. *Chem. Soc. Rev.* **2011**, *40*, 44–56. [CrossRef] [PubMed]
24. Khan, S.; Rizvi, S.M.D.; Avaish, M.; Arshad, M.; Bagga, P.; Khan, M.S. A novel process for size controlled biosynthesis of gold nanoparticles using bromelain. *Mater. Lett* **2011**, *159*, 373–376. [CrossRef]
25. Gomes, M.J.; Martins, S.; Ferreira, D.; Segundo, M.A.; Reis, S. Lipid nanoparticles for topical and transdermal application for alopecia treatment:Development, physicochemical characterization, and in vitro release and penetration studies. *Int. J. Nanomed.* **2014**, *9*, 1231–1242.
26. Shaikh, S.; Rizvi, S.M.D.; Shakil, S.; Hussain, T.; Alshammari, T.M.; Ahmad, W.; Tabrez, S.; Al-Qahtani, M.H.; Abuzenadah, A.M. Synthesis and Characterization of Cefotaxime Conjugated Gold Nanoparticles and Their Use to Target Drug-Resistant CTX-M-Producing Bacterial Pathogens. *J. Cell Biochem.* **2017**, *118*, 2802–2808. [CrossRef] [PubMed]
27. Majani Ayushi, V.; Paradkar Mansi, U. Development and Validation of UV Spectrophotometric Method for the Estimation of Ceftriaxone Sodium in Nanoparticles. *Der Pharma Chem.* **2018**, *10*, 151–157.
28. Ethiraj, R.; Thiruvengadam, E.; Sampath, V.S.; Vahid, A.; Raj, J. Development and Validation of Stability Indicating Spectroscopic Method for Content Analysis of Ceftriaxone Sodium in Pharmaceuticals. *Int. Schoraly Res. Not.* **2014**, *2014*, 278173. [CrossRef]

29. Pal, N.; Rao, A.S.; Hedi, M.A. HPLC method development and validation for the assay of ceftriaxone sodium injection. *Int. J. Pharma Sci.* **2012**, *2*, 84–90.
30. Perez, C.; Pauli, M.; Bazerque, P. An antibiotic assay by the well agar method. *Acta Biol. Med. Exp.* **1990**, *15*, 113–115.
31. Eloff, J.N. A sensitive and quick micro plate method to determine the minimal inhibitory concentration of plant extracts for bacteria. *Planta Med.* **1998**, *64*, 711–713. [CrossRef]
32. Von Maltzahn, G.; Centrone, A.; Park, J.-H.; Ramanathan, R.; Sailor, M.J.; Hatton, T.A.; Bhatia, S.N. SERS coded gold nanorods as a multifunctional platform for densely multiplexed near infrared imaging and photothermal heating. *Adv. Mater.* **2009**, *21*, 3175–3180. [CrossRef]
33. Fan, Y.; Pauer, A.C.; Gonzales, A.A.; Fenniri, H. Enhanced antibiotic activity of ampicillin conjugated to gold nanoparticles on PEGylated rosette nanotubes. *Int. J. Nanomed.* **2019**, *14*, 7281–7289. [CrossRef] [PubMed]
34. Bhattacharya, D.; Saha, B.; Mukherjee, A.; Santra, C.R.; Karmakar, P. Gold Nanoparticles Conjugated Antibiotics: Stability and Functional Evaluation. *Nanosci. Nanotechnol.* **2012**, *2*, 14–21. [CrossRef]
35. Fuller, M.; Whiley, H.; Köper, I. Antibiotic delivery using gold nanoparticles. *SN Appl. Sci.* **2020**, *2*, 1022. [CrossRef]
36. Apyari, V.V.; Arkhipova, V.V.; Dmitrienko, S.G.; Zolotov, Y.A. Using gold nanoparticles in spectrophotometry. *J. Anal. Chem.* **2014**, *69*, 111. [CrossRef]
37. Zhao, P.; Li, N.; Astruc, D. State of the art in gold nanoparticle synthesis. *Coord. Chem. Rev.* **2014**, *257*, 638–665. [CrossRef]
38. De Souza, C.D.; Nogueira, B.R.; Rostelato, M.E.C. Review of the methodologies used in the synthesis gold nanoparticles by chemical reduction. *J. Alloy. Compd.* **2019**, *798*, 714–740. [CrossRef]
39. Khan, S.; Rizvi, S.M.; Saeed, M.; Srivastava, A.K.; Khan, M. A Novel Approach for the synthesis of gold nanoparticles using Trypsin. *Adv. Sci. Lett.* **2014**, *20*, 1061–1065. [CrossRef]
40. Mangeney, C.; Ferrage, F.; Aujard, I.; Marchi-Artzner, V.; Jullien, L.; Ouari, O.; Rekai, E.D.; Laschewsky, A.; Vikholm, I.; Sadowski, J.W. Synthesis and properties of water-soluble gold colloids covalently derivatized with neutral polymer monolayers. *J. Am. Chem. Soc.* **2002**, *124*, 5811–5821. [CrossRef]
41. Mukherjee, P.; Bhattacharya, R.; Mukhopadhyay, D. Gold nanoparticles bearing functional anti cancer drug and anti-angiogenic agent: A "2 in 1" system with potential application in cancer therapeutics. *J. Biomed. Nanotech.* **2005**, *2*, 2224–2228. [CrossRef]
42. Khan, S.; Haseeb, M.; Baig, M.H.; Bagga, P.S.; Siddiqui, H.H.; Kamal, M.A.; Khan, M.S. Improved efficiency and stability of secnidazole—An ideal delivery system. *Saudi J. Biol. Sci.* **2015**, *22*, 42–49. [CrossRef] [PubMed]
43. Alba-Molina, D.; Santiago, A.R.; Giner-Casares, J.J.; Rodríguez-Castellón, E.; Martín-Romero, M.T.; Camacho, L.; Luque, R.; Cano, M. Tailoring the ORR and HER electrocatalytic performances of gold nanoparticles through metal–ligand interfaces. *J. Mater. Chem. A* **2019**, *7*, 20425–20434. [CrossRef]
44. Cano, M.; Núñez-Lozano, R.; Lumbreras, R.; González-Rodríguez, V.; Delgado-García, A.; Jiménez-Hoyuela, J.M.; de la Cueva-Méndez, G. Partial PEGylation of superparamagnetic iron oxide nanoparticles thinly coated with amine-silane as a source of ultrastable tunable nanosystems for biomedical applications. *Nanoscale* **2017**, *9*, 812–822. [CrossRef]
45. Xu, R.L. Progress in nanoparticles characterization: Sizing and zeta potential measurement. *Particuology* **2008**, *6*, 112–115. [CrossRef]
46. Tantra, R.; Schulze, P.; Quincey, P. Effect of nanoparticle concentration on zeta-potential measurement results and reproducibility. *Particuology* **2010**, *8*, 279–285. [CrossRef]
47. Baker, A.; Wahid, I.; Hassan Baig, M.; Alotaibi, S.S.; Khalid, M.; Uddin, I.; Dong, J.J.; Khan, M.S. Silk Cocoon-Derived Protein Bioinspired Gold Nanoparticles as a Formidable Anticancer Agent. *J. Biomed. Nanotechnol.* **2021**, *17*, 615–626.
48. Brown, A.N.; Smith, K.; Samuels, T.A.; Lu, J.; Obare, S.O.; Scott, M.E. Nanoparticles functionalized with ampicillin destroy multiple-antibiotic-resistant isolates of Pseudomonas aeruginosa and Enterobacter aerogenes and methicillin-resistant Staphylococcus aureus. *Appl. Env. Microbiol.* **2012**, *78*, 2768–2774. [CrossRef]
49. Tom, R.T.; Suryanarayanan, V.; Reddy, P.G.; Baskaran, S.; Pradeep, T. Ciprofloxacin-protected gold nanoparticles. *Langmuir* **2004**, *20*, 1909–1914. [CrossRef]
50. Yafout, M.; Ousaid, A.; Khayati, Y.; El Otmani, I.S. Gold nanoparticles as a drug delivery system for standard chemotherapeutics: A new lead for targeted pharmacological cancer treatments. *Sci. Afr.* **2021**, *11*, e00685.
51. Zhao, F.; Zhao, Y.; Liu, Y.; Chang, X.; Chen, C.; Zhao, Y. Cellular uptake, intracellular trafficking, and cytotoxicity of nanomaterials. *Small* **2011**, *7*, 1322–1337. [CrossRef]
52. Yu, Y. Resolving Endosome Rotation in Intracellular Trafficking. *Biophys. J.* **2018**, *114* (Suppl. S1), 630a. [CrossRef]
53. Foroozandeh, P.; Aziz, A.A. Insight into Cellular Uptake and Intracellular Trafficking of Nanoparticles. *Nanoscale Res. Lett.* **2018**, *13*, 339. [CrossRef] [PubMed]
54. Hillaireau, H.; Couvreur, P. Nanocarriers' entry into the cell: Relevance to drug delivery. *Cell. Mol. Life Sci.* **2009**, *66*, 2873–2896. [CrossRef] [PubMed]
55. Panariti, A.; Miserocchi, G.; Rivolta, I. The effect of nanoparticle uptake on cellular behavior: Disrupting or enabling functions? *Nanotechnol. Sci. Appl.* **2012**, *5*, 87. [PubMed]

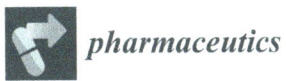

Article

Titanium Dioxide Nanoparticles Induce Inhibitory Effects against Planktonic Cells and Biofilms of Human Oral Cavity Isolates of *Rothia mucilaginosa*, *Georgenia* sp. and *Staphylococcus saprophyticus*

Saher Fatima [1], Khursheed Ali [1,*], Bilal Ahmed [2,*], Abdulaziz A. Al Kheraif [3], Asad Syed [4], Abdallah M. Elgorban [4], Javed Musarrat [1] and Jintae Lee [2]

[1] Faculty of Agricultural Sciences, Department of Agricultural Microbiology, Aligarh Muslim University, Aligarh 202002, India; saherfatima.amu@gmail.com (S.F.); musarratj1@yahoo.com (J.M.)
[2] School of Chemical Engineering, Yeungnam University, Gyeongsan 38541, Korea; jtlee@ynu.ac.kr
[3] Dental Health Department, College of Applied Medical Sciences, King Saud University, P.O. Box 10219, Riyadh 11433, Saudi Arabia; aalkhuraif@ksu.edu.sa
[4] Department of Botany and Microbiology, College of Science, King Saud University, P.O. Box 2455, Riyadh 11451, Saudi Arabia; assyed@ksu.edu.sa (A.S.); aelgorban@ksu.edu.sa (A.M.E.)
* Correspondence: khursheedamu@gmail.com (K.A.); bilal22000858@yu.ac.kr (B.A.)

Citation: Fatima, S.; Ali, K.; Ahmed, B.; Al Kheraif, A.A.; Syed, A.; Elgorban, A.M.; Musarrat, J.; Lee, J. Titanium Dioxide Nanoparticles Induce Inhibitory Effects against Planktonic Cells and Biofilms of Human Oral Cavity Isolates of *Rothia mucilaginosa*, *Georgenia* sp. and *Staphylococcus saprophyticus*. *Pharmaceutics* **2021**, *13*, 1564. https://doi.org/10.3390/pharmaceutics13101564

Academic Editor: Clive Prestidge

Received: 22 August 2021
Accepted: 23 September 2021
Published: 26 September 2021

Publisher's Note: MDPI stays neutral with regard to jurisdictional claims in published maps and institutional affiliations.

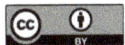

Copyright: © 2021 by the authors. Licensee MDPI, Basel, Switzerland. This article is an open access article distributed under the terms and conditions of the Creative Commons Attribution (CC BY) license (https://creativecommons.org/licenses/by/4.0/).

Abstract: Multi-drug resistant (MDR) bacterial cells embedded in biofilm matrices can lead to the development of chronic cariogenesis. Here, we isolated and identified three Gram-positive MDR oral cocci, (1) SJM-04, (2) SJM-38, and (3) SJM-65, and characterized them morphologically, biochemically, and by 16S rRNA gene-based phylogenetic analysis as *Georgenia* sp., *Staphylococcus saprophyticus*, and *Rothia mucilaginosa*, respectively. These three oral isolates exhibited antibiotic-resistance against nalidixic acid, tetracycline, cefuroxime, methicillin, and ceftazidime. Furthermore, these Gram positive MDR oral cocci showed significant ($p < 0.05$) variations in their biofilm forming ability under different physicochemical conditions, that is, at temperatures of 28, 30, and 42 °C, pH of 6.4, 7.4, and 8.4, and NaCl concentrations from 200 to 1000 µg/mL. Exposure of oral isolates to TiO$_2$NPs (14.7 nm) significantly ($p < 0.05$) reduced planktonic cell viability and biofilm formation in a concentration-dependent manner, which was confirmed by observing biofilm architecture by scanning electron microscopy (SEM) and optical microscopy. Overall, these results have important implications for the use of tetragonal anatase phase TiO$_2$NPs (size range 5–25 nm, crystalline size 13.7 nm, and spherical shape) as an oral antibiofilm agent against Gram positive cocci infections. We suggest that TiO$_2$NPs pave the way for further applications in oral mouthwash formulations and antibiofilm dental coatings.

Keywords: oral bacteria; *Rothia mucilaginosa*; TiO$_2$NPs; biofilm inhibition

1. Introduction

The enormously rich and complex salivary environment of the human oral cavity provides a uniquely structured habitat for a wide variety of commensal (aerobic/anaerobic) microorganisms, and more than an estimated 700 species [1] colonize the oral cavity and form biofilms to ensure their long-term survival. Moreover, notorious biofilm persisters, including streptococci and lactobacilli, live as mutual symbionts within biofilms [2]. Furthermore, it has often been speculated that oral microbiota (bacteria, yeasts, and viruses) promote biofilm formation by producing heterogeneous extracellular polymeric substances (EPS), proteins, and nucleic acids [3]. According to Tawakoli et al. [4], the most dominant oral diseases (caries and periodontitis) are caused by bacterial adherence and subsequent biofilm formation. Multi-layered bacterial biofilm matrices play a vital role in neutralizing the antimicrobial effects of various chemical agents by acquiring drug resistance against multiple antibiotics, which is sometimes >1000-fold greater than that of planktonic cells [5,6]. The metabolism of dietary sucrose/carbohydrates creates a highly acidic microenvironment on tooth surfaces during cariogenic biofilm accumulation, and the resulting tooth surface demineralization leads to periodontal disease and tooth decay, which affect up to 60–90% of humans [7]. The problems associated with oral biofilms and their clinical management also have significant adverse economic impacts. For example, the cumulative cost of treatments for oral biofilm-related diseases has been estimated to be around USD 81 billion per annum in the United States [8].

The clinical management of biofilm-induced cariogenesis using a variety of metal nanoparticles (NPs) is now being widely explored due to their potential antimicrobial and anti-adhesive characteristics [9–12]. Amongst the metal oxides investigated, nanoscale titanium dioxide (TiO_2) has a well-established antibacterial effect due to the production of reactive oxygen species (ROS) and cell membrane disrupting/penetrating, glutathione depleting, and toxic oxidative stress augmenting effects [13,14]. Furthermore, TiO_2NPs are normally applied at low concentrations and are widely considered to be bio-compatible [15], though opinions differ regarding inflammation generated by cytokine release [16]. As compared with their micro/bulk-sized counterparts, TiO_2NPs interact efficiently with a broad range of cell types (e.g., bacteria, fungi, and mammalian cells) due to their greater surface-to-volume ratios [17–19].

Because of its dynamic and open nature and the presence of highly complex mixes of biofilm microflora (due to host susceptibility and poor oral hygiene), the oral cavity has long been regarded as fertile ground for novel persistent biofilms. In the present study, from among ten oral isolates, we selected three Gram positive MDR cocci identified as *Georgenia* sp. (SJM-04), *S. saprophyticus* (SJM-38), and *R. mucilaginosa* (SJM-65) based on their Gram reaction, biochemical make-up, and 16S rRNA-based phylogenetic relatedness. These Gram positive MDR isolates were found resistant to nalidixic acid, tetracycline, cefuroxime, methicillin, and ceftazidime and also showed significant ($p < 0.05$) variations in biofilm formation under different experimental conditions viz., temperatures of 28, 30, or 42 °C, pH values of 6.4, 7.4, or 8.4, and NaCl concentrations of 200 to 1000 µg/mL. Exposure to TiO_2NPs ($\cong$14.7 nm) resulted in significant ($p < 0.05$) and concentration-dependent reductions in the viability of planktonic cells and the biofilm formation rates, and these reductions were subsequently confirmed by scanning electron and optical microscopy, respectively. Overall, these results have important implications regarding the use of TiO_2NPs to eradicate biofilms formed by these three species.

2. Materials and Methods

2.1. Ethics Statement

Human saliva samples were collected from patients regularly visiting the Outpatient Department (OPD) of the Dr. Ziauddin Ahmad Dental College and Hospital, Aligarh Muslim University, Uttar Pradesh, India for the project CST/372 dated 14 August 2017. The patient's consent was given before sampling. The use of saliva samples for isolation of bacteria was approved by the Internal Ethical Committee, Aligarh Muslim University, Uttar Pradesh, India.

2.2. Isolation and Culture Conditions

The Gram positive, oral coccoid strains, SJM-04, SJM-38, and SJM-65 were isolated from the Outpatient Department (OPD) of the Periodontics and Community Dentistry Clinic, Dr. Ziauddin Ahmad Dental College and Hospital, Aligarh Muslim University, India, by swab sampling as described by Papaioannou et al. [20]. In detail, sterile pure viscose swabs (PW043, Hi-media, Mumbai, India) were used to collect saliva samples from the floor, subgingival, and gingivae of the buccal cavities of patients. Swabs were then immediately immersed into 10 mL of sterile normal saline solution (NSS) for 30 min. Subsequently, 1000 µL samples were spread onto brain heart infusion (BHI) (Cat No. M210, Hi-media, Mumbai, India) agar plates and incubated for 24 h at 37 °C. Distinct colonies were isolated based on phenotypic characteristics (shape, size, color, margin, and colony elevation), purified, cultured, and preserved/stored in 20% glycerol at −80 °C.

2.3. Biochemical Characterization and Antibiotic Sensitivity Profiling of Oral Isolates

To determine the biochemical properties, IMViC, citrate, catalase, and sugar fermentation assays were performed as described in *Bergey's Manual of Systematic Bacteriology* [21]. Resistance to 1st, 2nd, 3rd, and 4th generation antibiotic discs, that is, nalidixic acid (NA, 30 µg) and tetracycline (TE, 30 µg); norfloxacin (NX, 10 µg) and cefuroxime (CXM, 30 µg); cefotaxime (CTX, 30 µg), levofloxacin (LE, 5 µg) and ceftazidime (CAZ, 30 µg); and methicillin (MET, 5 µg) (Hi-media, Mumbai, India) was investigated and interpreted as per the CLSI guidelines (2016).

2.4. Assessment of Biofilm Formation at Different pH Values, Temperatures, and Salinities

Biofilm formation by the three isolates was assessed at different temperatures, pH values, and salinities. *Georgenia* sp. (SJM-04), *S. saprophyticus* (SJM-38), or *R. mucilaginosa* (SJM-65) were exposed to these various conditions in 96-wells microtiter plates. To assess the effect of pH stress, BHI broth was adjusted to pH 6.4, 7.4, or 8.4 with 0.1 M HCl or 0.1 M NaOH. For salinity tolerance, the concentration of sodium chloride (NaCl) was increased from 200 to 1000 µg/mL, and to assess the effects of temperature, microtiter plates containing pristine BHI medium were subjected to 28 °C, 37 °C, or 42 °C. Wells were inoculated with 20 µL of freshly grown test strains ($\cong 1 \times 10^6$/mL) in BHI broth. All experiments were performed in triplicate using independent bacterial colonies and data were averaged.

2.5. Phylogenetic Characterization of Oral Bacteria

The 16S rRNA gene amplicons of the three Gram positive oral isolates were amplified by PCR using the primers: 16S-27F (5′ to 3′AGAGTTTGATCMTGGCTCAG, M = A or C) and 16S-1492R (5′ to 3′ACGGCTACCTTGTTACGA) (Sigma-Aldrich, St. Louis, MO, USA). Qiagen DNeasy kits (Valencia, CA, USA) were used for genomic DNA extraction. For polymerase chain reaction (PCR) amplification, reaction mixtures containing 2.5U Taq polymerase (Sigma Aldrich), 100 µM of each dNTP, 0.2 µM of each primer, and 3 µL of DNA template (substrate for Taq DNA polymerase) in 50 µL of 2 mM $MgCl_2$ solution were processed using a thermal cycler and the following program: 96 °C for 2 min (denaturation), followed by 30 amplification cycles of 95 °C for 15 s, 49 °C for 30 s, and 72 °C for 1 min, and a final extension at 72 °C for 1 min. PCR products were purified using the QIAquick-spin PCR Purification Kit (Qiagen, Chatsworth, CA, USA) and sequenced in a DNA sequencing facility using the BioEdit sequence alignment editor. Gene sequence homology was determined using archived 16S rRNA sequences in the GenBank server (www.ncbi.nlm.nih.gov/nucleotide) accessed on 24 January 2019, BLAST Multiple alignments of sequences, and Clustal W program. Phylogenetic trees were constructed using MEGA 6.0 and the neighbor-joining (NJ) DNA distance algorithm with bootstrap analysis (1000 replications).

2.6. Physicochemical Characterization of TiO_2NPs

The physicochemical characteristics of TiO_2NPs (Sigma-Aldrich, St. Louis, USA; product code 637254) were determined using: (i) a double beam UV-Visible spectrophotometer (UV 5704S from Electronics, India, Ltd., Panchkula, India), (ii) an X-ray diffractometer, (XRD, Rigaku Corporation, Tokyo, Japan), (iii) a transmission electron microscope, (iv) a scanning electron microscope (JSM 6510LV, SEM, Tokyo, Japan), and (v) by energy-dispersive X-ray (EDX) analyses (Oxford Instruments INCAx-sight EDX spectrometer, Concord, MA, USA). Details of the material characterization methods are provided in our earlier study [22]. Average TiO_2NP crystalline size was determined using the Debye–Scherrer's formula ($D = 0.9\lambda/\beta \cos \theta$; where D is crystal size, λ is X-ray wavelength, and β is the full-width at half-maximum (FWHM) of the diffraction peak).

2.7. TiO₂NP-Induced Cell Growth and Biofilm Inhibition

2.7.1. Dose-Dependent Anti-Planktonic Cell Activity of TiO$_2$NPs

The dose-dependent antibacterial effects of TiO$_2$NPs on isolated strains were determined. First, 100 µL of freshly grown (OD$_{600}$ = 0.01) SJM-04, SJM-38, or SJM-65 strains were added to microtiter wells containing 200 µL of BHI-TiO$_2$NPs (250, 500, 1000, or 2000 µg/mL) suspensions, and incubated at 37 °C in triplicate for 24 h. Untreated and treated bacterial cells were then diluted by a factor of 10^{-4} (OD$_{600}$ = 0.01) with sterile distilled water. To determine viable cell counts, 100 µL of diluted samples (OD$_{600}$ = 0.01) were spread on BHI agar plates and incubated at 37 °C for 24 h. The viabilities of test strains were determined by comparing the total plate counts (TPCs) of treated and untreated cells. Cells treated with or without TiO$_2$NPs (250 µg/mL) were also examined for TiO$_2$NP-induced morphological damage by SEM. Briefly, untreated and treated bacterial cells were spun at 3000 rpm for 5 min, fixed in glutaraldehyde (2.5%) at 4 °C for 4 h, and cell pellets were dehydrated in an ethanol series (30, 50, 70, and 90% ethanol for 15 min/step). A sample (100 µL) from each strain was mounted on a clean glass coverslip and coated with a thin layer of gold. Finally, the samples were examined under an SEM at 15 kV and 3000× [23].

2.7.2. Dose-Dependent Effect of TiO$_2$NPs on Biofilm Formation

The dose-dependent effects of TiO$_2$NPs on biofilm formation by the three isolates were quantified by measuring crystal violet (CV) absorbance, as described by Ahmed et al. [24]. In detail, 100µL ($\cong 1 \times 10^7$ cells) of freshly grown SJM-04, SJM-38, or SJM-65 cells were added to wells containing 250, 500, 1000, or 2000 µg/mL of TiO$_2$NPs in 200 µL of BHI broth per well. Cultures grown without TiO$_2$NPs and sterile BHI broth alone were used as positive and negative controls, respectively. Micro-well plates were incubated at 37 °C for 24 h, and then TiO$_2$NPs-BHI suspensions and loosely attached bacteria were carefully removed from the wells. Adherent biofilms on micro-well surfaces were then incubated with 200 µL of CV (1%) for 30 min, were washed with sterile PBS to remove non-absorbed CV, and air-dried. Biofilm bound CV was then solubilized with ethanol (95%) and absorbances (OD$_{620}$) were measured using a microplate reader (Thermo Scientific Multiskan EX, REF 51118170, Shanghai, China). In a similar manner, biofilms were formed in 96-well plate for 24 h and these mature biofilms were treated with TiO$_2$NPs to check the dispersal of mature biofilms by CV assay. In addition, TiO$_2$NP-induced reductions in biofilm formation were also assessed by microscopy as described by Ahmed et al. [25]. Briefly, using the same conditions mentioned above, biofilms adherent to glass coverslips were washed with PBS to remove loosely attached planktonic cells and then stained with CV (1%) for 30 min. Air-dried biofilms on cover glasses were examined under an optical microscope (Olympus BX60, Model BX60F5, Olympus Optical Co. Ltd. Tokyo, Japan) equipped with a digital camera (Sony, Model no. SSC-DC-58AP, Tokyo, Japan).

2.8. Statistical Analyses

Multiple comparisons versus controls were performed by one-way analysis of variance (ANOVA) using the Holm–Sidak method (Sigma Plot ver. 11.0, San Jose, CA, USA). Results are presented as the means ± SDs of at least two independent experiments performed in triplicate. Statistical significance was accepted for p values < 0.05.

3. Results and Discussion

3.1. Isolation and Characterization of Oral Bacteria

The diverse oral microbiota within biofilms obtain the proteins and glycoproteins (mucins) they require to thrive from saliva [26], which is produced at a rate of 1.5–2.0 mL/min [27] and normally supports bacterial proliferation of $\cong 10^9$ cells/mL [28]. Therefore, we collected human saliva with sterile swabs and subsequently added sterile saline solution enriched to near-physiological saline conditions, i.e., to millimolar concentrations of NaCl and Ca^{2+} ions. Figure 1 shows the primary characteristics of the colonies of oral isolates, such as color, elevation, margin (Figure 1(AI–AIII,BI–BIII)), morphologies, and antibiotic susceptibilities (Figure 1(CI–CIII)). The Gram reactions of *Georgenia* sp. (SJM-04), *S. saprophyticus* (SJM-38), and *R. mucilaginosa* (SJM-65) confirmed their primary identities as Gram positive rods (Figure 1(BI–BIII)) and cocci. Gram positive rod *Georgenia* sp. withstood nalidixic acid (NA), methicillin (MET), and ceftazidime (CAZ). Gram positive cocci *S. saprophyticus* was resistant to MET and CAZ, whereas *R. mucilaginosa* was resistant to tetracycline (TE), cefuroxime (CXM), MET, and CAZ (Table 1). Resistance against third-generation cephalosporin reflects the presence of single-nucleotide polymorphisms (SNPs) that directly increase CAZ hydrolysis by highly conserved class A β-lactamase [29] bacterial isolates. Similarly, Higashida et al. [30] in a study on eight *S. saprophyticus* strains also showed β-lactam resistance was due to *mecA* gene-mediated resistance. Moreover, transposon mutagenesis experiments have confirmed the role of *mecA* in conferring methicillin resistance [31]. Besides presenting as urinary tract infection bacterium, *S. saprophyticus* has been isolated from a variety of other samples such as different brands of minas cheese and beach water [32].

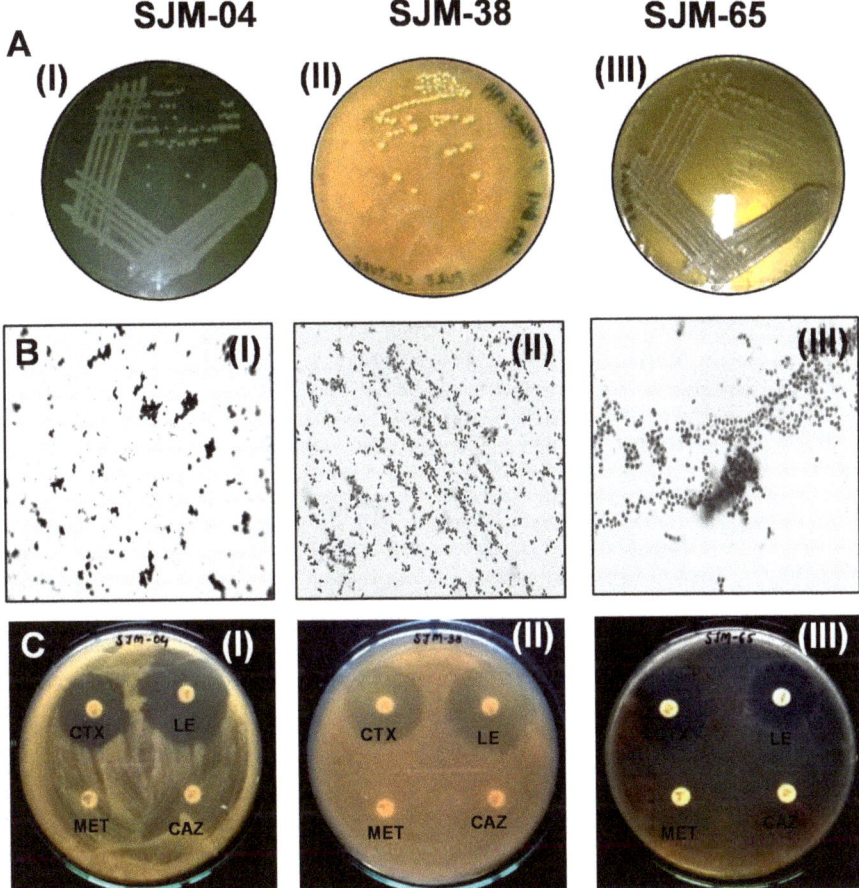

Figure 1. (**A,B**) show morphological characteristics of (**I**) SJM-04 (*Georgenia* sp.), (**II**) SJM-38 (*S. saprophyticus*), and (**III**) SJM-65 (*R. mucilaginosa*) grown onto their respective culture media. (**C**) shows representative images of the antibiotic sensitivity or resistance of (**I**) SJM-04 (*Georgenia* sp.), (**II**) SJM-65 (*S. saprophyticus*) and (**III**) SJM-38 (*R. mucilaginosa*) against multiple drugs.

Table 1. Antibiotic sensitivity profiling of Gram positive coccoid oral bacterial isolates.

Antibiotics	Concentration (µg/disc)	Zone of Inhibition (mm) ± S.D.		
		SJM-04	SJM-38	SJM-65
Nalidixic acid (NA)	30	0 ± 0 (R)	23 ± 2 (S)	15 ± 3 (S)
Tetracycline (TE)	10	25 ± 5 (S)	27 ± 3 (S)	0 ± 0 (R)
Norfloxacin (NX)	10	30 ± 3 (S)	27 ± 4 (S)	26 ± 4 (S)
Cefuroxime (CXM)	30	18 ± 2 (S)	32 ± 3 (S)	0 ± 0 (R)
Cefotaxime (CTX)	30	26 ± 4 (S)	30 ± 4 (S)	31 ± 2 (S)
Levofloxacin (LE)	5	32 ± 3 (S)	28 ± 5 (S)	29 ± 3 (S)
Methicillin (MET)	5	0 ± 0 (R)	0 ± 0 (R)	0 ± 0 (R)
Ceftazidime (CAZ)	30	0 ± 0 (R)	0 ± 0 (R)	0 ± 0 (R)

R = resistant and S = sensitive.

3.2. Biochemical Characterizations of the Three Oral Isolates

The survival of oral communities largely relies on the nature of the salivary environment (pH, temperature, and ionic strength) and the intrinsic metabolic responses of these communities to the salivary biochemical milieu. We subjected the oral isolates to 14 different biochemical tests. The biochemical abilities of SJM-04, SJM-38, and SJM-65, to metabolize monosaccharide and disaccharide and produce citrate, cytochrome oxidase, nitrate reductase, amylase, and lipase were determined using Voges–Proskauer (VP), sucrose fermentation, citrate, catalase, nitrate reductase, starch, and lipid hydrolysis assays, respectively (Table 2). According to Kampfer et al. [33], most strains of *Georgenia* species are able to utilize glucose and sucrose, and also showed that a Gram positive coccoid *Georgenia* sp. (~1–1.5 mm) isolate with a positive oxidase reaction demonstrated aerobic metabolism. The isolate SJM-38, identified as *S. saprophyticus*, a Gram positive cocci, is commonly found in the female urinary tract [34], but has also been isolated from meat, raw milk, cheese products [35], and the marine environment in polluted and recreational waters [32,36]. Recently, Uttatree and Charoenpanicha [37] reported certain biochemical properties of *S. saprophyticus* including fermentation and oxidation of glucose and sucrose, as we detected in the current study. Additionally, *S. saprophyticus* strains exhibited the production of citrate, catalase, amylase, and lipase (Table 2). The negative reaction of VP was well supported by the literature [38]. At least four types of nitrate-reducing enzymes have been reported in oral microflora, (i) periplasmic (NAP), (ii) membrane-bound (NAR), (iii) ferredoxin-dependent assimilatory (FdNAS), and (iv) flavin-dependent assimilatory (FAD-NAS), which exhibit distinct biochemical and catalytic properties of bacterial species including *R. mucilaginosa*, *R. dentocariosa*, and *S. epidermidis* [39]. Moreover, the isolate SJM-65 *R. mucilaginosa* was found to share a positive catalase reaction and a coccoid morphology with Staphylococci species [40]. Recently, Dhital et al. [41] reported a common starch hydrolytic reaction, whereby oral isolates secrete amylolytic enzymes that convert complex starch oligomers into simpler forms.

3.3. Phylogenetic Identification

Phylogenetic characterizations of the three bacterial isolates viz., SJM-04, SJM-38, and SJM-65 were carried out by analyzing 16S rRNA gene sequence homologies. PCR amplification (Figure 2A) and sequencing yielded partial nucleotide sequences of the 16S rRNA genes of SJM-04, SJM-38, and SJM-65, which were deposited in NCBI GenBank under accession nos. KT922165, KT922167, and KT922172, respectively. Phylogenetic analysis results of SJM-04, SJM-38, and SJM-65 concurred with the results of their presumptive identification as Gram positive cocci, and identified them as *Georgenia* sp. (accession no. KT922165), *S. saprophyticus* (accession no. KT922167), and *R. mucilaginosa* (accession no. KT922172), respectively. Furthermore, BLAST multiple alignments of the 16S rRNA sequence of isolate SJM-04 showed gene sequence homology with *Georgenia* sp. (accession no. KT922165) and close relatedness with the earlier recognized *Georgenia* species *Georgenia soli* strain CC-NMPT-T3 (FN356976) [33] and *G. daeguensis* strain 2C6-43 (HQ246163) [42], as shown in Figure 2B. Phylogenetic comparison of the *Staphylococcus* isolate (SJM-38) showed greatest similarity with *S. saprophyticus* strain ATCC 15305 (Figure 2B). In an identical manner, isolate SJM-65 was identified as *R. mucilaginosa* (accession no. KT922172) and showed close relatedness to all recognized species of genus Rhothia: *R. mucilaginosa* DSM 20746 and *R. dentocariosa* ATCC-17931 (Figure 2B).

Table 2. Biochemical characterization of Gram positive coccoid oral bacterial isolates.

Biochemical Assay	Bacterial Isolates		
	SJM-04	SJM-38	SJM-65
Indole test	−	−	−
Methyl red	−	−	−
Voges-Proskauer	+	+	−
Citrate	+	+	+
Sucrose fermentation	+	+	−
Lactose fermentation	−	−	−
Dextrose fermentation	−	+	+
Catalase	+	+	+
Oxidase	−	+	+
Nitrate reduction	+	−	+
Starch Hydrolysis	+	+	+
Lipid Hydrolysis	−	+	+
Urease	−	−	−

'−' and '+' signs denote a negative and positive reaction, respectively.

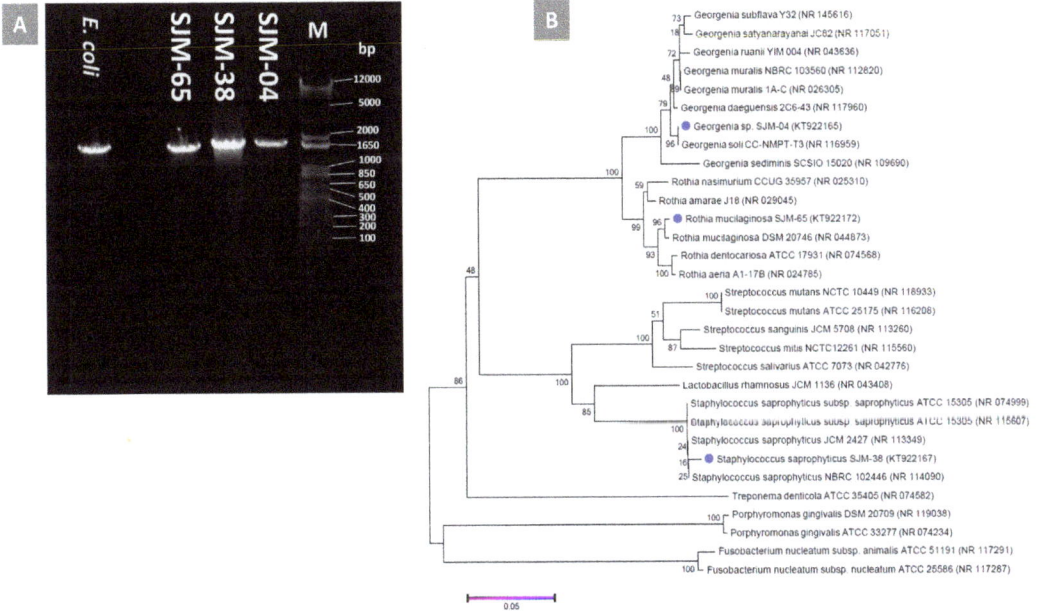

Figure 2. (A) shows an agarose gel electrophoresis result for purified 16S rDNA amplicons obtained after PCR amplification using genomic DNAs extracted from biofilm forming oral isolates as templates. (B) shows an unrooted neighbor-joined phylogenetic tree of closely related phylogenetic species based on 16S rRNA gene sequences of isolates SJM-04, SJM-38, and SJM-38 (marked with blue symbols). Sequences were aligned using the Clustal W sequence alignment tool in MEGA 7.0 software. The GenBank accession numbers of isolates and closely related species are presented in parenthesis. Bootstrap percentage values as obtained from 1000 replications of the data set are given at tree nodes. The scale bar represents the mean number of nucleotide substitutions per site.

3.4. Effects of Temperature, pH, and NaCl on Biofilm Formation

Growth patterns of bacterial cells proportionally affect the growths of biofilms, which are largely composed of non-replicating persister cells in an extracellular polysaccharide (EPS) matrix [43,44]. Unlike free planktonic cells, biofilm embedded/phenotypically altered cells become acclimatized to withstand microenvironmental stresses such as temperature, pH, and ionic strength changes. Hence, the present study primarily ascertains the optimal biofilm formation by modulating the physiochemical growth conditions for *Georgenia* sp. (SJM-04), *S. saprophyticus* (SJM-38), and *R. mucilaginosa* (SJM-65). Our results demonstrated (Figure 3A) that a lower temperature (28 °C) had a negligible effect on biofilm formation by bacterial strains as compared with the control temperature (37 °C). However, temperature elevation to 42 °C significantly limited biofilm adherence to $7.2 \pm 1.0\%$ ($p < 0.05$) for strain *Georgenia* sp. (SJM-04), and *S. saprophyticus* (SJM-38) and *R. mucilaginosa* (SJM-65) could not survive this temperature. It is widely accepted that the optimum temperature is directly related to the metabolic activities of microbial enzymes, and thus, nutrient metabolism [45] and biofilm formation [46].

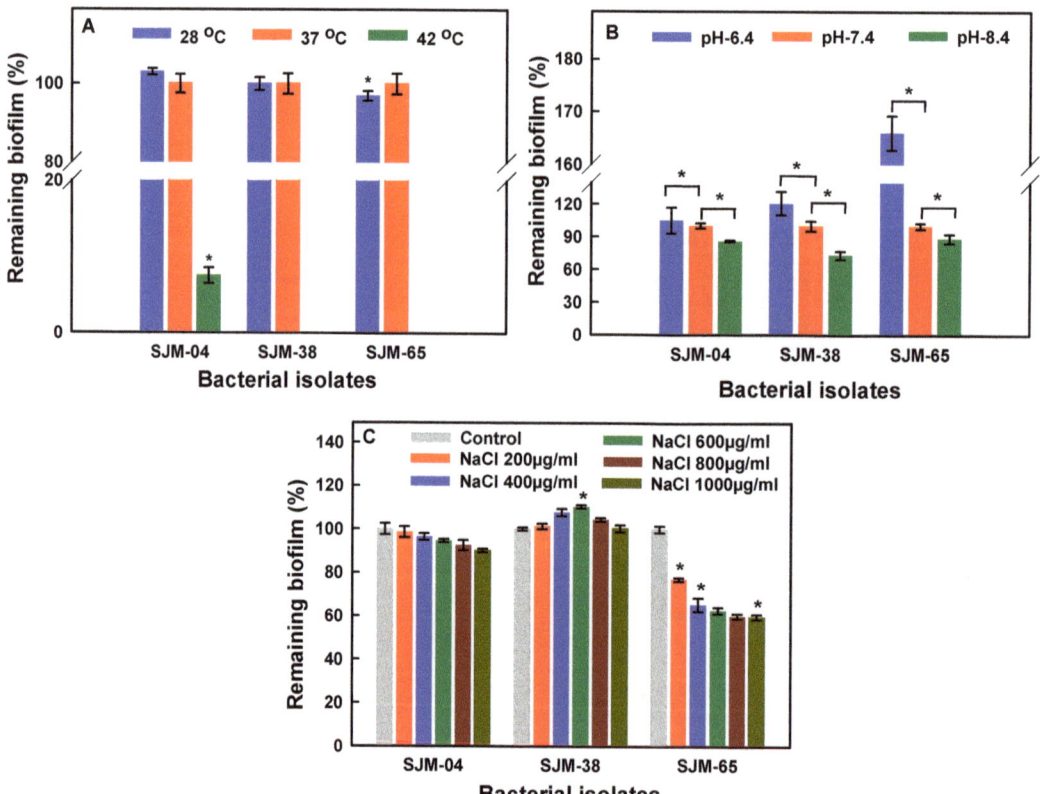

Figure 3. Assessment of biofilm formation as a function of temperature (**A**), pH (**B**), and NaCl concentration (**C**). '*' denotes the statistical difference at $p \leq 0.05$ between control and treated groups.

In the present study, an increase or decrease in one pH unit from the control level (pH—7.4) significantly ($p < 0.05$) affected the interaction between isolates *Georgenia* sp. (SJM-04), *S. saprophyticus* (SJM-38), and *R. mucilaginosa* (SJM-65) and glass surfaces (Figure 3B). At pH 6.4, significant ($p < 0.05$) increases in biofilm formation were observed for *Georgenia* sp. (SJM-04), *S. saprophyticus* (SJM-38), and *R. mucilaginosa* (SJM-65) strains by 105.2%,

120.7%, and 166%, respectively, as compared to 100% for controls at pH 7.4). Conversely, an increase in pH to 8.4 caused significant ($p < 0.05$) reductions in biofilm to 85.77 ± 0.80, 73.26 ± 3.6, and 88.57 ± 4.2%, respectively (Figure 3B). Thus, our results indicate that a slight change in external pH can overwhelm the cellular processes that support oral bacterial biofilms, which may include the synthesis of proteins [47] and polysaccharides [48] and the membrane electrochemical gradient [49]. Earlier studies on acyl-homoserine lactone (AHL) production in quorum sensing (QS) systems of marine bacteria demonstrated salinity dependence [50], and suggested that salinity is a significant factor for QS [51]. Therefore, we also investigated biofilm growth in the presence of different concentrations (200, 400, 600, 800, and 1000 μg/mL) of NaCl. Results demonstrated a dose-dependent decrease in biofilm formation from 98.5 ± 2.5% to 90.0 ± 8.7% and from 76.9 ± 2.8% to 59.7 ± 1.2% on increasing the NaCl concentration from 200–1000 μg/mL for *Georgenia* sp. (SJM-04) and *R. mucilaginosa* (SJM-65), respectively (Figure 3C). Interestingly, under identical conditions, biofilm formation by *S. saprophyticus* (SJM-38) slightly increased on increasing the NaCl (200–1000 μg/mL) concentration 101.3 ± 1.2%, 107.7 ± 1.6%, 110.3 ± 0.7%, 104.4 ± 0.7% and 100.4 ± 1.6%, respectively (Figure 3C). According to Moretro et al. [52], NaCl and glucose stimulate adherence and increase the stability of biofilms formed by *Staphylococci* genus due to the presence of the icaA gene, which is positively correlated with strong biofilm formation. Recently, Xu et al. [53] also reported that NaCl significantly increased biofilm formation by *S. aureus* in an concentration-dependent manner

3.5. Physicochemical Characteristics of TiO_2NPs

Surface plasmon resonance (SPR) happens due to the collective oscillations of electrons at the resonant frequency of metal NPs and results in absorption in the UV-Visible region [13]. In the present study, the appearance of a sharp peak at an absorption wavelength (λ_{max}) of 347 nm in the UV-Vis absorption spectrum is likely to be due to localized SPR of TiO_2NPs in aqueous suspension (Figure 4A). Furthermore, SPR frequencies of NPs are considered to be directly correlated with nanoparticle size, shape, and crystalline nature [54]. Therefore, we analyzed the morphology and composition and determined the size and crystallinity of TiO_2NPs. SEM analysis showed NPs had pleomorphic shapes, though the majority were spherical (Figure 4B). The EDX spectrum of TiO_2NPs revealed the presence of titanium (Ti) and oxygen (O) at elemental compositions of 32.74% and 67.26%, respectively (Figure 4C). TEM results showed TiO_2NPs shapes included spherical, oval, and hexagonal particles (Figure 4D) with sizes ranging from 5–25 nm (average diameter 14.7 nm) (Figure 4E). Furthermore, the XRD pattern of TiO_2NPs (Figure 4F), obtained by using cell parameters: a-3.8101 Å, b-3.8101 Å, and c-9.3632 Å; $\alpha = \beta = \gamma = 90°$ and centered tetragonal phase, showed the anatase phase TiO_2-NPs (JCPDS 21–1272) and peaks at 2θ values of 24.6°, 37.2°, 47.5°, 53.4°, 54.6°, and 62.2° corresponding to (101), (004), (200), (1050), (211), and (204) HKL miller indices, respectively. Average size by XRD was determined to be 13.7 nm based on full-width at half-maximum (FWHM) of the 101 reflection peak, which matched well with that of the TEM size.

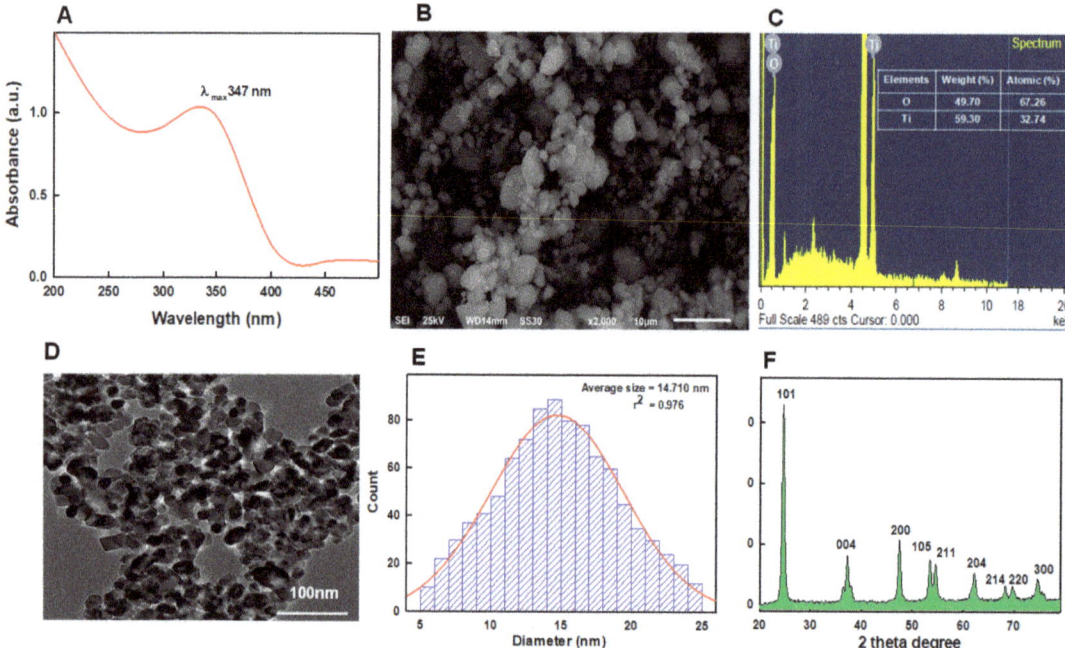

Figure 4. UV-Vis absorption spectrum of TiO$_2$NPs showing the characteristic SPR peak at 347 nm (**A**). (**B,C**) show the SEM image and energy dispersive X-ray analysis of TiO$_2$NPs, respectively. (**D**) shows a representative TEM micrograph of TiO$_2$NPs and (**E**) shows the TiO$_2$NP size distribution. (**F**) shows the X-ray diffraction pattern of TiO$_2$NPs.

The dose-dependent antibacterial effect of TiO$_2$NPs (250–2000 µg/mL) on oral bacterial strains: *Georgenia* sp. (SJM-04), *S. saprophyticus* (SJM-38), and *R. mucilaginosa* (SJM-65) exhibited significant growth inhibition over 24 h (Figure 5). We found that treatment with TiO$_2$NPs at 250, 500, 1000, and 2000 µg/mL for 24 h reduced the viability of *Georgenia* sp. (SJM-04), *S. saprophyticus* (SJM-38), and *R. mucilaginosa* (SJM-65) to 58.0 ± 5.2, 52.0 ± 3.8, 38.0 ± 4.5 and 4.5 ± 2.0% (Figure 5(AI)); 91.0 ± 3.8, 78.0 ± 5.2, 25.0 ± 4.5 and 5.0 ± 2.0% (Figure 5(BI)); and, 90.0 ± 5.2, 55.0 ± 4.8, 41.0 ± 4.5 and 38.0 ± 3.0% (Figure 5(CI)), respectively. The mechanisms responsible for the antibacterial activities of various metal-oxide NPs are unclear, though it is believed that the presence of dissolved metal ions on surfaces of NPs and/or NP-induced oxidative stress are involved [14]. Specifically, in the case of anatase TiO$_2$NPs, the photocatalytic activity of TiO$_2$ in aqueous environments results in the release of hydroxyl radicals (OH•) and the subsequent formation of superoxide radicals (O$_2^-$) [55]. Therefore, it could be argued that ROS may attack polyunsaturated phospholipids in bacteria and cause DNA damage [23,25]. Additionally, we treated *Georgenia* sp. (Figure 5(AIII)), *S. saprophyticus* (Figure 5(BIII)), and *R. mucilaginosa* (Figure 5(CIII)) with TiO$_2$NPs at 250 µg/mL and examined their effects by SEM. We observed that TiO$_2$NP–bacteria interactions caused morphological changes such as shrinkage and cell membrane damage, possibly because NPs penetrated bacterial membranes and compromised cell membrane permeability [56].

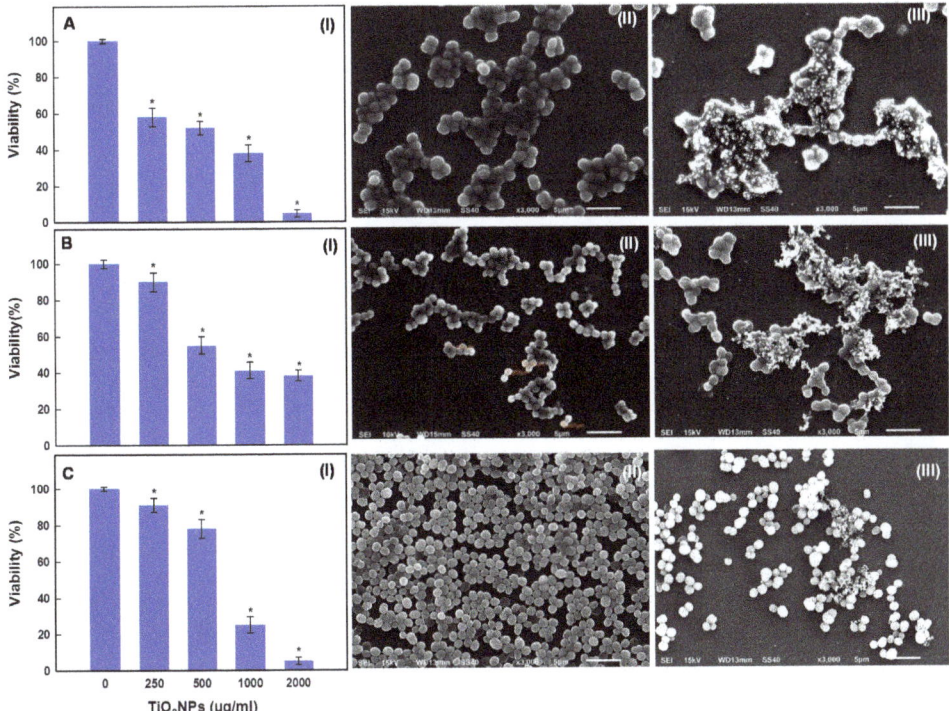

Figure 5. Reductions in the percentage viability of Gram positive SJM-04 (**AI**), SJM-38 (**BI**), and SJM-65 (**CI**) treated with 250, 500, 1000, or 2000 μg/mL concentrations of TiO$_2$NPs for 24h. SEM micrographs showing morphological changes in SJM-04 (**AIII**), SJM-38 (**BIII**), and SJM-65 (**CIII**) cells after treatment with TiO$_2$NPs at 250μg/mL vs. untreated control cells (**AII–CII**). '*' denotes the statistical difference at $p \leq 0.05$ between control and treated groups.

3.6. Dose-Dependent Effects of TiO$_2$NPs on Biofilm Formation

The effects of TiO$_2$NPs concentration (250–2000 μg/mL) on the adherence of the biofilms produced by the three oral strains were also examined. The biofilms produced by various bacterial species play decisive roles in the way they respond to their immediate surroundings. Treatment of *Georgenia* sp., *S. saprophyticus*, and *R. mucilaginosa* with TiO$_2$NPs at 250, 500, 1000, or 2000 μg/mL for 24 h significantly reduced biofilm adhesion on glass surfaces to 55.5 ± 3.2, 46.4 ± 4.1, 35.3 ± 4.2, and 13.1 ± 3.2%; 48.4 ± 3.2, 42.4 ± 4.1, 30.3 ± 1.9, and 18.1 ± 2.0%; and 68.3 ± 3.4, 50.2 ±3.3, 43.3 ± 3.2, and 33.3 ± 3.2%, respectively (Figure 6A). Taken together, these results show that TiO$_2$NPs reduced biofilm adherence in a concentration-dependent manner. Recently, Sodagar et al. [57] reported that treatment with 5% TiO$_2$NPs significantly inhibited biofilm formation by the Gram positive oral bacteria *S. mutans* and *S. sanguinis*. Additionally, the micrographs presented in Figure 6B–D show than TiO$_2$NPs reduced biofilm formation by *Georgenia* sp. (Figure 6(BII–BV)), *S. saprophyticus* (Figure 6(CII–CV)), and *R. Mucilaginosa* (Figure 6(DII–DV)) in a concentration-dependent manner versus untreated controls (Figure 6(BI,DI)). In assessing the reduction in mature (24 h) biofilms of the three tested strains of TiO$_2$NPs by CV assay, only 1000 or 2000 μg/mL resulted in significant destruction of mature biofilms, suggesting that TiO$_2$NPs are more efficient against developing biofilms at 250–500 μg/mL, but they can also destroy biofilms at higher concentrations of 1000 or 2000 μg/mL (Supplementary Materials, Figure S1).

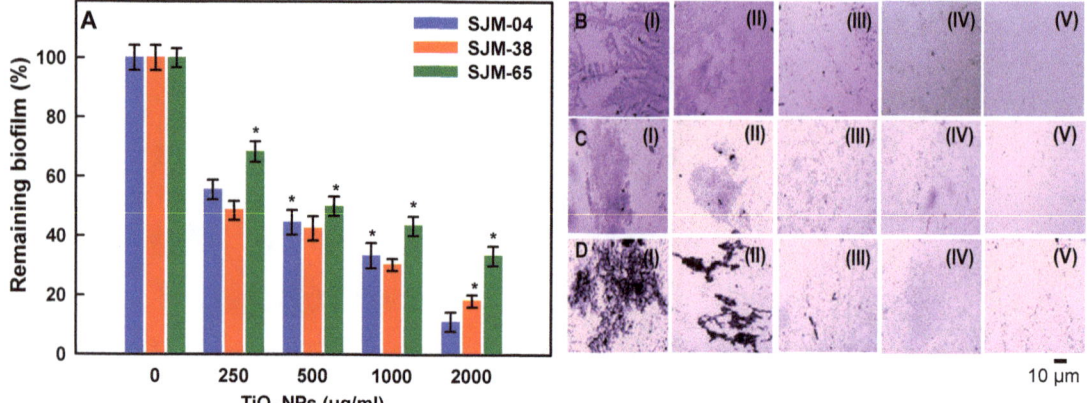

Figure 6. Reductions in biofilm formation after treatment with TiO$_2$NPs at 250, 500, 1000, or 2000 µg/mL for 24 h (Panel **A**). Error bars denote standard deviations of triplicate samples (**A**). Microscopic images showing reduced biofilm formation by SJM-04 (**B**), SJM-38 (**C**), and SJM-65 (**D**) after treatments with TiO$_2$NPs at 0 (**I**), 250 (**II**), 500 (**III**), 1000 (**IV**), or 2000µg/mL (**V**). '*' denotes the statistical difference at $p \leq 0.05$ between control and treated groups.

4. Conclusions

The MDR Gram positive cocci *Georgenia* sp., *R. mucilaginosa*, and *S. saprophyticus* isolated from oral cavity were successfully characterized for their morphologies, biochemical characteristics, phylogenetic relatedness, and biofilm formation at various pH, temperatures and salt concentrations. Exposure of these strains to crystalline TiO$_2$NPs (5> size <25 nm) significantly inhibited their planktonic cell growth and biofilm formation. Three exposure scenarios including low (250 µg/mL), moderate (500 µg/mL), and high (1000–2000 µg/mL) doses of TiO$_2$NPs decreased the biofilm in a dose-dependent manner, suggesting that the concentration of TiO$_2$NPs, apart from other factors, could be the main reason why they act as both an antibacterial and antibiofilm agent to the tested oral bacteria. Our results suggest that TiO$_2$NPs with the following physicochemical profile: absorption λ_{max} of 347 nm, diameter 5–25 nm, average crystalline size 13.7 nm, tetragonal anatase phase, and spherical shape might be a suitable choice for treating oral biofilms, can potentially be applied in orthodontics as a potential oral hygiene alternative to conventional rinses and for the suppression of cariogenic biofilm formation. Further in vivo biofilm studies on the interaction of TiO$_2$NPs with human saliva and the effect on NP's shape, size, and metal release are warranted for preparing the most effective antibiofilm formulations.

Supplementary Materials: The following are available online at https://www.mdpi.com/article/10.3390/pharmaceutics13101564/s1, Figure S1. Reduction in mature (24 h) biofilms of strain SJM-04, SJM-38, and SJM-65 by TiO2NPs. '*' represents statistical difference at $p \leq 0.05$.

Author Contributions: Conceptualization, J.M. and A.S.; methodology, S.F., K.A. and B.A.; software, J.M., S.F. and K.A.; validation, J.M., J.L. and A.M.E.; formal analysis, B.A., K.A. and A.A.A.K.; investigation, J.M., S.F., K.A. and B.A.; resources, J.M., A.M.E. and J.L.; data curation, S.F., K.A. and A.A.A.K.; writing—original draft preparation, K.A. and B.A.; writing—review and editing, J.M., K.A., B.A., A.S. and J.L.; supervision, J.M.; project administration, J.M. and B.A.; funding acquisition, J.M., A.M.E. and J.L. All authors have read and agreed to the published version of the manuscript.

Funding: This research was funded by the Priority Research Centers Program through the National Research Foundation of Korea (NRF) funded by the Ministry of Education (2014R1A6A1031189) and the Researchers Supporting Project Number (RSP-2021/31), King Saud University, Riyadh, Saudi Arabia.

Institutional Review Board Statement: The use of saliva samples for isolation of bacteria was approved by the Internal Ethical Committee, Aligarh Muslim University, Uttar Pradesh, India.

Informed Consent Statement: Informed consent was obtained from all subjects (patients) involved in the study.

Acknowledgments: This work was supported by the Priority Research Centers Program through the National Research Foundation of Korea (NRF) funded by the Ministry of Education (2014R1A6A1031189). The authors extend their appreciation to the Researchers Supporting Project Number (RSP-2021/31), King Saud University, Riyadh, Saudi Arabia.

Conflicts of Interest: The authors declare no conflict of interest.

References

1. Palmer, R.J., Jr. Composition and development of oral bacterial communities. *Periodontology 2000* **2014**, *64*, 20–39. [CrossRef]
2. Muñoz-González, I.; Thurnheer, T.; Bartolome, B.; Moreno-Arribas, M.V. Red wine and oenological extracts display antimicrobial effects in an oral bacteria biofilm model. *J. Agric. Food Chem.* **2014**, *62*, 4731–4737. [CrossRef] [PubMed]
3. Flemming, H.-C.; Wingender, J. The biofilm matrix. *Nat. Rev. Microbiol.* **2010**, *8*, 623–633. [CrossRef] [PubMed]
4. Tawakoli, P.N.; Al-Ahmad, A.; Hoth-Hannig, W.; Hannig, M.; Hannig, C. Comparison of different live/dead stainings for detection and quantification of adherent microorganisms in the initial oral biofilm. *Clin. Oral Investig.* **2013**, *17*, 841–850. [CrossRef] [PubMed]
5. Roberts, A.P.; Mullany, P. Oral biofilms: A reservoir of transferable, bacterial, antimicrobial resistance. *Expert Rev. Anti-Infect. Ther.* **2010**, *8*, 1441–1450. [CrossRef]
6. Potera, C. Antibiotic resistance: Biofilm dispersing agent rejuvenates older antibiotics. *Environ. Health Perspect.* **2010**, *118*, A288. [CrossRef]
7. Da Silva, B.R.; De Freitas, V.A.A.; Carneiro, V.A.; Arruda, F.V.S.; Lorenzón, E.N.; De Aguiar, A.S.W.; Cilli, E.M.; Cavada, B.S.; Teixeira, E.H. Antimicrobial activity of the synthetic peptide Lys-a1 against oral streptococci. *Peptides* **2013**, *42*, 78–83. [CrossRef]
8. Beikler, T.; Flemmig, T.F. Oral biofilm-associated diseases: Trends and implications for quality of life, systemic health and expenditures. *Periodontology 2000* **2011**, *55*, 87–103. [CrossRef]
9. Lu, M.; Ge, Y.; Qiu, J.; Shao, D.; Zhang, Y.; Bai, J.; Zheng, X.; Chang, Z.; Wang, Z.; Dong, W. Redox/pH dual-controlled release of chlorhexidine and silver ions from biodegradable mesoporous silica nanoparticles against oral biofilms. *Int. J. Nanomed.* **2018**, *13*, 7697. [CrossRef]
10. Liang, G.; Shi, H.; Qi, Y.; Li, J.; Jing, A.; Liu, Q.; Feng, W.; Li, G.; Gao, S. Specific Anti-biofilm Activity of Carbon Quantum Dots by Destroying, *P. gingivalis* Biofilm Related Genes. *Int. J. Nanomed.* **2020**, *15*, 5473. [CrossRef]
11. Coman, A.N.; Mare, A.; Tanase, C.; Bud, E.; Rusu, A. Silver-deposited nanoparticles on the titanium nanotubes surface as a promising antibacterial material into implants. *Metals* **2021**, *11*, 92. [CrossRef]
12. Tanase, C.; Berta, L.; Mare, A.; Man, A.; Talmaciu, A.I.; Roșca, I.; Mircia, E.; Volf, I.; Popa, V.I. Biosynthesis of silver nanoparticles using aqueous bark extract of *Picea abies* L. and their antibacterial activity. *Eur. J. Wood Wood Prod.* **2020**, *78*, 281–291. [CrossRef]
13. Zane, A.; Zuo, R.; Villamena, F.A.; Rockenbauer, A.; Foushee, A.M.D.; Flores, K.; Dutta, P.K.; Nagy, A. Biocompatibility and antibacterial activity of nitrogen-doped titanium dioxide nanoparticles for use in dental resin formulations. *Int. J. Nanomed.* **2016**, *11*, 6459. [CrossRef] [PubMed]
14. Khan, S.T.; Al-Khedhairy, A.A.; Musarrat, J. ZnO and TiO$_2$ nanoparticles as novel antimicrobial agents for oral hygiene: A review. *J. Nanopart. Res.* **2015**, *17*, 1–16. [CrossRef]
15. Allaker, R.P.; Memarzadeh, K. Nanoparticles and the control of oral infections. *Int. J. Antimicrob. Agents* **2014**, *43*, 95–104. [CrossRef]
16. Yazdi, A.S.; Guarda, G.; Riteau, N.; Drexler, S.K.; Tardivel, A.; Couillin, I.; Tschopp, J. Nanoparticles activate the NLR pyrin domain containing 3 (Nlrp3) inflammasome and cause pulmonary inflammation through release of IL-1α and IL-1β. *Proc. Natl. Acad. Sci. USA* **2010**, *107*, 19449–19454. [CrossRef] [PubMed]
17. Al-Shaeri, M.; Satar, R.; Ahmed, S.I.; Oves, M.; Ansari, S.A.; Chibber, S. Utilization of Doped Nanoparticles of ZnO and TiO$_2$ As Antimicrobial Agent. *Orient. J. Chem.* **2019**, *35*, 1235. [CrossRef]
18. Priyanka, K.P.; Harikumar, V.S.; Balakrishna, K.M.; Varghese, T. Inhibitory effect of TiO$_2$ NPs on symbiotic arbuscular mycorrhizal fungi in plant roots. *IET Nanobiotechnol.* **2017**, *11*, 66–70. [CrossRef]
19. de Dicastillo, C.L.; Correa, M.G.; Martínez, F.B.; Streitt, C.; Galotto, M.J. Antimicrobial effect of titanium dioxide nanoparticles. In *Titanium Dioxide*; IntechOpen: London, UK, 2020.
20. Papaioannou, W.; Gizani, S.; Haffajee, A.D.; Quirynen, M.; Mamai-Homata, E.; Papagiannoulis, L. The microbiota on different oral surfaces in healthy children. *Oral Microbiol. Immunol.* **2009**, *24*, 183–189. [CrossRef] [PubMed]
21. Vos, P.; Garrity, G.; Jones, D.; Krieg, N.R.; Ludwig, W.; Rainey, F.A.; Schleifer, K.-H.; Whitman, W.B. *Bergey's Manual of Systematic Bacteriology: Volume 3: The Firmicutes*; Springer Science & Business Media: New York, NY, USA, 2011; Volume 3, ISBN 0387684891.

22. Ali, K.; Abul Qais, F.; Dwivedi, S.; Abdel-Salam, E.M.; Ansari, S.M.; Saquib, Q.; Faisal, M.; Al-Khedhairy, A.A.; Al-Shaeri, M.; Musarrat, J. Titanium dioxide nanoparticles preferentially bind in subdomains IB, IIA of HSA and minor groove of DNA. *J. Biomol. Struct. Dyn.* **2018**, *36*, 2530–2542. [CrossRef] [PubMed]
23. Saleem, S.; Ahmed, B.; Khan, M.S.; Al-Shaeri, M.; Musarrat, J. Inhibition of growth and biofilm formation of clinical bacterial isolates by NiO nanoparticles synthesized from *Eucalyptus globulus* plants. *Microb. Pathog.* **2017**, *111*, 375–387. [CrossRef] [PubMed]
24. Ahmed, B.; Syed, A.; Ali, K.; Elgorban, A.M.; Khan, A.; Lee, J.; AL-Shwaiman, H.A. Synthesis of gallotannin capped iron oxide nanoparticles and their broad spectrum biological applications. *RSC Adv.* **2021**, *11*, 9880–9893. [CrossRef]
25. Ahmed, B.; Solanki, B.; Zaidi, A.; Khan, M.S.; Musarrat, J. Bacterial toxicity of biomimetic green zinc oxide nanoantibiotic: Insights into ZnONP uptake and nanocolloid-bacteria interface. *Toxicol. Res.* **2019**, *8*, 246–261. [CrossRef] [PubMed]
26. Marsh, P.D.; Devine, D.A. How is the development of dental biofilms influenced by the host? *J. Clin. Periodontol.* **2011**, *38*, 28–35. [CrossRef]
27. Holsinger, F.C.; Bui, D.T. Anatomy, function, and evaluation of the salivary glands. In *Salivary Gland Disorders*; Springer: Berlin/Heidelberg, Germany, 2007; pp. 1–16.
28. Dawes, C. Estimates, from salivary analyses, of the turnover time of the oral mucosal epithelium in humans and the number of bacteria in an edentulous mouth. *Arch. Oral Biol.* **2003**, *48*, 329–336. [CrossRef]
29. Sarovich, D.S.; Price, E.P.; Von Schulze, A.T.; Cook, J.M.; Mayo, M.; Watson, L.M.; Richardson, L.; Seymour, M.L.; Tuanyok, A.; Engelthaler, D.M. Characterization of ceftazidime resistance mechanisms in clinical isolates of *Burkholderia pseudomallei* from Australia. *PLoS ONE* **2012**, *7*, e30789. [CrossRef] [PubMed]
30. Higashide, M.; Kuroda, M.; Omura, C.T.N.; Kumano, M.; Ohkawa, S.; Ichimura, S.; Ohta, T. Methicillin-resistant *Staphylococcus saprophyticus* isolates carrying staphylococcal cassette chromosome mec have emerged in urogenital tract infections. *Antimicrob. Agents Chemother.* **2008**, *52*, 2061–2068. [CrossRef]
31. Matthews, P.; Tomasz, A. Insertional inactivation of the *mec* gene in a transposon mutant of a methicillin-resistant clinical isolate of *Staphylococcus aureus*. *Antimicrob. Agents Chemother.* **1990**, *34*, 1777–1779. [CrossRef] [PubMed]
32. de Sousa, V.S.; da-Silva, A.P.d.S.; Sorenson, L.; Paschoal, R.P.; Rabello, R.F.; Campana, E.H.; Pinheiro, M.S.; dos Santos, L.O.F.; Martins, N.; Botelho, A.C.N. *Staphylococcus saprophyticus* recovered from humans, food, and recreational waters in Rio de Janeiro, Brazil. *Int. J. Microbiol.* **2017**, *2017*, 4287547. [CrossRef]
33. Kämpfer, P.; Arun, A.B.; Busse, H.-J.; Langer, S.; Young, C.-C.; Chen, W.-M.; Schumann, P.; Syed, A.A.; Rekha, P.D. *Georgenia soli* sp. nov., isolated from iron-ore-contaminated soil in India. *Int. J. Syst. Evol. Microbiol.* **2010**, *60*, 1027–1030. [CrossRef]
34. Becker, K.; Heilmann, C.; Peters, G. Coagulase-negative staphylococci. *Clin. Microbiol. Rev.* **2014**, *27*, 870–926. [CrossRef]
35. Coton, E.; Desmonts, M.H.; Leroy, S.; Coton, M.; Jamet, E.; Christieans, S.; Donnio, P.Y.; Lebert, I.; Talon, R. Biodiversity of Coagulase-Negative Staphylococci in French cheeses, dry fermented sausages, processing environments and clinical samples. *Int. J. Food Microbiol.* **2010**. [CrossRef]
36. Basso, A.P.; Martins, P.D.; Nachtigall, G.; Sand, S.V.D.; Moura, T.M.; Frazzon, A.P.G. Antibiotic resistance and enterotoxin genes in *Staphylococcus* sp. isolates from polluted water in Southern Brazil. *An. Acad. Bras. Cienc.* **2014**, *86*, 1813–1820. [CrossRef] [PubMed]
37. Uttatree, S.; Charoenpanich, J. Purification and characterization of a harsh conditions-resistant protease from a new strain of *Staphylococcus saprophyticus*. *Agric. Nat. Resour.* **2018**, *52*, 16–23. [CrossRef]
38. Trivedi, M.K.; Branton, A.; Trivedi, D.; Nayak, G.; Mondal, S.C.; Jana, S. Antimicrobial sensitivity, biochemical characteristics and biotyping of *Staphylococcus saprophyticus*: An impact of biofield energy treatment. *J. Women's Health Care* **2015**, *4*, 1000271.
39. Doel, J.J.; Benjamin, N.; Hector, M.P.; Rogers, M.; Allaker, R.P. Evaluation of bacterial nitrate reduction in the human oral cavity. *Eur. J. Oral Sci.* **2005**, *113*, 14–19. [CrossRef]
40. Michels, F.; Colaert, J.; Gheysen, F.; Scheerlinck, T. Late prosthetic joint infection due to *Rothia mucilaginosa*. *Acta Orthop. Belg.* **2007**, *73*, 263.
41. Dhital, S.; Warren, F.J.; Butterworth, P.J.; Ellis, P.R.; Gidley, M.J. Mechanisms of starch digestion by α-amylase—Structural basis for kinetic properties. *Crit. Rev. Food Sci. Nutr.* **2017**, *57*, 875–892. [CrossRef]
42. Woo, S.-G.; Cui, Y.; Kang, M.-S.; Jin, L.; Kim, K.K.; Lee, S.-T.; Lee, M.; Park, J. *Georgenia daeguensis* sp. nov., isolated from 4-chlorophenol enrichment culture. *Int. J. Syst. Evol. Microbiol.* **2012**, *62*, 1703–1709. [CrossRef]
43. Fulaz, S.; Devlin, H.; Vitale, S.; Quinn, L.; O'Gara, J.P.; Casey, E. Tailoring nanoparticle-biofilm interactions to increase the efficacy of antimicrobial agents against *Staphylococcus aureus*. *Int. J. Nanomed.* **2020**, *15*, 4779. [CrossRef]
44. Ameen, F.; Alshehri, W.A.; Nadhari, S. Al Effect of electroactive biofilm formation on acetic acid production in anaerobic sludge driven microbial electrosynthesis. *ACS Sustain. Chem. Eng.* **2019**, *8*, 311–318. [CrossRef]
45. Lee, J.H.; Kim, Y.G.; Cho, M.H.; Lee, J. ZnO nanoparticles inhibit Pseudomonas aeruginosa biofilm formation and virulence factor production. *Microbiol. Res.* **2014**, *169*, 888–896. [CrossRef] [PubMed]
46. Stepanović, S.; Ćirković, I.; Mijač, V.; Švabić-Vlahović, M. Influence of the incubation temperature, atmosphere and dynamic conditions on biofilm formation by *Salmonella* spp. *Food Microbiol.* **2003**, *20*, 339–343. [CrossRef]
47. Olson, E.R. Influence of pH on bacterial gene expression. *Mol. Microbiol.* **1993**, *8*, 5–14. [CrossRef]
48. Oliveira, R.; Melo, L.F.; Oliveira, A.; Salgueiro, R. Polysaccharide production and biofilm formation by *Pseudomonas fluorescens*: Effects of pH and surface material. *Colloids Surf. B Biointerfaces* **1994**, *2*, 41–46. [CrossRef]

49. Rowland, B.M. Bacterial contamination of dental unit waterlines: What is your dentist spraying into your mouth? *Clin. Microbiol. Newsl.* **2003**, *25*, 73–77. [CrossRef]
50. Zhou, L.; Xia, S.; Zhang, Z.; Ye, B.; Xu, X.; Gu, Z.; Wang, X. Effects of pH, Temperature and Salinity on Extracellular Polymeric Substances of *Pseudomonas aeruginosa* Biofilm with N-(3-Oxooxtanoyl)-L-Homoserine Lactone Addition. *J. Water Sustain.* **2014**, *4*, 91.
51. Cai, T.; Ge, X.; Park, S.Y.; Li, Y. Comparison of Synechocystis sp. PCC6803 and Nannochloropsis salina for lipid production using artificial seawater and nutrients from anaerobic digestion effluent. *Bioresour. Technol.* **2013**, *144*, 255–260. [CrossRef]
52. Møretrø, T.; Hermansen, L.; Holck, A.L.; Sidhu, M.S.; Rudi, K.; Langsrud, S. Biofilm formation and the presence of the intercellular adhesion locus ica among staphylococci from food and food processing environments. *Appl. Environ. Microbiol.* **2003**, *69*, 5648–5655. [CrossRef] [PubMed]
53. Xu, H.; Zou, Y.; Lee, H.; Ahn, J. Effect of NaCl on the biofilm formation by foodborne pathogens. *J. Food Sci.* **2010**, *75*, M580–M585. [CrossRef]
54. Jensen, T.; Kelly, L.; Lazarides, A.; Schatz, G.C. Electrodynamics of noble metal nanoparticles and nanoparticle clusters. *J. Clust. Sci.* **1999**, *10*, 295–317. [CrossRef]
55. Linsebigler, A.L.; Lu, G.; Yates, J.T., Jr. Photocatalysis on TiO_2 surfaces: Principles, mechanisms, and selected results. *Chem. Rev.* **1995**, *95*, 735–758. [CrossRef]
56. Battin, T.J.; Kammer, F.V.D.; Weilhartner, A.; Ottofuelling, S.; Hofmann, T. Nanostructured TiO2: Transport behavior and effects on aquatic microbial communities under environmental conditions. *Environ. Sci. Technol.* **2009**, *43*, 8098–8104. [CrossRef] [PubMed]
57. Sodagar, A.; Akhoundi, M.S.A.; Bahador, A.; Jalali, Y.F.; Behzadi, Z.; Elhaminejad, F.; Mirhashemi, A.H. Effect of TiO_2 nanoparticles incorporation on antibacterial properties and shear bond strength of dental composite used in Orthodontics. *Dent. Press J. Orthod.* **2017**, *22*, 67–74.

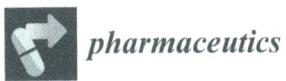

Article

Antimicrobial Properties of *Lepidium sativum* L. Facilitated Silver Nanoparticles

Samir Haj Bloukh [1,2], Zehra Edis [2,3,*], Hamid Abu Sara [1,3] and Mustafa Ameen Alhamaidah [1]

1. Department of Clinical Sciences, College of Pharmacy and Health Science, Ajman University, Ajman P.O. Box 346, United Arab Emirates; s.bloukh@ajman.ac.ae (S.H.B.); h.abusara@ajman.ac.ae (H.A.S.); mou.94.95@hotmail.com (M.A.A.)
2. Center of Medical and Bio-Allied Health Sciences Research, Ajman University, Ajman P.O. Box 346, United Arab Emirates
3. Department of Pharmaceutical Sciences, College of Pharmacy and Health Science, Ajman University, Ajman P.O. Box 346, United Arab Emirates
* Correspondence: z.edis@ajman.ac.ae

Abstract: Antibiotic resistance toward commonly used medicinal drugs is a dangerously growing threat to our existence. Plants are naturally equipped with a spectrum of biomolecules and metabolites with important biological activities. These natural compounds constitute a treasure in the fight against multidrug-resistant microorganisms. The development of plant-based antimicrobials through green synthesis may deliver alternatives to common drugs. *Lepidium sativum* L. (LS) is widely available throughout the world as a fast-growing herb known as garden cress. LS seed oil is interesting due to its antimicrobial, antioxidant, and anti-inflammatory activities. Nanotechnology offers a plethora of applications in the health sector. Silver nanoparticles (AgNP) are used due to their antimicrobial properties. We combined LS and AgNP to prevent microbial resistance through plant-based synergistic mechanisms within the nanomaterial. AgNP were prepared by a facile one-pot synthesis through plant-biomolecules-induced reduction of silver nitrate via a green method. The phytochemicals in the aqueous LS extract act as reducing, capping, and stabilizing agents of AgNP. The composition of the LS-AgNP biohybrids was confirmed by analytical methods. Antimicrobial testing against 10 reference strains of pathogens exhibited excellent to intermediate antimicrobial activity. The bio-nanohybrid LS-AgNP has potential uses as a broad-spectrum microbicide, disinfectant, and wound care product.

Keywords: antibiotic resistance; antimicrobial resistance; *Lepidium sativum* L.; silver nanoparticles; biomaterials; antimicrobial activity; synergism; green synthesis; surgical site infection; wound dressing

1. Introduction

Antibacterial resistance is according to the WHO causing increased morbidity and mortality throughout low- and medium-income countries due to a widespread, uncontrolled use of antibacterial agents [1]. The WHO report of 2020 "Prioritization of Pathogens to Guide Research and Development of New Antibiotics" mentions several pathogens as critical priority including the carbapenem-resistant *Pseudomonas aeruginosa* [1]. *Staphylococcus aureus* is listed as vancomycin and methicillin-resistant Gram-negative bacteria under the high-priority pathogens [1]. *Streptococcus pneumoniae* is not susceptible to penicillin and is considered a medium-priority pathogen [1]. Nosocomial infections acquired in hospital settings due to ESKAPE (*Enterococcus feacium*, *S. aureus*, *Klebsiella pneumoniae*, *Acinetobacter baumannii*, *P. aeruginosa*, *Enterobacter* species) pathogens lead to rising cases of morbidity and mortality everywhere in the world [2]. Increased treatment costs, duration, and delayed or no recovery are the outcomes of resistance [2–4]. Resistance against antibiotics during COVID-19 resulted in increased fatalities and serious setbacks [2–4]. Plant-based biomolecules and nanomaterials offer promising alternatives [2,5–11]. The use of carboxylic

Citation: Haj Bloukh, S.; Edis, Z.; Abu Sara, H.; Alhamaidah, M.A. Antimicrobial Properties of *Lepidium sativum* L. Facilitated Silver Nanoparticles. *Pharmaceutics* **2021**, 13, 1352. https://doi.org/10.3390/pharmaceutics13091352

Academic Editors: Aura Rusu, Valentina Uivarosi and Corneliu Tanase

Received: 29 July 2021
Accepted: 23 August 2021
Published: 27 August 2021

Publisher's Note: MDPI stays neutral with regard to jurisdictional claims in published maps and institutional affiliations.

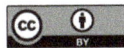

Copyright: © 2021 by the authors. Licensee MDPI, Basel, Switzerland. This article is an open access article distributed under the terms and conditions of the Creative Commons Attribution (CC BY) license (https://creativecommons.org/licenses/by/4.0/).

acids, polyphenols, and further phytochemicals against the coronavirus is discussed in recent papers [8–11]. Plant phytochemicals act also as reducing, stabilizing, and capping agents for bio-synthesized nanoparticles [12]. Nanoparticles can be prepared by green methods and are utilized as antimicrobials or drug carriers [2,12–14]. The mechanisms of antimicrobial activity of silver nanoparticles (AgNP) and gold nanoparticles were investigated in recent papers [15–17]. AgNP and silver ions may coexist and inhibit especially Gram-negative bacteria [18–21]. Once released by AgNP, they enter across the bacterial outer membrane through porin channels and ion transporter proteins [18]. Silver ions can cause oxidative stress and DNA strand damage through interaction with proteins [18]. Other mechanisms involve inhibiting proteins synthesis and DNA replication by interacting with ribosomal proteins and nucleic acids, respectively [18]. The mechanisms of antimicrobial inhibition by AgNP are not yet fully explained [18]. AgNP with sizes smaller than 17 nm can cause cell death by puncturing the cell membranes according to El-Kahky et al. [13]. Many factors determine the effectivity of AgNP against microorganisms [18]. The size of AgNP is determined by the stability and adsorption pattern of coating/capping agents on the Ag surface [18]. Strong reducing agents result in faster reaction rates, smaller, more stable NP with a narrow size distribution, and better microbial inhibition [17]. An agglomeration of AgNP reduces antimicrobial properties and is induced by the storing, aging, or degradation of the capping agent [18]. The size of AgNP depends on the pH level, concentration of silver ions, effectivity, and synergistic mechanisms of the available phytochemicals during the green synthesis [18–37]. The plant constituents can enhance the antimicrobial properties of the AgNP [17].

Medicinal/herbal plants are sources of phenolic acids, polyphenols, flavonoids, terpenoids, and further phytochemicals [3,6,8]. Phytochemicals can reduce biofilm formation, inhibit quorum sensing, prevent bacterial attachment on mucosal surfaces, influence cell surface hydrophobicity, and reduce glycolytic enzymes [23,24]. The antimicrobial activity of plant constituents is ruled by the morphology and structure of the target pathogen. This finding is in agreement with our previous investigations on complexes of "smart" triiodides, which were produced with the addition of molecular iodine (I_2) [37–41]. We utilized plant extracts of *Capsicum frutescens* (Paprika), *Zingiber officinale* (Ginger), *Aloe vera barbadensis* M. (AV), *Cinnamomum zeylanicum* (Cinn), and *Salvia officinalis* L. (Sage) in different formulations with AgNP and/or iodine [25,42–44]. The plant extracts contain *trans*-cinnamic acid (TCA), ferulic acid, caffeic acid, rosmarinic acid, carnosic acid, sagerinic acid, salvianolic acid, sage coumarin, and many other biocomponents [42–51]. These phytochemicals are also constituents in curly garden cress, which is also called *Lepidium sativum* L. (LS) [52].

Cress (LS) is a member of the *Brassicaceae* species (Cruciferae family) and is known as garden cress. LS is a fast-growing herbal plant, which grows in many regions of the world [52–61]. Many papers reported antimicrobial, antioxidant, and anti-inflammatory activities of LS seed oil [52–62]. The whole plant of LS contains cinnamic-, benzoic-, salicylic-, gallic-, ferulic-, caffeic-, *p*-coumaric-, chlorogenic-, vanilic acid, polysaccharides, and further biocompounds [54,57]. We encapsulated AgNP with LS extract to ameliorate the microbicidal activities. The nano-biohybrid LS-AgNP may prevent microbial resistance and biofilm formation by plant-based synergistic mechanisms [22–24]. Such properties are relevant for the treatment of wounds [63]. Effective antimicrobial agents help in faster wound closure, and they also reduce the time and costs of wound-treatment regimens [42,64]. The inability to control wound infections due to resistance and biofilm formation can result in chronic infections or even death [63]. Our investigations on polyvinylpyrrolidone (PVP) and povidone iodine (PI) stabilized TCA-AgNP, TCA-AgNP-PI, Cinn-AgNP, Cinn-AgNP-PI, AV-PVP-I_2, AV-PVP-I_2-NaI, and AV-PVP-Sage-I_2 showed promising results in disk diffusion studies [42–44]. The Sage biohybrid exhibited higher inhibitory action against *Candida albicans* and the Gram-positive bacteria compared to all the other formulations [42–44]. These studies confirm the antimicrobial action of phytochemicals in AV, Sage, and Cinn extracts [42–44]. The concerned plant constituents are TCA and cinnamaldehyde for the Cinn and TCA nanocolloids [43]. The AV-PVP-Sage-I_2 biohybrid consists mainly of sagerinic acid, salvianolic acid, sage coumarin, trans-rosmarinic acid, ferulic acid, vanilic acid, and caffeic acid [43]. The AV extract contains acemannan and cinnamic acid [43].

Relying on our previous investigations on plant constituents in "bio-antimicrobial" agents, we explored the effect of LS in combination with AgNP. We aimed to enhance the inhibitory activities of AgNP by utilizing LS as a reducing, stabilizing, and capping agent in different concentrations (5 and 10%) and pH levels (pH 7 and 8.5) in a time-dependent manner (fresh until 1 week old). We used these small concentrations in order to reduce the amount of AgNP within the biohybrid due to concerns related to bacterial resistance, cytotoxicity, environmental damage, and cost-effectiveness [65–70]. AgNP can initiate bacterial resistance to antibiotics through enhancing bacterial stress tolerance, which can be acquired by previous exposure to AgNP [18,65,68]. Another publication indicates rising AgNP and silver ion resistance of ESKAPE pathogens due to co-selection [67]. The exposure may be due to the manifold uses of AgNP in healthcare, consumer products, cosmetics, food packaging, textiles, and further uses in industry, as well as in agriculture [31,33,65,68]. Other concerns are due to environmental damage and cytotoxicity inflicted on living systems by AgNP [13,69]. These disadvantages of AgNP and Ag-ions encouraged us to utilize LS extract-mediated biosynthesis of AgNP with a low concentration of silver. Safety, sustainability, cost-effectiveness, and facile preparation by green synthesis are our main goals during our investigation of antimicrobial formulations of LS-AgNP.

AgNP were prepared in a one-pot synthesis by LS plant-biomolecules-induced reduction of silver nitrate via a green method. The biomolecules and metabolites in the aqueous LS extract act as reducing, capping, and stabilizing agents of AgNP. Scanning Electron Microscopy (SEM) and Energy-Dispersive X-ray Spectroscopy (EDX) were utilized to analyze the morphology, composition, and distribution of LS-AgNP. Fourier transform infrared spectroscopy (FT-IR), Ultraviolet-visible spectroscopy (UV-Vis), and X-ray Diffraction (XRD) confirmed the composition of the LS-AgNP biohybrids. Dynamic light scattering (DLS) was used to determine the size distribution and stability of the nanoparticles. Antimicrobial testing by the disc dilution method against a total of 10 reference strains of microorganisms verified excellent to intermediate antimicrobial activity. The Gram-negative pathogens *Escherichia coli* WDCM 00013 and *P. aeruginosa* WDCM 00026 were highly inhibited, which was followed by intermediate results for the Gram-positive bacteria *Bacillus subtilis* WDCM 00003, *S. pneumoniae* ATCC 49619, *S. aureus* ATCC 25923, *Streptococcus pyogenes* ATCC 19615, *E. faecalis* ATCC 29212, and the fungus *C. albicans* WDCM 00054. Our biohybrid LS-AgNP showed increased antimicrobial activity with potential uses as a disinfectant and wound care product.

2. Materials and Methods

2.1. Materials

Sabouraud Dextrose broth, Mueller–Hinton Broth (MHB), and silver nitrate were purchased from Sigma Aldrich (St. Louis, MO, USA). The microbial strains *E. coli* WDCM 00013 Vitroids, *P. aeruginosa* WDCM 00026 Vitroids, *K. pneumoniae* WDCM 00097 Vitroids, *C. albicans* WDCM 00054 Vitroids, and *Bacillus subtilis* WDCM 0003 Vitroids were purchased from Sigma-Aldrich Chemical Co. (St. Louis, MO, USA). Liofilchem (Roseto degli Abruzzi, Teramo, Italy) delivered *S. pneumoniae* ATCC 49619, *S. aureus* ATCC 25923, *E. faecalis* ATCC 29212, *S. pyogenes* ATCC 19615, and *P. mirabilis* ATCC 29906. Disposable sterilized Petri dishes with Mueller–Hinton II agar, McFarland standard sets, gentamicin (9125, 30 µg/disc), and nystatin (9078, 100 IU/disc) were obtained from Liofilchem Diagnostici (Roseto degli Abruzzi, Teramo, Italy). Sterile filter paper discs with 6 mm diameter were obtained from Himedia (Jaitala Nagpur, Maharashtra, India). Curly garden cress (*Lepidium sativum* L., (LS)) seeds were purchased from the local market. The seeds were planted and harvested during November 2020 to April 2021. Ultrapure water was used in the extraction and green synthesis instead of distilled water. All reagents were used as delivered and were of analytical grade.

2.2. Preparation of LS Extract

We obtained the seeds of LS from a local shop in Sharjah, UAE and planted them in November 2020. The plants grew up to 12 cm and were harvested from December 2020 to April 2021 in the morning hours. They were immediately transported to the research lab of the College of Pharmacy and Health Sciences, Ajman University, Ajman, UAE. The LS were rinsed several times with water to remove soil and impurities. Then, they were washed thoroughly three times with distilled water and finally with ultrapure water. The plants were left for drying at ambient temperature for 2 h until the remaining water evaporated. The extraction method was adapted partly from previous investigations [28,36]. 10 g of LS whole plants were added into a beaker with 100 mL of ultrapure water and heated to 60 °C. The covered beaker was kept for 30 min at 60 °C under continuous stirring. The green solution was allowed to cool down to room temperature. Then, 10 mL of LS extract was diluted with ultrapure water to 100 mL. For the investigation of the pH dependency, a few drops of 10% diluted NaOH solution were added until the pH was adjusted to 8.5 under continuous stirring. The other stock solution was adjusted to pH = 7. The light green color changed to greenish-yellow due to the dilution and change of pH. These stock solutions were immediately used for the preparation of LS-AgNP.

2.3. Preparation of LS-AgNP

Silver nitrate solution was prepared by adding 0.183 g (1.077 mmol) $AgNO_3$ into 100 mL of ultrapure water at 0 °C and stirring for 10 min. Then, 5 and 10 mL of the silver nitrate solution were added separately to the prepared LS stock solutions under continuous stirring for 30 min at 60 °C. The final products changed from greenish-yellow to yellowish-brown color. The colloids with the added silver nitrate concentrations of 5% (0.5386 µg/mL) and 10% (1.0773 µg/mL) were kept at 3 °C until further use.

2.4. Characterization of LS-AgNP

The nanocomposite LS-AgNP was analyzed by SEM/EDS, UV-vis, and FTIR, and X-ray diffraction (XRD). The results confirmed the composition and purity of LS-AgNP.

2.4.1. Scanning Electron Microscopy (SEM) and Energy-Dispersive X-ray Spectroscopy (EDX)

The scanning electron microscopy (SEM, VEGA3, Tescan, Brno, Czech Republic) analysis of LS-AgNP was used to study the morphology of the nanocomposite LS-AgNP. The elemental composition of our sample was investigated by energy-dispersive X-ray spectroscopy (EDS, VEGA3, Tescan, Brno, Czech Republic). The analysis was performed on VEGA3 from Tescan (Brno, Czech Republic) at 20 kV. The same instrument was used for the EDS analysis. The measurements were done by dispersing one drop of LS-AgNP into distilled water and placing this suspension onto a carbon-coated copper grid. After drying the sample under ambient conditions, it was coated by a Quorum Technology Mini Sputter Coater (Quorum Technologies, Laughton, East Sussex, UK) with a gold film.

2.4.2. Size and Zeta Potential Analysis

The calculation of the average size, size distribution, and the polydispersity index (PDI) was performed by dynamic light scattering (DLS) analysis with the model SZ-100 purchased from Horiba (Palaiseau, France). Dispersion and stability of the nanocolloidal biohybrid was undertaken at room temperature by zeta (ζ) potential measurement.

2.4.3. UV-Vis Spectrophotometry (UV-Vis)

The UV-Vis spectrophotometer model 2600i from Shimadzu (Kyoto, Japan) was utilized at a wavelength range from 195 to 800 nm in the analysis of LS-AgNP.

2.4.4. Fourier Transform Infrared Spectroscopy (FTIR)

An ATR IR spectrometer with a Diamond window from Shimadzu (Kyoto, Japan) was used for the FTIR analysis of LS-AgNP. The nanocomposite was freeze-dried and measured within the wavenumber range of 400 to 4000 cm^{-1}.

2.4.5. X-ray Diffraction (XRD)

A Bruker XRD (BRUKER, D8 Advance, Karlsruhe, Germany) was used to study the nanomaterial LS-AgNP. The Cu radiation had a wavelength of 1.54060 A. The analysis was done by coupled Two Theta/Theta with a time-step of 0.5 s and step size of 0.03.

2.5. Bacterial Strains and Culturing

The antimicrobial properties of LS-AgNP were studied against the reference strains of the pathogens *S. pneumoniae* ATCC 49619, *S. aureus* ATCC 25923, *E. faecalis* ATCC 29212, *S. pyogenes* ATCC 19615, *Bacillus subtilis* WDCM 0003 Vitroids, *P. mirabilis* ATCC 29906, *E. coli* WDCM 00013 Vitroids, *P. aeruginosa* WDCM 00026 Vitroids, *K. pneumoniae* WDCM 00097 Vitroids, and *C. albicans* WDCM 00054 Vitroids. These microorganisms were stored at −20 °C. MHB was inoculated by adding the fresh microbes and was kept at 4 °C until needed in the study.

2.6. Determination of Antimicrobial Properties of LS-AgNP

The antimicrobial properties of our title bio-nanocomposite were studied against nine reference bacterial strains and one fungal strain. The bacterial strains consisted of Gram-positive *S. pneumoniae* ATCC 49619, *S. aureus* ATCC 25923, *S. pyogenes* ATCC 19615, *E. faecalis* ATCC 29212, and *B. subtilis* WDCM 00003. Gram-negative bacteria were *P. mirabilis* ATCC 29906, *P. aeruginosa* WDCM 00026, *E. coli* WDCM 00013, and *K. pneumoniae* WDCM 00097. The antibiotic gentamycin was used as positive control for all the bacterial strains. The fungal reference strain *C. albicans* WDCM 00054 was compared to the antibiotic nystatin. Water was used as solvent and as negative control. The negative controls showed no inhibition zones and were not included in the discussion. All the antimicrobial tests were performed thrice, and their average was used in this investigation.

2.6.1. Zone of Inhibition Plate Studies

The microbial susceptibility against our nanocompound LS-AgNP was tested by zone of inhibition plate studies [70]. The selected bacterial strains were added into 10 mL of MHB and kept at 37 °C for an incubation period of 2 to 4 h. We used Sabouraud Dextrose broth to incubate *C. albicans* WDCM 00054 at 30 °C. Sterile Petri dishes with MHA were evenly seeded by sterile cotton swabs with a selected microbial culture of 100 µL conform to 0.5 McFarland standard. After a drying period of 10 min, the plates were ready for antimicrobial studies.

2.6.2. Disc Diffusion Method

We followed the descriptions of the Clinical and Laboratory Standards Institute (CLSI) to test the susceptibility of our 10 reference strains. We used the common antibiotic discs of nystatin and gentamycin as comparison [71]. Two mL of our nanocolloids with the 5% (0.54 µg/mL, 0.27 µg/mL, 0.14 µg/mL) and 10% (1.08 µg/mL, 0.54 µg/mL, 0.27 µg/mL) concentrations were used to impregnate sterile filter paper discs for 1 day. The soaked disks were dried for 24 h under ambient conditions. We incubated the fungal reference strain *C. albicans* WDCM 00054 on agar plates at 30 °C for 24 h. We used a ruler to measure the clear zone of inhibition (ZOI) diameter around the disc to the nearest millimeter. If there is no inhibition zone, the reference strain is not susceptible. In this case, the ZOI is equal to zero and the strain is resistant.

2.7. Statistical Analysis

The statistical analysis was done by SPSS software (version 17.0, SPSS Inc., Chicago, IL, USA). Mean values are presented as data, and one-way ANOVA was employed to calculate the statistical significance between groups. Values with $p < 0.05$ were noted as statistically significant.

3. Results and Discussion

The incidence of microbial resistance against common drugs and antimicrobial agents is a matter of concern. The future of mankind is at stake due to the notorious ESKAPE pathogens [1,2]. Medicinal plants may be an important alternative in the battle against resistant microorganisms [2,3,5–11]. Medicinal plants use synergistic mechanisms based on their antimicrobial constituents [3,5–11,23,24]. Plant constituents can inhibit biofilm formation, protein synthesis, and quorum sensing [3,5–11,23,24]. Silver ions and AgNP have similar antimicrobial properties [2,12–21]. Recent investigations on the green synthesis of AgNP gained popularity. Green methods are based on simple, cost-effective methods and sustainable, eco-friendly materials [15]. The use of biomass, waste materials, and plant constituents as reducing/stabilizing/capping agents is part of bio-silver nanoparticle synthesis [15]. Such methods encourage the development of nano-bio-antimicrobials, which can be used against resistant pathogens. Based on our experience on bio-synthesized antimicrobials, we investigated the use of curly garden cress (LS) extract. LS biocomponents acted as reducing and stabilizing agents in the green synthesis of AgNP. The facile one-pot synthesis of LS-AgNP produced cost-effective, sustainable antimicrobial agents in an eco-friendly way. The biohybrid LS-AgNP revealed pH, concentration, and time dependency. The alkaline pH of 8.5 during the synthesis produced stable LS-AgNP with a smaller size distribution and better antimicrobial activities. The same results are achieved when 10% silver ion concentration is used instead of 5%. The stability and antimicrobial action of LS-AgNP are inversely related to aging and decreased in a time-dependent pattern during storage after 7 days. The highest inhibitory action against the tested microorganisms was achieved by the 10% LS-AgNP prepared at pH of 8.5 with a concentration of 1.0773 µg/mL within the first 6 days. The UV-vis analysis supports this through a sharper surface plasmon peak for AgNP at λ-max = 447 nm. If not mentioned further, the analytical results are related to the 10% LS-AgNP colloid synthesized at a pH of 8.5 not older than 6 days.

3.1. Morphological Examination, Elemental Composition

3.1.1. Electron Microscope (SEM) and Energy-Dispersive X-ray Spectroscopic (EDS) Analysis

The composition, purity, and morphology of LS-AgNP were investigated by SEM and EDS (Figure 1).

The SEM analysis in Figure 1a depicts a microcrystalline, heterogeneous morphology. The purity of this sample is confirmed by the EDS analysis (Figure 1c). The sample LS-AgNP consists of 83.6% Ag, 11.6% C, 3.4% O, and 1.4% Cl (Figure 1c). The results confirm the purity of LS-AgNP. The layered EDS shows a homogenous presence of Ag in all the sample (Figure 1b,d). Carbon and oxygen are also uniformly distributed in the sample (Supplementary Materials, Figure S1). Cl ions are available in plant materials and form AgCl during the biosynthesis of AgNP [18,21,42]. Silver ions are released due to the oxidation of AgNP, moisture, or simply due to the equilibrium process [29,42]. The formation of a AgCl secondary phase was also observed during the preparation of Cinn-AgNP-PI in our previous investigations [42].

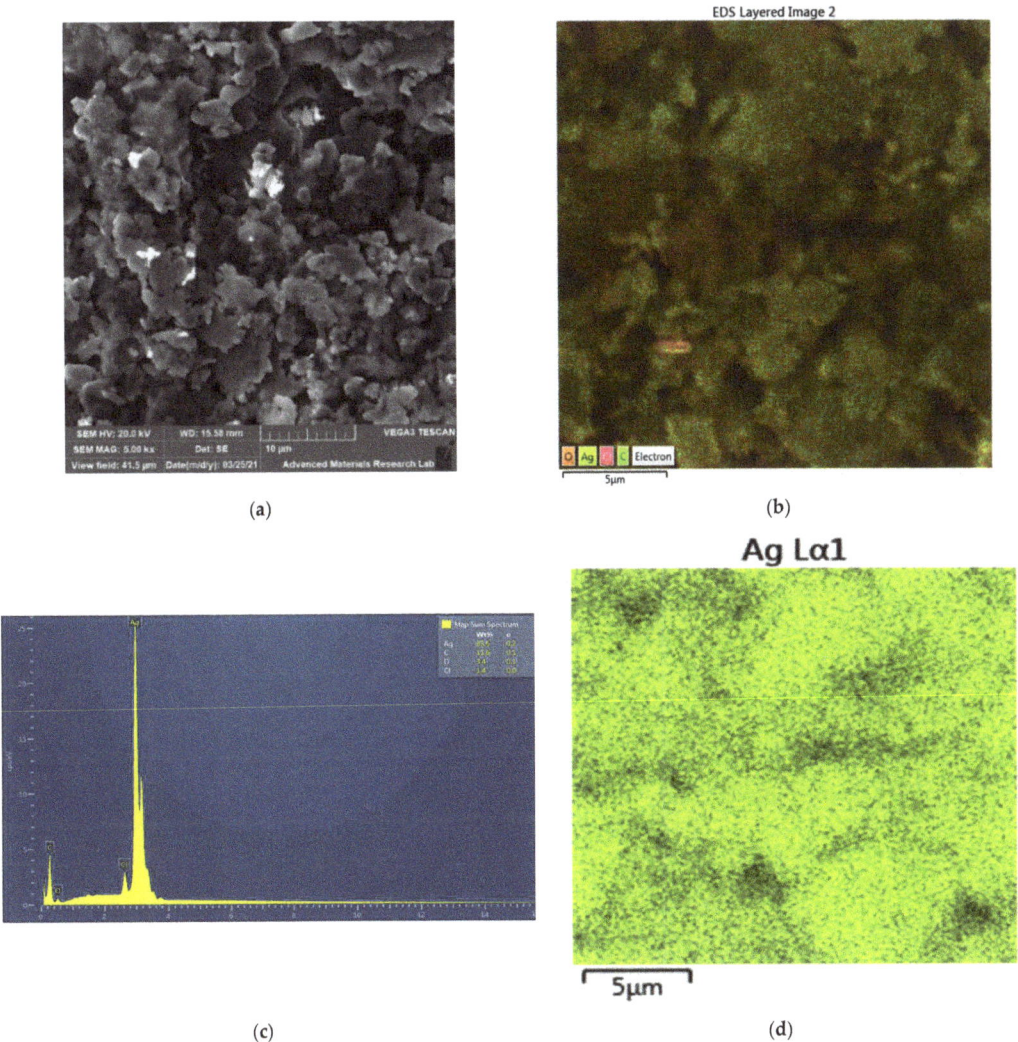

Figure 1. Scanning electron microscopy (SEM) (**a**); energy-dispersive spectroscopy (EDS) (**b**); layered EDS (**c**); EDS analysis; and (**d**) layered EDS of LS-AgNP.

3.1.2. Dynamic Light Scattering (DLS) and Zeta Potential Analysis

The DLS analysis confirms the unimodal size distribution of LS-AgNP, which is in agreement with the SEM results (Figure 1). Table 1 shows the results of the DLS measurements.

Table 1. Zeta potential measurements and DLS results for each sample of LS-AgNP.

Sample	Zeta Potential (mV)	Particle Size Mean (nm)	Z-Average (nm)	Polydispersity Index (PDI)
5% LS-AgNP	−0.1	20.3 ± 11.5	65.5	0.735
10% LS-AgNP	−0.2	36.1 ± 12.3	57.9	0.388

The zeta (ζ) potential of 10% LS-AgNP shows a small negative charge of −0.2 mV (Table 1).

The zeta potential is an indicator of the stability of a colloidal suspension. The small negative charge of −0.2 mV reveals rapid coagulation of the 10% LS-AgNP biohybrid. The PDI value highlights the size distribution of the molecules within the given sample. The 5% LS-AgNP has a higher PDI compared to the 10% sample (Table 1). This result indicates a broader size distribution in the 5% LS-AgNP sample due to agglomeration. The 10% LS-AgNP biohybrid shows a smaller PDI of 0.388 due to its smaller size distribution and less agglomeration (Table 1). The 10% LS-AgNP sample contains more stable, smaller, and polydisperse AgNPs. The Z-average for the 5% and the 10% LS-AgNP samples are 65.5 and 57.9 nm, respectively (Table 1). The Z-average for the 10% LS-AgNP is smaller compared to the 5% sample and confirms the same findings of the PDI values (Table 1). The particle mean sizes of the 5% LS-AgNP is smaller than the 10% LS-AgNP sample, but the PDI of the latter is more favorable regarding stability, size distribution, and agglomeration.

The DLS analysis of the 10% LS-AgNP biocolloid indicates a homogenous size distribution around 36.1 nm (Supplementary Materials, Figure S2). In the spectrum, there are no other peak intensities available. In other reports, the prevalence of bulky aggregates with a wide size distribution is observed [30,32]. The low polydispersion index of 0.388 confirms the presence of a uniform dispersion of LS-AgNP. The phytochemicals in the LS extract acted effectively as reducing and stabilizing agents, resulting in small, homogenous, and narrow size distribution [32]. Zeta (ζ) potential analysis renders further information about AgNP stability, size distribution, and agglomeration profiles in solution. The ζ-potential value of LS-AgNP is −0.2 mV and indicates a negatively charged AgNP surface (Table 1). The results verify the presence of a stable, small sized, homogenous biocolloid LS-AgNP. There are no aggregates, because the biomolecules within LS rapidly reduced the silver ions to Ag nanoparticles and prevented a secondary nucleation on the silver surface by forming a monolayer [15,17]. Silver ions were reduced by the hydroxyl and carbonyl moieties within the biomolecules of LS consisting of phenolic acids, polyphenols, flavonoids, terpenoids, and proteins [15,54,56,57]. The monolayer of plant biomolecules counteracts agglomeration and improves the antimicrobial activities of AgNP [15,17].

3.2. Spectroscopical Characterization

The composition of the LS-AgNP can be elucidated by spectroscopical characterization. We used UV-vis, FT-IR, and X-ray diffraction techniques.

3.2.1. UV-Vis Spectroscopy

UV-vis spectroscopy can be utilized to assess the formation and size of AgNP in the biocolloidal LS-AgNP. The presence of different biocompounds originating from the LS extract can be elucidated. The synthesis of the biocomposite LS-AgNP was analyzed by UV-vis spectroscopy at two different concentrations and times (Figure 2).

AgNP formation is confirmed in UV-vis analysis with a plasmonic peak in the range of around 400–500 nm (Figure 2). The peak is available at λ-max = 447 nm in the 10% LS-AgNP sample (Figure 2, red curve). After 7 days, the 10% LS-AgNP sample reveals a lower intensity band around 435 nm for AgNP (Figure 2, light blue curve). The lower intensity absorption after one week infers an increased encapsulation of AgNP by the biomolecules. Chromophores cannot absorb due to the lower availability of π-electrons. The molecular structure of LS-AgNP is coiled, resulting in a smaller size. Both of the 5% LS-AgNP formulations show a lower intensity small, broad band at around 412 nm (Figure 2). This broad peak comes in form of a shoulder with lower absorption intensity and is blue-shifted compared to the 10% sample. The blue shift from 447 to 412 nm and the hypochromic effect indicate a smaller NP size (Supplementary Materials, Figure S2). Lower intensity absorptions indicate the adsorption of an increased number of biomolecules on the AgNP. This reduces the size of the AgNP by encapsulating the primary Ag layer and preventing a secondary layer of attached Ag nuclei [15,17]. The sharpness of the peak in the 10% LS-AgNP indicates a faster reduction rate of silver ions compared to the 5% formulation. The doubling of silver ion concentration from 5% to 10% resulted in a red shift and slightly bigger sizes of the NP in the latter. The DLS analysis confirmed the findings. The bathochromic effect means an increase in conjugated systems, chromophores, and solvent effect due to the phytochemicals in 10% LS-AgNP. The red shift indicates a change in the phytochemicals from C–O bonds to C=O and C–C to C=C. This leads to inner-particle interactions such as repulsion, steric hindrance, and crowding between adsorbed biomolecules through their conjugated, bulky phenolic groups on the surroundings of the Ag surface [42]. As a result, AgNP in 10% LS-AgNP are more stable because agglomeration is prevented by inner-particle interactions.

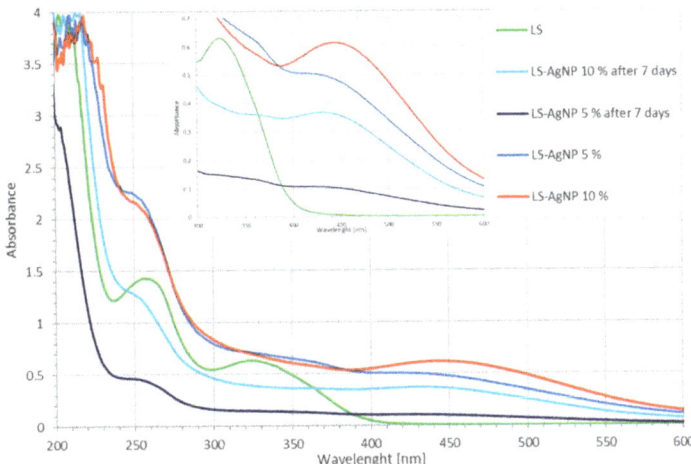

Figure 2. UV-vis analysis of LS and LS-AgNP: with inset of 300–600 nm (LS extract: dark green; LS-AgNP: dark blue; 5% LS-AgNP: black; 5% LS-AgNP after 7 days: red; 10% LS-AgNP: light blue; 10% LS-AgNP after 7 days).

In the green synthesis of AgNP by *Cinnamomum zeylanicum* (Cinn) bark extract and trans-cinnamic acid (TCA), the UV-vis analysis showed surface plasmon peaks at 390–415 nm (broad) and 400 nm (sharp), respectively [42]. Soni et al. mentioned a broad peak at 480 nm for AgNP biosynthesized by *Cinnamomum zeylanicum* [34]. These results infer the availability of cinnamic acid and its derivatives caffeic acid, rosmarinic acid, coumaric acid, chicoric acid, ferulic acid, and further polyphenols [8,42]. AgNP bio-synthesis is a complex phenomenon and has an impact on the antimicrobial properties of the biocolloid. The best results in this work were achieved by the AgNP synthesis at pH 8.5 with an initial silver ion concentration of 10% at pH 8.5 (Figure 2, red curve).

The entity of the biomolecules responsible for the reduction of silver ions can be identified by UV-vis-spectroscopic analysis through comparative observation of absorption peaks. In general, phenolic compounds appear in the region around 320–380 nm and flavonoids appear in the region around 280–315 nm. These compound classes are represented in the green curve depicting the LS-extract (Figure 2). In Figure 2, the LS extract shows broad absorption intensities between 230 and 290 nm and 295–400 nm related to flavonoids and phenolic compounds, respectively.

This is in agreement with our investigations on TCA-AgNP, Cinn-AgNP, as well as TCA-AgNP-, Cinn-AgNP-, AV-PVP-, and AV-PVP-Sage-iodine formulations [42,43]. Pure TCA absorbs at 265 nm, which suggests the presence of trans-cinnamic acid in the LS-extract [42]. The broadness of the absorption infers the availability of other hydroxycinnamic acid derivatives as well. Pure Sage biomolecules show absorptions around 200–230 nm (high intensity), 260–300 nm (broad shoulder), as well as low-intensity absorption bands at 310–480 nm and 400–450 nm [43,45,50]. The spectrum of AV-PVP-Sage reveals strong absorption peaks at 283 and 338 nm, which are Sage and AV phenolic compounds [43–45]. The LS extract shows comparable broad bands around 200–220 nm, 240 to 290 nm (λ-max = 257 nm), and 300 to 350 nm (λ-max = 322 nm) (Figure 3). The two latter broad absorption bands belong to trans-rosmarinic acid and caffeic acid, which appear at 280/330 nm and 328 nm, respectively [43,50]. We reported in our AV-PVP-iodine formulations a peak at 331 nm originating from caffeic acid and rosmarinic acid previously [43]. The absorption at around 270 nm in pure LS may be due to rosmarinic, ferulic, caffeic, carnosic, and cinnamic acid [43,47]. The broad band around 320 nm suggests the availability of quercetin, chlorogenic acid, chicoric acid, p-coumaric acid, catechin, kaempferol, cirsimaritin, apigenin, luteolin, hesperidine, and thymol [8,26,50].

The UV-vis absorption pattern of pure LS changes, when silver ions are added into the plant extract. A red shift is seen around 200–220 nm toward 205–235 nm in the 10% LS-AgNP formulation (Figure 2, red curve). All the spectra show the same red shift except the 7-day-old 5% LS-AgNP (Figure 2, black curve). The biomolecules undergo a change to higher conjugation with more absorption by chromophores from C–O to C=O. This can be an indicator for the reduction of silver ions to AgNP. The reduction happens by the deprotonated hydroxyl-groups within the polyphenols in the slightly alkaline solution at pH 8.5 [26]:

$$Ag^+ + R\text{-}C\text{-}O^- \leftrightarrows Ag + R\text{-}C\text{=}O \quad (1)$$

with a high-intensity absorption at 219 and a shoulder at 228 nm. The related absorptions were available at 200 and 220 nm in the LS extract. The same reduction is indicated by the blue shift from 257 nm in the pure LS extract toward 248 nm in all the other spectra (Figure 2). The LS-bio-constituents absorbing at this range are rosmarinic, ferulic, caffeic, carnosic, and cinnamic acid. All phenolic acids except cinnamic acid contain hydroxyl groups and reduce the silver ions, as indicated in Equation (1). The reduction decreases the availability of π-electrons and reduces the conjugation in the ring systems. This is reflected in the lower absorption intensity of the older LS-AgNP biohybrids. The lower absorption intensity indicates higher encapsulation, more hydrogen bonding, and less availability of the chromophores within the phenolic acids. After 6 days and above, phenolic acids are fixed within an extended molecular network due to inner-particle interactions. The fresher samples of 5% and 10% LS-AgNP show up to 6 days higher absorption intensities from 230 to 800 nm compared to the pure LS sample. The stability and antimicrobial properties are directly related to the availability of conjugated systems, free π-electrons, and less hydrogen bonding. The two samples contain intact phenolic acids (rosmarinic, ferulic, caffeic, carnosic, and cinnamic acid), which stabilize the AgNP by capping. The capping counteracts agglomeration of the AgNP [42]. In this process,

$$AgNP + R\text{-}C\text{-}O^- \leftrightarrows R\text{-}C\text{-}O^- \cdots\cdots AgNP \quad (2)$$

where negatively charged oxygen atoms originating from carbonyl groups and deprotonated hydroxyl groups adsorb on the AgNP surface [42]. The AgNP surface increases its negative charge by this adsorption [42]. Electrostatic interactions between oxygen atoms in carbonyl- and hydroxyl-π-electrons

$$AgNP + R\text{-}C\text{=}O \leftrightarrows R\text{-}C\text{=}O \cdots\cdots AgNP \quad (3)$$

with the positively charged naked AgNP lead to adsorption onto the AgNP surface as well [42]. The same mechanisms are valid for the bioconstitutents absorbing around 320 nm in the LS-AgNP samples up to 6 days. Quercetin, chlorogenic acid, catechin, kaempferol, cirsimaritin, apigenin, luteolin, hesperidine, and thymol may act as capping and stabilizing agents by adsorbing on the AgNP surface through their negatively charged oxygen atoms [26,42,50].

3.2.2. Fourier Transform Infrared (FTIR) Spectroscopy

FTIR analysis was employed to analyze the composition of the LS extract and the biocomposite LS-AgNP (Table 2, Supplementary Figures S3 and S4).

Table 2. Fourier transform infrared (FTIR) spectroscopic analysis of LS and LS-AgNP (cm^{-1}).

Group	LS	LS-AgNP
(O–H)ν	3100–3600	3100–3600
(H-C=O)ν	2750	2750↑
(O–H)ν	2990 2850	2980↑ 2850
(C=O)ν$_{as}$	1663	1679
(C=O)ν$_{as}$		1659
(C=O)ν$_s$	1418 1448 1458 1385, 1379	1419↓ 1449↓ 1456↓ 1379
(C–O–C)ν$_s$	1330	1330
(C–OH)ν (C–O)ν	1103 1275 1085 1050 1030 804 656	1097↓ 1275 1085↑ 1050↑ 1030↓ 804↑ 656↑
(CH–CH)ν	880	880↑

ν = vibrational stretching, s = symmetric, a = asymmetric. ↑ = increased absorption intensity, ↓ = reduced absorption intensity.

The two FTIR spectra show similarities in most of the regions (Table 2, Supplementary Materials, Figures S3 and S4). The phenolic acids from LS are rosmarinic, caffeic, cinnamic, *p*-coumaric, carnosic, and ferulic acid [35,42–44,72]. These compounds are represented in the FTIR absorption spectrum of both title compounds by the bands around 3500–3100, 2980, 2850, 1659, 1456, 1449, 1420, 1379, 1331, 1275, 1097, 1085, and 1050 cm^{-1} Table 2, Supplementary Materials, Figures S3 and S4) [43]. Both spectra show broad bands around 3500 to 3100 cm^{-1} for the hydrogen bonded alcohol, carboxylic acid-OH, and amide NH groups originating from the biomolecules within LS Table 2, Supplementary Materials, Figures S3 and S4). Carboxylate groups with their carbonyl C=O asymmetric stretching vibration appear in the spectrum around 1700 to 1600 cm^{-1} (Table 2, Supplementary Materials, Figures S3 and S4). The pure LS extract shows very low absorption peaks at around 1663 cm^{-1} (Supplementary Figure S3). LS-AgNP absorbs with slightly higher intensity at 1679 cm^{-1} (Table 2, Supplementary Figure S4). The increase in absorption intensity combined with a shift to a higher wavenumber of 1679 cm^{-1} verifies the emergence of asymmetric carboxylate moieties. These groups appear due to the reduction of silver ions by deprotonated hydroxyl groups (Equation (1)). The symmetric stretching vibrations of the carboxylate groups absorb at 1419, 1449, 1456, and 1379 cm^{-1} (Table 2, Supplementary Materials, Figure S4). These bands except the band at 1379 cm^{-1} absorb at lower intensities in the LS-AgNP in comparison to the pure LS (Table 2, Supplementary Materials, Figures S3 and S4). When silver ions are reduced to AgNP,

$$Ag + R\text{-}COO^- \leftrightarrows R\text{-}COO^-; \cdots\cdots Ag \quad (4)$$

these groups adsorb on the AgNP surface. The band at 1379 cm^{-1} became narrower (Supplementary Figure S4). The Ag–OOC interaction is clearly verified and is in agreement with previous reports for the bands at 1419, 1449, 1456, and 1379 cm^{-1} [42,73].

The C–OH groups reveal absorption bands for the C–O stretching vibration at 1275, 1030 (phenols), around 1085 cm^{-1} (secondary alcohols), and 1050 cm^{-1} (primary alcohols) Table 2, Supplementary Materials, Figures S3 and S4). The latter are showing higher absorption intensities in the LS-AgNP biohybrid (Table 2). The absorption band for the C–O stretching vibration at 1103 cm^{-1} in pure LS is found at 1094 cm^{-1} in LS-AgNP (Table 2, Supplementary Figures S3 and S4). This band is accompanied by O–H stretching vibrations around 3350 cm^{-1} as well as two O–H bending at 1330 and 656 cm^{-1} (Table 2, Supplementary Materials, Figures S3 and S4). The red shift from 1103 to smaller frequency and lower energy at 1094 cm^{-1} combined with the reduced absorption intensity suggests an increase in the mass of the concerned secondary alcohols by higher encapsulation and hydrogen bonding interactions. This is in agreement with previous reports of another Ag–O–C interaction on the silver surface by secondary deprotonated hydroxyl groups (Equation (2)). The absorption bands of the phenolic C–O stretching vibrations at 1275 cm^{-1} are both the same in intensity and appearance in both spectra Table 2, Supplementary Materials, Figures S3 and S4). We can assume that the phenolic hydroxyl groups do not encapsulate the AgNP due to their bulky, hydrophobic phenolic groups. Instead, the carboxylate C–O and C=O are adsorbed, while the phenolic groups are pointing outwards [42]. The intensity in both figures remains the same, because the concentration of phenolic hydroxyl groups remains equal. Phenolic hydroxyl groups assist in reducing the silver ions, as seen in the reduced absorption intensity in LS-AgNP at 1030 cm^{-1} (Supplementary Figure S4). This is confirmed by the decrease of conjugation around the aromatic ring CH-CH bonds through increased absorption intensity at 880 cm^{-1} Table 2, Supplementary Materials, Figures S3 and S4). The same results were reported for the AV and Sage biomolecules in our previous investigation on AV-Sage formulations [43]. C=O groups are reduced back to C–OH in order to reinstate the stable conjugated system within the molecules and to maintain equilibrium.

The band at 1085 cm^{-1} is related to C–O stretching vibrations of ester and secondary alcohol groups (Table 2, Supplementary Materials, Figures S3 and S4). The higher absorption intensity in LS-AgNP reveals that these groups are not encapsulating the AgNP and do not form hydrogen bonding (Table 2, Supplementary Materials, Figures S3 and S4). The very small intensity band related to esters at 1730 cm^{-1} indicates a very low amount of intact rosmarinic acid in the sample. The very low absorption intensities for carbonyl C=O in esters confirm this assumption. The ester bond may have been broken to produce caffeic acid and 3,4-dihydroxyphenyllactic acid. The latter compound is the only polyphenol with a primary alcohol group.

The C–O stretching bands for primary alcohols appear around 1075–1000 cm^{-1} (Table 2, Supplementary Materials, Figures S3 and S4). These confirm the availability of 3,4-dihydroxyphenyllactic acid and the solvent ethanol in the samples. After adding silver ions, the C–O stretching vibration absorption intensities for primary and secondary alcohols increase around 1045 to 1100 cm^{-1} (Supplementary Materials, Figures S3 and S4). The increase may refer to reduced conjugation by reduction from C=O to C–O, less encapsulation, and reduced hydrogen bonding interactions. Primary alcohol groups are within ethanol and 3,4-dihydroxyphenyllactic acid. Ethanol molecules had dipol–dipol interactions and hydrogen bonding with the bioconstituents in the pure LS extract. After the AgNP synthesis, the biomolecules acted as reducing and capping agents. Ethanol molecules were removed from the biomolecules due to steric hindrance and crowding on the AgNP surface. Ethanol molecules were set free, while 3,4-dihydroxyphenyllactic acid is produced by breaking the ester bond in rosmarinic acid molecules.

The broad shoulder around 2750 cm^{-1} is related to an aldehyde H–C=O stretching vibration (Table 2, Supplementary Materials, Figures S3 and S4). This band belongs to cinnamaldehyde in both of the samples according to previous reports (Figure 4) [42,74]. Cinnamaldehyde reduces silver ions and is oxidized to cinnamic acid [42].

As a conclusion, primary, secondary alcohol, and phenolic hydroxyl groups do not adsorb readily on the AgNP surface. The reduction of silver ions happens through cinnamaldehyde and phenol OH-groups producing cinnamic acid and carbonyl groups, respectively (Equation (1)). The increase of C=O groups is confirmed by the absorption band with increased intensity at 1659 cm^{-1} (Figure 4b). The adsorption to the metallic surface happens through the carboxylate groups and the carbonyl C=O entities in the biomolecules (Equations (2)–(4)) [42]. This hints at the availability of hydroxycinnamic acids (caffeic, cinnamic, p-coumaric, ferulic, chlorogenic, sinapic acid). These molecules form a layer on the AgNP surface with the carboxylate groups adsorbed on the metallic silver surface and the phenol groups pointing outwards. The encapsulation stabilizes the AgNP and prevents agglomeration. Silver ions are released during this process, which reinstates the concentration and stability of the resonance system of the phenolic acid groups during equilibrium.

3.2.3. X-ray Diffraction (XRD)

The examination of composition and purity of LS-AgNP was investigated by XRD analysis. The spectrum reveals peaks at 2θ = 23.3°, 27°, 27.6°, 29.2°, 29.6°, 31.7°, 32°, and 46° (Figure 3).

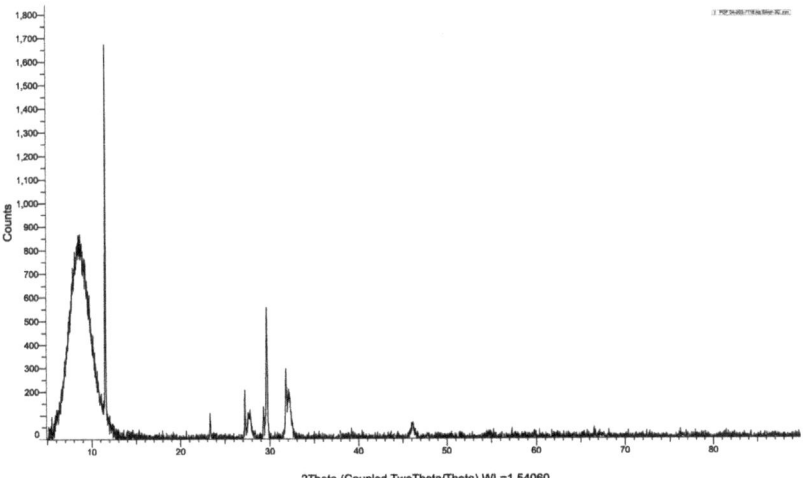

Figure 3. X-ray diffraction (XRD) analysis of LS-AgNP.

The XRD spectrum of LS-AgNP shows sharp peaks around 2θ = 23.3° (001), 27° (001), 29.6° (003), 31.7° (003), and 46° (200) (Figure 3). The broad bands from 2θ = 0° to 13°, 27° to 28°, and 32° to 33°, as well as the peak at 12° are due to the biomolecules in LS (Figure 3). These broad bands reveal amorphous phases related to the biocomponents of LS, as mentioned in previous reports [42]. The peaks around 27.6° and 29.2° originate from AgCl (Figure 3) [19–21,35]. Oxidation of AgNP, moisture, the equilibrium process itself, and degradation of the capping/stabilizing agents adsorbed on the AgNP surface cause the release of silver ions [18,29,42]. Cl ions are available in the plant material itself and could be the result of uptake from our UAE soil during plantation. The sharp peaks confirm the presence of crystalline phases in agreement with investigations on other bio-synthesized AgNPs [13,21,28,35,42]. The biohybrid LS-AgNP incorporates semicrystalline morphology with amorphous phases originating from LS biocomponents.

The XRD analysis of LS-AgNP verifies by the lack of other phases the purity of the nanocolloid (Figure 3).

3.2.4. Antimicrobial Activities of LS-AgNP

The phenomenon of resistance is aggravating the need to develop new antimicrobials for a better future. The survival of mankind depends on new strategies to combat nosocomial infections, morbidity, and mortality due to unsuccessful treatment [1–4]. These factors impacted severely ill patients and caused unnecessary suffering, treatment failure, and fatal outcomes during the COVID-19 pandemic [2–4].

Investigations on the antimicrobial activities of NP and phytochemicals are raising steadily the benchmarks to achieve the set targets [8–14,18–21]. Silver ions released from AgNP are known to inhibit especially Gram-negative microorganisms due to their interaction with different parts of the bacterial cells [18]. They prevent protein synthesis, DNA replication, and biofilm formation by entering through the porin channels of Gram-negative pathogens [18]. Plant phytochemicals such as polyphenols, hydroxy-cinnamic acids, flavonoids, and further constituents have inhibitory action against microorganisms [8–11,23,24]. Phytochemicals are a rich source of natural antimicrobials, which can be utilized as microbicides [24]. Such molecules can enhance the antimicrobial properties of any formulation [24]. In this work, we reported the effect of LS extract on the antimicrobial action of AgNP.

The antimicrobial properties of LS-AgNP were investigated by agar well (AW) and disc diffusion assay (DD) against 10 reference microorganisms. The concerned Gram-positive strains included *S. pneumoniae* ATCC 49619, *S. aureus* ATCC 25923, *S. pyogenes* ATCC 19615, *E. faecalis* ATCC 29212, and *B. subtilis* WDCM 0003. The tested Gram-negative bacteria were *E. coli* WDCM 00013 Vitroids, *P. mirabilis* ATCC 29906, *P. aeruginosa* WDCM 00026 Vitroids, and *K. pneumoniae* WDCM 00097 Vitroids. The yeast *C. albicans* WDCM 00054 Vitroids was also utilized against LS and LS-AgNP. Gentamicin and nystatin were used as positive control antibiotics for bacterial strains and the fungus, respectively. The results of the antibiotics were compared to the inhibitory action of LS and LS-AgNP by measuring the zone of inhibition (ZOI) in mm. Ethanol and water were utilized as negative controls and showed no zone of inhibition (ZOI). The results of the negative controls are not mentioned in any table. The results of agar well (AW) and disk dilution (DD) studies of pure LS, AW of 10% LS-AgNP at pH 8.5 (10-AW), and AW of 10% LS-AgNP at pH 7 (10-AW-7) are represented in Table 3.

Table 3. Antimicrobial testing of antibiotics (A), LS by disc dilution studies (1, 2, 3), LS (LS-AW), 10% LS-AgNP at pH 8.5 (10-AW), and 10% LS-AgNP at pH 7 (10-AW-7) by agar well method. Microbial strain susceptibility indicated by ZOI (mm).

Strain	Antibiotic	A	LS1 [+]	LS2 [+]	LS3 [+]	LS-AW	10-AW	10-AW-7
S. pneumoniae ATCC 49619	G	18	12	11	10	12	15	14
S. aureus ATCC 25923	G	28	14	13	13	0	20	19
S. pyogenes ATCC 19615	G	25	11	10	9	10	15	14
E. faecalis ATCC 29212	G	25	0	0	0	12	15	14
B. subtilis WDCM 00003	G	21	13	12	10	0	18	18
P. mirabilis ATCC 29906	G	30	0	0	0	0	10	10
P. aeruginosa WDCM 00026	G	23	17	16	15	0	22	22
E. coli WDCM 00013	G	23	15	14	13	0	17	17
K. pneumoniae WDCM 00097	G	30	14	13	12	0	20	20
C. albicans WDCM 00054	NY	16	0	0	0	0	13	12

[+] Disc diffusion studies (6 mm disc impregnated with 2 mL of 0.01 g/mL (LS1), 2 mL of 0.005 g/mL (LS2), and 2 mL of 0.0025 g/mL (LS3)) of LS. LS-AW = Agar method with LS extract of 0.01 g/mL. 10-AW = Agar well method with 10% LS-AgNP (1.08 µg/mL) at pH = 8.5. 10-AW-7 = Agar well method with 10% LS-AgNP (1.08 µg/mL) at pH = 7. A = G Gentamicin (30 µg/disc). NY (Nystatin) (100 IU). The gray shaded area represents Gram-negative bacteria. 0 = Resistant. No statistically significant differences ($p > 0.05$) between row-based values through Pearson correlation.

The pure LS extract inhibits in AW studies only three Gram-positive pathogens intermediately, while the rest of the tested pathogens are resistant (Table 3). DD studies at concentrations of 0.01 g/mL reveal higher antibacterial action against the Gram-negative *P. aeruginosa* (17 mm), which is followed by *E. coli* (15 mm) and *K. pneumoniae* (14 mm) (Table 3, Figure 4a–c).

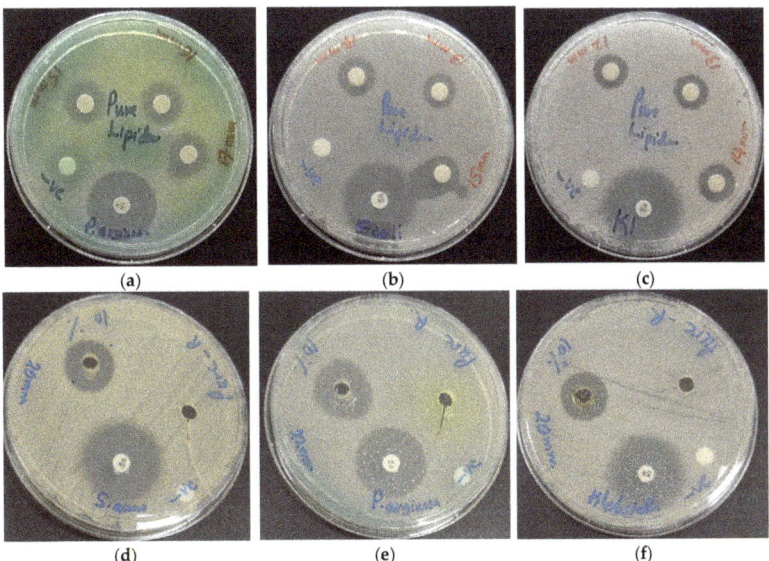

Figure 4. Susceptibility of reference strains against LS pure (0.01, 0.005, 0.0025 g/mL) and LS-AgNP (10%, 1.08 µg/mL) by disc diffusion assay (DD) and agar well method (AW) with positive control antibiotic gentamicin (30 µg/disc). From left to right: DD LS against (**a**) *P. aeruginosa* WDCM 00026; (**b**) *E. coli* WDCM00013; (**c**) *K. pneumoniae* WDCM 00097; AW LS and LS-AgNP against (**d**) *S. aureus* ATCC 25932; (**e**) *P. aeruginosa* WDCM 00026; (**f**) *K. pneumoniae* WDCM 00097.

The bioconstituents caffeic, ferulic, and cinnamic acid as well as other hydroxycinnamic acids are not supported by the AW method due to their low solubility in water. The AW method diminishes the antimicrobial action of the hydroxycinnamic acids against most of the utilized microorganisms due to their hydrophobic properties (Table 3, Figure 4d–f).

The DD method is more suitable for the pure LS extract (Table 3). Gram-negative pathogens were more inhibited than Gram-positive (Table 3). Gram-positive pathogens showed intermediate results with *S. aureus* (14 mm), which is followed by *B. subtilis* (13 mm), *S. pneumoniae* (12 mm), and *S. pyogenes* (11 mm) at a concentration of 0.01 g/mL (Table 3). Pure Sage extract with its bioconstituents did not inhibit Gram-positive bacteria in previous investigations at a concentration of 1 g/mL [42]. The tests revealed antibacterial action against the Gram-positive microorganisms *S. aureus* (13 mm), *B. subtilis* (13 mm), and *S. pyogenes* (11 mm) [43]. The pure LS extract was more efficient against the selected bacteria in comparison to Sage extract [43].

The AW method augmented the antimicrobial properties of the 10% LS-AgNP (pH = 8.5) compared to all other tests (Table 3). The highest inhibition was seen in *P. aeruginosa* (22 mm), which is followed by *K. pneumoniae* (20 mm), *S. aureus* (20 mm), *B. subtilis* (18 mm), *E. coli* (17 mm), *S. pneumoniae* (15 mm), *S. pyogenes* (15 mm), *E. faecalis* (15 mm), and *C. albicans* (13 mm) (Table 3, Figure 4d–f). Pure LS had no inhibitory action against Gram-negative pathogens in AW studies. The inhibitory action in AW seems to depend on the release of silver ions from LS-AgNP [18]. The best results in this study were recorded for the AW method of 10% LS-AgNP (pH = 8.5), which was followed by the DD method of the same formulation. Further DD studies revealed decreasing inhibitory action in the following order: pure LS, 5% LS-AgNP (pH = 8.5), 1-week-old 10% LS-AgNP (pH = 8.5), and lastly 10% LS-AgNP (pH = 7) (Table 4).

Table 4. Antimicrobial testing by disc diffusion (1, 2, 3) of antibiotics (A), LS-AgNP (5 and 10%, pH = 7 and 8.5, up to 5 days to 1-week-old sample). Microbial strain susceptibility indicated by ZOI (mm).

Strain	Antibiotic	A	5-1 [+]	5-2 [+]	5-3 [+]	10-1 [+]	10-2 [+]	10-3 [+]	10 *-1 [+]	10 *-2 [+]	10 *-3 [+]	10-7-1 [+]	10-7-2 [+]	10-7-3 [+]
S. pneumoniae ATCC 49619	G	18	10	0	0	15	13	12	11	0	0	14	13	0
S. aureus ATCC 25923	G	28	13	12	10	14	13	12	13	12	11	12	10	0
S. pyogenes ATCC 19615	G	25	11	10	9	13	12	11	11	9	0	11	10	0
E. faecalis ATCC 29212	G	25	0	0	0	13	12	11	9	0	0	0	0	0
B. subtilis WDCM 00003	G	21	9	0	0	13	11	10	10	0	0	14	13	0
P. mirabilis ATCC 29906	G	30	0	0	0	0	0	0	0	0	0	0	0	0
P. aeruginosa WDCM 00026	G	23	15	14	12	20	18	15	15	12	11	18	15	0
E. coli WDCM 00013	G	23	14	13	9	15	14	13	12	10	9	16	15	0
K. pneumoniae WDCM 00097	G	30	14	13	10	15	14	12	13	12	11	15	11	0
C. albicans WDCM 00054	NY	16	0	0	0	0	0	0	0	0	0	14	0	0

[+] Disc diffusion studies (6 mm disc impregnated with: 5% LS-AgNP 2 mL of 0.54 µg/mL (5-1), 2 mL of 0.27 µg/mL (5-2) and 2 mL of 0.14 µg/mL (5-3). 10% LS-AgNP 2 mL of 1.08 µg/mL (10-1), 2 mL of 0.54 µg/mL (10-2), and 2 mL of 0.27 µg/mL (10-3). 10% LS-AgNP 2 mL of 1.08 µg/mL at pH = 7 (10-7-1), 2 mL of 0.54 µg/mL (10-7-2), and 2 mL of 0.27 µg/mL (10-7-3). * One-week-old 10% LS-AgNP 2 mL of 1.08 µg/mL (10 *-1), 2 mL of 0.54 µg/mL (10 *-2), and 2 mL of 0.27 µg/mL (10 *-3). A = G Gentamicin (30 µg/disc). NY (Nystatin) (100 IU). The gray shaded area represents Gram-negative bacteria. 0 = Resistant. No statistically significant differences ($p > 0.05$) between row-based values through Pearson correlation.

The DD studies of 10% LS-AgNP (pH = 8.5) show the highest inhibition zones for the Gram-negative *P. aeruginosa* (20/18/15 mm), which is followed by *E. coli* (15/14/13 mm) and *K. pneumoniae* (15/14/12 mm) (Table 4, Figure 4). The Gram-positive pathogens can be arranged with slightly lower results in the order *S. pneumoniae* (15/13/12 mm), *S. aureus* (14/13/12 mm), *S. pyogenes* (13/12/11 mm), and *E. faecalis* (13/12/11 mm) (Table 4, Figure 5).

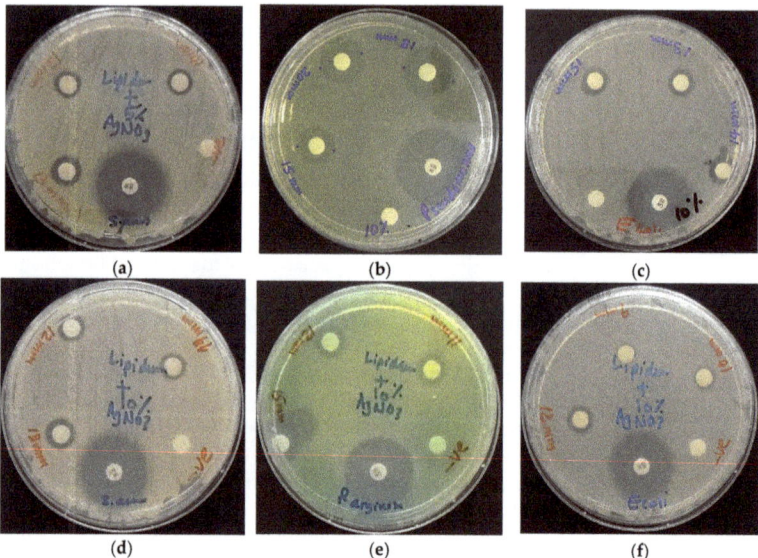

Figure 5. LS-AgNP with positive control antibiotic gentamicin. From left to right: (**a**) 5% LS-AgNP (0.54 µg/mL, 0.27 µg/mL, and 0.14 µg/mL) against *S. aureus* ATCC 25932; 10% LS-AgNP (1.08 µg/mL, 0.54 µg/mL, and 0.27 µg/mL) against: (**b**) *P. aeruginosa* WDCM 00026; (**c**) *E. coli* WDCM 00013; (**c**) *E. coli* WDCM 00013; 1-week-old, aged 10% LS-AgNP (1.08 µg/mL, 0.54 µg/mL and 0.27 µg/mL) against (**d**) *S. aureus* ATCC 25932; (**e**) *P. aeruginosa* WDCM 00026; (**f**) *E. coli* WDCM 00013.

Other groups reported recently similar results with plant biosynthesized AgNP [13,25–29]. Gram-positive and Gram-negative pathogens are susceptible to reported AgNP biohybrids [13,25–29]. DD studies showed similar zones of inhibition for *S. aureus* (13/14 mm), *E. coli* (12 mm), and *P. aeruginosa* (9 mm) [13]. AgNP synthesis by *Aaronsohnia factorovskyi* revealed antibacterial action against *S. aureus* (19 mm), which is followed by *P. aeruginosa* (15.33 mm), *E. coli*, and *B. subtilis* with 13.83 mm in descending order [28]. Cinn-AgNP showed much lower antimicrobial properties compared to LS-AgNP at the same concentration with the same reference strains [42]. The susceptible bacteria were *E. coli* (11 mm), *P. aeruginosa* (10 mm), and *S. aureus* (10 mm) [42]. The LS extract ameliorated the antimicrobial properties of AgNP in comparison to Cinn bark extract [42].

DD studies with LS-AgNP synthesized at pH = 8.5 of fresh 5% and 1-week-old 10% samples showed lower inhibitory action on the selected Gram-positive pathogens except *S. aureus* (Table 4). The 10% LS-AgNP synthesized at pH 7 inhibited the microorganisms intermediately at concentrations of 1.08 µg/mL and 0.54 µg/mL (Table 4). The pathogens were resistant at a concentration of 0.27 µg/mL (Table 4). These results are in agreement with recent investigations on the time, pH, and concentration dependence of AgNP [26]. Our samples did not inhibit *C. albicans* except in the AW study of 10% LS-AgNP (pH = 8.5) and the DD study of 10% LS-AgNP (pH = 8.5).

As a conclusion, the antimicrobial action of LS-AgNP is concentration-, time- and pH-dependent. Our samples inhibited all the selected reference strains under given conditions. Remarkable results are the broad spectrum antimicrobial activity against ESKAPE pathogens. Best results were achieved by 10% LS-AgNP at a concentration of 1.08 µg/mL, synthesized with a 10% content of silver ions, at pH 8.5 and not stored longer than 6 days.

The increased number of adsorbed biomolecules did not enhance the antimicrobial properties in any of the cases except for the 10% LS-AgNP formulation for up to 6 days. The best antimicrobial results were achieved by fresh 10% LS-AgNP prepared at a pH of 8.5. The same finding was presented by Fanoro et al. recently [17]. AgNP releases silver ions during the equilibrium process by oxidation and increases the antimicrobial properties of the LS-AgNP [17,18,21]. AgCl molecules are confirmed by the XRD analysis (Figure 5). The pure LS extract showed no antimicrobial action in AW studies against the Gram-negative pathogens. This finding confirms the antimicrobial action of released silver ions in the AW studies of LS-AgNP. The released silver ions move through the porin channels of the Gram-negative bacteria and exert their antibacterial action. The plant biocompounds are not able to move through the porin channels in AW studies.

Gram-negative pathogens were more susceptible. Noteworthy is the high inhibition of the multidrug-resistant *P. aeruginosa*. The zone of inhibition was 22 mm in AW studies of 10% LS-AgNP compared to the antibiotic gentamicin with 23 mm (Table 3). The multiple drug efflux systems of these rod shaped, motile bacilli were highly susceptible against all our samples except in the AW study of pure LS.

P. mirabilis is the only resistant Gram-negative bacteria in this series. It is a rod-shaped bacillus with multiple *flagellae* and swarming motility. This morphology enables *P. mirabilis* resistance against our title compounds except in both AW studies of 10% LS-AgNP at pH 8.5 and 7 with ZOI = 10 mm (Table 3).

The title compounds exhibit the highest antimicrobial properties against rod-shaped, motile bacilli, which is followed by round *strepto-* and *staphylococci*. The round-shaped cocci can be ordered according to the impact of our samples and their morphology. Clustered cocci are more susceptible than chains and pairs of bacteria.

Gram-negative bacteria with their small peptidoglycan layers, less crosslinking, and highly negatively charged outer cell membranes with lipopolysaccharides are more susceptible due to their porin channels [8,44,72]. Silver ions, AgNP, smaller, lipophilic hydroxycinnamic acids and further phytochemicals move through these channels or puncture the outer cell membrane [8,13,18,42–44]. They disrupt protein synthesis, inhibit DNA replication, cancel efflux systems, and result in cell death [8,13,18,22–24,28,42–44,75].

Gram-positive bacteria are inhibited by our title compounds as well. These pathogens consist of a lower negatively charged outer cell membrane. The Gram-positive bacteria have a thick peptidoglycan layer crosslinked by peptides and inclusions of lipoteichoic as well as teichoic acid [8,44,72]. The phytochemicals in our samples interact with the partial negatively charged atoms in the cell membranes and crosslinked peptides to destabilize the cell wall structure by intermolecular interactions [43]. Phytochemicals prevent bacterial attachment on mucosal surfaces, reduce biofilm formation, inhibit quorum sensing, influence cell surface hydrophobicity, and reduce glycolytic enzymes [23,24].

4. Conclusions

Increasing cases of microbial resistance to drugs and antimicrobials endanger the future of mankind. Plants developed mechanisms to defend themselves against harmful pathogens since the beginning of their existence. Many civilizations utilized phytochemicals in medicinal plants, herbs, spices, and agricultural products as antimicrobial agents. Silver is known and has been used for centuries by mankind against microorganisms. There is an increasing number of publications on phytochemicals and the plant-based synthesis of silver nanoparticles (AgNP). We investigated the antimicrobial properties of the widespread plant LS, which is also known as curly garden cress. Our aim was to ameliorate these properties by utilizing the LS in the green synthesis of AgNP. The combination of LS with AgNP enhanced the inhibitory action against notorious ESKAPE pathogens. The LS-AgNP bio-composites revealed pH, time, and concentration dependencies related to their antimicrobial action. The stability and antimicrobial properties are directly related to the availability of conjugated systems within the bio-compounds and inversely related to agglomeration. LS phytochemicals acted as reducing, stabilizing, and capping agents for AgNP. Carbonyl C=O groups adsorbed on the metallic silver surface and encapsulated the AgNP, resulting in small sizes around 36.1 nm. Silver ions are released by AgNP into the colloidal suspension due to the equilibrium, moisture, and oxidation of AgNP, as well as degradation of the plant-based capping agents. Silver ions increase the inhibitory action against Gram-negative bacteria by moving through their porin channels. Pure LS extract and the 10% LS-AgNP formulations at concentrations of 1.08 µg/mL, 0.54 µg/mL, and 0.27 µg/mL showed very good to intermediate antimicrobial actions on the selection of 10 microorganisms. Gram-negative strains of *P. aeruginosa*, *K. pneumoniae*, and *E. coli* are susceptible, as well as Gram-positive *S. aureus*, the spore-forming *B. subtilis*, *S. pneumoniae*, *S. pyogenes*, and *E. faecalis*. Antifungal activity against *C. albicans* was detected in agar well and disc diffusion studies of two of our 10% LS-AgNP samples. The results confirm the potential uses of LS-AgNP as broad-spectrum microbicides, disinfectants, and wound care products.

Supplementary Materials: The following are available online at https://www.mdpi.com/article/10.3390/pharmaceutics13091352/s1, Figure S1: Layered EDS, Figure S2: DLS, Figure S3: FTIR-Pure LS extract in ethanol, Figure S4: FTIR-LS-AgNP in ethanol.

Author Contributions: Conceptualization, Z.E., S.H.B. and M.A.A.; methodology, S.H.B.; software, Z.E.; validation, Z.E., S.H.B. and H.A.S.; formal analysis, H.A.S. and M.A.A.; investigation, Z.E., S.H.B., M.A.A. and H.A.S.; resources, Z.E. and S.H.B.; data curation, H.A.S. and M.A.A.; writing—original draft preparation, Z.E. and S.H.B.; writing—review and editing, Z.E. and S.H.B.; visualization, Z.E. and S.H.B.; supervision, S.H.B. and Z.E.; project administration, S.H.B. and Z.E.; funding acquisition, Z.E. All authors have read and agreed to the published version of the manuscript.

Funding: This work was kindly supported by the Deanship of Graduate Studies and Research, AU, Ajman, United Arab Emirates (Project ID No: Ref. # IRG-2018-A-PH-09).

Acknowledgments: We are extremely grateful to Sohaib Khan for his excellent efforts during the whole investigation for performing FTIR and his tremendous support in every aspect of the study. We express our gratitude to May Reda Ibrahim and her important input into this investigation. We are also thankful to Hussain Alawadhi, Mohammad Shameer, and Muhammed Irshad from

Sharjah University for performing the SEM, EDS, and XRD analysis. We also like to thank the artist "@art_by_amie_" for providing us with a digital art image as a graphical abstract.

Conflicts of Interest: The authors declare no conflict of interest.

References

1. World Health Organization (WHO). 2020 Antibacterial Agents in Clinical and Preclinical Development: An Overview and Analysis. Available online: https://www.who.int/publications/i/item/9789240021303 (accessed on 13 June 2021).
2. Mulani, M.S.; Kamble, E.E.; Kumkar, S.N.; Tawre, M.S.; Pardesi, K.R. Emerging Strategies to Combat ESKAPE Pathogens in the Era of Antimicrobial Resistance: A Review. *Front. Microbiol.* **2019**, *10*, 539–563. [CrossRef]
3. Bhatia, P.; Sharma, A.; George, A.J.; Anvitha, D.; Kumar, P.; Dwivedi, V.P.; Chandra, N.S. Antibacterial activity of medicinal plants against ESKAPE: An update. *Heliyon* **2021**, *7*, e06310. [CrossRef] [PubMed]
4. Bloukh, S.H.; Edis, Z.; Shaikh, A.A.; Pathan, H.M. A Look Behind the Scenes at COVID-19: National Strategies of Infection Control and Their Impact on Mortality. *Int. J. Environ. Res. Public Health* **2020**, *17*, 5616. [CrossRef]
5. Barranco, R.; Du Tremoul, L.; Ventura, F. Hospital-Acquired SARS-Cov-2 Infections in Patients: Inevitable Conditions or Medical Malpractice? *Int. J. Environ. Res. Public Health* **2021**, *18*, 489. [CrossRef]
6. Anand, U.; Jacobo-Herrera, N.; Altemimi, A.; Lakhssassi, N. A Comprehensive Review on Medicinal Plants as Antimicrobial Therapeutics: Potential Avenues of Biocompatible Drug Discovery. *Metabolites* **2019**, *9*, 258. [CrossRef]
7. Eleraky, N.E.; Allam, A.; Hassan, S.B.; Omar, M.M. Nanomedicine Fight against Antibacterial Resistance: An Overview of the Recent Pharmaceutical Innovations. *Pharmaceutics* **2020**, *12*, 142. [CrossRef]
8. Godlewska-Żyłkiewicz, B.; Świsłocka, R.; Kalinowska, M.; Golonko, A.; Świderski, G.; Arciszewska, Ż.; Nalewajko-Sieliwoniuk, E.; Naumowicz, M.; Lewandowski, W. Biologically Active Compounds of Plants: Structure-Related Antioxidant, Microbiological and Cytotoxic Activity of Selected Carboxylic Acids. *Materials* **2020**, *13*, 4454. [CrossRef]
9. Piccolella, S.; Crescente, G.; Faramarzi, S.; Formato, M.; Pecoraro, M.T.; Pacifico, S. Polyphenols vs. Coronaviruses: How Far Has Research Moved Forward? *Molecules* **2020**, *25*, 4103. [CrossRef]
10. Mani, J.S.; Johnson, J.B.; Steel, J.C.; Broszczak, D.A.; Neilsen, P.M.; Walsh, K.B.; Naiker, M. Natural product-derived phytochemicals as potential agents against coronaviruses: A review. *Virus Res.* **2020**, *284*, 197989. [CrossRef] [PubMed]
11. Paraiso, I.L.; Revel, J.S.; Stevens, J.F. Potential use of polyphenols in the battle against COVID-19. *Curr. Opin. Food Sci.* **2020**, *32*, 149–155. [CrossRef] [PubMed]
12. Wahab, M.A.; Li, L.; Li, H.; Abdala, A. Silver Nanoparticle-Based Nanocomposites for Combating Infectious Pathogens: Recent Advances and Future Prospects. *Nanomaterials* **2021**, *11*, 581. [CrossRef] [PubMed]
13. El-Kahky, D.; Attia, M.; Easa, S.M.; Awad, N.M.; Helmy, E.A. Interactive Effects of Biosynthesized Nanocomposites and Their Antimicrobial and Cytotoxic Potentials. *Nanomaterials* **2021**, *11*, 903. [CrossRef] [PubMed]
14. Edis, Z.; Haj Bloukh, S.; Ashames, A.; Ibrahim, M. Copper-based Nanoparticles, their chemistry and Antibacterial properties: A review. In *Chemistry for a Clean and Healthy Planet*, 1st ed.; Ramasami, P., Gupta Bhowon, M., Jhaumeer Laulloo, S., Li Kam Wah, H., Eds.; Springer: Cham, Switzerland, 2019; pp. 401–428. ISBN 13-978-3-030-20282-8.
15. Rónavári, A.; Igaz, N.; Adamecz, D.I.; Szerencsés, B.; Molnar, C.; Kónya, Z.; Pfeiffer, I.; Kiricsi, M. Green Silver and Gold Nanoparticles: Biological Synthesis Approaches and Potentials for Biomedical Applications. *Molecules* **2021**, *26*, 844. [CrossRef]
16. Castillo-Henríquez, L.; Alfaro-Aguilar, K.; Ugalde-Álvarez, J.; Vega-Fernández, L.; Montes de Oca-Vásquez, G.; Vega-Baudrit, J.R. Green Synthesis of Gold and Silver Nanoparticles from Plant Extracts and Their Possible Applications as Antimicrobial Agents in the Agricultural Area. *Nanomaterials* **2020**, *10*, 1763. [CrossRef] [PubMed]
17. Fanoro, O.T.; Oluwafemi, O.S. Bactericidal Antibacterial Mechanism of Plant Synthesized Silver, Gold and Bimetallic Nanoparticles. *Pharmaceutics* **2020**, *12*, 1044. [CrossRef]
18. Kędziora, A.; Speruda, M.; Krzyżewska, E.; Rybka, J.; Łukowiak, A.; Bugla-Płoskońska, G. Similarities and Differences between Silver Ions and Silver in Nanoforms as Antibacterial Agents. *Int. J. Mol. Sci.* **2018**, *19*, 444. [CrossRef] [PubMed]
19. Hamed, S.M.; Mostafa, A.M.A.; Abdel-Raouf, N.; Ibraheem, I.B.M. Biosynthesis of silver and silver chloride nanoparticles by Parachlorella kessleri SAG 211-11 and evaluation of its nematicidal potential against the root-knot nematode; Meloidogyne incognita. *Aust. J. Basic Appl. Sci.* **2016**, *10*, 354–364.
20. Kumar, V.A.; Uchida, T.; Mizuki, T.; Nakajima, Y.; Katsube, Y.; Hanajiri, T.; Maekawa, T. Synthesis of nanoparticles composed of silver and silver chloride for a plasmonic photocatalyst using an extract from a weed *Solidago altissima* (goldenrod). *Adv. Nat. Sci. Nanosci. Nanotechnol.* **2016**, *7*, 015002. [CrossRef]
21. Al Aboody, M.S. Silver/silver chloride (Ag/AgCl) nanoparticles synthesized from *Azadirachta indica* lalex and its antibiofilm activity against fluconazole resistant *Candida tropicalis*. *Artif. Cells Nanomed. Biotechnol.* **2019**, *47*, 2107–2113. [CrossRef]
22. Zhao, Q.; Luan, X.; Zheng, M.; Tian, X.-H.; Zhao, J.; Zhang, W.-D.; Ma, B.-L. Synergistic Mechanisms of Constituents in Herbal Extracts during Intestinal Absorption: Focus on Natural Occurring Nanoparticles. *Pharmaceutics* **2020**, *12*, 128. [CrossRef]
23. Abachi, S.; Lee, S.; Rupasinghe, H.P.V. Molecular Mechanisms of Inhibition of *Streptococcus* Species by Phytochemicals. *Molecules* **2016**, *21*, 215. [CrossRef]
24. Malheiro, J.F.; Maillard, J.-Y.; Borges, F.; Simões, M. Biocide Potentiation Using Cinnamic Phytochemicals and Derivatives. *Molecules* **2019**, *24*, 3918. [CrossRef]

25. Reda, M.; Ashames, A.; Edis, Z.; Bloukh, S.; Bhandare, R.; Abu Sara, H. Green Synthesis of Potent Antimicrobial Silver Nanoparticles Using Different Plant Extracts and Their Mixtures. *Processes* **2019**, *7*, 510. [CrossRef]
26. Miljković, M.; Lazić, V.; Davidović, S.; Milivojević, A.; Papan, J.; Fernandes, M.M.; Lanceros-Mendez, S.; Ahrenkiel, S.P.; Nedeljković, J.M. Selective Antimicrobial Performance of Biosynthesized Silver Nanoparticles by Horsetail Extract Against. *E. coli*. *J. Inorg. Organomet. Polym. Mater.* **2020**, *30*, 2598–2607. [CrossRef]
27. Ankegowda, V.M.; Kollur, S.P.; Prasad, S.K.; Pradeep, S.; Dhramashekara, C.; Jain, A.S.; Prasad, A.; Srinivasa, C.; Sridhara Setty, P.B.; Gopinath, S.M.; et al. Phyto-Mediated Synthesis of Silver Nanoparticles Using *Terminalia chebula* Fruit Extract and Evaluation of Its Cytotoxic and Antimicrobial Potential. *Molecules* **2020**, *25*, 5042. [CrossRef] [PubMed]
28. Al-Otibi, F.; Al-Ahaidib, R.A.; Alharbi, R.I.; Al-Otaibi, R.M.; Albasher, G. Antimicrobial Potential of Biosynthesized Silver Nanoparticles by *Aaronsohnia factorovskyi* Extract. *Molecules* **2021**, *26*, 130. [CrossRef] [PubMed]
29. Samuggam, S.; Chinni, S.V.; Mutusamy, P.; Gopinath, S.C.B.; Anbu, P.; Venugopal, V.; Reddy, L.V.; Enugutti, B. Green Synthesis and Characterization of Silver Nanoparticles Using *Spondias mombin* Extract and Their Antimicrobial Activity against Biofilm-Producing Bacteria. *Molecules* **2021**, *26*, 2681. [CrossRef]
30. Küünal, S.; Rauwel, P.; Rauwel, E. Plant extract mediated synthesis of nanoparticles. In *Emerging Applications of Nanoparticles and Architecture Nanostructures: Current Prospects and Future Trends, Micro and Nano Technologies*, 1st ed.; Makhlouf, A.S.H., Barhoum, A., Eds.; Elsevier: Amsterdam, The Netherlands, 2018; ISBN 9780128135167.
31. Sang Hun Lee, S.H.; Jun, B.-H. Silver Nanoparticles: Synthesis and Application for Nanomedicine. *Int. J. Mol. Sci.* **2019**, *20*, 865. [CrossRef]
32. Logaranjan, K.; Raiza, A.J.; Gopinath, S.C.B.; Chen, Y.; Pandian, K. Shape- and Size-Controlled Synthesis of Silver Nanoparticles Using Aloe vera Plant Extract and Their Antimicrobial Activity. *Nanoscale Res. Lett.* **2016**, *11*, 520–529. [CrossRef] [PubMed]
33. Riau, A.K.; Aung, T.T.; Setiawan, M.; Yang, L.; Yam, G.H.F.; Beuerman, R.W.; Venkatraman, S.S.; Mehta, J.S. Surface Immobilization of Nano-Silver on Polymeric Medical Devices to Prevent Bacterial Biofilm Formation. *Pathogens* **2019**, *8*, 93. [CrossRef]
34. Soni, N.; Prakash, S. Green Nanoparticles for Mosquito Control. *Sci. World J.* **2014**, *2014*, 496362. [CrossRef]
35. Premkumar, J.; Sudhakar, T.; Dhakal, A.; Shrestha, J.B.; Krishnakumar, S.; Balashanmugam, P. Synthesis of silver nanoparticles (AgNPs) from cinnamon against bacterial Pathogens. *Biocatal. Agric. Biotechnol.* **2018**, *15*, 311–316. [CrossRef]
36. Singh, P.; Kim, Y.J.; Wang, C.; Mathiyalagan, R.; Yang, D.C. The development of a green approach for the biosynthesis of silver and gold nanoparticles by using *Panax ginseng* root extract, and their biological applications. *Artif. Cells Nanomed. Biotechnol.* **2016**, *44*, 1150–1157. [CrossRef]
37. Mamatha, G.; Rajulu, A.V.; Madhukar, K. Development and analysis of cellulose nanocomposite films with in situ generated silver nanoparticles using tamarind nut powder as a reducing agent. *Int. J. Polym. A Charact.* **2019**, *24*, 219–226. [CrossRef]
38. Edis, Z.; Bloukh, S.H.; Abu Sara, H.; Bhakhoa, H.; Rhyman, L.; Ramasami, P. "Smart" triiodide compounds: Does halogen bonding influence antimicrobial activities? *Pathogens* **2019**, *8*, 182. [CrossRef] [PubMed]
39. Edis, Z.; Raheja, R.; Bloukh, S.H.; Bhandare, R.R.; Sara, H.A.; Reiss, G.J. Antimicrobial Hexaaquacopper(II) Complexes with Novel Polyiodide Chains. *Polymers* **2021**, *13*, 1005. [CrossRef]
40. Bloukh, S.H.; Edis, Z. Halogen bonding in Crystal structure of bis(1,4,7,10-tetraoxacyclododecane-κ^4O,O',O'',O''')cesium triiodide, $C_{16}H_{32}CsI_3O_8$. *Z. Krist. NCS* **2020**, *235*, 717–719. [CrossRef]
41. Edis, Z.; Bloukh, S.H. Preparation and structural and spectroscopic characterization of triiodides [M(12-crown-4)$_2$]I$_3$ with M = Na and Rb. *Z. Nat.* **2014**, *69*, 995–1002. [CrossRef]
42. Bloukh, S.H.; Edis, Z.; Ibrahim, M.R.; Abu Sara, H. "Smart" antimicrobial nanocomplexes with potential to decrease surgical site infections (SSI). *Pharmaceutics* **2020**, *12*, 361. [CrossRef]
43. Edis, Z.; Bloukh, S.H. Facile Synthesis of Bio-Antimicrobials with "Smart" Triiodides. *Molecules* **2021**, *26*, 3553. [CrossRef]
44. Edis, Z.; Bloukh, S.H. Facile Synthesis of Antimicrobial Aloe Vera- "Smart" Triiodide-PVP Biomaterials. *Biomimetics* **2020**, *5*, 45. [CrossRef] [PubMed]
45. Martins, N.; Barros, L.; Santos-Buelga, C.; Henriques, M.; Silva, S.; Ferreira, I.C.F.R. Evaluation of bioactive properties and phenolic compounds in different extracts prepared from *Salvia officinalis* L. *Food Chem.* **2015**, *170*, 378–385. [CrossRef] [PubMed]
46. Pavić, V.; Jakovljević, M.; Molnar, M.; Jokić, S. Extraction of Carnosic Acid and Carnosol from Sage (*Salvia officinalis* L.) Leaves by Supercritical Fluid Extraction and Their Antioxidant and Antibacterial Activity. *Plants* **2019**, *8*, 16. [CrossRef]
47. Boufadi, M.Y.; Keddari, S.; Moulai-Hacene, F.; Chaa, S. Chemical Composition, Antioxidant and Anti-Inflammatory Properties of *Salvia officinalis* Extract from Algeria. *Pharm. J.* **2021**, *13*, 506–515. [CrossRef]
48. Vieira, S.F.; Ferreira, H.; Neves, N.M. Antioxidant and Anti-Inflammatory Activities of Cytocompatible *Salvia officinalis* Extracts: A Comparison between Traditional and Soxhlet Extraction. *Antioxidants* **2020**, *9*, 1157. [CrossRef]
49. Zaccardelli, M.; Pane, C.; Caputo, M.; Durazzo, A.; Lucarini, M.; Silva, A.M.; Severino, P.; Souto, E.B.; Santini, A.; De Feo, V. Sage Species Case Study on a Spontaneous Mediterranean Plant to Control Phytopathogenic Fungi and Bacteria. *Forests* **2020**, *11*, 704. [CrossRef]
50. Sik, B.; Kapcsándi, V.; Székelyhidi, R.; Hanczné, E.L.; Ajtony, Z. Recent Advances in the Analysis of Rosmarinic Acid From Herbs in the Lamiaceae Family. *Nat. Prod. Commun.* **2019**, *14*, 1934578X1986421. [CrossRef]
51. Sánchez, M.; González-Burgos, E.; Iglesias, I.; Gómez-Serranillos, M.P. Pharmacological Update Properties of *Aloe vera* and its Major Active Constituents. *Molecules* **2020**, *25*, 1324. [CrossRef]

52. Gokavi, S.S.; Malleshi, N.G.; Guo, M. Chemical Composition of Garden Cress (*Lepidium sativum*) Seeds and Its Fractions and use of Bran as a Functional Ingredient. *Plant Foods Hum. Nutr.* **2004**, *59*, 105–111. [CrossRef]
53. Alkahtani, J.; Elshikh, M.S.; Almaary, K.S.; Ali, S.; Imtiyaz, Z.; Ahmad, S.B. Anti-bacterial, anti-scavenging and cytotoxic activity of garden cress polysaccharides. *Saudi J. Biol. Sci.* **2020**, *27*, 2929–2935. [CrossRef]
54. Alqahtani, F.Y.; Aleanizy, F.S.; Mahmoud, A.Z.; Farshori, N.N.; Alfaraj, R.; Al-sheddi, E.S.; Alsarra, I.A. Chemical composition and antimicrobial, antioxidant, and anti-inflammatory activities of *Lepidium sativum* seed oil. *Saudi J. Biol. Sci.* **2019**, *26*, 1089–1092. [CrossRef] [PubMed]
55. Jain, T.; Grover, K. A Comprehensive Review on the Nutritional and Nutraceutical Aspects of Garden Cress (*Lepidium sativum* Linn). *Proc. Natl. Acad. Sci. India Sect. B Biol. Sci.* **2018**, *88*, 829–836. [CrossRef]
56. Rafińska, K.; Pomastowski, P.; Rudnicka, J.; Krakowska, A.; Maruśka, A.; Narkute, M.; Buszewski, B. Effect of solvent and extraction technique on composition and biological activity of *Lepidium sativum* extracts. *Food Chem.* **2019**, *289*, 16–25. [CrossRef]
57. Elguera, J.C.T.; Barrientos, E.Y.; Wrobel, K.; Wrobel, K. Effect of cadmium (Cd(II)), selenium (Se(IV)) and their mixtures on phenolic compounds and antioxidant capacity in *Lepidium sativum*. *Acta Physiol. Plant.* **2013**, *35*, 431–441. [CrossRef]
58. Keutgen, N.; Hausknecht, M.; Tomaszewska-Sowa, M.; Keutgen, A.J. Nutritional and Sensory Quality of Two Types of Cress Microgreens Depending on the Mineral Nutrition. *Agronomy* **2021**, *11*, 1110. [CrossRef]
59. Ciesielska, K.; Ciesielski, W.; Kulawik, D.; Oszczęda, Z.; Tomasik, P. Cultivation of Cress Involving Water Treated Under Different Atmospheres with Low-Temperature, Low-Pressure Glow Plasma of Low Frequency. *Water* **2020**, *12*, 2152. [CrossRef]
60. Pignattelli, S.; Broccoli, A.; Renzi, M. Physiological responses of garden cress (*L. sativum*) to different types of microplastics. *Sci. Total Environ.* **2020**, *727*, 138609. [CrossRef]
61. Razmkhah, S.; Mohammadifar, M.A.; Razavi, S.M.A.; Ale, M.T. Purification of cress seed (*Lepidium sativum*) gum: Physicochemical characterization and functional properties. *Carbohydr. Polym.* **2016**, *141*, 166–174. [CrossRef]
62. Ibrahim, E.H.; Ghramh, H.A.; Alshehri, A.; Kilany, M.; Khalofah, A.; El-Mekkawy, H.I.; Sayed, M.A.; Alothaid, H.; Taha, R. *Lepidium sativum* and Its Biogenic Silver Nanoparticles Activate Immune Cells and Induce Apoptosis and Cell Cycle Arrest in HT-29 Colon Cancer Cells. *J. Biomater. Tissue Eng.* **2021**, *11*, 195–209. [CrossRef]
63. Granados, A.; Pleixats, R.; Vallribera, A. Recent Advances on Antimicrobial and Anti-Inflammatory Cotton Fabrics Containing Nanostructures. *Molecules* **2021**, *26*, 3008. [CrossRef] [PubMed]
64. Sunitha, S.; Adinarayana, K.; Sravanthi, R.P.; Sonia, G.; Nagarjun, R.; Pankaj, T.; Veerabhadra, S.C.; Sujatha, D. Fabrication of Surgical Sutures Coated with Curcumin Loaded Gold Nanoparticles. *Pharm. Anal. Acta* **2017**, *8*, 1–12. [CrossRef]
65. Amaro, F.; Morón, Á.; Díaz, S.; Martín-González, A.; Gutiérrez, J.C. Metallic Nanoparticles-Friends or Foes in the Battle against Antibiotic-Resistant Bacteria? *Microorganisms* **2021**, *9*, 364. [CrossRef]
66. McNeilly, O.; Mann, R.; Hamidian, M.; Gunawan, C. Emerging Concern for Silver Nanoparticle Resistance in Acinetobacter Baumannii and Other Bacteria. *Front. Microbiol.* **2021**, *12*, 894. [CrossRef]
67. Panáček, A.; Kvítek, L.; Smékalová, M.; Večeřová, R.; Kolář, M.; Röderová, M.; Dyčka, F.; Šebela, M.; Prucek, R.; Tomanec, O.; et al. Bacterial Resistance to Silver Nanoparticles and How to Overcome It. *Nat. Nanotechnol.* **2018**, *13*, 65–71. [CrossRef]
68. Kaweeteerawat, C.; Na Ubol, P.; Sangmuang, S.; Aueviriyavit, S.; Maniratanachote, R. Mechanisms of Antibiotic Resistance in Bacteria Mediated by Silver Nanoparticles. *J. Toxicol. Environ. Health A* **2017**, *80*, 1276–1289. [CrossRef] [PubMed]
69. Liao, C.; Li, Y.; Tjong, S.C. Bactericidal and Cytotoxic Properties of Silver Nanoparticles. *Int. J. Mol. Sci.* **2019**, *20*, 449. [CrossRef] [PubMed]
70. Bauer, A.W.; Perry, D.M.; Kirby, W.M.M. Single-disk antibiotic-sensitivity testing of staphylococci: An analysis of technique and results. *AMA Arch. Intern. Med.* **1959**, *104*, 208–216. [CrossRef] [PubMed]
71. Clinical and Laboratory Standards Institute (CLSI). *Performance Standards for Antimicrobial Disk Susceptibility Testing*, 28th ed.; M100S; CLSI: Wayne, PA, USA, 2018; Volume 38.
72. Jakovljević, M.; Jokić, S.; Molnar, M.; Jašić, M.; Babić, J.; Jukić, H.; Banjari, I. Bioactive Profile of Various *Salvia officinalis* L. Preparations. *Plants* **2019**, *8*, 55. [CrossRef]
73. Aguilar-Hernández, I.; Afseth, N.K.; López-Luke, T.; Contreras-Torres, F.F.; Wold, J.P.; Ornelas-Soto, N. Surface enhanced Raman spectroscopy of phenolic antioxidants: A systematic evaluation of ferulic acid, *p*-coumaric acid, caffeic acid and sinapic acid. *Vib. Spectr.* **2017**, *89*, 113–122. [CrossRef]
74. Doyle, A.A.; Stephens, J.C. A review of cinnamaldehyde and its derivatives as antibacterial agents. *Fitoterapia* **2019**, *139*, 104405. [CrossRef]
75. Mohamed, D.S.; El-Baky, R.M.A.; Sandle, T.; Mandour, S.A.; Ahmed, E.F. Antimicrobial Activity of Silver-Treated Bacteria against other Multi-Drug Resistant Pathogens in Their Environment. *Antibiotics* **2020**, *9*, 181. [CrossRef] [PubMed]

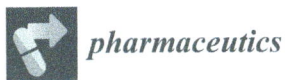

Article

Characterization and Genome Analysis of *Arthrobacter bangladeshi* sp. nov., Applied for the Green Synthesis of Silver Nanoparticles and Their Antibacterial Efficacy against Drug-Resistant Human Pathogens

Md. Amdadul Huq [1,*] and Shahina Akter [2,*]

1 Department of Food and Nutrition, College of Biotechnology and Natural Resource, Chung-Ang University, Anseong 17546, Korea
2 Department of Food Science and Biotechnology, Gachon University, Seongnam 461-701, Korea
* Correspondence: amdadbge@gmail.com or amdadbge100@cau.ac.kr (M.A.H.); shahinabristy16@gmail.com (S.A.); Tel.: +82-031-670-4568 (M.A.H.)

Abstract: The present study describes the isolation and characterization of novel bacterial species *Arthrobacter bangladeshi* sp. nov., applied for the green synthesis of AgNPs, and investigates its antibacterial efficacy against drug-resistant pathogenic *Salmonella* Typhimurium and *Yersinia enterocolitica*. Novel strain MAHUQ-56[T] is Gram-positive, aerobic, non-motile, and rod-shaped. Colonies were spherical and milky white. The strain showed positive activity for catalase and nitrate reductase, and the hydrolysis of starch, L-tyrosine, casein, and Tween 20. On the basis of the 16S rRNA gene sequence, strain MAHUQ-56[T] belongs to the *Arthrobacter* genus and is most closely related to *Arthrobacter pokkalii* P3B162[T] (98.6%). *Arthrobacter bangladeshi* MAHUQ-56[T] has a genome 4,566,112 bp long (26 contigs) with 4125 protein-coding genes, 51 tRNA and 6 rRNA genes. The culture supernatant of *Arthrobacter bangladeshi* MAHUQ-56[T] was used for the easy and green synthesis of AgNPs. Synthesized AgNPs were characterized by UV–vis spectroscopy, FE-TEM, XRD, DLS, and FT-IR. Synthesized AgNPs were spherical and 12–50 nm in size. FT-IR analysis revealed various biomolecules that may be involved in the synthesis process. Synthesized AgNPs showed strong antibacterial activity against multidrug-resistant pathogenic *S. typhimurium* and *Y. enterocolitica*. MIC values of the synthesized AgNPs against *S. typhimurium* and *Y. enterocolitica* were 6.2 and 3.1 ug/mL, respectively. The MBC of synthesized AgNPs for both pathogens was 12.5 ug/mL. FE-SEM analysis revealed the morphological and structural alterations, and damage of pathogens treated by AgNPs. These changes might disturb normal cellular functions, which ultimately leads to the death of cells.

Keywords: *Arthrobacter bangladeshi* MAHUQ-56[T]; AgNPs; green synthesis; *S. typhimurium*; *Y. enterocolitica*

Citation: Huq, M.A.; Akter, S. Characterization and Genome Analysis of *Arthrobacter bangladeshi* sp. nov., Applied for the Green Synthesis of Silver Nanoparticles and Their Antibacterial Efficacy against Drug-Resistant Human Pathogens. *Pharmaceutics* **2021**, *13*, 1691. https://doi.org/10.3390/pharmaceutics13101691

Academic Editor: Teresa Cerchiara

Received: 30 August 2021
Accepted: 12 October 2021
Published: 15 October 2021

Publisher's Note: MDPI stays neutral with regard to jurisdictional claims in published maps and institutional affiliations.

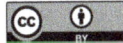

Copyright: © 2021 by the authors. Licensee MDPI, Basel, Switzerland. This article is an open access article distributed under the terms and conditions of the Creative Commons Attribution (CC BY) license (https://creativecommons.org/licenses/by/4.0/).

1. Introduction

The *Arthrobacter* genus within the *Micrococcaceae* family was first proposed by Conn and Dimmick [1]. The *Arthrobacter* genus comprises 54 validly published species at the time of writing (https://lpsn.dsmz.de/genus/Arthrobacter (accessed on 28 August 2021)). Members of this genus are Gram-positive, aerobic (requiring oxygen for growth), non-motile, rod-coccus-shaped, with negative acidification of glucose, catalase-positive, and contain $C_{15:0\ anteiso}$, $C_{15:0\ iso}$, $C_{16:0\ iso}$ and $C_{17:0\ anteiso}$ as the major fatty acids, MK-9 (H2) or MK-8/MK-9 as the predominant respiratory quinone, and high DNA G + C content [2,3]. The *Arthrobacter* genus is one of the most divergent heterotrophic bacterial groups because of metabolic versatility. Members of the *Arthrobacter* genus were isolated from various environments, such as sewage, soil, water, ice, rhizosphere, marsh, sediment, and pests [4–8]. Many species of this genus were utilized for beneficial purposes [4,5,7]. Here, a novel species of *Arthrobacter* was isolated from the soil sample of a rice field and applied for the green synthesis of silver nanoparticles (AgNPs). On the basis of the phylogenetic analysis of 16S rRNA gene sequence, genome sequence analysis, digital DNA–DNA hybridization analysis, and physiological and chemotaxonomic characteristics, we demonstrate that strain MAHUQ-56^T represents a novel species of the *Arthrobacter* genus, for which the name *Arthrobacter bangladeshi* sp. nov. (type strain MAHUQ-56^T) is proposed.

Nanotechnology deals with the design, synthesis, and application of nanosized particles in the range of 1–100 nm. There are different kinds of metallic nanoparticles, such as gold, silver, iron, and zinc. Among them, AgNPs are widely used nanoparticles due to their various applications in biological fields such as antimicrobial, anticancer, drug delivery, catalysis, and biomolecular detection [9–11]. Due to the various applications of metal nanoparticles in different scientific fields, researchers have devoted extensive efforts to develop easy and ecofriendly techniques for the rapid and mass production of nanoparticles. Chemical, physical, and biological methods are available for the synthesis of nanoparticles [12]. Chemical and physical methods are commonly used for the synthesis of well-characterized nanoparticles. However, these two method types need enormous energy amounts and hazardous chemicals, and produce toxic byproducts that make them unsuitable approaches [13,14]. Therefore, the development of a green approach for the synthesis of nanoparticles is an emerging demand to avoid the drawbacks of conventional physical and chemical methods. Biological methods are an important route for the synthesis of nanoparticles because of their nontoxic, cost-effective, and ecofriendly properties [15,16]. For the ecofriendly synthesis of nanoparticles, various biological resources could be used, such as plants or plant products, and microorganisms such as bacteria, fungi, and algae [13,16–19]. Among different natural resources, bacteria are mostly chosen for the biosynthesis of nanoparticles because of their easy handling and growth, and large-scale production [20,21].

The emergence of multidrug-resistant bacteria is a major concern for public health. Antibiotic-resistant microorganisms cause life-threatening diseases in humans. *Salmonella* Typhimurium is a rod-shaped, aerobic, flagellated, Gram-negative bacterium, and a primary enteric pathogen for both humans and animals. Infection begins with the ingestion of contaminated food or water. After consuming the contaminated food or water, the pathogen reaches the intestinal epithelium and triggers gastrointestinal disease [22]. *Yersinia enterocolitica* is a Gram-negative, rod-shaped bacterium within the *Yersiniaceae* family. Yersiniosis disease is developed by *Y. enterocolitica* infection, which is an animal-borne disease occurring in humans and different animals such as cattle, pigs, deer, and birds [23]. Both *S. typhimurium* and *Y. enterocolitica* showed resistance against various drugs [24,25]. The development of a novel antibacterial agent is the key solution for this issue. Therefore, green synthesized AgNPs are a promising agent to control these multidrug-resistant bacteria. The present study isolates and characterizes novel bacterial species *Arthrobacter bangladeshi* sp. nov., used for the easy and ecofriendly extracellular synthesis of AgNPs, and investigates its antibacterial efficacy against drug-resistant pathogenic *S. typhimurium* and *Y. enterocolitica*.

2. Materials and Methods

2.1. Materials

Silver nitrate (AgNO$_3$) and bacterial growth media were obtained from Sigma-Aldrich Chemicals (St. Louis, MO, USA). Pathogenic strains *Salmonella* Typhimurium (ATCC 14028) and *Yersinia enterocolitica* (ATCC 9610) were collected from American Type Culture Collection (ATCC).

2.2. Isolation of AgNP-Producing Bacteria

Strains were isolated from the soil sample of a rice field located in Dighalgram, Magura, Bangladesh. Samples were collected in 15 mL conical tubes and suspended in sterile NaCl solution (0.85%, w/v). Strains were isolated through a serial dilution technique using an R2A agar medium after incubation for 3 days at 30 °C according to a previous study [18]. To check the AgNPs' synthesis ability, all isolated strains were separately cultured in 5 mL R2A broth media for 72 h at 30 °C. Then, the culture supernatant was collected and incubated with 1 mM AgNO$_3$ solution (final concentration) in a shaking incubator for 72 h at 30 °C. On the basis of AgNO$_3$ reduction efficacy to AgNPs, strain MAHUQ-56^T was selected as the perfect candidate. Strain MAHUQ-56^T was stored at −80 °C in R2A broth containing 30% (v/v) glycerol. Strain MAHUQ-56^T was deposited into the Korean Agriculture Culture Collection (KACC) and China General Microbiological Culture Collection Center (CGMCC).

2.3. Phenotypic, Physiological, and Biochemical Characteristics

The growth of strain MAHUQ-56^T was investigated at 30 °C for 5 days on several agar media, namely, R2A agar, nutrient agar (NA), MacConkey agar, Luria–Bertani (LB) agar, and trypticase soy agar (TSA). To determine the optimal growth temperature, strain MAHUQ-56^T was cultivated at different temperatures (5–45 °C with 5 °C intervals) on R2A agar. To investigate the optimal growth pH, strain MAHUQ-56^T was cultivated at different pH values (3.0–11.0 at intervals of 0.5 pH unit) in an R2A broth medium. NaCl tolerance was examined in R2A broth medium (0–5% (w/v)). Gram staining (bioMérieux) was examined according to the manufacturer's instructions. Cell morphology was assessed by transmission electron microscopy after culturing the strain for 2 days at 30 °C on an R2A agar medium. The cell motility and anaerobic growth ability of strain MAHUQ-56^T were established according to a previous description [18]. The production of flexirubin-type pigments was checked according to Sheu et al. [26]. The activities of DNase, oxidase, urease, and catalase, and the hydrolysis of starch, gelatin, casein, and Tweens 20 and 80 were found according to a previous description [18]. Additional biochemical and physiological characterization of strain MAHUQ-56^T and close relatives was investigated using the API ZYM and API 20NE kits (bioMérieux). Close type strains *Arthrobacter pokkalii* KCTC 29498^T, *Pseudarthrobacter defluvii* KCTC 19209^T, *Pseudarthrobacter niigatensis* CCTCC AB 206012^T, *Pseudarthrobacter phenanthrenivorans* DSM 18606^T, and *Pseudarthrobacter enclensis* DSM 25279^T were used as reference strains, and grown under the same experimental conditions to compare phenotypic properties and fatty acid compositions.

2.4. 16S rRNA Gene Sequencing and Phylogenetic Analysis

Phylogenetic analysis of isolated strain MAHUQ-56^T was conducted using the 16S rRNA gene sequence. Having extracted the genomic DNA of strain MAHUQ-56^T, the 16S rRNA gene was amplified by PCR using bacterial universal primers 27F and 1492R [27]. The PCR product was purified and sequenced by Biofact Co. Ltd. (Daejeon, South Korea). The 16S rRNA sequence similarity was checked and compared with validly published type strains from the EzTaxon database (http://www.ezbiocloud.net/eztaxon (accessed on 28 August 2021)) [28]. Phylogenic trees were constructed using neighbor-joining and maximum-likelihood algorithms [26] in MEGA software, Version 6 [29] with bootstrap values of 1000 replications [30].

2.5. Genomic Sequence Analysis

The draft genomic sequence of strain MAHUQ-56^T was analyzed by Illumina HiSeq X Ten (Illumina, Inc., San Diego, CA, USA), and assembly was carried out using a de novo assembler (SOAPdenovo v. 3.10.1). The NCBI prokaryotic genome annotation pipeline (PGAP) was used for genome annotation. DNA G + C content of strain MAHUQ-56^T was directly calculated from its genomic sequence. Average nucleotide identity (ANI) values were analyzed to investigate the level of pairwise relatedness between MAHUQ-56^T and close type strains using the EzTaxon-e server (https://www.ezbio cloud.net/tools/ani (accessed on 28 August 2021)) [28]. Digital DNA–DNA hybridization (dDDH) values were determined using the genome-to-genome distance calculator (http://ggdc.dsmz.de/ggdc.php (accessed on 28 August 2021)) [31]. For functional analysis, the genome of strain MAHUQ-56^T was annotated using the Rapid Annotation Subsystems Technology (RAST) server (https://rast.nmpdr.org (accessed on 28 August 2021)) [32].

2.6. Cellular Fatty Acid and Respiratory Quinones Analysis

To identify fatty acid compositions, strain MAHUQ-56^T and reference strains were cultured on an R2A agar medium at 30 °C for 48 h. Extraction, purification, and analysis of cellular fatty acids were performed according to a previous description [18,33]. The respiratory quinones of strain MAHUQ-56^T were extracted, purified, and analyzed by HPLC using the method of Collins [34].

2.7. Biosynthesis of AgNPs Using Arthrobacter bangladeshi sp. nov.

The green synthesis of AgNPs was performed using the culture supernatant of strain MAHUQ-56^T. Briefly, strain MAHUQ-56^T was cultured in 100 mL R2A broth medium for 3 days at 30 °C with 180 rpm. Then, the bacterial culture was spun down at 9000 rpm for 10 min to obtain a cell-free supernatant. We added 1 mM of AgNO$_3$ solution (final concentration) to the 100 mL cell-free culture supernatant and incubated it again in dark shaking condition (180 rpm, 35 °C) for 48–72 h. The reaction mixture was observed continuously for the synthesis of nanoparticles by visual inspection and UV–vis spectral analysis. Synthesized AgNPs were collected by high-speed centrifugation (14,000 rpm for 20 min). Collected AgNPs were washed several times with distilled water and obtained in precipitate form. Precipitated AgNPs were air-dried, and used for characterization and antimicrobial application.

2.8. Characterization of Synthesized AgNPs

The UV–vis spectrum of synthesized AgNPs was analyzed by UV–vis spectrophotometer (Optizen POP, Mecasys, Daejeon, South Korea) in the range of 300–800 nm. To investigate the morphology, composition, and metallic nature of synthesized AgNPs, field emission-transmission electron microscopy (FE-TEM) analysis was conducted, operated with voltage of 200 kV (JEM 2100F, JEOL, Tokyo, Japan). An AgNP sample for TEM was prepared by dissolving in distilled water, and spotting onto carbon-coated TEM grid, followed by air-drying at room temperature. The air-dried AgNP sample was used for X-ray diffraction (XRD) analysis using an X-ray diffractometer (D8 Advance, Bruker, Germany) over a 2θ value in the range of 30°–90°. The hydrodynamic diameters and polydispersity index of green synthesized AgNPs were investigated by dynamic light scattering (DLS, Otsuka Electronics, Osaka, Japan) (Malvern Zetasizer Nano ZS90) according to a previous description [35]. Fourier transform-infrared (FTIR, PerkinElmer Inc., Waltham, MA, USA) analysis was performed by scanning the air-dried purified AgNPs using FTIR spectroscopy over the range of 4000–500 cm^{-1}.

2.9. Antimicrobial Activity of Synthesized AgNPs

The antibacterial properties of green synthesized AgNPs against pathogenic *S. typhimurium* and *Y. enterocolitica* were investigated by the disc diffusion method. In brief, the tested pathogens were grown overnight in Mueller–Hinton (MH) broth. Then, 100 μL culture suspensions of both *S. typhimurium* and *Y. enterocolitica* were spread onto MH agar plates, and 8 mm sterile paper discs were placed on the surface of MH agar plates. Then, 30 and 60 μL (1000 ppm) of green synthesized AgNPs solutions (AgNPs were dissolved in water) were placed onto the paper discs. Plates were incubated at 37 °C for 24 h to observe the inhibition zones. The inhibition zone was calculated in millimeters (mm) after 24 h of incubation. This test was performed three times.

2.10. MIC and MBC Investigation

The bacteriostatic activity of green synthesized AgNPs was determined by measuring minimum inhibitory concentration (MIC) using microdilution assay as follows. Pathogenic strains *S. typhimurium* and *Y. enterocolitica* were grown in MH broth medium at 37 °C overnight; then, the culture was diluted to approximately 1×10^6 CFUs/mL. Then, 100 uL of diluted bacterial culture was added into 96-well ELISA plate, followed by an equal volume of AgNPs solutions (AgNPs were dissolved in MH broth medium) with various concentrations (3.1, 6.2, 12.5, 25, 50, 100, and 200 µg/mL). As a control, only MH broth was used instead of an AgNP solution. Samples were incubated at 37 °C for 24 h. Every 3 h of the interval, bacterial growth was calculated using an ELISA plate reader (LabTech 4000, BMG LABTECH, Ortenberg, Germany) by recording OD_{600}. Minimum bactericidal concentration (MBC) was defined as the lowest concentration of synthesized AgNPs that was required to kill the tested pathogenic strains. For measuring MBC, 10 µL of the above mixtures was streaked on MH agar plates and incubated at 37 °C for 24 h. Lastly, MBC was evaluated by determining the lowest concentration that killed the bacteria [36].

2.11. Investigation of Morphological Changes by FE-SEM

Bacterial strains of *S. typhimurium* and *Y. enterocolitica* (approximately 1×10^7 CFU/mL) were each incubated with and without biosynthesized AgNPs (at MBC concentration) at 37 °C overnight. Upon the end of the incubation period, samples were processed for FE SEM analysis to investigate structural changes according to a previous report [36]. AgNP-treated cells were collected by centrifugation at 8000 rpm for 5 min. Then, cells were washed by PBS (pH 7.0) and fixed by 2.5% glutaraldehyde for 4 h at room temperature. Cells were again washed by PBS and serially dehydrated by various concentrations of ethanol (from 30% to 100%) in 10 min intervals at room temperature. Subsequently, dehydrated cells were dried using a desiccator, and samples were lastly coated with gold for the investigation of structural changes by FE-SEM (S-4700, Hitachi, Tokyo, Japan).

3. Results and Discussion

3.1. Phenotypic, Physiological, and Biochemical Characteristics

Cells of strain MAHUQ-56^T were Gram-positive, aerobic, non-motile, and rod-shaped, 0.6–1.0 µm wide and 1.3–2.5 µm long (Figure 1). Strain MAHUQ-56^T grew on R2A agar, NA, TSA, and LB agar media, but not on MacConkey agar. Colonies were spherical, milky white, and 0.4–0.9 mm in diameter when grown on R2A agar medium for 2 days. The strain showed positive activity for catalase, but negative for oxidase- and flexirubin-type pigments. Cells could hydrolyze starch, L-tyrosine, casein and Tween 20, but were negative for DNA, gelatin, esculin, urea, and Tween 80. Strain MAHUQ-56^T was positive for the assimilation of glucose, mannose, arabinose, maltose, gluconate, N-acetyl-glucosamine, malate, citrate, mannitol, adipate, and phenyl-acetate (API 20NE). Based on the API ZYM kit, strain MAHUQ-56^T was positive for valine arylamidase, esterase, acid phosphatase, esterase lipase (C8), trypsin, alkaline phosphatase, leucine arylamidase, cystine arylamidase, β-glucosidase, naphthol-AS-BI-phosphohydrolase, β-galactosidase, α-glucosidase, α-mannosidase, α-galactosidase, α-chymotrypsin, α-fucosidase, β-glucuronidase and lipase (C14). Strain MAHUQ-56^T showed many different phenotypic characteristics from its close relatives, including different growth conditions, and enzymatic and assimilation activities (Table 1). Strain MAHUQ-56 was deposited into KACC (KACC 22003^T) and CGMCC (CGMCC 1.18517^T).

3.2. 16S rRNA Gene Sequence and Phylogenetic Analysis

The 16S rRNA gene sequence (1451 bp, GenBank accession number, MT514504) similarities showed that strain MAHUQ-56^T was most closely related to *Arthrobacter pokkalii* P3B162^T (98.6%), *Pseudarthrobacter defluvii* 4C1-a^T (98.5%), *Pseudarthrobacter niigatensis* LC4^T (98.2%), *Pseudarthrobacter phenanthrenivorans* Sphe3^T (98.2%), and *Pseudarthrobacter enclensis* NIO-1008^T (98.0%). Phylogenetic analysis based on 16S rRNA gene sequences using neighbor-joining (NJ) (Figure 2) and maximum-likelihood (ML) (Supplementary Figure S1) phylogenetic trees revealed that strain MAHUQ-56^T clustered within the *Arthrobacter* genus and formed a monophyletic clade to *Arthrobacter pokkalii*. From 16s rRNA gene sequence and phylogenetic analysis, it is clear that strain MAHUQ-56^T is a new member of the *Arthrobacter* genus.

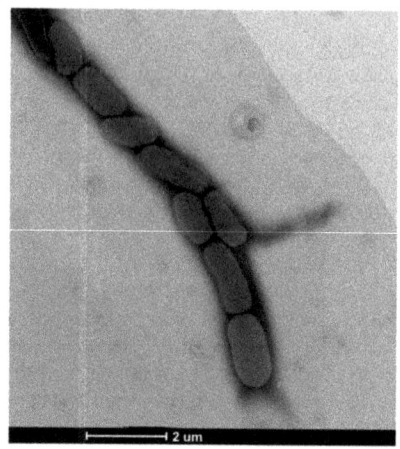

Figure 1. Transmission electron micrograph of cells of *Arthrobacter bangladeshi* MAHUQ-56[T] after negative staining with uranyl acetate; Bar, 2.0 μm.

Table 1. Differential characteristics of *Arthrobacter bangladeshi* MAHUQ-56[T] and phylogenetically closely related species.

Characteristics	1	2	3	4	5	6
Isolation source	Soil of rice field	Pokkali rice	Sewage	Filtration substrate from trass	Creosote-contaminated soil	Marine sediments
Cell morphology	Rod	Rod	Rod–coccus	Rod–coccus	Rod–coccus	Rod–coccus
Colony color	Milky white	Yellow	Creamy white	Light yellow	Cream to yellow	Cream to light grey
Growth temperature (°C)	10–40	18–37 [a]	5–37 [b]	5–40 [c]	4–37 [d]	10–45 [e]
Growth pH	5.0–10.0	5.5–8.0 [a]	6.0–10.0 [b]	6.0–11.0 [c]	6.5–8.5 [d]	5.0–9.0 [e]
Hydrolysis of:						
Gelatin (API 20 NE)	-	-	-	+	-	-
Urea (API 20 NE)	-	-	-	W	-	-
Enzyme activity (API ZYM):						
Esterase (C4)	+	+	W	+	W	+
Alkaline phosphatase	+	+	-	+	W	+
Esterase lipase (C8)	W	+	-	+	W	+
Acid phosphatase	+	-	+	+	W	-
Valine arylamidase	W	+	-	W	W	+
Trypsin	+	+	-	+	W	-
β-glucuronidase	+	+	+	+	+	-
α-glucosidase	+	+	+	+	W	-
β-galactosidase	+	+	+	+	W	-
α-fucosidase	+	+	+	-	-	-
Assimilation of (API 20 NE):						
D-glucose	+	-	+	+	-	+
D-maltose	+	+	+	-	-	+
D-mannose	+	-	+	-	-	+
D-mannitol	+	+	+	-	W	-
Malic acid	+	+	+	W	W	+
DNA G + C content (mol%)	66.0	64.0 [a]	64.4 [b]	70.8 [c]	65.7 [d]	61.3 [e]

Strains: 1, *A. bangladeshi* MAHUQ-56[T]; 2, *A. pokkalii* KCTC 29498[T]; 3, *P. defluvii* KCTC 19209[T]; 4, *P. niigatensis* CCTCC AB 206012[T]; 5, *P. phenanthrenivorans* DSM 18606[T] and 6, *P. enclensis* DSM 25279[T]. All data were obtained in this study, except [a–d] and [e], which were taken from Krishnan et al. [4], Kim et al. [5], Ding et al. [6], Kallimanis et al. [7], and Dastager et al. [8], respectively. All strains were aerobic and nonmotile. All strains were positive for catalase, reduction of nitrate, leucine arylamidase and naphthol-AS-BI-phosphohydrolase. All strains were negative for oxidase. +, positive; W, weakly positive; -, negative.

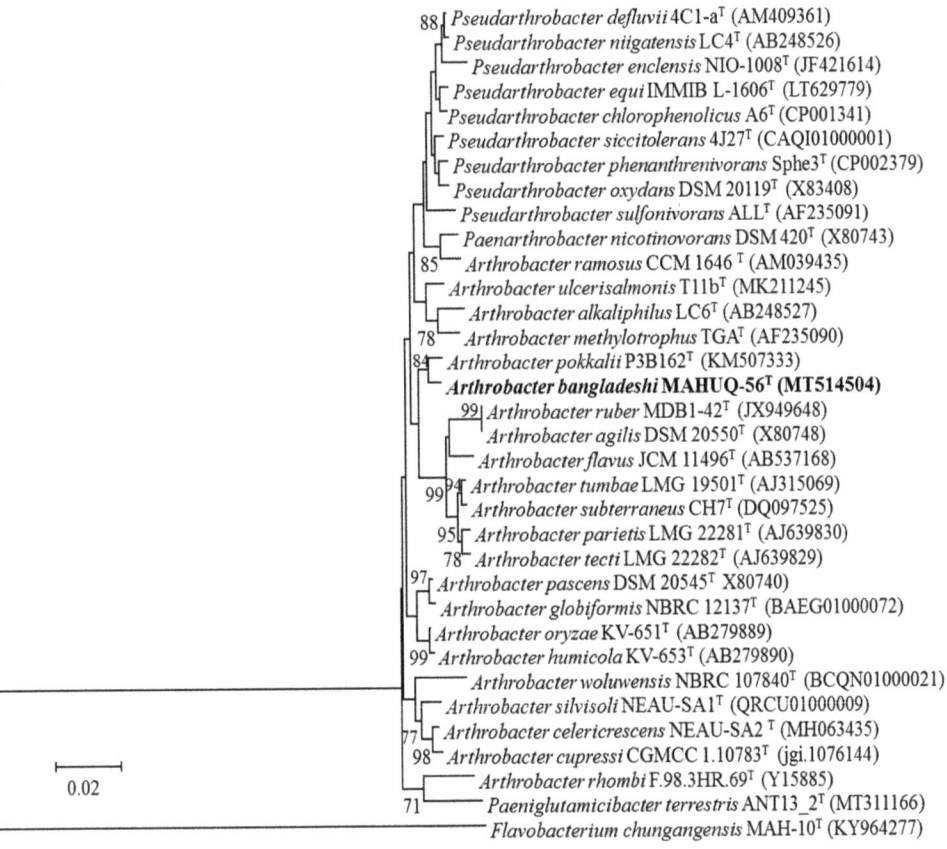

Figure 2. Neighbor-joining (NJ) tree based on 16S rRNA gene sequence analysis showing phylogenetic relationships of strain MAHUQ-56 and the related type strains. Bootstrap values more than 70% based on 1000 replications shown at branching points. Scale bar, 0.02 substitutions per nucleotide position.

3.3. Draft Genome and DNA G + C Content Analysis

The draft genome of strain MAHUQ-56^T contains 26 contigs with an N50 size of 360,503 bp. Total genome size was 4,566,112 bp, with an average G + C content of 66.0 mol%. Gene annotation by PGAP revealed 4125 protein-encoding genes, 51 tRNA genes, and 6 rRNA genes (NCBI accession number, JAIFZQ000000000). The common features of the genome sequence of strain MAHUQ-56^T are shown in Table 2. Characterization of novel species is increasingly dependent on genomic sequence [37]. Functional annotation by the RAST server showed that 172 genes were involved with the metabolism of proteins, 83 genes were associated with the metabolism of nucleosides and nucleotides, 343 genes were linked with amino acids and derivatives, and 408 genes were involved with carbohydrate metabolism (Figure 3). The closest type strain, *Arthrobacter pokkalii* GZK-1 contains a 4,415,912 bp long genome with 65.9 mol% GC, 4091 protein-encoding genes, 15 rRNA genes, and 51 tRNA genes (https://www.ezbiocloud.net/genome/explore?puid=230640 (accessed on 28 August 2021)). Genomic ANI values between strain MAHUQ-56^T and close type strains *A. pokkalii* GZK-1^T, *P. phenanthrenivorans* Sphe3^T and *P. enclensis* NIO-1008^T were 84.0%, 81.5%, and 82.0%, respectively (Supplementary Table S1), which were well below ($\geq$95–96%) suggesting a novel species. The dDDH values based on the draft genomes between strain MAHUQ-56^T and close relatives *A. pokkalii* GZK-1^T, *P. phenanthrenivorans* Sphe3^T and *P. enclensis* NIO-1008^T were 27.5%, 24.5%, and 24.8%, respectively (Supplementary Table S1), which were also far below the threshold value (70%) for species delineation.

Table 2. Genome sequence features of *Arthrobacter bangladeshi* MAHUQ-56^T.

Features	Strain MAHUQ-56^T
Accession no.	JAIFZQ000000000
Biosample	SAMN20721218
BioProject	PRJNA754020
Total sequence length (nt)	4,566,112
Scaffold N50	360,503
Scaffold N75	196,969
Number of scaffold	26
Sequencing method	de novo (illumina XTen)
Annotation pipeline	NCBI Prokaryotic Genome
DNA G + C content (mol%)	66.0
Total genes	4233
Genes (coding)	4125
Number of RNAs	60
tRNAs	51
rRNAs	6

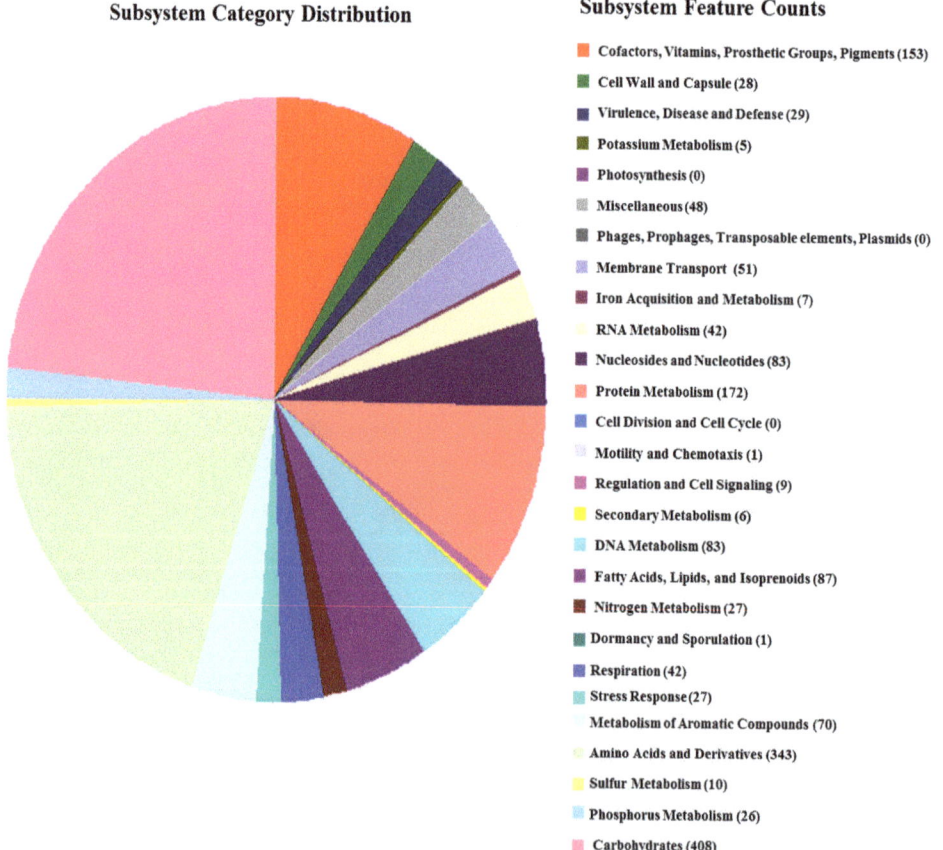

Figure 3. COG functional genes of *Arthrobacter bangladeshi* MAHUQ-56^T.

3.4. Cellular Fatty Acid and Respiratory Quinones Analysis

The predominant fatty acids of strain MAHUQ-56^T were $C_{15:0\ anteiso}$ (47.8%), $C_{15:0\ iso}$ (11.9%), $C_{16:0\ iso}$ (15.8%), and $C_{17:0\ anteiso}$ (11.7%). Overall fatty acid composition was similar to those of close type strains. However, there were some clear quantitative and qualitative differences in the fatty acid profiles (Table 3). The major respiratory quinone of strain MAHUQ-56^T was MK-9(H2). Closest type strain *Arthrobacter pokkalii* P3B162^T also showed the same major respiratory quinone [4].

Table 3. Cellular fatty acid composition of *Arthrobacter bangladeshi* MAHUQ-56^T and phylogenetically closely related species.

Fatty Acid	1	2	3	4	5	6
$C_{14:0}$	2.3	1.4	1.5	1.3	1.6	2.0
$C_{14:0\ iso}$	3.5	1.6	3.4	1.5	ND	2.2
$C_{15:0\ iso}$	11.9	8.1	13.8	7.8	15.1	14.5
$C_{15:0\ anteiso}$	47.8	54.5	55.6	52.0	37.7	48.3
$C_{16:1}\ w7c$	ND	ND	ND	ND	2.6	ND
$C_{16:0\ iso}$	15.8	8.5	11.9	12.2	16.0	11.2
$C_{16:0}$	3.8	7.2	4.0	6.0	7.9	6.2
$C_{17:0\ iso}$	1.6	1.5	1.1	2.0	4.2	2.0
$C_{17:0\ anteiso}$	11.7	13.8	5.9	13.9	13.1	11.3

Strains: 1, *A. bangladeshi* MAHUQ-56^T; 2, *A. pokkalii* KCTC 29498^T; 3, *P. defluvii* KCTC 19209^T; 4, *P. niigatensis* CCTCC AB 206012^T; 5, *P. phenanthrenivorans* DSM 18606^T and 6, *P. enclensis* DSM 25279^T. All data were collected from this study. Tr, trace (less than 1.0%); ND, not detected.

3.5. Taxonomic Conclusions

Phenotypic, chemotaxonomic, and biochemical characteristics, and phylogenetic inference and genomic features support that strain MAHUQ-56^T represents a novel species of the *Arthrobacter* genus, for which the name *Arthrobacter bangladeshi* sp. nov. is proposed.

3.6. Description of Arthrobacter bangladeshi sp. nov.

Arthrobacter bangladeshi (bangla.desh'i. N.L. gen. n. *bangladeshi* pertaining to Bangladesh, where the rice field is located and the type strain was isolated).

Cells are Gram-stain-positive, aerobic, non-motile, and rod-shaped, 0.6–1.0 μm wide and 1.3–2.5 μm long. Strain MAHUQ-56^T grew on R2A agar, NA, TSA, and LB agar media, but not on MacConkey agar. Colonies were spherical, milky white, and 0.4–0.9 mm in diameter when grown on R2A agar medium for 2 days. Growth occurs at 10–40 °C (optimum, 30 °C), at pH 5.0–10.0 (optimum, pH 7.0) and with 0–2% NaCl (optimum, 0%). Positive for catalase activity and the hydrolysis of starch, L-tyrosine, casein and Tween 20. Negative for oxidase, flexirubin-type pigments production, glucose fermentation, and the hydrolysis of DNA, gelatin, esculin, urea, and Tween 80. Nitrate is reduced to nitrite. Strain MAHUQ-56^T was positive for the assimilation of glucose, mannose, arabinose, maltose, gluconate, N-acetyl-glucosamine, malate, citrate, mannitol, adipate and phenyl-acetate, but negative for the assimilation of caprate (API 20NE). In API ZYM tests, valine arylamidase, C4 esterase, acid phosphatase, esterase lipase (C8), trypsin, alkaline phosphatase, leucine arylamidase, cystine arylamidase, β-glucosidase, naphthol-AS-BI-phosphohydrolase, β-galactosidase, α-glucosidase, α-mannosidase, α-galactosidase, α-chymotrypsin, α-fucosidase, β-glucuronidase and lipase (C14) activities were present, but N-acetyl-β-glucosaminidase activities were absent. Major fatty acids were $C_{15:0\ anteiso}$, $C_{15:0\ iso}$, $C_{16:0\ iso}$ and $C_{17:0\ anteiso}$. The predominant respiratory quinone was MK-9(H2). The DNA G + C content of the type strain MAHUQ-56^T was 66.0 mol%.

Type strain was MAHUQ-56^T (=KACC 22003^T = CGMCC 1.18517^T), isolated from soil sample of a rice field, Magura, Bangladesh.

3.7. Green Synthesis of AgNPs Using Arthrobacter bangladeshi sp. nov.

The culture supernatant of *Arthrobacter bangladeshi* MAHUQ-56^T was supplemented with 1 mM AgNO$_3$ for the green synthesis of AgNPs. The synthesis of AgNPs by strain MAHUQ-56^T was initially confirmed by visual observation. The color of the reaction mixture changed into deep brown from pale yellow within 72 h of incubation (Figure 4B). The change in color is attributed to the surface plasmon resonance of AgNPs, and indicated the formation of AgNPs [38,39]. There was no color change in the control (Figure 4A). Intracellular and extracellular methods are available for the bacteria-mediated synthesis of AgNPs. The extracellular method is easier and more rapid compared to the intracellular method, which needs complex purification steps [40]. In the current study, a facile and convenient extracellular process was used for the biosynthesis of AgNPs using *Arthrobacter bangladeshi* MAHUQ-56^T.

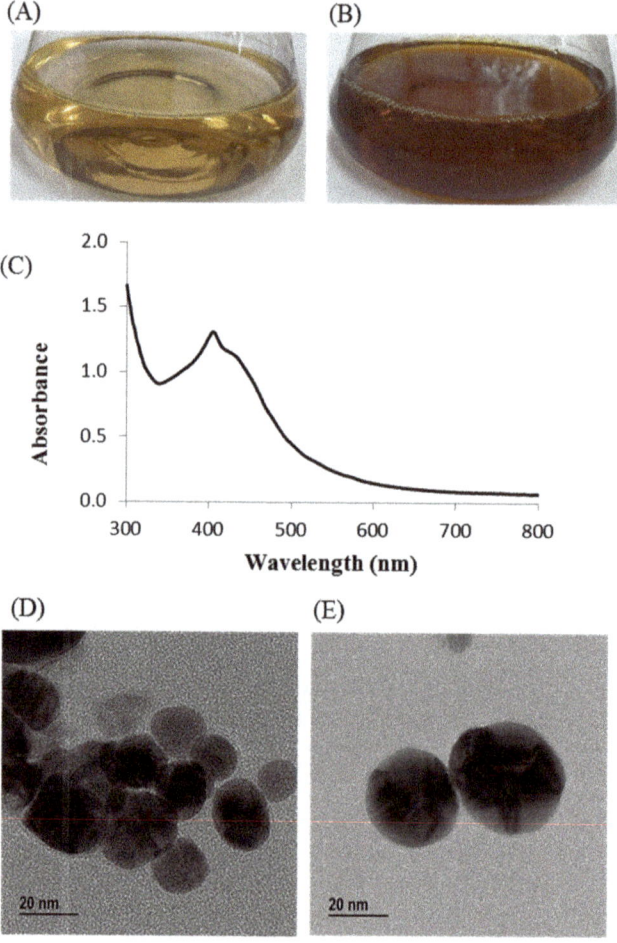

Figure 4. (**A**) R2A broth with AgNO$_3$ as control, (**B**) biosynthesized AgNPs, (**C**) UV–vis spectra, and (**D,E**) FE-TEM images of synthesized AgNPs.

3.8. Characterization of Green Synthesized AgNPs

The biosynthesis of AgNPs was further confirmed by UV–visible spectral analysis in the range of 300–800 nm. A strong peak appeared at 405 nm (Figure 4C), which ensured the synthesis of AgNPs [41]. Our results agree with those of Du et al., who reported that AgNPs synthesized by *Novosphingobium* sp. THG-C3 showed an SPR band at 406 nm [35]. The standard SPR peak of biosynthesized Ag-NPs generally shows within 400 to 450 nm [42]. The morphology of synthesized AgNPs was investigated by FE-TEM, which revealed a spherical shape. The size of *Arthrobacter bangladeshi* MAHUQ-56^T-mediated synthesized AgNPs was determined to the range of 12 to 50 nm (Figure 4D,E). Singh et al. reported a similar particle size (10–40 nm) of AgNPs that was synthesized by *Cedecea* sp. [43]. The elemental composition and purity of synthesized AgNPs was examined by EDX, as shown in Figure 5. The EDX spectrum revealed a strong peak for silver at 3 keV, which ensures the synthesis of metallic AgNPs [44]. Some extra peaks were also found in the EDX spectrum due to the use of copper grids (Figure 5A). Elemental mapping results showed the highest distribution of silver elements in the sample (Figure 5B,C, Table 4). To investigate the phase of AgNPs, selected area electron diffraction (SAED) analysis was performed (Figure 5D). SAED analysis showed a sharp rings corresponding to the following reflections at 111, 200, 220, and 311 of lattice planes (Figure 5D), which indicated the crystalline nature of biosynthesized AgNPs. X-ray diffraction (XRD) analysis was conducted to determine the crystalline property of synthesized AgNPs. The XRD pattern showed four distinct peaks at 2θ values of 38.21°, 46.42°, 64.69°, and 77.41° corresponding to the intensities of 111, 200, 220, and 311 for the reflections of metallic silver (Figure 5E). Some recently reported studies showed similar XRD patterns of AgNPs synthesized by microorganisms [35,45].

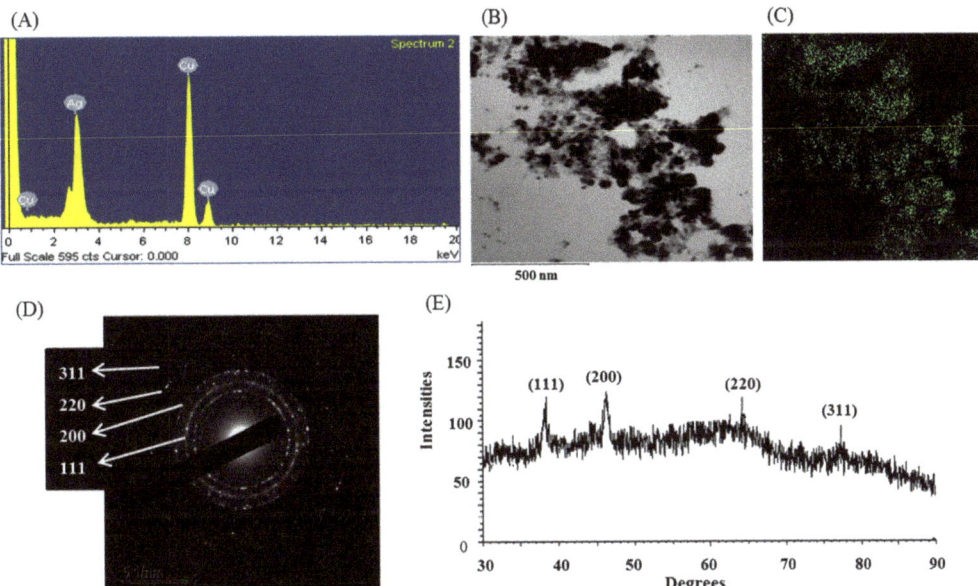

Figure 5. (**A**) EDX spectrum of synthesized AgNPs, (**B**) TEM image used for mapping, (**C**) distribution of silver in elemental mapping, (**D**) SAED pattern, and (**E**) X-ray diffraction pattern of biosynthesized AgNPs.

Table 4. Number and percentage of chemical elements present in EDX spectrum of *Arthrobacter bangladeshi* MAHUQ-56^T-mediated synthesized AgNPs.

Element	Weight %	Atomic %
Cu K	50.66	63.54
Ag L	49.34	36.46
Totals	100.00	100.00

The size and polydispersity value of the synthesized AgNPs was investigated by DLS. The average hydrodynamic diameter was 122.5 nm, with a polydispersity index of 0.286 (Supplementary Figure S2). The possible role of biomolecules presence in bacterial culture supernatant for the synthesis and stabilization of AgNPs was identified by Fourier transform infrared (FT-IR) analysis. The FTIR spectrum revealed major intense absorbance peaks at 3438.60, 2921.32, 2848.50, 2352.20, 2330.50, and 1645.20 cm^{-1} (Figure 6). The vibration peak at 3438.60 cm^{-1} may have been due to the presence of an O–H (alcohol) and/or N–H (amine) group with synthesized AgNPs. The bands at 2921.32 and 2848.50 cm^{-1} were due to the stretching vibration of C-H (alkane) group. Absorbance peaks at 2352.20 and 2330.50 cm^{-1} could have been the presence of O=C=O (carbonyl bond group). The band located at 1645.20 cm^{-1} may have been due to the presence of a C=O (ester) or –C=C bond. FT-IR data identified the presence of biomolecules, which may have been responsible for the synthesis and stabilization of AgNPs. Some previous studies showed a similar FT-IR spectrum of AgNPs synthesized using microorganisms [43,46]. Supplementary Table S2 shows the physicochemical properties of AgNPs synthesized by *Arthrobacter bangladeshi* and some other bacterial strains.

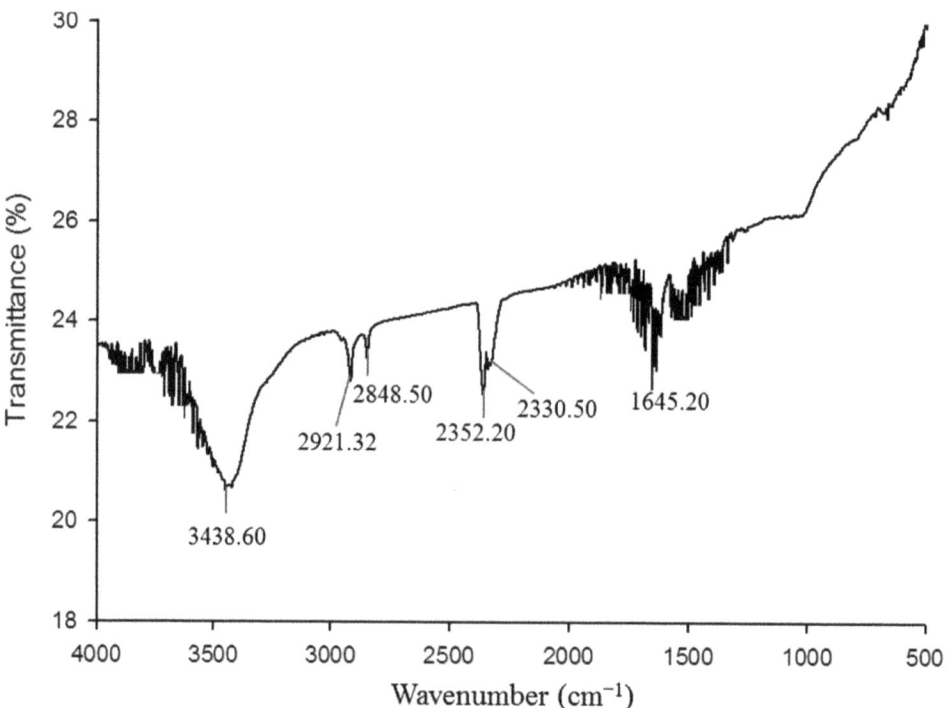

Figure 6. FT-IR spectra of *Arthrobacter bangladeshi* MAHUQ-56^T-mediated synthesized AgNPs.

3.9. Antimicrobial Activity of Synthesized AgNPs

In the present study, the antibacterial activity of *Arthrobacter bangladeshi* MAHUQ-56^T-mediated synthesized AgNPs was investigated against multidrug-resistant pathogenic *S. typhimurium* and *Y. enterocolitica*. Synthesized AgNPs exhibited strong antibacterial activity against both tested pathogens *S. typhimurium* and *Y. enterocolitica*. The potential antibacterial activity of synthesized AgNPs against pathogenic microorganisms was confirmed by the formation of an inhibition zone (Figure 7). Figure 7 reveals a clear zone of inhibition (ZOI) around the paper discs treated by synthesized AgNPs. The diameters of the ZOI of biosynthesized AgNPs *against S. typhimurium* and *Y. enterocolitica* were 18.3 ± 0.6 and 20.4 ± 0.8 mm, respectively, and are shown in Table 5. The biosynthesized AgNPs showed the highest activity against multidrug-resistant *Y. enterocolitica*, followed by *S. typhimurium*. These results suggest that *Arthrobacter bangladeshi* MAHUQ-56^T-mediated synthesized AgNPs could be useful as an antibacterial agent to control multidrug-resistant *S. typhimurium* and *Y. enterocolitica*. These findings were consistent with those of previous studies [35,45].

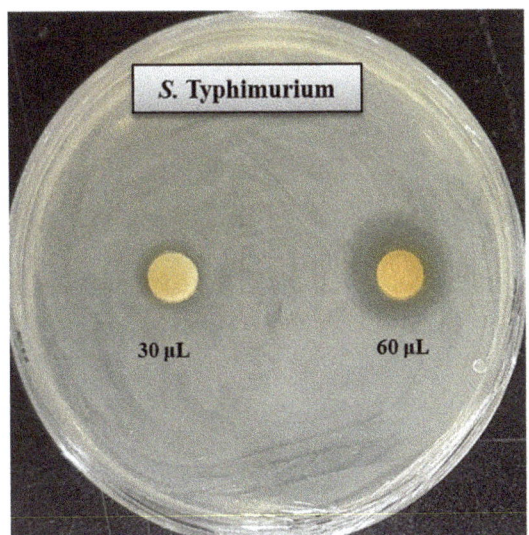 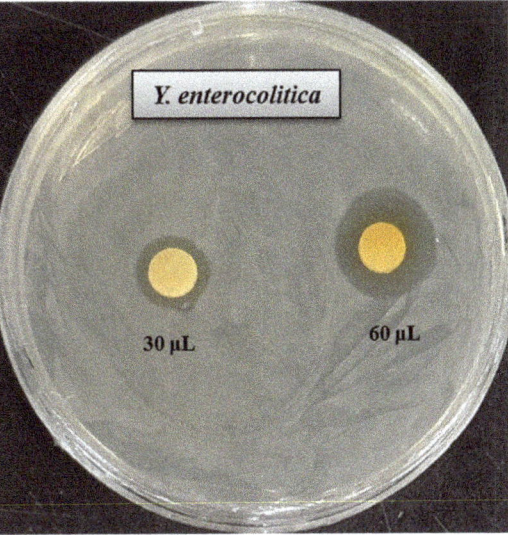

Figure 7. Zones of inhibition of 30 and 60 µL of biosynthesized AgNPs at 1000 ppm concentrations in water against *S. typhimurium* and *Y. enterocolitica*.

Table 5. Antibacterial efficacy of *Arthrobacter bangladeshi* MAHUQ-56^T-mediated synthesized AgNPs against *S. typhimurium* and *Y. enterocolitica*.

Pathogenic Species	Zone of Inhibition (mm)	
	AgNPs (30 µL)	AgNPs (60 µL)
Salmonella Typhimurium (ATCC 14028)	11.5 ± 0.5	18.3 ± 0.6
Yersinia enterocolitica (ATCC 9610)	13.5 ± 0.7	20.4 ± 0.8

3.10. MIC and MBC Investigation

The MIC was defined as the lowest concentration of AgNPs that fully inhibited the growth of bacteria. The MIC was determined by a microdilution assay using 96-well plates. The MICs of *Arthrobacter bangladeshi* MAHUQ-56^T-mediated synthesized AgNPs for *S. typhimurium* and *Y. enterocolitica* were 6.2 and 3.1 ug/mL, respectively (Figure 8, Table 6). These MIC values were significantly lower than those of some other antibacterial agents, including biosynthesized nanoparticles against both *S. typhimurium* and *Y. enterocolitica*. Several studies reported that the MIC values of olive-oil polyphenol extract and Licochalcone A against *S. typhimurium* were 625 and 62.5–1000 ug/mL, respectively [47,48]. Similarly, the MIC values of chitosan nanoparticles and *Parrotia persica* leaf extract against *Y. enterocolitica* were 1500 and 750 ug/mL, respectively [49,50]. MBC is the lowest concentration of antimicrobial agents that fully kills the tested pathogens. The MBC of *Arthrobacter bangladeshi* MAHUQ-56^T-mediated synthesized AgNPs for both *S. typhimurium* and *Y. enterocolitica* was 12.5 ug/mL (Figure 9, Table 6). This MBC value was also significantly lower than that of some other antibacterial agents against both *S. typhimurium* and *Y. enterocolitica* [47–50].

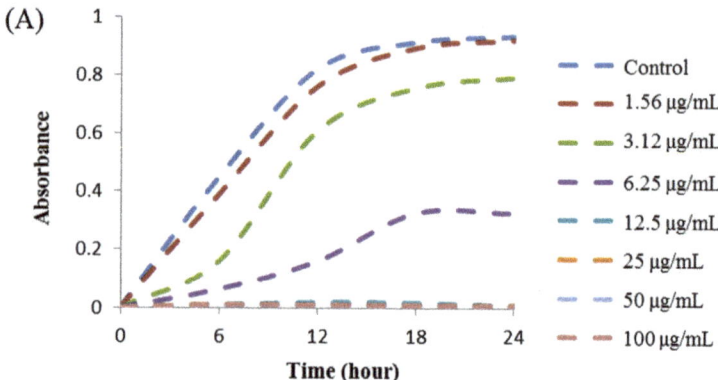

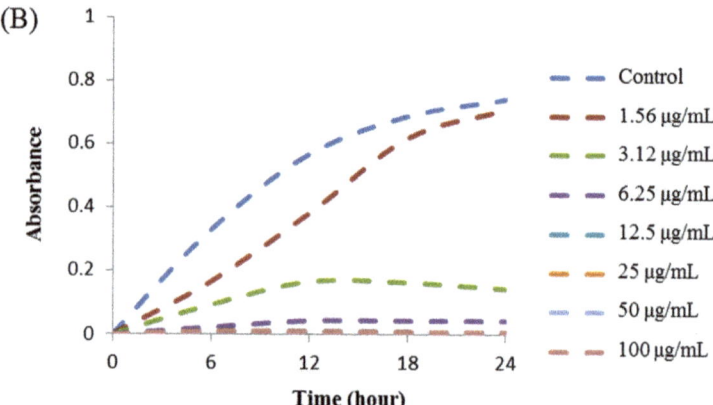

Figure 8. Growth curves of (**A**) *S. typhimurium* and (**B**) *Y. enterocolitica* cultured in MHB with different concentrations of biosynthesized AgNPs to determine MIC.

Table 6. Minimum inhibitory concentration (MIC) and minimum bactericidal concentration (MBC) of biosynthesized AgNPs against *S. typhimurium* and *Yersinia enterocolitica*.

Pathogenic Species	MIC (µg/mL)	MBC (µg/mL)
Salmonella Typhimurium (ATCC 14028)	6.2	12.5
Yersinia enterocolitica (ATCC 9610)	3.1	12.5

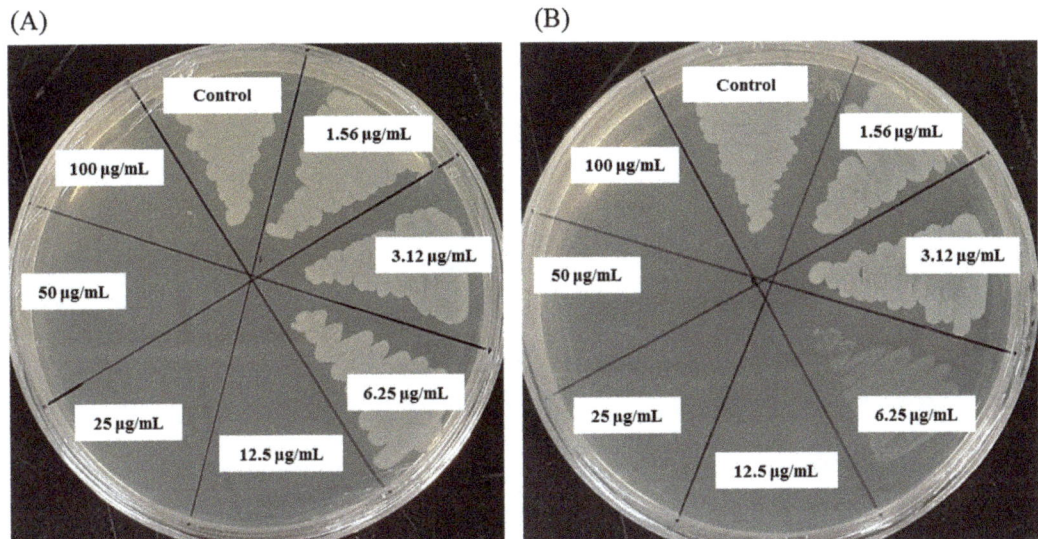

Figure 9. MBC of biosynthesized AgNPs against (**A**) *S. typhimurium* and (**B**) *Y. enterocolitica*.

3.11. Investigation of Morphological Changes by FE-SEM

Morphological changes in AgNP-treated *S. typhimurium* and *Y. enterocolitica* cells were observed by FE-SEM. FE-SEM images showed the nature and degree of the structural alteration of both tested pathogens (Figure 10). Untreated *S. typhimurium* cells displayed normal morphology and structure without any damage to the cell surface (Figure 10A). However, *S. typhimurium* cells treated with *Arthrobacter bangladeshi* MAHUQ-56^T-mediated synthesized AgNPs displayed structural changes with abnormal, wrinkled, damaged, and collapsed cell surface and membrane (Figure 10B). Similar results were found for *Y. enterocolitica*. Untreated *Y. enterocolitica* cells exhibited normal rod-shaped structure without any damage to the cell surface (Figure 10C). However, AgNP-treated *Y. enterocolitica* cells exhibited structural changes with abnormal, damaged, and collapsed cell walls and membrane (Figure 10D). The morphological and structural alterations, and damage indicated that the *Arthrobacter bangladeshi* MAHUQ-56^T-mediated synthesized AgNPs might disturb the normal cellular functions of multidrug-resistant *S. typhimurium* and *Y. enterocolitica*, ultimately leading to the death of cells [44,51].

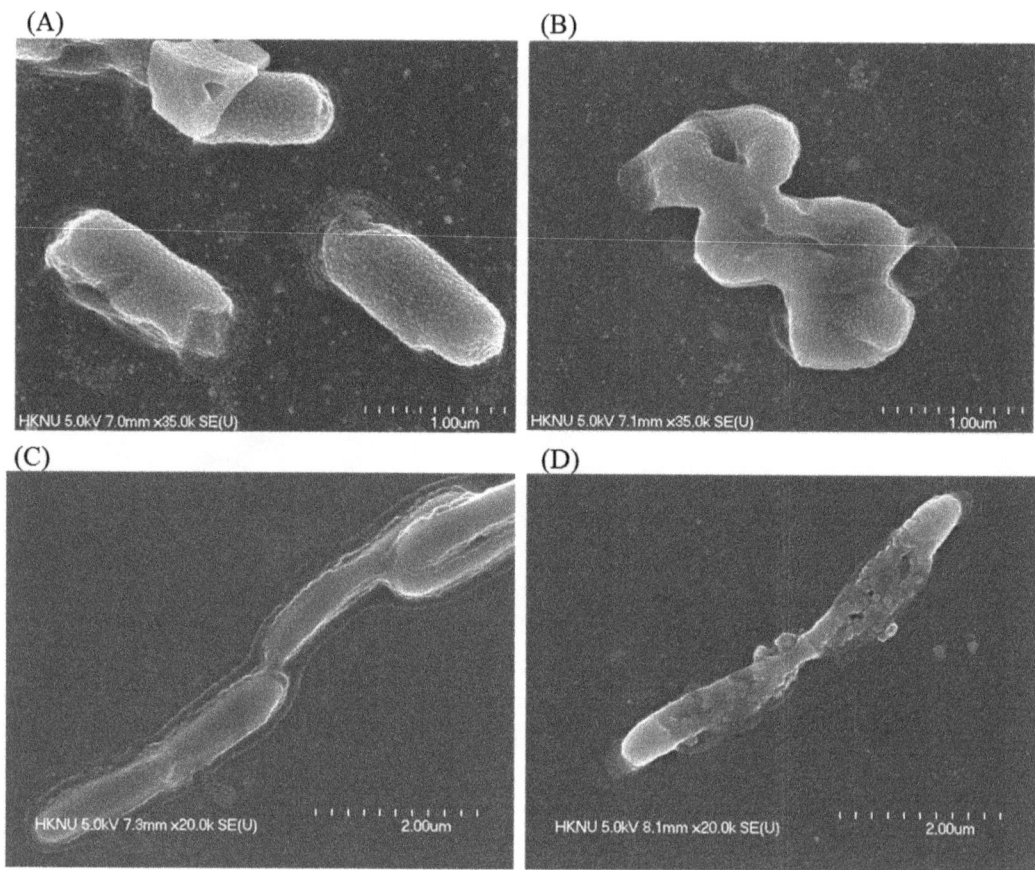

Figure 10. SEM images of (**A**) normal *S. typhimurium* cells, (**B**) 1 × MBC AgNPs treated *S. typhimurium* cells, (**C**) normal *Y. enterocolitica* cells, (**D**) 1 × MBC AgNPs treated *Y. enterocolitica* cells.

4. Conclusions

The present study described the isolation and characterization of novel bacterial species *Arthrobacter bangladeshi* sp. nov., used for the easy and ecofriendly extracellular synthesis of AgNPs, and investigated its antibacterial efficacy against drug-resistant pathogenic *S. typhimurium* and *Y. enterocolitica*. A facile and convenient extracellular process was used for the biosynthesis of AgNPs using *Arthrobacter bangladeshi* MAHUQ-56[T]. Synthesized AgNPs were characterized by UV-Vis spectroscopy, FE-TEM, XRD, DLS, and FT-IR. Synthesized AgNPs were spherical with a size range of 12–50 nm. FT-IR analysis revealed various biomolecules that may be involved in the synthesis and capping of AgNPs. Biosynthesized AgNPs showed strong antibacterial activity against multidrug-resistant pathogenic *S. typhimurium* and *Y. enterocolitica*. AgNPs showed a ZOI of 18.3 ± 0.6 and 20.4 ± 0.8 mm against *S. typhimurium* and *Y. enterocolitica*, respectively. MIC values of synthesized AgNPs against *S. typhimurium* and *Y. enterocolitica* were 6.2 and 3.1 ug/mL, respectively. The MBC of synthesized AgNPs for both pathogens was 12.5 ug/mL. FE-SEM analysis revealed the morphological and structural alterations, and damage of *S. typhimurium* and *Y. enterocolitica* cells treated by synthesized AgNPs. These changes might disturb the normal cellular functions of multidrug-resistant *S. typhimurium* and *Y. enterocolitica*, ultimately leading to the death of cells. Results of the present study suggest that novel bacterial species *Arthrobacter bangladeshi* MAHUQ-56[T] could be used for the rapid and mass production of AgNPs, and the synthesized AgNPs could be used as an alternative antibacterial agent to treat multidrug-resistant *S. typhimurium* and *Y. enterocolitica*.

Supplementary Materials: The following are available online at https://www.mdpi.com/article/10.3390/pharmaceutics13101691/s1, Figure S1: The maximum-likelihood (ML) tree based on 16S rRNA gene sequence analysis showing phylogenetic relationships of strain MAHUQ-56T and the related type strains. Values less than 50 % were not shown. Scale bar, 0.05 substitutions per nucleotide position, Figure S2: Particles size distribution of biosynthesized AgNPs according to intensity (A), number (B) and volume (C), Table S1: dDDH and ANI values between proposed novel strain MAHUQ-56T and the closest type strains, Table S2: The physicochemical properties of AgNPs synthesized by *Arthrobacter bangladeshi* and some other bacterial strains.

Author Contributions: M.A.H. conceived the original screening and research plans, and wrote the article. M.A.H. and S.A. performed all experiments. All authors have read and agreed to the published version of the manuscript.

Funding: This study was performed with the support of the National Research Foundation (NRF) of Korea grant (project no. NRF-2018R1C1B5041386, grant recipient: Md. Amdadul Huq) funded by Korean government, Republic of Korea.

Institutional Review Board Statement: Not applicable.

Informed Consent Statement: Not applicable.

Data Availability Statement: Not applicable.

Acknowledgments: Special thanks to the GM 10K project for analyzing the draft genomic sequence of strain MAHUQ-56[T] (GCM60020060).

Conflicts of Interest: The authors declare that they have no conflict of interest.

References

1. Conn, H.J.; Dimmick, I. Soil bacteria similar in morphology to *Mycobacterium* and *Corynebacterium*. *J. Bacteriol.* **1947**, *54*, 291–303. [CrossRef]
2. Chen, Y.G.; Tang, S.K.; Zhang, Y.Q.; Li, Z.Y.; Yi, L.B.; Wang, Y.X.; Li, W.J.; Cui, X.L. *Arthrobacter halodurans* sp. nov., a new halotolerant bacterium isolated from sea water. *Antonie Van Leeuwenhoek* **2009**, *96*, 63–70. [CrossRef]
3. Yan, R.; Liu, D.; Fu, Y.; Zhang, Y.; Ju, H.; Zhao, J.; Wang, X.; Zhang, J.; Xiang, W. *Arthrobacter celericrescens* sp. nov., isolated from forest soil. *Int. J. Syst. Evol. Microbiol.* **2019**, *69*, 3093–3099. [CrossRef]
4. Krishnan, R.; Menon, R.R.; Tanaka, N.; Busse, H.J.; Krishnamurthi, S.; Rameshkumar, N. *Arthrobacter pokkalii* sp nov, a Novel Plant Associated *Actinobacterium* with Plant Beneficial Properties, Isolated from Saline Tolerant Pokkali Rice, Kerala, India. *PLoS ONE* **2016**, *11*, e0150322. [CrossRef]
5. Kim, K.K.; Lee, K.C.; Oh, H.M.; Kim, M.J.; Eom, M.K.; Lee, J.S. *Arthrobacter defluvii* sp. nov., 4-chlorophenoldegrading bacteria isolated from sewage. *Int. J. Syst. Evol. Microbiol.* **2008**, *58*, 1916–1921. [CrossRef] [PubMed]
6. Ding, L.; Hirose, T.; Yokota, A. Four novel *Arthrobacter* species isolated from filtration substrate. *Int. J. Syst. Evol. Microbiol.* **2009**, *59*, 856–862. [CrossRef] [PubMed]
7. Kallimanis, A.; Kavakiotis, K.; Perisynakis, A.; Spröer, C.; Drainas, C.; Koukkou, A.I. *Arthrobacter phenanthrenivorans* sp. nov., to accommodate the phenanthrene-degrading bacterium *Arthrobacter* sp. strain Sphe3. *Int. J. Syst. Evol. Microbiol.* **2009**, *59*, 275–279. [CrossRef] [PubMed]
8. Dastager, S.G.; Qin, L.; Tang, S.K.; Krishnamurthi, S.; Lee, J.C.; Li, W.J. *Arthrobacter enclensis* sp. nov., isolated from sediment sample. *Arch. Microbiol.* **2014**, *196*, 775–782. [CrossRef] [PubMed]
9. Burdusel, A.C.; Gherasim, O.; Grumezescu, A.M.; Mogoanta, L.; Ficai, A.; Andronescu, E. Biomedical applications of silver nanoparticles: An up-to-date overview. *Nanomaterials* **2018**, *8*, 681. [CrossRef] [PubMed]
10. Rai, M.; Yadav, A.; Gade, A. Silver nanoparticles as a new generation of antimicrobials. *Biotechnol. Adv.* **2009**, *27*, 76–83. [CrossRef]
11. Akter, S.; Huq, M.A. Biologically rapid synthesis of silver nanoparticles by *Sphingobium* sp. MAH-11[T] and their antibacterial activity and mechanisms investigation against drug-resistant pathogenic microbes. *Artif. Cells Nanomed. Biotechnol.* **2020**, *48*, 672–682. [CrossRef]
12. Iravani, S.; Korbekandi, H.; Mirmohammadi, S.V.; Zolfaghari, B. Synthesis of silver nanoparticles: Chemical, physical and biological methods. *Res. Pharm. Sci.* **2014**, *9*, 385.
13. Thakkar, K.N.; Mhatre, S.S.; Parikh, R.Y. Biological synthesis of metallic nanoparticles. *Nanome. Nanotechnol. Biol. Med.* **2010**, *6*, 257–262. [CrossRef]
14. Binupriya, A.; Sathishkumar, M.; Yun, S.-I. Biocrystallization of silver and gold ions by inactive cell filtrate of *Rhizopus stolonifer*. *Colloids Surf. B Biointerfaces* **2010**, *79*, 531–534. [CrossRef]

15. Narayanan, K.B.; Sakthivel, N. Biological synthesis of metal nanoparticles by microbes. *Adv. Colloids Interface Sci.* **2010**, *156*, 1–13. [CrossRef] [PubMed]
16. Li, X.; Xu, H.; Chen, Z.-S.; Chen, G. Biosynthesis of nanoparticles by microorganisms and their applications. *J. Nanomater.* **2011**, *8*, 1–16. [CrossRef]
17. Roy, A.; Bulut, O.; Some, S.; Mandal, A.K.; Yilmaz, M.D. Green synthesis of silver nanoparticles: Biomolecule-nanoparticle organizations targeting antimicrobial activity. *RSC Adv.* **2019**, *9*, 2673–2702. [CrossRef]
18. Huq, M.A. *Paenibacillus anseongense* sp. nov. a Silver Nanoparticle Producing Bacterium Isolated from Rhizospheric Soil. *Curr. Microbiol.* **2020**, *77*, 2023–2030. [CrossRef]
19. Huq, M.A. *Microvirga rosea* sp. nov.: A nanoparticle producing bacterium isolated from soil of rose garden. *Arch. Microbiol.* **2018**, *200*, 1439–1445. [CrossRef] [PubMed]
20. Vaidyanathan, R.; Gopalram, S.; Kalishwaralal, K.; Deepak, V.; Pandian, S.R.K.; Gurunathan, S. Enhanced silver nanoparticle synthesis by optimization of nitrate reductase activity. *Colloids Surf. B Biointerfaces* **2010**, *75*, 335–341. [CrossRef]
21. Gopinath, V.; Velusamy, P. Extracellular biosynthesis of silver nanoparticles using *Bacillus* sp. Gp-23 and evaluation of their antifungal activity towards fusarium oxysporum. *Spectrochim. Acta A Mol. Biomol. Spectrosc.* **2013**, *106*, 170–174. [CrossRef] [PubMed]
22. Galán, J.E. *Salmonella Typhimurium* and inflammation: A pathogen-centric affair. *Nat. Rev. Microbiol.* **2021**, *19*, 716–725. [CrossRef] [PubMed]
23. Raymond, P.; Houard, E.; Denis, M.; Esnault, E. Diversity of *Yersinia enterocolitica* isolated from pigs in a French slaughterhouse over 2 years. *MicrobiologyOpen* **2019**, *8*, e00751. [CrossRef] [PubMed]
24. Nair, D.V.T.; Venkitanarayanan, K.; Johny, A.K. Antibiotic-Resistant *Salmonella* in the Food Supply and the Potential Role of Antibiotic Alternatives for Control. *Foods* **2018**, *7*, 167. [CrossRef]
25. Younis, G.; Mady, M.; Awad, A. *Yersinia enterocolitica*: Prevalence, virulence, and antimicrobial resistance from retail and processed meat in Egypt. *Vet. World* **2019**, *12*, 1078–1084. [CrossRef]
26. Sheu, S.Y.; Su, C.L.; Kwon, S.W.; Chen, W.M. *Flavobacterium amniphilum* sp. nov., isolated from a stream. *Int. J. Syst. Evol. Microbiol.* **2017**, *67*, 5179–5186. [CrossRef]
27. Weisburg, W.G.; Barns, S.M.; Pelletier, D.A.; Lane, D.J. 16S ribosomal DNA amplification for phylogenetic study. *J. Bacteriol.* **1991**, *173*, 697–703. [CrossRef]
28. Yoon, S.H.; Ha, S.M.; Kwon, S.; Lim, J.; Kim, Y. Introducing EzBioCloud: A taxonomically united database of 16S rRNA gene sequences and whole-genome assemblies. *Int. J. Syst. Evol. Microbiol.* **2017**, *67*, 1613–1617. [CrossRef]
29. Tamura, K.; Stecher, G.; Peterson, D.; Filipski, A.; Kumar, S. MEGA6: Molecular evolutionary genetics analysis version 6.0. *Mol. Biol. Evol.* **2013**, *30*, 2725–2729. [CrossRef]
30. Felsenstein, J. Confidence limits on phylogenies: An approach using the bootstrap. *Evolution* **1985**, *39*, 783–791. [CrossRef]
31. Meier-Kolthoff, J.P.; Auch, A.F.; Klenk, H.P.; Göker, M. Genome sequence-based species delimitation with confidence intervals and improved distance functions. *BMC Bioinform.* **2013**, *14*, 60. [CrossRef]
32. Aziz, R.K.; Bartels, D.; Best, A.A.; DeJongh, M.; Disz, T.; Edwards, R.A.; Formsma, K.; Gerdes, S.; Glas, E.M.; Kubal, M. The RAST server: Rapid annotations using subsystems technology. *BMC Genome* **2008**, *9*, 1–15. [CrossRef]
33. Sasser, M. *Identification of Bacteria by Gas Chromatography of Cellular Fatty Acids*; MIDI Technical Note 101; MIDI Inc.: Newark, DE, USA, 1990.
34. Collins, M.D. Isoprenoid quinones. In *Chemical Methods in Prokaryotic Systematics Chichester*; Goodfellow, M., O'Donnell, A.G., Eds.; Wiley: Hoboken, NJ, USA, 1994; pp. 265–309.
35. Du, J.; Sing, H.; Yi, T.H. Biosynthesis of silver nanoparticles by *Novosphingobium* sp. THG-C3 and their antimicrobial potential. *Artif. Cells Nanomed. Biotechnol.* **2017**, *45*, 211–217. [CrossRef]
36. Ansari, M.A.; Baykal, A.; Asiri, S. Synthesis and characterization of antibacterial activity of spinel chromium-substituted copper ferrite nanoparticles for biomedical application. *J. Inorg. Organomet. Polym. Mater.* **2018**, *28*, 2316–2327. [CrossRef]
37. Shi, W.; Sun, Q.; Fan, G.; Hideaki, S.; Moriya, O.; Itoh, T.; Zhou, Y.; Cai, M.; Kim, S.G.; Lee, J.S. gcType: A high-quality type strain genome database for microbial phylogenetic and functional research. *Nucleic Acids Res.* **2021**, *49*, D694–D705. [CrossRef]
38. Huq, M.A. Green Synthesis of Silver Nanoparticles Using *Pseudoduganella eburnean* MAHUQ-39 and Their Antimicrobial Mechanisms Investigation against Drug Resistant Human Pathogens. *Int. J. Mol. Sci.* **2020**, *21*, 1510. [CrossRef]
39. Zhang, X.F.; Liu, Z.G.; Shen, W.; Gurunathan, S. Silver nanoparticles: Synthesis, characterization, properties, applications, and therapeutic approaches. *Int. J. Mol. Sci.* **2016**, *17*, 1534. [CrossRef] [PubMed]
40. Ganesh-Babu, M.M.; Gunasekaran, P. Production and structural characterization of crystalline silver nanoparticles from Bacillus cereus isolate. *Colloids Surf. B Biointerfaces* **2009**, *74*, 191–195. [CrossRef] [PubMed]
41. Singh, N.; Khanna, P.K. In situ synthesis of silver nano-particles in polymethylmethacrylate. *Mater. Chem. Phys.* **2007**, *104*, 367–372. [CrossRef]
42. Dong, Z.Y.; Rao, N.; Prabhu, M.; Xiao, M.; Wang, H.F.; Hozzein, W.N.; Chen, W.; Li, W.J. Antibacterial activity of silver nanoparticles against *Staphylococcus warneri* synthesized using endophytic bacteria by photo-irradiation. *Front. Microbiol.* **2017**, *8*, 1090. [CrossRef] [PubMed]
43. Singh, P.; Pandit, S.; Jers, C.; Abhayraj, S.; Garnæs, J.; Mijakovic, I. Silver nanoparticles produced from *Cedecea* sp. exhibit antibiofilm activity and remarkable stability. *Sci. Rep.* **2021**, *11*, 12619. [CrossRef] [PubMed]

44. Shankar, S.; Rhim, J.W. Amino acid mediated synthesis of silver nanoparticles and preparation of antimicrobial agar/silver nanoparticles composite films. *Carbohydr. Polym.* **2015**, *130*, 353–363. [CrossRef] [PubMed]
45. Huq, M.A.; Akter, S. Bacterial Mediated Rapid and Facile Synthesis of Silver Nanoparticles and Their Antimicrobial Efficacy against Pathogenic Microorganisms. *Materials* **2021**, *14*, 2615. [CrossRef] [PubMed]
46. Akter, S.; Lee, S.-Y.; Siddiqi, M.Z.; Balusamy, S.R.; Ashrafudoulla, M.; Rupa, E.J.; Huq, M.A. Ecofriendly synthesis of silver nanoparticles by *Terrabacter humi* sp. nov. and their antibacterial application against antibiotic-resistant pathogens. *Int. J. Mol. Sci.* **2020**, *21*, 9746. [CrossRef]
47. Guo, L.; Gong, S.; Wang, Y.; Sun, Q.; Duo, K.; Fei, P. Antibacterial Activity of Olive Oil Polyphenol Extract Against *Salmonella Typhimurium* and *Staphylococcus aureus*: Possible Mechanisms. *Foodborne Pathog. Dis.* **2020**, *17*. [CrossRef]
48. Hosseinzadeh, S.; Saei, H.D.; Ahmadi, M.; Salehi, T.Z. Antimicrobial effect of Licochalcone A and Epigallocatechin-3-gallate against *Salmonella Typhimurium* isolated from poultry flocks. *Iran. J. Microbiol.* **2018**, *10*, 51–58.
49. Polinarski, M.A.; Ana, L.B.; Silva, F.E.B.; Bernardi-Wenzel, J. New Perspectives of Using Chitosan, Silver, and Chitosan–Silver Nanoparticles against Multidrug-Resistant Bacteria. *Part. Part. Syst. Charact.* **2021**, *38*, 2100009. [CrossRef]
50. Khan, S.U.; Ansarid, M.J.; Khan, M.H.U. Antimicrobial potentials of medicinal plant's extract and their derived silver nanoparticles: A focus on honey bee pathogen. *Saudi J. Biol. Sci.* **2019**, *26*, 1815–1834. [CrossRef]
51. Kim, J.S.; Kuk, E.; Yu, K.N. Antimicrobial effects of silver nanoparticles. *Nanomed. Nanotechnol. Biol. Med.* **2007**, *3*, 95–101. [CrossRef]

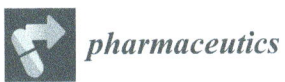

Review

Myxobacteria as a Source of New Bioactive Compounds: A Perspective Study

Mudasir Ahmad Bhat [1,†], Awdhesh Kumar Mishra [2,†], Mujtaba Aamir Bhat [3,†], Mohammad Iqbal Banday [4], Ommer Bashir [5], Irfan A. Rather [6], Safikur Rahman [7], Ali Asghar Shah [1,*] and Arif Tasleem Jan [3,*]

1. Department of Biotechnology, Baba Ghulam Shah Badshah University, Rajouri 185234, Jammu and Kashmir, India; mudasirbiotech@bgsbu.ac.in
2. Department of Biotechnology, Yeungnam University, Gyeongsan 38541, Korea; awdhesh@ynu.ac.kr
3. Department of Botany, Baba Ghulam Shah Badshah University, Rajouri 185234, Jammu and Kashmir, India; mujtaba@bgsbu.ac.in
4. Department of Microbiology, Baba Ghulam Shah Badshah University, Rajouri 185234, Jammu and Kashmir, India; bandayiqbal.1000@gmail.com
5. Department of School Education, Jammu 181205, Jammu and Kashmir, India; ommerbashir@gmail.com
6. Department of Biological Sciences, Faculty of Science, King Abdulaziz University (KAU), Jeddah 21589, Saudi Arabia; ammm@kau.edu.sa
7. Department of Botany, MS College, BR Ambedkar Bihar University, Muzaffarpur 845401, Bihar, India; shafique2@gmail.com
* Correspondence: aashah@bgsbu.ac.in (A.A.S.); atasleem@bgsbu.ac.in (A.T.J.)
† These authors contributed equally to this work.

Abstract: Myxobacteria are unicellular, Gram-negative, soil-dwelling, gliding bacteria that belong to class δ-proteobacteria and order *Myxococcales*. They grow and proliferate by transverse fission under normal conditions, but form fruiting bodies which contain myxospores during unfavorable conditions. In view of the escalating problem of antibiotic resistance among disease-causing pathogens, it becomes mandatory to search for new antibiotics effective against such pathogens from natural sources. Among the different approaches, Myxobacteria, having a rich armor of secondary metabolites, preferably derivatives of polyketide synthases (PKSs) along with non-ribosomal peptide synthases (NRPSs) and their hybrids, are currently being explored as producers of new antibiotics. The *Myxobacterial* species are functionally characterized to assess their ability to produce antibacterial, antifungal, anticancer, antimalarial, immunosuppressive, cytotoxic and antioxidative bioactive compounds. In our study, we have found their compounds to be effective against a wide range of pathogens associated with the concurrence of different infectious diseases.

Keywords: antibiotics; bioactive compounds; medication; Myxobacteria; human diseases

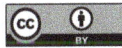

1. Introduction

Myxobacteria, bacteria belonging to family δ-proteobacteria and order Myxococcales, are unicellular, soil-dwelling, rod-shaped bacteria that display gliding motility on attachment to solid surfaces. They are omnipresent, with habitats ranging from tundra to hot deserts and from acidic soils to alkaline conditions [1–3]. The source for their isolation ranges from soil to decaying wood and leaves of trees up to excreta of herbivorous creatures [4,5]. Under nutrient-deficient conditions, they produce species-explicit structures (fruiting bodies) that exhibit myxospores (arisen from vegetative cells) within themselves to pass decades of unfavorable environmental conditions [6]. Withstanding regular confinement endeavors, myxospores sprout with the onset of favorable conditions into full-fledged structures, with the exception of depicted facultative anaerobic species, *Anaeromyxobacter dehalogenans* [7]. Recently, a large number of studies have been performed to gain a detailed account of the *Myxobacterial* properties along with types, dynamics and biogenesis of Myxobacteria-derived secondary metabolites [8–12].

The rise in resistance to armor of available antibiotic regimes represents a problem of global magnitude [13–16]. With increases in mortality and morbidity rates, it becomes imperative to have a strategic management plan to monitor the impact of resistance development and means for exploration of new molecules that can combat the emergence of different diseases among humans [12,17]. *Myxobacterial* species, despite exhibiting sensitiveness to tetracycline, kanamycin, erythromycin, streptomycin, neomycin and actinomycin, produce a variety of chemically different structures that in due course were found effective in combatting the growing problem of drug resistance. The present study highlights the potential of Myxobacteria as a source of new bioactive molecules, with strong emphasis on the production and screening of secondary metabolites, their effect observed in overcoming the odyssey associated with different diseases, as well as having updated information of the current development of their exploitation as a source of effective molecules with potential to compliment available drugs in the control of different diseases.

2. Distribution

Myxobacteria are largely cosmopolitan. Besides inhabiting terrestrial conditions, they mark their presence in extreme habitats, such as anaerobic/microaerophilic, freshwater, acidic soils, saline waters and others [12]. Since maximum populations of Myxobacteria predominantly inhabit terrestrial ecosystems, a large proportion of their secretions (secondary metabolites) are derived from terrestrial *Myxobacterial* species. On the basis of habitats, their distribution is studied under the following.

2.1. Terrestrial Habitats

Adaptation of Myxobacteria to terrestrial habitats manifests their existence in wide phenotypic characteristics, such as social swarming and gliding, resting myxospores, etc., capable of producing secondary metabolites with a wide range of antibiotic or antifungal activity as well as predation or cellulose decomposition [18]. With the help of different probes and primers, Wu et al. explored a wide range of Myxobacteria, mostly Myxococcales, from the soil samples [19]. Mohr revealed greater presentation of *Myxococcus* and *Corallococcus* genera by standardized cultivation techniques as compared to cultivation-independent clone libraries [12].

2.2. Acidic and Alkaline Habitats

Generally, Myxobacteria inhabit the soils which are neutral or slightly alkaline and show a narrow range in their pH, i.e., approximately 6.5–8.5 [12]. Myxobacteria species isolated from the alkaline bogs include *Myxococcus, Archangium* and *Sorangium*, along with others such as *Melittangium* [20]. *Corallococcus coralloides* (formerly *Myxococcus coralloides*) dominated in slightly acidic soils, while *M. fulvus* dominated in soils with a pH range in between 3.0 and 3.5 [21]. Ruckert reported that *Myxobacterial* diversity decreases with the decrease in the pH of the soil at alpine regions [21].

2.3. Freshwater Habitats

Freshwater-dwelling Myxobacteria share some characteristic features with soil inhabitants, which justifies that these Myxobacteria have been blown away or washed from soil into the freshwater bodies [22]. Research related to freshwater habitats of Myxobacteria reveal that in lake mud, Myxobacteria were the dominant bacterial groups [23].

2.4. Marine/Saline Environments

Though Myxobacteria are less adapted to saline environments, their existence in salty conditions was reported by Brockman in 1963, who observed *Myxobacterial* fruiting bodies in sand dunes from an ocean beach of South Carolina [24]. Marine Myxobacteria are represented by four different genera: Salimabromide [25], Enhygrolides [26], Haliangicin [27] and Haliamide [28]. *Haliangium tepidum* and *H. ochraceum* are the representative members of Myxobacteria from coastal salt marshes. They differ from members of the terrestrial genus with respect to the presence of anteiso-branched fatty acids, that help them to survive in greater salt concentrations (2–3% NaCl) [29]. Some genera of Myxobacteria, including Enhygromyxa [30], Plesiocystis [31] and Pseudenhygromyxa [32], are entirely detected in the saline environments. Brinkhoff et al. reported a cluster of marine Myxobacteria (MMB) from sediments of the North Sea [33,34]. Zhang et al. studied 58 species of Myxobacteria from the saline soils of Xinjiang, China [35], and Li et al. observed that species such as *Sorangium, Cystobacter, Myxococcus, Polyangium, Corallococcus* and *Nannocystis* show better survival in elevated salt conditions [36].

2.5. Facultative Anaerobic Myxobacteria

Myxobacteria are strictly aerobes, with the exception of *Anaeromyxobacter dehalogenans*, which is a facultative anaerobe. This strain of Myxobacteria was studied from sediments of the stream and grows with 2-chlorophenol (2-CPh) as an electron acceptor and acetate as an electron donor [7]. Later, different strains of this Myxobacteria were isolated from uranium-contaminated soils [37], flooded paddy fields [38], corrosive material of water pipelines [39] and arsenic-polluted environments [40].

2.6. Myxobacteria Inhabiting Moderate to Extreme Environments

Most of the *Myxobacterial* species are mesophilic, i.e., they survive in the range of 4–44 °C. However, they are also reported to survive in the extreme temperature range. Myxospores liberated by bacteria inhabiting extreme environments act as a means of sexual reproduction and can survive with temperature extremes of 58–60 °C. Production of myxospores differentiates these organisms from the rest of the faunal diversity [22]. Brockman analyzed greater diversity among Myxobacteria from regions that received greater annual rainfall (400–800 mm) as compared to the normal range of 200–400 mm [41]. Gerth and Müller [42] reported that Cystobacterineae and Sorangiineae-*Myxobacterial* suborders show greater morphogenesis at temperatures of 42–48 °C. Mohr et al. reported that *N. konarekensis*, which was studied from an Iranian desert, exhibits the best growth at 37 °C, compared with *N. pusilla* and *N. exedens*, which show optimal growth at 30 °C [43]. Though hot springs are not considered suitable for the growth of mesophilic Myxobacteria, Iizuka et al. reported four different strains of Myxobacteria that grow in geothermal conditions (optimum 45–49 °C) from Japan [44].

3. *Myxobacterial* Secondary Metabolites

Secondary metabolites represent incredible gathering of characteristically differing molecules blended among different creatures, such as microorganisms, plants, etc. Though they are not actively involved in development or any type of advancement, their absence prompts a long-haul disability in the survivability of living beings [45]. Production of secondary metabolites has been reported from a large number of *Myxobacterial* species, but a major proportion of them are reported among *Myxococcus xanthus*, *Sorangium cellulosum* and *Chondromyces* species [46]. In addition to ribosomally produced secondary metabolites, a major proportion of *Myxobacterial* metabolites were found to be derivatives of polyketide synthases (PKSs), non-ribosomal peptide synthetases (NRPSs) or hybrids of PK-NRPS systems [3,6,47]. The synthesis module in both cases proceeds through buildup of monomeric blocks: acyl CoA thioester (in case of PK metabolites) and amino acids (both proteinogenic and non-proteinogenic in case of NRPs), in a stepwise manner, followed by modification either during assembly of reaction intermediates or at the end after release from the multienzyme complex [3]. Over the past 3 decades, more than 100 secondary metabolites with over 600 analogs were reportedly isolated from more than 9000 *Myxobacterial* strains [48]. The production of unique metabolites among *Myxobacterial* strains reflects a strong correlation between genome size and the biosynthetic pathway [49,50].

Considered as a rich source of secondary metabolites, the production of a large number (>80 distinctive and 350 structural variants) of bioactive compounds by Myxobacteria puts it on par with *Pseudomonas* for being a rich source of antibiotics [51]. A large number of

Myxobacterial secondary metabolites show similarity to those produced by *Pseudomonas* and *Bacillus* spp. Antibiotics produced as bioactive secondary metabolites have been observed for about 55% and 95% of *Myxobacterial* spp. that exhibit bacteriolytic and cellulolytic properties [52]. With greater potential for use in clinical settings, compounds isolated from Myxobacteria are found either as macrocyclic lactones or linear cyclic peptides [51,52]. Information on different aspects of secondary metabolites produced by different strains of Myxobacteria along with their uses is summarized in Table 1.

Table 1. Categorization of *Myxobacterial*-derived secondary metabolites based on their function.

Bioactive Compound	Chemical Structure	Classification	Myxobacterial sp.	Uses	References
Bioactive compounds exerting antimicrobial effect					
Ajudazol		Depsipeptides	*Chondromyces crocatus*	Acts as inhibitor of mitochondrial electron transport. More effective against yeast and fungi.	[3,47,53]
Althiomycin		Polyketide, peptide	*Myxococcus xanthus*	Disrupts translocation of tRNA for peptide bond formation by peptidyltransferase. It is effective in treatment of injury and sepsis associated with *Yersinia pestis* infection.	[54]
Angiolactone		Furanone	*Angiococcus* sp.	Exhibits siderophore production which enables its antibacterial and antiproliferative activity.	[55]
Antalid		Depsipeptide	*Polyangium* sp.	NA	[56]
Aurachins E		Quinoline alkaloids	*Stigmatella aurantiaca*	Exhibits antimalarial activity (effective against *Plasmodium falciparum*).	[57]
Carolacton		Macrolactone	*Sorangium cellulosum*	Effective in regulating the growth of biofilm-producing microbes such as *Streptococcus mutans* and *pneumococci*.	[58]
Chlorotonil		Macrolactone	*Sorangium cellulosum*	Antibacterial and antimalarial activity.	[59]

Table 1. Cont.

Bioactive Compound	Chemical Structure	Classification	*Myxobacterial sp.*	Uses	References
Corallopyronin A		α-Pyrone	*Corallococcus (Myxococcus) coralloides*	Exhibits antibacterial action, effective in treating filariasis.	[60]
Corallorazine		Piperazine	*Corallococcus coralloides*	Exhibits antibacterial activity.	[61]
Crocacin		Depsipeptides	*Chondromyces crocatus*	Antibacterial. Inhibits electron transport system.	[62]
Cystobactamid		Peptide	*Cystobacter* sp.	Broad-spectrum antibacterial; topoisomerase (gyrase) inhibition.	[63]
Cytochromone		Polyketide, chromone	*Proteus mirabilis*	Essential in mitochondrial electron transport and intrinsic type II apoptosis.	[64]
Cystomanamide		Lipopeptide	*Cystobacter fuscus*	Exhibits strong antifungal and antibacterial activity.	[65]
Cystothiazol		Heterocyclic alkaloid	*Cystobacter fuscus*	Antifungal/cytostatic. Inhibits sub-mitochondrial NADH oxidation.	[66]
Disciformycin		Macrolide	*Pyxidicoccus fallax*	Exhibits antibacterial activity.	[67]
Enhygrolide A		Furanone	*Enhygromyxa salina*	Effective in inhibiting the growth of *Arthrobacter crystallopoietes*.	[68]

Table 1. Cont.

Bioactive Compound	Chemical Structure	Classification	Myxobacterial sp.	Uses	References
Etnangien		Polyketides	*Sorangium cellulosum*	Works as an inhibitor of eubacterial DNA polymerase.	[3,47,53]
Gulmirecin		Macrolide	*Pyxidicoccus fallax*	Exhibits antibacterial activity.	[69]
Haliangicin		Polyketide	*Haliangium luteum*	Effective against fungi *Aspergillus niger* and *Fusarium* sp. at very low concentrations of 6–12 µg/mL.	[70]
Hyalachelin		Catechol	*Hyalangium minutum*	Shows sidrophore, i.e., iron-chelating activity, and cytotoxic activity is minor.	[71]
Hyaladione		Quinone	*Hyalangium minutum*	Exhibits antimicrobial and cytotoxic activity.	[72]
Hyapyrroline		Polyketide, pyrrole	*Hyalangium minutum*	NA	[73]
Hyapyrone		Polyketide, pyrone	*Hyalangium minutum*	Exhibits weak antibacterial and antifungal activity.	[73]
p-Hydroxyacetophenone amide		Amide	*Cystobacter ferrugineus*	Shows marginal activity against microalgae (P. simplex).	[74]

Table 1. Cont.

Bioactive Compound	Chemical Structure	Classification	Myxobacterial sp.	Uses	References
1-Hydroxyphenazin-6-yl-a-Darabinofuranoside		Glycoside	Nannocystis pusilla	Exhibits weak antimicrobial activity.	[75]
Icumazol		Polyketide	Sorangium cellulosum	Effective antifungal. Inhibition of NADH oxidation.	[76]
Indiacen		Indole	Sandaracinus amylolyticus	Exhibits antibacterial and antifungal activity.	[77,78]
Indothiazinone		Indole	Ohtaekwangia kribbensis	Weak antimicrobial and cytotoxic activity.	[75]
Kulkenon		Macrolactone	Sorangium cellulosum	Exhibits antibacterial activity.	[79]
Leupyrrins		Macrolides	Sorangium cellulosum	Exhibits antibacterial activity.	[80]
Macyranone		Peptide	Cystobacter fuscus	Shows moderate cytotoxic activity; antiparasitic (L. donovani); proteasome inhibitor (CT-L activity).	[81]

Table 1. Cont.

Bioactive Compound	Chemical Structure	Classification	Myxobacterial sp.	Uses	References
Maltepolid		Macrolactone		Exhibits moderate cytotoxic activity.	[82]
Methyl indole-3-carboxylate		Indole	*Sorangium cellulosum*	NA	[75]
Melithiazols		Heterocyclic alkaloid	*Archangium gephyra*	Antibacterial. Inhibits NADH oxidation.	[83]
Microsclerodermin		Cyclic peptide	*Microscleroderma, theonella*	Exhibits antifungal activity, NF-kB inhibition and induction of apoptosis.	[84,85]
Myxalamids		Amide	*Myxococcus xanthus*	Exhibits antibacterial and antifungal activity; inhibits electron transport system.	[3,47,53]
Myxochelin		Peptide	*Angiococcus disciformis*	Shows siderophore production. Exhibits antibacterial, antitumor and antiproliferative activities: inhibits 5-lipoxygenase.	[86,87]
Myxocoumarin		Coumarin	*Stigmatella aurantiaca*	Exhibits antifungal activity.	[88]

Table 1. Cont.

Bioactive Compound	Chemical Structure	Classification	*Myxobacterial* sp.	Uses	References
Myxoprincomide		Peptide	*Myxococcus xanthus*	NA	[89–91]
Myxopyronin B		Peptide	*Myxococcus fulvus*	Effective in combating diseases caused by *Staphylococcus aureus*.	[92]
Myxothiazol		Macrocyclic	*Myxococcus fulvus*	Inhibits mitochondrial cytochrome c reductase.	[3,47,53]
Myxovalargin		Lipopeptide	*Myxococcus fulvus*	Exhibits antibacterial activity against *Micrococcus luteus* and *Corynebacterium Mediolanum*. Disrupts memebrane integrity and aminoacyl-tRNA binding to site A during translation.	[93]
Myxovirescin		Macrocyclic	*Myxococcus xanthus*	Exhibits antibacterial activity. Blocks bacterial cell wall synthesis via interference in lipid-disaccharide pentapeptide polymerization, as well as targeting type II signal peptidase LspA.	[94,95]
Nannozinone		Pyrrolopyrazinoe	*Nannocystis pusilla*	Exhibits weak antimicrobial and cytotoxic activity.	[75]
Noricumazol		Polyketide	*Sorangium cellulosum*	Inhibits conductance of potassium channel KscA. Exhibits antiviral (EBOV, HCV) activity.	[76,96,97]
Phenoxan		Lipopeptide	*Polyganium* sp.	Effective as an inhibitor of eukaryotic respiratory chain (blocks Complex I). Exhibits antifungal activity.	[3,47,53]

Table 1. Cont.

Bioactive Compound	Chemical Structure	Classification	Myxobacterial sp.	Uses	References
Phoxalone		Macrolides	*Sorangium cellulosum*	Exhibits antimicrobial activity.	[98]
Pyrronazol		Pyrrole	*Nannocystis pusilla*	Shows weak antifungal activity.	[75]
Ripostatin B		Polyketide	*Sorangium cellulosum*	Effective in treating tuberculosis.	[99]
Roimatacene		Cyclic peptide	*Cystobacter ferrugineus*	Exhibits antibacterial activity.	[74]
Saframycin Mx1		α-cyanoamine	*Myxococcus xanthus*	Acts as a broad-spectrum inhibitor for a wide range of Gram-positive and halobacteria. Shows week activity against Gram-negative bacteria.	[3,47,53]
Salimyxin A and Salimabromide		Sterol, Furano lactone	*Enhygromyxa salina*	Effective against *Arthrobacter cristallopoietes*.	[100]
Sesqiterpene		Terpenes	*Sorangium cellulosum*	Exhibits antimicrobial activity.	[101,102]

226

Table 1. Cont.

Bioactive Compound	Chemical Structure	Classification	*Myxobacterial* sp.	Uses	References
Sorangicin		Macrolides	*Sorangium cellulosum*	Exhibits antimicrobial activity.	[82]
Sorangiadenosine		Macrolides	*Sorangium cellulosum*	Exhibits antimicrobial activity.	[101]
Soraphinol		Macrolides	*Sorangium cellulosum*	Exhibits antimicrobial activity.	[103]
Sorazinnone		Pyrazinone	*Pyxidicoccus fallax*	Siderophore production. Exhibits antibacterial activity.	[75]
Sorazolon		Indole	*Sorangium cellulosum*	Weak activity against Gram-positive bacteria.	[104]
Stigmatellin		Macrolactone	*Stigmatella aurantica*	Exhibits strong antifungal activity. Inhibits quinol oxidation of mitochondrial cytochrome bc1 complex.	[3,47,53]
Sulfangolid		Macrolactone	*Sorangium cellulosum*	Exhibits antiviral (HIV-1) activity.	[105,106]

Table 1. Cont.

Bioactive Compound	Chemical Structure	Classification	Myxobacterial sp.	Uses	References
Thuggacin		Macrolactone	Sorangium cellulosum	Effective against Mycobacterium tuberculosis.	[107,108]
Bioactive compounds exerting cytotoxic effects					
Aetheramide		Cyclic peptide	Atherobacter rufus	Shows cytotoxic and moderate antifungal activity.	[109–111]
Archazolid		Macrolactone	Archangium gephyra, Cystobacter violaceus	Exhibits cytotoxic and antitumor activity. Inhibits V-ATPase.	[112]
Argyrin		Peptolide	Archangium gephyra	Acts as a potential inhibitor of antibody formation by murine B-cells. Exhibits antibacterial and cytotoxic activity.	[113]
Bengamide		Caprolactam	Myxococcus virescens	Shows cytotoxic, antitumor, antibacterial and anthelmintic activity. Inhibits MetAP. Acts as an anti-inflammatory.	[114]

Table 1. Cont.

Bioactive Compound	Chemical Structure	Classification	Myxobacterial sp.	Uses	References
Chivosazol		Peptide	Sorangium cellulosum	Effective antifungal activity at higher concentration. Exhibits strong cytotoxic activity. Destroys cyto-skeleton.	[3,47,53]
Chrondramide		Depsipeptide	Chondromyces crocatus	Exhibits strong cytotoxic activity; effective against breast cancer metastasis.	[3,47,53]
Cystodienoic acid		Terpene	Cystobacter ferrugineus	Exhibits cytotoxic activity.	[115]
Disorazol		Peptide	Sorangium cellulosum	Exhibits strong antifungal activity; inhibits proliferation of different cancer cell lines.	[116]
Eliamid		polyketide	Sorangium cellulosum	Exhibits cytotoxic activity; shows moderate anthelmintic and antifungal activity; acts as a respiratory chain inhibitor.	[117]
Epothilone		Peptide	Sorangium cellulosum	Acts as an inhibitor of microtubule function concerning cell division.	[118]

Table 1. Cont.

Bioactive Compound	Chemical Structure	Classification	Myxobacterial sp.	Uses	References
Haliamide		Polyene	*Haliangium ochraceum*	Exhibits moderate cytotoxic activity.	[28]
Hyafurone		Polyketide, furanone	*Hyalangium minutum*	Exhibits moderate cytotoxic activity, as well as showing marginal antiparasitic activity.	[73]
Miuraenamide		cyclic depsipeptides	*Paraliomyxa miuraensis*	Exhibits antibacterial and cytotoxic activity.	[119]
Nannocystin		Macrocyclic epoxyamide	*Nannocystis* sp.	Exhibits strong antifungal and cytotoxic activity; inhibits eukaryotic translation elongation factor 1α.	[120,121]
Pellasoren		Polyketide	*Sorangium cellulosum*	Exhibits cytotoxic activity.	[51,122]
Ratjadone A		α-pyrone	*Sorangium cellulosum*	Acts as an antiviral drug. Inhibits HIV infection by ceasing the Rev/CRM1-mediated nuclear export.	[106]
Rhizopodin		Amide	*Myxococcus stipitatus*	Effective against cancer cell lines. Interferes with cytoskeleton assembly. Acts as a strong antiviral.	[3,123]

Table 1. Cont.

Bioactive Compound	Chemical Structure	Classification	*Myxobacterial* sp.	Uses	References
Spirangien		Polyketide	*Sorangium cellulosum*	Exhibits antifungal, cytotoxic, antiviral (HIV) and anti-inflamatory activity.	[124]
Tubulysin		Peptide	*Archangium gephyra* and *Angiococcus disciformis*	It has been found to be effective in treating the cancer associated with Luteinizing Hormone-releasing hormone receptor. Effective in cell cycle arrest at G2/M phase.	[125]
Bioactive compounds exerting beneficial effects in agriculture					
Ambruticin		Polyketide	*Sorangium cellulosum*	Acts as a fungicide, effective against *Hansenula anomala* and other plant pathogens such as *Botrytis cinerea*, via interference in osmoregulation system.	[126]
Pyrrolnitrin		Pyrrole	*Myxococcus fulvus, Carallococcus exiguous, Cystobacter ferrugineus*	Exhibits strong antifungal activity.	[3,47,53]
Tartrolon		Pilyketide	*Sorangium cellulosum*	Effective against Gram-positive bacteria and mammalian cells.	[127]
Thiangazol		Amide	*Polyangium* sp.	Exhibits strong antifungal, acaricidal and insecticidal activities, as well as having anti-HIV activity.	[128]

Table 1. Cont.

Bioactive Compound	Chemical Structure	Classification	Myxobacterial sp.	Uses	References
Soraphen A		Polyketide	Sorangium cellulosum	Effective as a plant disease control agent. Possesses strong antifungal activity. Acts as a broad-spectrum antiviral (effective against HIV and Hepatitis C Virus).	[129,130]

4. Pharmacological Effects of Myxobacteria-Derived Bioactive Compounds

Myxobacteria, an adaptable cosmopolitan, produces a wide range of bioactive molecules. About 40% of Myxobacteria-derived compounds represent novel (mostly non-glycosylated) chemical structures that act against targets often not covered by compounds derived from *Actinomycetes*, *Bacillus* and *Pseudomonas*. A variety of bioactive compounds produced by *Myxobacterial* spp. play a vital role in biological activities, and mostly, their activities are antifungal, antibacterial, anti-cancerous, antiparasitic and immunomodulatory.

4.1. Myxobacteria and Infectious Diseases

Before the advent of an era of widely accessible anti-infectious agents, mankind was considered vulnerable to infections such as cholera, which reached the extent of epidemics that caused a huge loss of human lives [131]. With the passage of time, the period of anti-infectious agents moved along from quinine (utilized against fever), to Salvarsan (arsenic compound used against syphilis) and Sulpha drugs such as Protonsil (utilized against diseases caused by Gram-positive *cocci*). The circumstances profoundly improved with the discovery of the β-lactam drug Penicillin, from *Penicillium* spp. [132]. The era of antibiotics moved on to aminoglycosides [133], macrolides [134] and so on to treat ailments that were considered untreatable. Inaccurate recommendation and wrong use of antibiotics in human medication, veterinary and horticulture expanded portability, and as such, quick spread of microbes, that raised alarm regarding the use of multi-tranquilize safe microbes. Many pharmaceutical companies withdrew from manufacturing new drugs due to high-cost screening systems developed for nosocomial infections caused by ESKAPE (*Enterococcus faecium*, *Staphylococcus aureus*, *Klebsiella pneumoniae*, *Acinetobacter baumannii*, *Pseudomonas aeruginosa* and *Enterobacter* spp.) pathogens [135]. With less new medications, the dying antimicrobial pipeline caused by an absence in development and inefficient ways of screening bioactive substances presented a dreadful situation that led to obstruction in the production of drugs [136,137]. The bottlenecks that choked the production of anti-infective agents prompted qualified countermeasures to be implemented regarding improvements in the production of engineered medications, proper screening of the metabolite markers, followed by assessment of the rediscovered drugs. At this instance, exploration of new genera and species are of extraordinary intrigue [138] as it may involve the creation of auxiliary metabolites in scaleup forms or fitting hardware for maturation and release of substances from fermenter stock for resolving biotic and abiotic conditions of the maker strain.

Myxobacteria, together with *actinomycetes* [139] and *Bacillus* spp., are considered as the best producers of bioactive compounds [140]. A large proportion of Myxobacteria-derived bioactive compounds (29%) displaying antibacterial properties reflect their competitiveness for existence in their natural habitats. These characteristic products demonstrate a more extensive scope of biological activities which are regularly less direct to rationalize, as the production of regular objects from different *Myxobacterial* spp. requires regular screening and enormous scaleup development [6].

4.2. Myxobacteria and Viral Diseases

4.2.1. Human Immunodeficiency Virus (HIV)

Human Immunodeficiency Virus is a single-strand RNA (ssRNA) lentivirus which targets human immune cells, and integrates into host DNA by reverse transcription. Secondary metabolites extracted from different *Myxobacterial* strains are reported to play crucial roles against HIV. The Sulfangolids are an important class of antiviral secondary metabolites secreted by different strains of *Sorangium cellulosum* [105]. *Myxobacterial* extracts such as spirangien B, sulfangolid C, soraphen F and epothilon D at different concentrations showed impressive activity against HIV [124]. Soraphens exert antiviral activity by inhibiting acetyl-CoA carboxylate transferase [141], while epothilones stabilize the activity of macrophage microtubuli in a parallel way to Taxol® [142,143]. Ixabepilone®, an FDA-registered anticancer drug, is derived from epothilone B [144]. Epothilon D and spirangien B are believed to decrease the phosphorylation, and as such degradation of inhibitor of kappa B (IkBS) [143,145]. Rhizopodin, a well-known actin inhibitor, extracted from *Myxococcus stipitatus* [124], interferes in virus synapses and hence blocks the virological synapse arrangement. Stigmatellin extracted from *Stiginatella aurantiaca* Sga15, disorazol extracted from *Sorangium cellulosum* Soce 56 and tubulysin extracted from *Archangium gephyrs* strain Ar315 shows mild anti-HIV activity [124], while Phenalamide A1, phenoxan and thiangazole separated from *Polyangium* sp. and *Myxococcus stipitatus* strain Mxs40 suppress HIV-1-mediated cell death in the MT-4 cell assay, thereby exhibiting high anti-HIV activity [146]. Aetheramide A and B isolated from the genus *Aetherobacter*, that inhibits HIV-1 infection, show IC_{50} values of 0.015 and 0.018 M, respectively [109,147,148]. Similarly, Ratjadon A (a compound isolated from *Sorangium cellulosum* Soce 360), capable of blocking the Rev/CRM1-mediated nuclear export, inhibits HIV infectivity; however, its toxicity and low SI value becomes a limiting factor for its exploitation as a potential therapeutic molecule [106,149].

4.2.2. Human Cytomegalovirus (HCMV)

Infections of Human Cytomegalovirus are associated with diseases such as glandular fever and pneumonia. Myxochelin, a secondary metabolite obtained from different *Myxobacterial* strains, responsible for iron uptake during iron-limiting circumstances, was found to be a potent antitumor agent [87,150,151]. The ability of nannochelins and hylachelins (siderophores of *Myxobacterial* source) in inhibiting the human 5-lipoxygenase (5-LO, a gene associated with the proliferation of cancerous cells) were found exerting antitumor activity [87,142–154]. It is believed that a similar pathway of inhibiting 5-LO is associated with the strong anticancer activity of myxochelin [153,155]. Of the different Myxochelins, which are either isolated from *Angiococcus disciformis* (strain And30) or synthesized [155,156], Myxochelin C is capable of inhibiting HCMV (IC_{50} value of 0.7 g/mL) [150,157]. It opens avenues for testing other known siderophores, such as nannochelins, hylachelins and myxochelin analogues, in the future for their possible role in inhibiting HCMV [158]. Additionally, structure–activity relationships of the siderophores need to be studied for possible discovery of more potent antivirals [123].

4.2.3. Ebola Virus Disease (EVD)

Ebola virus (EBOV) is a single-stranded RNA virus which causes hemorrhagic fever. Different metabolites extracted from Myxobacteria were analyzed for their possible activity in inhibiting the Ebola virus using GP-pseudo-typed lentiviral vectors expressing Ebola envelope glycoprotein [97]. Chondramides extracted from the genus Chondromyces [159] of Myxobacteria were found capable of inhibiting the EBOV-GP-mediated transduction [123]. Noricumazole, a polyketide extracted from *Sorangium cellulosum*, exerts an EBOV-GP inhibitory effect with an IC_{50} value of 0.33 M. [97]. The secondary metabolite is believed to lower the virulence of EBOV via blocking of the potassium channels [76,97].

4.2.4. Hepatitis C Virus (HCV)

Hepatitis C virus, a single-stranded RNA virus, undergoes transmission through blood transfusions. Heterocyclic metabolites such as labindoles A and B [160], 3-chloro-9H-carbazole and 4-hydroxymethyl-quinoline extracted from *Myxobacterial* strain *Labilithrix luteola*, exert potent antiviral activity, and thereby help to overcome the effects of HCV [160]. Of the different macrolactones, Soraphens A obtained from *Myxobacterial* species was found to inhibit HCV replication in in vitro HCV culture models (cells in sub-genomic and full-length replicons) and in cell culture-adapted virus with an IC_{50} value of 5 nM [96,161–163]. Lanyamycin, a macrolide obtained from *Sorangium cellulosum* (strain Soce 481) that exhibits similarity to bafilomycins of actinobacteria effective against influenza A virus (IC_{50} value of 0.1 nM), was found to moderately inhibit HCV [96,160,164].

4.3. Myxobacterial Metabolites as Anti-Neurodegenerative Diseases

Inside the cell, the endoplasmic reticulum (ER) helps in the processing of proteins before their transport to the target sites. However, any kind of ER dysfunction due to protein misfolding may lead to neurodegenerative disorder or cell death [165–167]. *Myxobacterial* secondary metabolites act on protein GRP78/Bip, which helps to release any kind of stress created in the ER [168]. It also decreases the release of apoptosis-inducing factor (AIF) and cytochrome C (an apoptosis-related marker proteins). Therefore, *Myxobacterial* secondary metabolites help in combating the Parkinson's disease (PD) pathology via decreasing the ER stress, which contributes to inhibition of cell apoptosis [169]. Microtubules play a major role in the axoplasmic transport of different constituents of the cell (mitochondria, synaptic vesicles, lipids, proteins) [170]. Neurodegenerative diseases such as Alzheimer's disease (AD), Amyotrophic lateral Sclerosis (ALS) and PD arise by distraction in the axoplasmic transport due to microtubules linked to tau proteins—the phenomenon known as tauopathy [171–175]. Epothilones (A–F) are a particular class of secondary metabolites produced by *Sorangium cellulosum* strain So ce90 that exhibit antifungal and anti-cancerous potential [176]. These compounds bind to microtubules and help them in stabilization, hence resulting in the elevation of axoplasmic transport in neurodegenerative disorders [177]. Of the different Epothilones, Epothilone D plays an important role in improving the axonal transport, as well as protecting cognitive deficits in a mouse tauopathy model having overexpression of P301S (a mutant tau), thereby contributing to inhibition of tau pathology [178]. Epothilone D also plays an active role in alleviating the microtubule defects in a C57Bl model of PD [179].

Neurodegenerative diseases such as PD, AD and Huntington's Disease (HD) are the outcomes of different mitochondrial dysfunctions [180]. Earlier studies predicted that certain prokaryotes have the ability to synthesize PUFAs, however, these predictions failed as some extremophilic bacteria which inhabit extreme environments of seas and oceans invalidated this hypothesis [181,182]. Among different terrestrial prokaryotes, Myxobacteria are considered as a major contributor of PUFAs [183]. In the studies employing the genome mining approach, two *Myxobacterial* species, *Sorangium* and *Aetherobacter*, were found, having different organization of gene clusters associated with biosynthetic PUFA compared with their marine counterparts [184]. *Myxobacterial* omega 3 PUFAs play an antagonistic role against prenatal stress, which arises from mitochondrial abnormalities such as changes in mitochondrial complexes, DNA damage and memory deficiency [185,186]. Having a remarkable effect regarding the phospholipid profile, and as such fluidity of the mitochondrial membrane, DHA was observed to play a critical role in maintaining stability of the structure, and as such functions of the mitochondrial membrane, and thereby in non-amyloidogenic processing of APP in the HEK-APP cell line [187].

Immune Modulating *Myxobacterial* Compounds

Employment of *Myxobacterial* secondary metabolites such as Soraphen A, bengamide A and B and Spirangiens as immune-enhancing compounds has attracted the attention of different researchers throughout the world [188]. Castro et al. worked out the immune-enhancing responses of Soraphen A [189]. Acting on the biotin carboxylase (BC) domain, Soraphen A extracted from *Sorangium cellulosum* So ce26 was found to exert an inhibitory effect on acetyl-CoA carboxylase (ACC) [141]. Bengamides, an important class of secondary metabolites produced by *Myxococcus virescens*, exert both anti-inflammatory as well as immune-boosting effects via regulation of the nuclear factor-ΚB (NF-ΚB) and pro-inflammatory cytokines (IL-6, TNFα and MCP-1) [190]. Spirangien A produced by *Sorangium cellulosum* strain So ce90 shows antifungal activity, as well as suppressing transcription of IL-8 in response to IL-1 (cytotoxic activity). The compound along with its derivative, spirangien M522, were found effective in inhibiting IL-8 gene expression in the HeLa cell line [145].

4.4. Myxobacterial Compounds Attributing Cytotoxic Effects

Myxobacterial secondary metabolites display unique structural properties and exhibit novel modes of action. These metabolites mainly target the cellular structures that are rarely hit by metabolites from other sources.

4.4.1. Compounds Targeting Electron Transport

Myxobacterial compounds such as crocacins [191] and aurachin C [192,193], along with a group of closely related bithiazole derivatives, particularly myxothiazol, cystothiazol and melithiazole [66,194–196], were found effective in inhibiting mitochondrial respiration through interference in the functioning of complex-I (NADH-Ubiquinone oxidoreductase) and complex-III (Cyt b–C1 complex). Stigmatellin was found to exert its inhibitory effect at complex III of the mitochondria [6] and Cyt b6/f of the photosynthetic apparatus in plants [197–199].

4.4.2. Compounds Targeting RNA and Protein Synthesis

With enormous potential to lead as building blocks for drug development, compounds of Myxobacteria origin such as saframycin tie to DNA [200], ambruticin helps in osmoregulation of fungi [126] and gephyronic acid [201] and myxovalargin [93,202] repress eukaryotic and prokaryotic protein synthesis, respectively [83]. Etnangien is a metabolite that targets protein synthetic machinery via inhibition of the eubacterial RNA polymerases. In addition to rifampicins utilized maximally in clinics, other inhibitors of RNA polymerase of *Myxobacterial* origin include thiolutin [203,204], streptolydigin [205] and holomycin [206]. These molecules (ripostatin and corallopyronin) show no cross-resistance with rifamycin, and likewise concentrate on the commencement of RNA synthesis [207]. Acting in an alternate way to rifamycin, it is believed that these metabolites can potentially be used to overcome rifamycin resistance in bacteria [208,209]. Inhibition of the protein synthetic machinery is mediated by both naturally occurring compounds such as sorangicins and ripostatins that exert their effect during initiation (sorangicins) [210,211] and chain elongation (ripostatins) [212,213], as well as by chemically related myxopyronins [93] and corallopyronins [214].

Compounds of *Myxobacterial* origin (10% of *Myxobacterial* compounds), that interfere with the microtubule assembly (cytoskeleton) and thereby hinder cell proliferation and promote apoptosis, are currently being used in cancer chemotherapies. Similar to notorious fungal toxins obtained from mushrooms (preferably green and white cap mushrooms), *Myxobacterial* compounds such as rhizopodin [215,216] and chondramides [159,217,218] are reported to work explicitly on the actin [214]. Though all chondramide variants exert similar effects, chondramide C was found to be most effective in its action on actin [217]. Of the different compounds, a few compounds, such as epothilones [219,220], play important roles in retaining tubular polymerization under in vitro conditions, while others, such as tubulysins [221,222], favor depolymerization events of the tubulin. Epothilones and their analogs have shown antitumor activity towards multidrug-resistant and paclitaxel-safe tumor cell lines [223]. In 2007, the FDA recommended Ixabepilone (IxempraTM)—a derivative of epothilone—for the treatment of metastatic breast cancer, while epothilones B and D are currently undergoing clinical trials [224]. From the tubulysins class, tubulysin D displays action that surpasses other tubulin modifiers, such as taxol, epothilones and vinblastine, by 20–100-fold [225,226]. Additionally, tubulysin A is currently explored for its pharmacological properties related to its use as an antiangiogenic and antiproliferative agent [227].

4.4.3. Other Activities

Soraphen A from *Sorangium cellulosum* was found to hinder normal functioning of acetyl-CoA carboxylase through interference with its biotin carboxylase (BC) domain. With its novel modus operandi, Soraphen A has explicit utility as a promising therapeutic (novel inhibitor of ACCs) in the treatment of cancers [3,228]. Its utility as a potent inhibitor in cancers hindered by its poor water solubility and less bioavailability is overruled through generation of either structural variants of this metabolite or through the genetic engineering approach, upholding its bioactivity.

4.5. Myxobacteria and Plant Diseases of Bacterial and Fungal Origin

Although the contribution of Myxobacteria to plant health remains largely unexplored, studies have assessed the role of *Myxobacterial* secondary metabolites in the predation of microorganisms and other plant pathogens. Based on their ability to degrade biomolecules, two groups of *Myxobacterial* spp., i.e., bacteriolytic and cellulolytic, have been formed [229]. The Myxobacteria of the bacteriolytic category produce a large number of agriculturally important compounds such as pyrrolnitrin, a thiangazoletic that acts as an antagonistic in the control of phytopathogens that destroy crops [230]. Pyrrolnitrin produced by *Myxobacterial* spp. (*Myxococcus fulvus*, *Cystobacter ferrugineus* and *Corallococcus exiguous*) was found effective in controlling the damping-off of diseases of cotton caused by *Rhizoctonia solani* [229,230]. The ability of Myxobacteria to utilize cellulose categorizes them into two groups: Group I, capable of utilizing inorganic nitrogen compounds during their growth on cellulose and glucose sources (members of the Sorangineae suborder), and Group II, unable to make direct use of cellulose (majority of *Myxobacterial* spp.) and as such, dependent on enzymatic degradative products of proteins (peptides and amino acids) as their source of nitrogen [230]. Under natural conditions, Group II *Myxobacterial* spp. causes lysis of other organisms, such as eubacteria, via secretion of exoenzymes (proteases, lipases, xylanases, etc.). The lysate generated thereof is used as a nutrient by these *Myxobacterial* spp., and tags them with the name "micro-predators" [231], *Myxobacterial* proteolytic enzymes exhibiting both cellulolytic (genus *Sorangium*) and predatory roles (genus *Myxococcus*). These proteases are believed to perform lysis of prey, cellular membrane disruption for cytoplasmic content release and protein hydrolysis for supplying amino acids to the Myxobacteria-like functions [232]. Lipids containing fatty acids c16:1ω5c, utilized along with proteins as an energy and carbon source during the growth of myxobacteria, play pivotal roles in the predation by acting as chemo-attractants for the prey. In *Myxococcus xanthus*, lipolytic enzymes belonging to three families—α/β hydrolases, patatin and GDSL lipases—disintegrate the membrane barrier, thereby releasing fatty acids and cytoplasmic contents of the prey. Genus *Polyangium* was found perforating, and as such lysing, the conidia of *Cochliobolus miyabeanus* and hyphae of *R. solani*. Genus *Sorangium* reduces damping-off of conifers in addition to lysis of microorganisms under culture conditions [231,232]. Additionally, the production of unsaturated fats by *Myxoxoccus xanthus* was found to exert an inhibitory effect on the growth of Fusarium roseum [233]. Taken together, the production of agriculturally important compounds along with a series of lytic enzymes show that Myxobacteria have potential for use as biocontrol agents.

5. Techniques for Exploring *Myxobacterial* Metabolites

As emerging endeavors of whole-genome sequencing together with metabolic profiling of *Myxobacterial* species revealed high profundity of secondary metabolites, it becomes necessary to have information on mining genomes of both terrestrial and marine Myxobacteria for novel metabolites [234]. It becomes obligatory to have a strategic plan regarding the methodology (in terms of media composition, temperature, pH, along with others) adopted for identification of secondary metabolites from cultivated strains under standard research laboratory conditions. One such strategy is OSMAC (one strain many compounds), initially introduced in Actinomycetes and fungi during isolation of new secondary metabolites [235]. Traditional but untested strategies for isolation of secondary metabolites include inoculation of microorganisms into the culture, much like induction of cytotoxic compounds [236].

Optimization of the growth conditions along with addition of the explicit precursors would be a way to support generation and expansion of the metabolite yield [234]. The adoption of the genetic engineering techniques for producing a strain with desired characters can be achieved. For instance, overexpression of a particular gene activator regulating biosynthesis of a cryptic gene cluster might be activated, as recently illustrated for the fungus *Aspergillus nidulans* [237]. The irregular transposon mutagenesis approach was adopted to obtain genetic information regarding gene clusters of metabolites produced from a prepared cosmid library of the strain [238]. The methodology helped in obtaining information of the gene clusters for ambruticin/jerangolid [239,240], aurachin [240,241], disorazol [242] and tubulysin [243] metabolites. In *Cystobacter fuscus* Cb f17, irregular transposon mutation helped in the recognition of a particular regulatory element for a metabolite [244]. The adopted methodology helped in unravelling information of the biosynthetic gene cluster with two components (StiR) associated with the synthesis of the polyketide stigmatellin. Recognition of ChiR protein following detachment of the promoter binding protein by the biomagnetic bead assay revealed its role in the biosynthesis of the metabolite chivosazol in *Sorangium cellulosum* So ce56, as its overexpression led to a 5-fold increase in the production of chivosazol [245]. Alternatively, intentional inactivation of the gene cluster followed by screening of mutants for non-production of the explicit metabolite compared with the wild phenotypes helped in the recognition of myxochelins, myxochromides and aurafurones [246,247]. Additionally, shot-gun genome sequencing can be adopted to obtain information of the gene clusters for the identification of different metabolites, as observed for phosphoglycolipid moenomycin A [248,249].

To overcome the problem of recalcitrance of a strain for manipulation, heterologous expression of gene clusters (both orphan and known) in a suitable host that offers advantages for genetic manipulation seems a suitable alternative for exploring the function of genes [247]. Using specific hosts such as *Myxococcus xanthus* and a few other bacterial strains such as *Pseudomonas*, it is possible to arrange different gene sets in a codon-optimized manner for heterologous expression that abolishes the requirement for genetic engineering of the host [250]. Though *Myxococcus xanthus* shares codon usage and other physiological parameters with a majority of the *Myxobacterial* species, *Pseudomonads* offers the advantage of a growth rate on par with *E. coli*, with plasmids harboring inducible promoters. Examples of heterologous expression of gene clusters for metabolites, such as epothilone in *M. Xanthus* [251], *Streptomyces coelicolor* [252] and *E. coli* [253], myxochromide S in *Pseudomonas putida* [247,254], soraphen in *Streptomyces lividans* [255], myxothiazol in both *M. Xanthus* [256] and *P. putida* [257] and flaviolin in three *Pseudomonas* strains [257], are available. Employment of Red/ET recombination technology has overcome the limitation of cluster reconstruction associated with the heterologous gene expression by enabling reconstruction of gene clusters onto a suitable vector [258]. Recently, an approach of combining *Myxobacterial* biosynthetic machineries has been explored for production of novel metabolites in a so-called combinatorial biosynthesis approach [259].

6. Conclusions and Future Perspectives

The escalating problem of resistance against the current regime of antibiotics has increased concern, particularly related to treatment of human diseases. It has resulted in a community crisis, necessitating the requirement to undertake studies towards development of effective alternatives that could replace or supplement the antibiotics in counteracting occurrence at a global scale. Based on this scenario, studies were undertaken to explore natural resources towards the development of potent products that offer promise for treatment of different diseases. Exhibiting potent antimicrobial activity, secondary metabolites of microbial origin (in particular Myxobacteria) were investigated for possible use in the prevention and treatment of diseases. Myxobacteria, a highly adaptable and cosmopolitan group of microorganisms, were screened at genome and metabolome levels for identification and characterization of metabolites that can serve as potent lead structures for drug development. Evaluation of the rich repertoire of *Myxobacterial* metabolites for safety, specificity, distribution, immune modulation and anti-infectivity potential revealed information of novel antimicrobials that offer great potential to be utilized in the manufacturing of drugs. Despite the fact that *Myxobacterials* exhibit survival under different habitats and extreme climatic conditions, secondary metabolites of *Myxobacterial* origin were found effective in the treatment of a wide range of diseases. Studies need to be undertaken to gain insight into the production mechanism that holds promise in elucidating the regulatory circuit of different secondary metabolites towards optimal design of a strategic plan for enhancing their production. Alongside strategic approaches for elucidating the potency of the secondary metabolites using recently developed techniques that offer flexibility to approval strategies, consistency in safety, efficacy and delivery methods need to be adapted to broaden exploration, and as such adoption of the secondary metabolites of *Myxobacterial* origin.

Author Contributions: Conceptualization, A.A.S. and A.T.J.; writing—original draft preparation, M.A.B. (Mudasir Ahmad Bhat), M.A.B. (Mujtaba Aamir Bhat) and A.K.M.; writing—editing, M.I.B., S.R., I.A.R. and A.T.J.; structures, O.B.; supervision, A.A.S. and A.T.J.; funding acquisition, A.K.M., I.A.R. and A.T.J. All authors have read and agreed to the published version of the manuscript.

Funding: This work was supported by the Department of Science and Technology, India, under the Science and Engineering Research Board (DST-SERB), grant no. CRG/2019/004106.

Institutional Review Board Statement: Not applicable.

Informed Consent Statement: Not applicable.

Data Availability Statement: Not applicable.

Acknowledgments: The authors extend their appreciation to their fellow colleagues, whose helped in improving the contents of the manuscript.

Conflicts of Interest: The authors declare that they have no conflict of interest.

References

1. Gerth, K.; Pradella, S.; Perlova, O.; Beyer, S.; Müller, R. Myxobacteria: Proficient producers of novel natural products with various biological activities-Past and future biotechnological aspects with the focus on the genus *Sorangium*. *J. Biotechnol.* **2003**, *106*, 233–253. [CrossRef] [PubMed]
2. Kim, Y.S.; Bae, W.C.; Back, S.J. Bioactive substances from myxobacteria. *Korean J. Microbiol. Biotechnol.* **2003**, *31*, 1–12.
3. Weissman, K.J.; Muller, R. Myxobacterial secondary metabolites: Bioactivities and modes-of-action. *Nat. Prod. Rep.* **2010**, *27*, 1276–1295. [CrossRef] [PubMed]
4. Dawid, W. Biology and global distribution of myxobacteria in soils. *FEMS Microbiol. Rev.* **2000**, *24*, 403–427. [CrossRef]
5. Shimkets, L.J.; Dworkin, M.; Reichenbach, H. The myxobacteria. In *The Prokaryotes*; Springer: New York, NY, USA, 2006; pp. 31–115.
6. Reichenbach, H. Myxobacteria, producers of novel bioactive substances. *J. Ind. Microbiol. Biotech.* **2001**, *27*, 149–156. [CrossRef] [PubMed]
7. Sanford, R.A.; Cole, J.R.; Tiedje, J.M. Characterization and Description of *Anaeromyxobacter dehalogenans* gen. nov., sp. nov., an Aryl-Halorespiring Facultative Anaerobic Myxobacterium. *Appl. Environ. Microbiol.* **2002**, *68*, 893–900. [CrossRef]
8. Sharma, G.; Yao, A.I.; Smaldone, G.T.; Liang, J.; Long, M.; Facciotti, M.T.; Singer, M. Global gene expression analysis of the *Myxococcus xanthus* developmental time course. *Genomics* **2021**, *113*, 120–134. [CrossRef]
9. Wrótniak-Drzewiecka, W.; Brzezińska, A.J.; Dahm, H.; Ingle, A.P.; Rai, M. Current trends in myxobacteria research. *Ann. Microbiol.* **2016**, *66*, 17–33. [CrossRef]

10. Livingstone, P.G.; Morphew, R.M.; Whitworth, D.E. Genome Sequencing and Pan-Genome Analysis of 23 Corallococcus spp. Strains Reveal Unexpected Diversity, With Particular Plasticity of Predatory Gene Sets. *Front. Microbiol.* **2018**, *9*, 3187. [CrossRef]
11. Sajedi, H.; Mohammadipanah, F.; Pashaei, A. Automated identification of Myxobacterial genera using Convolutional Neural Network. *Sci. Rep.* **2019**, *9*, 18238. [CrossRef]
12. Mohr, K.I. Diversity of Myxobacteria-We Only See the Tip of the Iceberg. *Microorganisms* **2018**, *6*, 84. [CrossRef]
13. Azam, M.; Jan, A.T.; Haq, Q.M.R. blaCTX-M-152, a Novel Variant of CTX-M-group-25, Identified in a Study Performed on the Prevalence of Multidrug Resistance among Natural Inhabitants of River Yamuna, India. *Front. Microbiol.* **2016**, *7*, 176. [CrossRef]
14. Hemlata; Jan, A.T.; Tiwari, A. The Ever-*Changing* Face of Antibiotic Resistance: Prevailing Problems and Preventive Measures. *Curr. Drug Metab.* **2017**, *18*, 69–77. [CrossRef]
15. Hemlata; Bhat, M.A.; Kumar, V.; Ahmed, M.Z.; Alqahtani, A.S.; Alqahtani, M.S.; Jan, A.T.; Rahman, S.; Tiwari, A. Screening of natural compounds for identification of novel inhibitors against β-lactamase CTX-M-152 reported among *Kluyvera georgiana* isolates: An in vitro and in silico study. *Microb. Pathog.* **2021**, *150*, 104688. [CrossRef] [PubMed]
16. Sultan, I.; Rahman, S.; Jan, A.T.; Siddiqui, M.T.; Mondal, A.H.; Haq, Q.M.R. Antibiotics, Resistome and Resistance Mechanisms: A Bacterial Perspective. *Front. Microbiol.* **2018**, *9*, 2066. [CrossRef] [PubMed]
17. AlSheikh, H.M.A.; Sultan, I.; Kumar, V.; Rather, I.A.; Al-Sheikh, H.; Tasleem Jan, A.; Haq, Q.M.R. Plant-Based Phytochemicals as Possible Alternative to Antibiotics in Combating Bacterial Drug Resistance. *Antibiotics* **2020**, *9*, 480. [CrossRef] [PubMed]
18. Ringel, S.M.; Greenough, R.C.; Roemer, S.; Connor, D.; Gutt, A.L.; Blair, B.; Kanter, G.; von Strandtmann, M. Ambruticin (W7783), a new antifungal antibiotic. *J. Antibiot.* **1977**, *30*, 371–375. [CrossRef]
19. Wu, Z.H.; Jiang, D.M.; Li, P.; Li, Y.Z. Exploring the diversity of myxobacteria in a soil niche by myxobacteria-specific primers and probes. *Environ. Microbiol.* **2005**, *7*, 1602–1610. [CrossRef]
20. Hook, L.A. Distribution of Myxobacters in Aquatic Habitats of an Alkaline Bog. *Appl. Environ. Microbiol.* **1977**, *34*, 333–335. [CrossRef] [PubMed]
21. Rückert, G. Myxobakterien-Artenspektren von Boden in Abhängigkeit von bodenbildenden Faktoren unterbesonderer Berücksichtigung der Bodenreaktion. *Z. Pflanzenernaehr. Bodenkd.* **1979**, *142*, 330–343. [CrossRef]
22. Reichenbach, H. The ecology of the myxobacteria. *Environ. Microbiol.* **1999**, *1*, 15–21. [CrossRef]
23. Li, S.G.; Zhou, X.W.; Li, P.F.; Han, K.; Li, W.; Li, Z.F.; Wu, Z.H.; Li, Y.Z. The existence and diversity of myxobacteria in lake mud-A previously unexplored myxobacteria habitat. *Environ. Microbiol. Rep.* **2012**, *4*, 587–595. [CrossRef] [PubMed]
24. Brockman, E.R. Fruiting myxobacteria from the South Carolina coast. *J. Bacteriol.* **1963**, *94*, 1253–1254. [CrossRef]
25. Felder, S.; Dreisigacker, S.; Kehraus, S.; Neu, E.; Bierbaum, G.; Wright, P.R.; Menche, D.; Schäberle, T.F.; König, G.M. Salimabromide: Unexpected chemistry from the obligate marine myxobacterium *Enhygromxya salina*. *Chemistry* **2013**, *19*, 9319–9324. [CrossRef]
26. Felder, S.; Kehraus, S.; Neu, E.; Bierbaum, G.; Schäberle, T.F.; König, G.M. Salimyxins and enhygrolides: Antibiotic, sponge-related metabolites from the obligate marine myxobacterium *Enhygromyxa salina*. *Chem. Bio. Chem.* **2013**, *14*, 1363–1371. [CrossRef]
27. Fudou, R.; Iizuka, T.; Sato, S.; Ando, T.; Shimba, N.; Yamanaka, S. Haliangicin, a novel antifungal metabolite produced by a marine myxobacterium. 2. Isolation and structural elucidation. *J. Antibiot.* **2001**, *54*, 153–156. [CrossRef] [PubMed]
28. Sun, Y.; Tomura, T.; Sato, J.; Iizuka, T.; Fudou, R.; Ojika, M. Isolation and Biosynthetic Analysis of Haliamide, a New PKS-NRPS Hybrid Metabolite from the Marine Myxobacterium *Haliangium ochraceum*. *Molecules* **2016**, *21*, 59. [CrossRef] [PubMed]
29. Fudou, R.; Jojima, Y.; Iizuka, T.; Yamanaka, S. *Haliangium ochraceum* gen. nov., sp. nov. and *Haliangium tepidum* sp. nov.: Novel moderately halophilic myxobacteria isolated from coastal saline environments. *J. Gen. Appl. Microbiol.* **2002**, *48*, 109–116. [CrossRef]
30. Iizuka, T.; Jojima, Y.; Fudou, R.; Tokura, M.; Hiraishi, A.; Yamanaka, S. *Enhygromyxa salina* gen. nov.; sp. nov., a slightly halophilic myxobacterium isolated from the coastal areas of Japan. *Syst. Appl. Microbiol.* **2003**, *26*, 189–196. [CrossRef]
31. Iizuka, T.; Jojima, Y.; Fudou, R.; Hiraishi, A.; Ahn, J.W.; Yamanaka, S. *Plesiocystis pacifica* gen. nov.; sp. nov.; a marine myxobacterium that contains dihydrogenated menaquinone, isolated from the Pacific coasts of Japan. *Int. J. Syst. Evol. Microbiol.* **2003**, *53*, 189–195. [CrossRef]
32. Iizuka, T.; Jojima, Y.; Hayakawa, A.; Fujii, T.; Yamanaka, S.; Fudou, R. *Pseudenhygromyxa salsuginis* gen. nov., sp. nov., a myxobacterium isolated from an estuarine marsh. *Int. J. Syst. Evol. Microbiol.* **2013**, *63*, 1360–1369. [CrossRef] [PubMed]
33. Brinkhoff, T.; Fischer, D.; Vollmers, J.; Voget, S.; Beardsley, C.; Thole, S.; Mussmann, M.; Kunze, B.; Wagner-Döbler, I.; Daniel, R.; et al. Biogeography and phylogenetic diversity of a cluster of exclusively marine myxobacteria. *Int. J. Syst. Evol. Microbiol.* **2012**, *6*, 1260–1272. [CrossRef]
34. Tian, F.; Yong, Y.; Chen, B.; Li, H.; Yao, Y.F.; Guo, X.K. Bacterial, archaeal and eukaryotic diversity in Arctic sediment as revealed by 16S rRNA and 18S rRNA gene clone libraries analysis. *Polar Biol.* **2009**, *32*, 93–103. [CrossRef]
35. Zhang, X.; Yao, Q.; Cai, Z.; Xie, X.; Zhu, H. Isolation and Identification of Myxobacteria from Saline-Alkaline Soils in Xinjiang, China. *PLoS ONE* **2013**, *8*, e70466. [CrossRef] [PubMed]
36. Li, B.; Yao, Q.; Zhu, H. Approach to analyze the diversity of myxobacteria in soil by semi-nested PCR-denaturing gradient gel electrophoresis (DGGE) based on taxon-specific gene. *PLoS ONE* **2014**, *9*, e108877. [CrossRef]

37. Thomas, S.H.; Padilla-Crespo, E.; Jardine, P.M.; Sanford, R.A.; Löffler, F.E. Diversity and distribution of anaeromyxobacter strains in a uranium-contaminated subsurface environment with a nonuniform groundwater flow. *Appl. Environ. Microbiol.* **2009**, *75*, 3679–3687. [CrossRef]
38. Treude, N.; Rosencrantz, D.; Liesack, W.; Schnell, S. Strain FAc12, a dissimilatory iron-reducing member of the Anaeromyxobacter subgroup of Myxococcales. *FEMS Microbiol. Ecol.* **2003**, *44*, 261–269. [CrossRef]
39. Lin, J.; Ratering, S.; Schnell, S. Microbial iron cylce in corrosion material of drinking water pipelines. *Ann. Agrar. Sci.* **2011**, *9*, 18–25.
40. Kudo, K.; Yamaguchi, N.; Makino, T.; Ohtsuka, T.; Kimura, K.; Dong, D.T.; Amachi, S. Release of arsenic from soil by a novel dissimilatory arsenate reducing bacterium, Anaeromyxobacter sp. strain PSR-1. *Appl. Environ. Microbiol.* **2013**, *79*, 4635–4642. [CrossRef]
41. Brockman, E.R. Myxobacters from Arid Mexican Soil. *Appl. Environ. Microbiol.* **1976**, *32*, 642–644. [CrossRef]
42. Gerth, K.; Müller, R. Moderately thermophilic Myxobacteria: Novel potential for the production of natural products isolation and characterization. *Environ. Microbiol.* **2005**, *7*, 874–880. [CrossRef]
43. Mohr, K.I.; Moradi, A.; Glaeser, S.P.; Kämpfer, P.; Gemperlein, K.; Nübel, U.; Schumann, P.; Müller, R.; Wink, J. *Nannocystis konarekensis* sp. nov.; a novel myxobacterium from an Iranian desert. *Int. J. Syst. Evol. Microbiol.* **2018**, *68*, 721–729. [CrossRef] [PubMed]
44. Reichenbach, H. The Myxococcales. In *Bergey's Manual of Systematic Bacteriology*, 2nd ed.; Garrity, G.M., Ed.; Springer: New York, NY, USA, 2005.
45. Mohiuddin, A.K. Chemistry of Secondary Metabolites. *Ann. Clin. Toxicol.* **2019**, *2*, 1014.
46. Xiao, Y.; Wei, X.; Ebright, R.; Wall, D. Antibiotic production by myxobacteria plays a role in predation. *J. Bacteriol.* **2011**, *193*, 4626–4633. [CrossRef] [PubMed]
47. Wenzel, S.C.; Muller, R. Myxobacteria-Microbial factories for the production of bioactive secondary metabolites. *Mol. BioSyst.* **2009**, *5*, 567–574. [CrossRef]
48. Herrmann, J.; Fayad, A.A.; Müller, R. Natural products from myxobacteria: Novel metabolites and bioactivities. *Nat. Prod. Rep.* **2017**, *34*, 135–160. [CrossRef] [PubMed]
49. Korp, J.; Gurovic, M.S.V.; Nett, M. Antibiotics from predatory bacteria. *Beilstein J. Org. Chem.* **2016**, *12*, 594–607. [CrossRef] [PubMed]
50. Albataineh, H.; Stevens, D.C. Marine Myxobacteria: A Few Good Halophiles. *Mar. Drugs* **2018**, *16*, 209. [CrossRef]
51. Reichenbach, H.; Höfle, G. Myxobacteria as Producers of Secondary Metabolites. In *Drug Discovery from Nature*; Grabley, S., Thiericke, R., Eds.; Springer: Berlin, Germany, 1999; pp. 149–179.
52. Reichenbach, H.; Höfle, G. Biologically active secondary metabolites from myxobacteria. *Biotechnol. Adv.* **1993**, *11*, 219–277. [CrossRef]
53. Kaur, R.; Singh, S.K.; Kaur, R.; Kumari, A.; Kaur, R. *Myxococcus xanthus*: A source of antimicrobials and natural bio-control agent. *Pharm. Innov.* **2017**, *6*, 260–262.
54. Wilson, C.N. Endacea Inc. Methods for Preventing and Treating Tissue Injury and Sepsis Associated with *Yersinia pestis* Infection. U.S. Patent 12/220,377, 19 February 2009.
55. Raju, R.; Garcia, R.; Müller, R. Angiolactone, a new Butyrolactone isolated from the terrestrial myxobacterium, Angiococcus sp. *J. Antibiot* **2014**, *67*, 725–726. [CrossRef]
56. Tautz, T.; Hoffmann, J.; Hoffmann, T.; Steinmetz, H.; Washausen, P.; Kunze, B.; Huch, V.; Kitsche, A.; Reichenbach, H.; Muller, R.; et al. Isolation, structure elucidation, biosynthesis, and synthesis of Antalid, a secondary metabolite from *Polyangium species*. *Org. Lett.* **2016**, *18*, 2560–2563. [CrossRef]
57. Hofle, G.; Böhlendorf, B.; Fecker, T.; Sasse, F.; Kunze, B. Semisynthesis and antiplasmodial activity of the quinoline alkaloid aurachin E. *J. Nat. Prod.* **2008**, *71*, 1967–1969. [CrossRef] [PubMed]
58. Kunze, B.; Reck, M.; Dötsch, A.; Lemme, A.; Schummer, D.; Irschik, H.; Steinmetz, H.; Wagner-Döbler, I. Damage of *Streptococcus mutans* biofilms by carolacton, a secondary metabolite from the myxobacterium *Sorangium cellulosum*. *BMC Microbiol.* **2010**, *10*, 199. [CrossRef]
59. Jungmann, K.; Jansen, R.; Gerth, K.; Huch, V.; Krug, D.; Fenical, W.; Müller, R. Two of a Kind-The Biosynthetic Pathways of Chlorotonil and Anthracimycin. *ACS Chem. Biol.* **2015**, *10*, 2480–2490. [CrossRef] [PubMed]
60. Schiefer, A.; Schmitz, A.; Schäberle, T.F.; Specht, S.; Lämmer, C.; Johnston, K.L.; Vassylyev, D.G.; König, G.M.; Hoerauf, A.; Pfarr, K. Corallopyronin A specifically targets and depletes essential obligate *Wolbachia endobacteria* from filarial nematodes in vivo. *J. Infect. Dis.* **2012**, *206*, 249–257. [CrossRef]
61. Schmitz, A.; Kehraus, S.; Schaberle, T.F.; Neu, E.; Almeida, C.; Roth, M.; König, G.M. Corallorazines from the Myxobacterium *Corallococcus coralloides*. *J. Nat. Prod.* **2014**, *77*, 159–163. [CrossRef] [PubMed]
62. Kunze, B.; Jansen, R.; Höfle, G.; Reichenbach, H. Crocacin, a new electron transport inhibitor from *Chondromyces crocatus* (myxobacteria). Production, isolation, physico-chemical and biological properties. *J. Antibiot.* **1994**, *47*, 881–886. [CrossRef]
63. Baumann, S.; Herrmann, J.; Raju, R.; Steinmetz, H.; Mohr, K.I.; Huttel, S.; Harmrolfs, K.; Stadler, M.; Muller, R. Cystobactamids: Myxobacterial topoisomerase inhibitors exhibiting potent antibacterial activity. *Angew. Chem. Int. Ed.* **2014**, *53*, 14605–14609. [CrossRef] [PubMed]

64. Nadmid, S.; Plaza, A.; Garcia, R.; Müller, R. Cystochromones, Unusual Chromone-Containing Polyketides from the Myxobacterium *Cystobacter* sp. MCy9104. *J. Nat. Prod.* **2015**, *78*, 2023–2028. [CrossRef] [PubMed]
65. Etzbach, L.; Plaza, A.; Garcia, R.; Baumann, S.; Müller, R. Cystomanamides: Structure and biosynthetic pathway of a family of glycosylated lipopeptides from myxobacteria. *Org. Lett.* **2014**, *16*, 2414–2417. [CrossRef]
66. Ojika, M.; Suzuki, Y.; Tsukamoto, A.; Sakagami, Y.; Fudou, R.; Yoshimura, T.; Yamanaka, S. Cystothiazoles A and B, new bithiazole-type antibiotics from the myxobacterium *Cystobacter fuscus*. *J. Antibiot.* **1998**, *51*, 275–281. [CrossRef] [PubMed]
67. Surup, F.; Viehrig, K.; Mohr, K.I.; Herrmann, J.; Jansen, R.; Müller, R. Disciformycins A and B: 12-membered macrolide glycoside antibiotics from the myxobacterium *Pyxidicoccus fallax* active against multiresistant *staphylococci*. *Angewandte Chemie* (International ed. in English). *Angew. Chem. Int. Ed. Engl.* **2014**, *53*, 13588–13591. [CrossRef]
68. Muddala, R.; Acosta, J.A.; Barbosa, L.C.; Boukouvalas, J. Synthesis of the Marine Myxobacterial Antibiotic Enhygrolide A. *J. Nat. Prod.* **2017**, *80*, 2166–2169. [CrossRef]
69. Schieferdecker, S.; König, S.; Weigel, C.; Dahse, H.M.; Werz, O.; Nett, M. Structure and biosynthetic assembly of gulmirecins, macrolide antibiotics from the predatory bacterium *Pyxidicoccus fallax*. *Chemistry* **2014**, *20*, 15933–15940. [CrossRef] [PubMed]
70. Dávila-Céspedes, A.; Hufendiek, P.; Crüsemann, M.; Schäberle, T.F.; König, G.M. Marine-derived myxobacteria of the suborder Nannocystineae: An underexplored source of structurally intriguing and biologically active metabolites. *Beilstein J. Org. Chem.* **2016**, *12*, 969. [CrossRef] [PubMed]
71. Nadmid, S.; Plaza, A.; Lauro, G.; Garcia, R.; Bifulco, G.; Müller, R. Hyalachelins A-C, unusual siderophores isolated from the terrestrial myxobacterium *Hyalangium minutum*. *Org. Lett.* **2014**, *16*, 4130–4133. [CrossRef]
72. Okanya, P.W.; Mohr, K.I.; Gerth, K.; Steinmetz, H.; Huch, V.; Jansen, R.; Müller, R. Hyaladione, an S-methyl cyclohexadiene-dione from *Hyalangium minutum*. *J. Nat. Prod.* **2012**, *75*, 768–770. [CrossRef]
73. Okanya, P.; Mohr, K.; Gerth, K.; Kessler, W.; Jansen, R.; Stadler, M.; Müller, R. Hyafurones, hyapyrrolines and hyapyrones: Polyketides from *Hyalangium minutum*. *J. Nat. Prod.* **2014**, *77*, 1420–1429. [CrossRef]
74. Zander, W.; Mohr, K.I.; Gerth, K.; Jansen, R.; Müller, R. P-hydroxyacetophenone amides from *cystobacter ferrugineus*, strain Cb G35. *J. Nat. Prod.* **2011**, *74*, 1358–1363. [CrossRef]
75. Jansen, R.; Sood, S.; Huch, V.; Kunze, B.; Stadler, M.; Müller, R. Pyrronazols, metabolites from the mxobacteria *Nannocystis pusilla* and *N. exedens* are unusual chlorinated pyrone-oxazole-pyrroles. *J. Nat. Prod.* **2014**, *77*, 320–326. [CrossRef]
76. Barbier, J.; Jansen, R.; Irschik, H.; Benson, S.; Gerth, K.; Böhlendorf, B.; Höfle, G.; Reichenbach, H.; Wegner, J.; Zeilinger, C.; et al. Isolation and total synthesis of icumazoles and noricumazoles-Antifungal antibiotics and cation-channel blockers from *Sorangium cellulosum*. *Angew. Chem. Int. Ed.* **2012**, *51*, 1256–1260. [CrossRef]
77. Steinmetz, H.; Mohr, K.; Zander, W.; Jansen, R.; Müller, R. Indiacens A and B: Prenyl indoles from the myxobacterium *Sandaracinus amylolyticus*. *J. Nat. Prod.* **2012**, *75*, 1803–1805. [CrossRef] [PubMed]
78. Marsch, N.; Jones, P.G.; Lindel, T. SmI2-mediated dimerization of indolylbutenones and synthesis of the myxobacterial natural product indiacen B. *Beilstein J. Org. Chem.* **2015**, *11*, 1700–1706. [CrossRef] [PubMed]
79. Symkenberg, G.; Kalesse, M. Structure elucidation and total synthesis of kulkenon. *Angew. Chem. Int. Ed.* **2014**, *53*, 1795–1798. [CrossRef]
80. Kopp, M.; Irschik, H.; Gemperlein, K.; Buntin, K.; Meiser, P.; Weissman, K.J.; Bode, H.B.; Müller, R. Insights into the complex biosynthesis of the leupyrrins in *Sorangium cellulosum* So ce690. *Mol. Biosyst.* **2011**, *7*, 1549–1563. [CrossRef] [PubMed]
81. Keller, L.; Plaza, A.; Dubiella, C.; Groll, M.; Kaiser, M.; Müller, R. Macyranones: Structure, Biosynthesis, and Binding Mode of an Unprecedented Epoxyketone that Targets the 20S Proteasome. *J. Am. Chem. Soc.* **2015**, *137*, 8121–8130. [CrossRef] [PubMed]
82. Irschik, H.; Washausen, P.; Sasse, F.; Fohrer, J.; Huch, V.; Müller, R.; Prusov, E.V. Isolation, structure elucidation, and biological activity of maltepolides: Remarkable macrolides from myxobacteria. *Angew. Chem. Int. Ed.* **2013**, *52*, 5402–5405. [CrossRef]
83. Irschik, H.; Schummer, D.; Höfle, G.; Reichenbach, H.; Steinmetz, H.; Jansen, R. Etnangien, a macrolide-polyene antibiotic from *Sorangium cellulosum* that inhibits nucleic acid polymerases. *J. Nat. Prod.* **2007**, *70*, 1060–1063. [CrossRef]
84. Hoffmann, T.; Müller, S.; Nadmid, S.; Garcia, R.; Müller, R. Microsclerodermins from terrestrial myxobacteria: An intriguing biosynthesis likely connected to a sponge symbiont. *J. Am. Chem. Soc.* **2013**, *135*, 16904–16911. [CrossRef]
85. Guzman, E.A.; Maers, K.; Roberts, J.; Kemami-Wangun, H.V.; Harmody, D.; Wright, A.E. The marine natural product microsclerodermin A is a novel inhibitor of the nuclear factor kappa B and induces apoptosis in pancreatic cancer cells. *Invest. New Drugs* **2015**, *33*, 86–94. [CrossRef] [PubMed]
86. Kunze, B.; Bedorf, N.; Kohl, W.; Höfle, G.; Reichenbach, H. Myxochelin A, a new iron-chelating compound from *Angiococcus disciformis* (Myxobacterales). Production, isolation, physico-chemical and biological properties. *J. Antibiot.* **1989**, *42*, 14–17. [CrossRef]
87. Schieferdecker, S.; König, S.; Koeberle, A.; Dahse, H.M.; Werz, O.; Nett, M. Myxochelins target human 5-lipoxygenase. *J. Nat. Prod.* **2015**, *78*, 335–338. [CrossRef]
88. Gulder, T.A.; Neff, S.; Schüz, T.; Winkler, T.; Gees, R.; Böhlendorf, B. The myxocoumarins A and B from *Stigmatella aurantiaca* strain MYX-030. *Beilstein J. Org. Chem.* **2013**, *9*, 2579–2585. [CrossRef] [PubMed]
89. Cortina, N.S.; Krug, D.; Plaza, A.; Revermann, O.; Müller, R. Myxoprincomide: A natural product from *Myxococcus xanthus* discovered by comprehensive analysis of the secondary metabolome. *Angew. Chem. Int. Ed.* **2012**, *51*, 811–816. [CrossRef]

90. Goldman, B.S.; Nierman, W.C.; Kaiser, D.; Slater, S.C.; Durkin, A.S.; Eisen, J.A.; Ronning, C.M.; Barbazuk, W.B.; Blanchard, M.; Field, C.; et al. Evolution of sensory complexity recorded in a myxobacterial genome. *Proc. Natl. Acad. Sci. USA* **2006**, *103*, 15200–15205. [CrossRef] [PubMed]
91. Schley, C.; Altmeyer, M.O.; Swart, R.; Müller, R.; Huber, C.G. Proteome analysis of *Myxococcus xanthus* by off-line two-dimensional chromatographic separation using monolithic poly-(styrene-divinylbenzene) columns combined with ion-trap tandem mass spectrometry. *J. Proteome Res.* **2006**, *5*, 2760–2768. [CrossRef]
92. Moy, T.I.; Daniel, A.; Hardy, C.; Jackson, A.; Rehrauer, O.; Hwang, Y.S.; Zou, D.; Nguyen, K.; Silverman, J.A.; Li, Q.; et al. Evaluating the activity of the RNA polymerase inhibitor myxopyronin B against Staphylococcus aureus. *FEMS Microbiol. Lett.* **2011**, *319*, 176–179. [CrossRef]
93. Irschik, H.; Gerth, K.; Kemmer, T.; Steinmetz, H.; Reichenbach, H. The myxovalargins, new peptide antibiotics from *Myxococcus fulvus* (myxobacterales). I. cultivation, isolation, and some chemical and biological properties. *J. Antibiot.* **1983**, *36*, 6–12. [CrossRef]
94. Gerth, K.; Irschik, H.; Reichenbach, H.; Trowitzsch, W. The myxovirescins, a family of antibiotics from *Myxococcus virescens* (Myxobacterales). *J. Antibiot.* **1982**, *35*, 1454–1459. [CrossRef]
95. Vogeley, L.; El-Arnaout, T.; Bailey, J. Structural basis of lipoprotein signal peptidase II action and inhibition by the antibiotic globomycin. *Science* **2016**, *351*, 876–880. [CrossRef] [PubMed]
96. Gentzsch, J.; Hinkelmann, B.; Kaderali, L.; Irschik, H.; Jansen, R.; Sasse, F.; Frank, R.; Pietschmann, T. Hepatitis C virus complete life cycle screen for identification of small molecules with pro- or antiviral activity. *Antivir. Res.* **2011**, *89*, 136–148. [CrossRef]
97. Beck, S.; Henß, L.; Weidner, T.; Herrmann, J.; Müller, R.; Chao, Y.; Weber, C.; Sliva, K.; Schnierle, S. Identification of inhibitors of Ebola virus pseudotyped vectors from a myxobacterial compound library. *Antivir. Res.* **2016**, *132*, 85–91. [CrossRef]
98. Guo, W.J.; Tao, W.Y. Phoxalone, a novel macrolide from *Sorangium cellulosum*: Structure identification and its anti-tumor bioactivity in vitro. *Biotechnol. Lett.* **2008**, *30*, 349–356. [CrossRef]
99. Glaus, F.; Dedić, D.; Tare, P.; Nagaraja, V.; Rodrigues, L.; Aínsa, J.A.; Kunze, J.; Schneider, G.; Hartkoorn, R.C.; Cole, S.T.; et al. Total Synthesis of Ripostatin B and Structure–Activity Relationship Studies on Ripostatin Analogs. *J. Org. Chem.* **2018**, *83*, 7150–7172. [CrossRef] [PubMed]
100. Blunt, J.W.; Copp, B.R.; Keyzers, R.A.; Munro, M.H.; Prinsep, M.R. Marine natural products. *Nat. Prod. Rep.* **2015**, *32*, 116–211. [CrossRef]
101. Ahn, J.W.; Jang, K.H.; Chung, S.C.; Oh, K.B.; Shin, J. Sorangiadenosine, a new sesquiterpene adenoside from the myxobacterium *Sorangium cellulosum*. *Org. Lett.* **2008**, *10*, 1167–1169. [CrossRef] [PubMed]
102. Okoth, D.A.; Hug, J.J.; Garcia, R.; Spröer, C.; Overmann, J.; Müller, R. 2-Hydroxysorangiadenosine: Structure and Biosynthesis of a Myxobacterial Sesquiterpene-Nucleoside. *Molecules* **2020**, *25*, 2676. [CrossRef] [PubMed]
103. Li, Y.; Weissman, K.J.; Müller, R. Myxochelin biosynthesis: Direct evidence for two- and four-electron reduction of a carrier protein-bound thioester. *J. Am. Chem Soc.* **2008**, *130*, 7554–7555. [CrossRef]
104. Karwehl, S.; Jansen, R.; Huch, V.; Stadler, M. Sorazolons, Carbazole Alkaloids from Sorangium cellulosum Strain Soce375. *J. Nat. Prod.* **2016**, *79*, 369–375. [CrossRef]
105. Zander, W.; Irschik, H.; Augustiniak, H.; Herrmann, M.; Jansen, R.; Steinmetz, H.; Gerth, K.; Kessler, W.; Kalesse, M.; Hofle, G.; et al. Sulfangolids, macrolide sulfate esters from *Sorangium cellulosum*. *Chemistry* **2012**, *18*, 6264–6271. [CrossRef]
106. Fleta-Soriano, E.; Martinez, J.P.; Hinkelmann, B.; Gerth, K.; Washausen, P.; Diez, J.; Frank, R.; Sasse, F.; Meyerhans, A. The myxobacterial metabolite ratjadone A inhibits HIV infection by blocking the Rev/CRM1-mediated nuclear export pathway. *Microb. Cell Factories* **2014**, *13*, 17. [CrossRef]
107. Steinmetz, H.; Irschik, H.; Kunze, B.; Reichenbach, H.; Hoefle, G.; Jansen, R. Thuggacins, macrolide antibiotics active against *Mycobacterium tuberculosis*: Isolation from myxobacteria, structure elucidation, conformation analysis and biosynthesis. *Chemistry* **2007**, *13*, 5822–5832. [CrossRef] [PubMed]
108. Mdluli, K.; Kaneko, T.; Upton, A. The tuberculosis drug discovery and development pipeline and emerging drug targets. *Cold Spring Harb. Perspect. Med.* **2015**, *5*, a021154. [CrossRef]
109. Plaza, A.; Garcia, R.; Bifulco, G.; Martinez, J.P.; Hüttel, S.; Sasse, F.; Meyerhans, A.; Stadler, M.; Müller, R. Aetheramides A and B, potent HIV-inhibitory depsipeptides from a myxobacterium of the new genus "Aetherobacter". *Org. Lett.* **2012**, *14*, 2854–2857. [CrossRef]
110. Ghosh, A.K.; Rao, K.V.; Akasapu, S. An Enantioselective Synthesis of a MEM-Protected Aetheramide a Derivative. *Tetrahedron Lett.* **2014**, *55*, 5191–5194. [CrossRef] [PubMed]
111. Gerstmann, L.; Kalesse, M. Total Synthesis of Aetheramide A. *Chemistry* **2016**, *22*, 11210–11212. [CrossRef]
112. Zhang, S.; Schneider, L.S.; Vick, B.; Grunert, M.; Jeremias, I.; Menche, D.; Müller, R.; Vollmar, A.M.; Liebl, J. Anti-leukemic effects of the V-ATPase inhibitor Archazolid A. *Oncotarget* **2015**, *6*, 43508–43528. [CrossRef] [PubMed]
113. Sasse, F.; Steinmetz, H.; Schupp, T.; Petersen, F.; Memmert, K.; Hofmann, H.; Heusser, C.; Brinkmann, V.; Von-matt, P.; Hofle, G.; et al. Argyrins, immunosuppressive cyclic peptides from myxobacteria. I. Production, isolation, physico-chemical and biological properties. *J. Antibiot.* **2002**, *55*, 543–551.
114. Wenzel, S.C.; Hoffmann, H.; Zhang, J.; Debussche, L.; Haag-Richter, S.; Kurz, M.; Nardi, F.; Lukat, P.; Kochems, I.; Tietgen, H.; et al. Production of the Bengamide Class of Marine Natural Products in Myxobacteria: Biosynthesis and Structure-Activity Relationships. *Angew. Chem. Int. Ed. Engl.* **2015**, *54*, 15560–15564. [CrossRef]

115. Raju, R.; Mohr, K.; Bernecker, S.; Herrmann, J.; Müller, R. Cystodienoic acid: A new diterpene isolated from the myxobacterium *Cystobacter* sp. *J. Antibiot.* **2015**, *68*, 473–475. [CrossRef] [PubMed]
116. Elnakady, Y.; Sasse, F.; Lünsdorf, H.; Reichenbach, H. Disorazol A(1), a highly effective antimitotic agent acting on tubulin polymerization and inducing apoptosis in mammalian cells. *Biochem. Pharmacol.* **2004**, *67*, 927–935. [CrossRef] [PubMed]
117. Höfle, G.; Gerth, K.; Reichenbach, H.; Kunze, B.; Sasse, F.; Forche, E.; Prusov, E.V. Isolation, biological activity evaluation, structure elucidation, and total synthesis of eliamid: A novel complex I inhibitor. *Chemistry* **2012**, *18*, 11362–11370. [CrossRef]
118. Altmann, K.H.; Pfeiffer, B.; Arseniyadis, S.; Pratt, B.; Nicolaou, K. The Chemistry and Biology of Epothilones—The Wheel Keeps Turning. *Chem. Med. Chem.* **2007**, *2*, 396–423. [CrossRef]
119. Ojima, D.; Yasui, A.; Tohyama, K.; Tokuzumi, K.; Toriihara, E.; Ito, K.; Iwasaki, A.; Tomura, T.; Ojika, M.; Suenaga, K. Total Synthesis of Miuraenamides A and D. *J. Org. Chem.* **2016**, *81*, 9886–9894. [CrossRef] [PubMed]
120. Hoffmann, H.; Kogler, H.; Heyse, W.; Matter, H.; Caspers, M.; Schummer, D.; Klemke-Jahn, C.; Bauer, A.; Penarier, G.; Debussche, L.; et al. Discovery, Structure Elucidation, and Biological Characterization of Nannocystin A, a Macrocyclic Myxobacterial Metabolite with Potent Antiproliferative Properties. *Angew. Chem. Int. Ed. Engl.* **2015**, *54*, 10145–10148. [CrossRef]
121. Krastel, P.; Roggo, S.; Schirle, M.; Ross, N.; Perruccio, F.; Aspesi, P.; Aust, T.; Buntin, K.; Estoppey, D.; Liechty, B.; et al. Nannocystin A: An Elongation Factor 1 Inhibitor from Myxobacteria with Differential Anti-Cancer Properties. *Angew. Chem. Int. Ed. Engl.* **2015**, *54*, 10149–10154. [CrossRef]
122. Jahns, C.; Hoffmann, T.; Müller, S.; Gerth, K.; Washausen, P.; Höfle, G.; Reichenbach, H.; Kalesse, M.; Müller, R. Pellasoren: Structure elucidation, biosynthesis, and total synthesis of a cytotoxic secondary metabolite from *Sorangium cellulosum*. *Angew. Chem. Int. Ed. Engl.* **2012**, *51*, 5239–5243. [CrossRef]
123. Mulwa, L.S.; Stadler, M. Antiviral compounds from Myxobacteria. *Microorganisms* **2018**, *6*, 73. [CrossRef]
124. Martinez, J.P.; Hinkelmann, B.; Fleta-Soriano, E.; Steinmetz, H.; Jansen, R.; Diez, J.; Frank, R.; Sasse, F.; Meyerhans, A. Identification of myxobacteria-derived HIV inhibitors by a high-throughput two-step infectivity assay. *Microb. Cell Factories* **2013**, *12*, 85. [CrossRef] [PubMed]
125. Roy, J.; Kaake, M.; Srinivasarao, M.; Low, P.S. Targeted Tubulysin B Hydrazide Conjugate for the Treatment of Luteinizing Hormone-Releasing Hormone Receptor-Positive Cancers. *Bioconjug. Chem.* **2018**, *29*, 2208–2214. [CrossRef] [PubMed]
126. Knauth, P.; Reichenbach, H. On the mechanism of action of the myxobacterial fungicide ambruticin. *J. Antibiot.* **2000**, *53*, 1182–1190. [CrossRef] [PubMed]
127. Irschik, H.; Schummer, D.; Gerth, K.; Höfle, G.; Reichenbach, H. ChemInform Abstract: The Tartrolons, New Boron-Containing Antibiotics from a Myxobacterium, *Sorangium cellulosum*. *J. Antibiot.* **2010**, *48*, 26–30. [CrossRef] [PubMed]
128. Kunze, B.; Jansen, R.; Pridzun, L.; Jurkiewicz, E.; Hunsmann, G.; Höfle, G.; Reichenbach, H. Thiangazole, a new thiazoline antibiotic from Polyangium sp. (myxobacteria): Production, antimicrobial activity and mechanism of action. *J. Antibiot.* **1993**, *46*, 1752–1755. [CrossRef] [PubMed]
129. Gerth, K.; Bedorf, N.; Irschik, H.; Höfle, G.; Reichenbach, H. The soraphens: A family of novel antifungal compounds from *Sorangium cellulosum* (Myxobacteria). *J. Antibiot.* **1994**, *47*, 23–31. [CrossRef]
130. Fleta-Soriano, E.; Smutná, K.; Martinez, J.P.; Oró, C.L.; Sadiq, S.K.; Mirambeau, G.; Lopez-Iglesias, C.; Bosch, M.; Pol, A.; Brönstrup, M.; et al. The myxobacterial metabolite soraphen A inhibits HIV-1 by reducing virus production and altering virion composition. *Antimicrob. Agents Chemother.* **2017**, *61*, e00739-17. [CrossRef]
131. Mohr, K.I.; Zindler, T.; Wink, J.; Wilharm, E.; Stadler, M. Myxobacteria in high moor and fen: An astonishing diversity in a neglected extreme habitat. *MicrobiologyOpen* **2017**, *6*, e00464. [CrossRef]
132. Houbraken, J.; Frisvad, J.C.; Samson, R.A. Fleming's penicillin producing strain is not *Penicillium chrysogenum* but *P. rubens*. *IMA Fungus* **2011**, *1*, 87–95. [CrossRef]
133. Schatz, A.; Bugie, E.; Waksman, S. Streptomycin: A substance exhibiting antibiotic activity against gram positive and gram-*negative* bacteria. *Proc. Exp. Biol. Med.* **1944**, *55*, 66–69. [CrossRef]
134. McGuire, J.M.; Bunch, R.L.; Anderson, R.C.; Boaz, H.E.; Flynn, E.H.; Powell, H.M.; Smith, J.W. Ilotycin a new antibiotic. *Antibiot. Chemother.* **1952**, *2*, 281–283.
135. Bartlett, J.G.; Gilbert, D.N.; Spellberg, B. Seven ways to preserve the miracle of antibiotics. *Clin. Infect. Dis.* **2013**, *56*, 1445–1450. [CrossRef]
136. Ventola, C.L. The Antibiotic Resistance Crisis: Part 1: Causes and Threats. *Pharm. Ther.* **2015**, *40*, 277–283.
137. Hesterkamp, T. Antibiotics Clinical Development and Pipeline. In *How to Overcome the Antibiotic Crisis-Facts, Challenges, Technologies and Future Perspective*; Stadler, M., Dersch, P., Eds.; Springer: Berlin, Germany, 2016; pp. 447–474.
138. Hoffmann, T.; Krug, D.; Bozkurt, N.; Duddela, S.; Jansen, R.; Garcia, R.; Gerth, K.; Steinmetz, H.; Müller, R. Correlating chemical diversity with taxonomic distance for discovery of natural products in myxobacteria. *Nat. Commun.* **2018**, *9*, 803. [CrossRef]
139. Landwehr, W.; Wolf, C.; Wink, J. Actinobacteria and Myxobacteria-Two of the Most Important Bacterial Resources for Novel Antibiotics. In *How to Overcome the Antibiotic Crisis-Facts, Challenges, Technologies & Future Perspective*; Stadler, M., Dersch, P., Eds.; Springer: Berlin, Germany, 2016.
140. Sansinenea, E.; Ortiz, A. Secondary metabolites of soil *Bacillus* spp. *Biotechnol. Lett.* **2011**, *33*, 1523–1538. [CrossRef] [PubMed]
141. Shen, Y.; Volrath, S.L.; Weatherly, S.C.; Elich, T.D.; Tong, L. A mechanism for the potent inhibition of eukaryotic acetyl-coenzyme A carboxylase by soraphen A, a macrocyclic polyketide natural product. *Mol. Cell* **2004**, *16*, 881–891. [CrossRef] [PubMed]

142. Mühlradt, P.F.; Sasse, F. Epothilone B stabilizes microtubuli of macrophages like taxol without showing taxol-like endotoxin activity. *Cancer Res.* **1997**, *57*, 3344–3346.
143. Goodin, S.; Kane, M.P.; Rubin, E.H. Epothilones: Mechanism of action and biologic activity. *J. Clin. Oncol.* **2004**, *22*, 2015–2025. [CrossRef]
144. Peterson, J.K.; Tucker, C.; Favours, E.; Cheshire, P.J.; Creech, J.; Billups, C.A.; Smykla, R.; Lee, F.Y.F.; Houghton, P.J. In vivo evaluation of Ixabepilone (BMS247550), A novel epothilone B derivative, against pediatric cancer models. *Clin. Cancer Res.* **2005**, *11*, 6950–6958. [CrossRef] [PubMed]
145. Reboll, M.R.; Ritter, B.; Sasse, F.; Niggemann, J.; Frank, R.; Nourbakhsh, M. The myxobacterial compounds spirangien A and spirangien M522 are potent inhibitors of IL-8 expression. *Chem. Bio. Chem.* **2012**, *13*, 409–415. [CrossRef]
146. Jurkliewicz, E.; Jansen, R.; Kunze, B.; Trowitzsch-Klenast, W.; Porche, E.; Reichenbach, H.; Höfle, G.; Hunsmann, G. Three new potent HIV-1 inhibitors from myxobacteria. *Antivir. Chem. Chemother.* **1992**, *3*, 189–193. [CrossRef]
147. Trowitzsch-Kienast, W.; Forche, E.; Wray, V.; Reichenbach, H.; Jurkiewicz, E.; Hunsmann, G.; Höfle, G. Phenalamide, neue HIV-1-Inhibitoren aus *Myxococcus stipitatus* Mx s40. *Liebigs Ann. Chem.* **1992**, *1992*, 659–664. [CrossRef]
148. Garcia, R.; Stadler, M.; Gemperlein, K.; Müller, R. *Aetherobacter fasciculatus* gen. nov.; sp. nov. and *Aetherobacter rufus* sp. nov.; novel myxobacteria with promising biotechnological applications. *Int. J. Syst. Evol. Microbiol.* **2016**, *66*, 928–938. [CrossRef]
149. Gerth, K.; Schummer, D.; Höfle, G.; Irschik, H.; Reichenbach, H. Ratjadon: A new antifungal compound from *Sorangium cellulosum* (Myxobacteria) Production, physico-chemical and biological properties. *J. Antibiot.* **1995**, *48*, 787–792. [CrossRef]
150. Kaul, D.R.; Stoelben, S.; Cober, E.; Ojo, T.; Sandusky, E.; Lischka, P.; Zimmermann, H.; Rübsamen-Schaeff, H. First report of successful treatment of multidrug-resistant cytomegalovirus disease with the novel anti-CMV compound AIC246. *Am. J. Transpl.* **2011**, *11*, 1079–1084. [CrossRef] [PubMed]
151. Nagoba, B.; Vedpathak, D. Medical applications of siderophores. *Eur. J. Gen. Med.* **2011**, *8*, 229–235. [CrossRef]
152. Miyanaga, S.; Obata, Y.; Onaka, H.; Fujita, T.; Saito, N.; Sakurai, H.; Saiki, I.; Furumai, T.; Igarashi, Y. Absolute configuration and antitumor activity of myxochelin a produced by *Nonomuraea pusilla* TP-A0861. *J. Antibiot.* **2006**, *59*, 698–703. [CrossRef]
153. Korp, J.; König, S.; Schieferdecker, S.; Dahse, H.M.; König, G.M.; Werz, O.; Nett, M. Harnessing enzymatic promiscuity in myxochelins biosynthesis for the production of 5-lipoxygenase inhibitors. *Chem. Bio. Chem.* **2015**, *16*, 2445–2450. [CrossRef] [PubMed]
154. Schieferdecker, S.; König, S.; Simona Pace, S.; Werz, O.; Nett, M. Myxochelin-inspired 5-lipoxygenase inhibitors: Synthesis and biological evaluation. *Chem. Med. Chem.* **2017**, *12*, 23–27. [CrossRef]
155. Miyanga, S.; Sakurai, H.; Saiki, I.; Onaka, H.; Igarashi, Y. Synthesis and evaluation of myxochelins analogues as antimetastatic agents. *Biol. Med. Chem.* **2009**, *17*, 2724–2732. [CrossRef]
156. Ambrosi, H.D.; Hartmann, V.; Pistorius, D.; Reissbrodt, R.; Trowitzsch-Kienast, W. Myxochelins B, C, D, E and F: A new structural principle for powerful siderophores imitating Nature. *Eur. J. Org. Chem.* **1998**, *1998*, 541–551. [CrossRef]
157. Britt, W.J.; Vugler, L.; Butfiloski, E.D.; Stevens, E.B. Cell surface expression of Human Cytomegalovirus (HCMV): Use of HCMV-recombinant vaccinia virus-infected cells in analysis of the human neutralizing antibody response. *J. Virol.* **1990**, *64*, 1079–1085. [CrossRef] [PubMed]
158. Saha, M.; Sarkar, S.; Sarkar, B.; Sharma, B.K.; Bhattacharjee, S.; Prosun, T. Microbial siderophores and their potential applications: A review. *Environ. Sci. Pollut. Res.* **2016**, *23*, 3984–3999. [CrossRef] [PubMed]
159. Kunze, B.; Jansen, R.; Sasse, F.; Höfle, G.; Reichenbach, H. Chondramides A-D, new antifungal and cytostatic depsipeptides from *Chondromyces crocatus* (Myxobacteria). Production, physicochemical and biological properties. *J. Antibiot.* **1995**, *48*, 1262–1266. [CrossRef] [PubMed]
160. Mulwa, L.; Jansen, R.; Praditya, D.; Mohr, K.; Wink, J.; Steinmann, E.; Stadler, M. Six heterocyclic metabolites from the Myxobacterium *Labilithrix luteola*. *Molecules* **2018**, *23*, 542. [CrossRef]
161. Bedorf, N.; Schomburg, D.; Gerth, K.; Reichenbach, H.; Höfle, G.; Bedorf, N.; Schomburg, D.; Gerth, K.; Reichenbach, H.; Höfle, G. Isolation and structure elucidation of soraphen A1, a novel antifungal macrolide from *Sorangium cellulosum*. *Liebigs Ann. Chem.* **1993**, *1993*, 1017–1021. [CrossRef]
162. Singaravelu, R.; Desrochers, G.F.; Srinivasan, P.; O'Hara, S.; Lyn, R.; Müller, R.; Jones, D.M.; Russell, R.; Pezacki, J.P. Soraphen A: A probe for investigating the role of de novo lipogenesis during viral infection. *ACS Infect. Dis.* **2015**, *1*, 130–134. [CrossRef]
163. Koutsoudakis, G.; Romero-Brey, I.; Berger, C.; Pérez-Vilaró, G.; Monteiro, P.P.; Vondran, F.W.R.; Kalesse, M.; Harmrolfs, K.; Müller, R.; Martinez, J.P.; et al. Soraphen A: A broad-spectrum antiviral natural product with potent anti-hepatitis C virus activity. *J. Hepatol.* **2015**, *63*, 813–821. [CrossRef]
164. Yeganeh, B.; Ghavami, S.; Kroeker, A.L.; Mahood, T.H.; Stelmack, G.L.; Klonisch, T.; Coombs, K.M.; Halayko, A.J. Suppression of influenza A virus replication in human lung epithelial cells by noncytotoxic concentrations bafilomycin A1. *Am. J. Physiol. Lung Cell. Mol. Physiol.* **2015**, *308*, 270–286. [CrossRef]
165. Oslowski, C.M.; Urano, F. Measuring ER stress and the unfolded protein response using mammalian tissue culture system. *Methods Enzymol.* **2011**, *490*, 71.
166. Rahman, S.; Jan, A.T.; Ayyagari, A.; Kim, J.; Kim, J.; Minakshi, R. Entanglement of UPRER in Aging Driven Neurodegenerative Diseases. *Front. Aging Neurosci.* **2017**, *9*, 341. [CrossRef]
167. Rahman, S.; Archana, A.; Jan, A.T.; Minakshi, R. Dissecting Endoplasmic Reticulum Unfolded Protein Response (UPRER) in Managing Clandestine Modus Operandi of Alzheimer's Disease. *Front. Aging Neurosci.* **2018**, *10*, 30. [CrossRef]

168. Dehhaghi, M.; Mohammadipanah, F.; Guillemin, G.J. Myxobacterial natural products: An under-valued source of products for drug discovery for neurological disorders. *NeuroToxicology* **2018**, *66*, 195–203. [CrossRef]
169. Kim, S.J.; Lee, Y.-J.; Kim, J.-B. Myxobacterial metabolites enhance cell proliferation and reduce intracellular stress in cells from a Parkinson's disease mouse model. *Gene* **2013**, *514*, 36–40. [CrossRef]
170. Sabry, J.; O'Connor, T.P.; Kirschner, M.W. Axonal transport of tubulin in tit pioneer neurons in situ. *Neuron* **1995**, *14*, 1247–1256. [CrossRef]
171. Chu, Y.; Morfini, G.A.; Langhamer, L.B.; He, Y.; Brady, S.T.; Kordower, J.H. Alterations in axonal transport motor proteins in sporadic and experimental Parkinson's disease. *Brain* **2012**, *135*, 2058–2073. [CrossRef] [PubMed]
172. Ikenaka, K.; Katsuno, M.; Kawai, K.; Ishigaki, S.; Tanaka, F.; Sobue, G. Disruption of axonal transport in motor neuron diseases. *Int. J. Mol. Sci.* **2012**, *13*, 1225–1238. [CrossRef]
173. Ye, X.; Tai, W.; Zhang, D. The early events of Alzheimer's disease pathology: From mitochondrial dysfunction to BDNF axonal transport deficits. *Neurobiol. Aging* **2012**, *33*, 1122.e1-10. [CrossRef] [PubMed]
174. Magen, I.; Gozes, I. Microtubule-stabilizing peptides and small molecules protecting axonal transport and brain function: Focus on davunetide (NAP). *Neuropeptides* **2013**, *47*, 489–495. [CrossRef] [PubMed]
175. Saman, S.; Kim, W.; Raya, M.; Visnick, Y.; Miro, S.; Saman, S.; Jackson, B.; McKee, A.C.; Alvarez, V.E.; Lee, N.C. Exosome-associated tau is secreted in tauopathy models and is selectively phosphorylated in cerebrospinal fluid in early Alzheimer disease. *J. Biol. Chem.* **2012**, *287*, 3842–3849. [CrossRef]
176. Gerth, K.; Bedorf, N.; Höfle, G.; Irschik, H.; Reichenbach, H. Epothilons A and B: Antifungal and cytotoxic compounds from *Sorangium cellulosum* (Myxobacteria). *J. Antibiot.* **1996**, *49*, 560–563. [CrossRef]
177. De Vos, K.J.; Grierson, A.; Ackerley, S.; Miller, C. Role of axonal transport in neurodegenerative diseases. *Annu. Rev. Neurosci.* **2008**, *31*, 151–173. [CrossRef]
178. Zhang, B.; Carroll, J.; Trojanowski, J.Q.; Yao, Y.; Iba, M.; Potuzak, J.S.; Hogan, A.-M.L.; Xie, S.X.; Ballatore, C.; Smith, A.B.; et al. The microtubule-stabilizing agent, epothilone D, reduces axonal dysfunction, neurotoxicity, cognitive deficits, and Alzheimer-like pathology in an interventional study with aged tau transgenic mice. *J. Neurosci.* **2012**, *32*, 3601–3611. [CrossRef] [PubMed]
179. Cartelli, D.; Casagrande, F.; Busceti, C.L.; Bucci, D.; Molinaro, G.; Traficante, A.; Passarella, D.; Giavini, E.; Pezzoli, G.; Battaglia, G.; et al. Microtubule alterations occur early in experimental parkinsonism and the microtubule stabilizer epothilone D is neuroprotective. *Sci. Rep.* **2013**, *3*, 1837. [CrossRef] [PubMed]
180. Eckert, G.P.; Lipka, U.; Muller, W.E. Omega-3 fatty acids in neurodegenerative diseases: Focus on mitochondria. *Prostaglandins Leukotrienes Essent. Fat. Acids (PLEFA)* **2013**, *88*, 105–114. [CrossRef]
181. Nichols, D.S.; McMeekin, T.A. Biomarker techniques to screen for bacteria that produce polyunsaturated fatty acids. *J. Microbiol. Methods* **2002**, *48*, 161–170. [CrossRef]
182. Yano, Y.; Nakayama, A.; Yoshida, K. Distribution of polyunsaturated fatty acids in bacteria present in intestines of deep-sea fish and shallow-sea poikilothermic animals. *Appl. Environ. Microbiol.* **1997**, *63*, 2572–2577. [CrossRef]
183. Hayashi, S.; Satoh, Y.; Ujihara, T.; Takata, Y.; Dairi, T. Enhanced production of polyunsaturated fatty acids by enzyme engineering of tandem acyl carrier proteins. *Sci. Rep.* **2016**, *6*, 35441. [CrossRef]
184. Gemperlein, K.; Rachid, S.; Garcia, R.O.; Wenzel, S.C.; Müller, R. Polyunsaturated fatty acid biosynthesis in myxobacteria: Different PUFA synthases and their product diversity. *Chem. Sci.* **2014**, *5*, 1733–1741. [CrossRef]
185. Feng, Z.; Zou, X.; Jia, H.; Li, X.; Zhu, X.; Liu, X.; Bucheli, P.; Ballevre, O.; Hou, Y.; Zhang, W.; et al. Maternal docosahexaenoic acid feeding protects against impairment of learning and memory and oxidative stress in prenatally stressed rats: Possible role of neuronal mitochondria metabolism. *Antioxid. Redox. Signal.* **2012**, *16*, 275–289. [CrossRef]
186. Song, L.; Zheng, J.; Li, H.; Jia, N.; Suo, Z.; Cai, Q.; Bai, Z.; Cheng, D.; Zhu, Z. Prenatal stress causes oxidative damage to mitochondrial DNA in hippocampus of offspring rats. *Neurochem. Res.* **2009**, *34*, 739–745. [CrossRef]
187. Eckert, G.P.; Zheng, J.; Li, H.; Jia, N.; Suo, Z.; Cai, Q.; Bai, Z.; Cheng, D.; Zhu, Z. Liposome-incorporated DHA increases neuronal survival by enhancing non-amyloidogenic APP processing. *Biochim Biophys Acta BBA Biomembr* **2011**, *1808*, 236–243. [CrossRef]
188. White, K.N.; Tenney, K.; Crews, P. The Bengamides: A Mini-Review of Natural Sources, Analogues, Biological Properties, Biosynthetic Origins, and Future Prospects. *J. Nat. Prod.* **2017**, *80*, 740–755. [CrossRef] [PubMed]
189. Castro, C.; Freitag, L.; Berod, L.; Lochner, M.; Sparwasser, T. Microbe-associated immunomodulatory metabolites: Influence on T cell fate and function. *Mol. Immunol.* **2015**, *68*, 575–584. [CrossRef]
190. Johnson, T.A.; Sohn, J.; Vaske, Y.M.; White, K.N.; Cohen, T.L.; Vervoort, H.C.; Tenney, K.; Valeriote, F.A.; Bjeldanes, L.F.; Crews, P. Myxobacteria versus sponge-derived alkaloids: The bengamide family identified as potent immune modulating agents by scrutiny of LC MS/ELSD libraries. *Bioorg. Med. Chem.* **2012**, *20*, 4348–4355. [CrossRef] [PubMed]
191. Jansen, R.; Washausen, P.; Kunze, B.; Reichenbach, H.; Höfle, G. ChemInform Abstract: Antibiotics from Gliding Bacteria. Part 83. The Crocacins, Novel Antifungal and Cytotoxic Antibiotics from *Chondromyces crocatus* and *Chondromyces pediculatus* (Myxobacteria): Isolation and Structure Elucidation. *Cheminform* **2010**, *30*. [CrossRef]
192. Kunze, B.; Hofle, G.; Reichenbach, H. The aurachins, new quinoline antibiotics from myxobacteria: Production, physico-chemical and biological properties. *J. Antibiot.* **1987**, *40*, 258–265. [CrossRef] [PubMed]
193. Miyoshi, H.; Takegami, K.; Sakamoto, K.; Mogi, T.; Iwamura, H. Characterization of the ubiquinol oxidation sites in cytochromes bo and bd from *Escherichia coli* using aurachin C analogues. *J. Biochem.* **1999**, *125*, 138–142. [CrossRef]

194. Gerth, K.; Irschik, H.; Reichenbach, H.; Trowitzsch, W. Myxothiazol, an antibiotic from *Myxococcus fulvus* (Myxobacterales). *J. Antibiot.* **1980**, *33*, 1474–1479. [CrossRef] [PubMed]
195. Thierbach, G.; Reichenbach, H. Myxothiazol, a new antibiotic interfering with respiration. *Antimicrob. Agents Chemother.* **1981**, *19*, 504–507. [CrossRef]
196. Sasse, F.; Böhlendorf, B.; Herrmann, M.; Kunze, B.; Forche, E.; Steinmetz, H.; Höfle, G.; Reichenbach, H. Melithiazols, new beta-methoxyacrylate inhibitors of the respiratory chain isolated from myxobacteria. Production, isolation, physico-chemical and biological properties. *J. Antibiot.* **1999**, *52*, 721–729. [CrossRef]
197. Oettmeier, W.; Godde, D.; Höfle, G. Stigmatellin. A dual type inhibitor of photosynthetic electron transport. *Biochim. Biophys. Acta.* **1985**, *807*, 216–219. [CrossRef]
198. Yamashita, E.; Zhang, H.; Cramer, W.A. Structure of the cytochrome b6f complex: Quinone analogue inhibitors as ligands of heme cn. *J. Mol. Biol.* **2007**, *370*, 39–52. [CrossRef]
199. Dejon, L.; Speicher, A. Synthesis of aurachin D and isoprenoid analogues from the myxobacterium *Stigmatella aurantiaca*. *Tetrahedron Lett.* **2013**, *54*, 6700–6702. [CrossRef]
200. Irschik, H.; Trowitzsch-Kienast, W.; Gerth, K.; Hofle, G.; Reichenbach, H. Saframycin Mx1, a new natural saframycin isolated from a myxobacterium. *J. Antibiot.* **1988**, *41*, 993–998. [CrossRef] [PubMed]
201. Sasse, F.; Steinmetz, H.; Höfle, G.; Reichenbach, H. Gephyronic acid, a novel inhibitor of eukaryotic protein synthesis from *Archangium gephyra* (myxobacteria). Production, isolation, physico-chemical and biological properties, and mechanism of action. *J. Antibiot.* **1995**, *48*, 21–25. [CrossRef]
202. Irschik, H.; Reichenbach, H. The mechanism of action of myxovalargin A, a peptide antibiotic from *Myxococcus fulvus*. *J. Antibiot.* **1985**, *38*, 1237–1245. [CrossRef] [PubMed]
203. Jimenez, A.; Tipper, D.J.; Davies, J. Mode of action of thiolutin, an inhibitor of macromolecular synthesis in *Saccharomyces cerevisiae*. *Antimicrob. Agents Chemother.* **1973**, *3*, 729–738. [CrossRef] [PubMed]
204. Tipper, D.J. Inhibition of yeast ribonucleic acid polymerases by thiolutin. *J. Bacteriol.* **1973**, *116*, 245–256. [CrossRef]
205. Tuske, S.; Sarafianos, S.G.; Wang, X.; Hudson, B.; Sineva, E.; Mukhopadhyay, J.; Birktoft, J.J.; Leroy, O.; Ismail, S.; Clark, A.D., Jr.; et al. Inhibition of bacterial RNA polymerase by streptolydigin: Stabilization of a straight-bridge-helix active-center conformation. *Cell* **2005**, *122*, 541–552. [CrossRef]
206. Oliva, B.; O'Neill, A.; Wilson, J.M.; O'Hanlon, P.J.; Chopra, I. Antimicrobial properties and mode of action of the pyrrothine holomycin. *Antimicrob. Agents Chemother.* **2001**, *45*, 532–539. [CrossRef]
207. Artsimovitch, I.; Vassylyeva, M.N.; Svetlov, D.; Svetlov, V.; Perederina, A.; Igarashi, N.; Matsugaki, N.; Wakatsuki, S.; Tahirov, T.H.; Vassylyev, D.G. Allosteric modulation of the RNA polymerase catalytic reaction is an essential component of transcription control by rifamycins. *Cell* **2005**, *122*, 351–363. [CrossRef]
208. O'Neill, A.J.; Huovinen, T.; Fishwick, C.W.; Chopra, I. Molecular genetics and structural modeling studies of *Staphylococcus aureus* RNA polymerase and the fitness of rifampin resistance genotypes in relation to clinical prevalence. *Antimicrob. Agents Chemother.* **2006**, *50*, 298–309. [CrossRef]
209. O'Neill, A.; Oliva, B.; Storey, C.; Hoyle, A.; Fishwick, C.; Chopra, I. RNA polymerase inhibitors with activity against rifampin-resistant mutants of *Staphylococcus aureus*. *Antimicrob. Agents Chemother.* **2000**, *44*, 3163–3166. [CrossRef]
210. Campbell, E.A.; Pavlova, O.; Zenkin, N.; Leon, F.; Irschik, H.; Jansen, R.; Severinov, K.; Darst, S.A. Structural, functional, and genetic analysis of sorangicin inhibition of bacterial RNA polymerase. *EMBO J.* **2005**, *24*, 674–682. [CrossRef] [PubMed]
211. Irschik, H.; Jansen, R.; Gerth, K.; Höfle, G.; Reichenbach, H. The sorangicins, novel and powerful inhibitors of eubacterial RNA polymerase isolated from myxobacteria. *J. Antibiot.* **1987**, *40*, 7–13. [CrossRef] [PubMed]
212. Augustiniak, H.; Höfle, G.; Irschik, H.; Reichenbach, H. Antibiotics from gliding bacteria, LXXVIII. Isolation and structure and structure elucidation of novel metabolites from *Sorangium cellulosum*. *Liebigs Ann.* **1996**, *1996*, 1657–1663. [CrossRef]
213. Irschik, H.; Augustiniak, H.; Gerth, K.; Höfle, G.; Reichenbach, H. Antibiotics from gliding bacteria. No. 68. The Ripostatins, Novel Inhibitors of Eubacterial RNA Polymerase Isolated from myxobacteria. *J. Antibiot.* **1995**, *48*, 787–792. [CrossRef] [PubMed]
214. Irschik, H.; Jansen, R.; Höfle, G.; Gerth, K.; Reichenbach, H. The corallopyronins, new inhibitors of bacterial RNA synthesis from Myxobacteria. *J. Antibiot.* **1985**, *38*, 145–152. [CrossRef] [PubMed]
215. Gronewold, T.; Sasse, F.; Lünsdorf, H.; Reichenbach, H. Effects of rhizopodin and latrunculin B on the morphology and on the actin cytoskeleton of mammalian cells. *Cell Tissue Res.* **1999**, *295*, 121–129. [CrossRef]
216. Sasse, F.; Steinmetz, H.; Höfle, G.; Reichenbach, H. Rhizopodin, a new compound from *Myxococcus stipitatus* (Myxobacteria) causes formation of rhizopodia-like structures in animal cell cultures. Production, isolation, physico-chemical and biological properties. *J. Antibiot.* **1993**, *46*, 741–748. [CrossRef]
217. Holzinger, A.; Lütz-Meindl, U. Chondramides, novel cyclodepsipeptides from myxobacteria, influence cell development and induce actin filament polymerization in the green alga Micrasterias. *Cell Motil. Cytoskelet.* **2001**, *48*, 87–95. [CrossRef]
218. Sasse, F.; Kunze, B.; Gronewold, T.; Reichenbach, H. The chondramides: Cytostatic agents from myxobacteria acting on the actin cytoskeleton. *J. Natl Cancer Inst.* **1998**, *90*, 48–52. [CrossRef]
219. Bollag, D.M.; McQueney, P.A.; Zhu, J.; Hensens, O.; Koupal, L.; Liesch, J.; Goetz, M.; Lazarides, E.; Woods, C.M. Epothilones, a new class of microtubule-stabilizing agents with a taxol-like mechanism of action. *Cancer Res.* **1995**, *55*, 2325–2333. [PubMed]

220. Höfle, G.; Bedorf, N.; Steinmetz, H.; Schomburg, D.; Gerth, K.; Reichenbach, H. Epothilone A and B-Novel 16-membered macrolides with cytotoxic activity: Isolation, crystal structure, and conformation in solution. *Angew. Chem. Int. Ed. Engl.* 1996, 35, 1567–1569. [CrossRef]
221. Khalil, M.W.; Sasse, F.; Lünsdorf, H.; Elnakady, Y.A.; Reichenbach, H. Mechanism of action of tubulysin, an antimitotic peptide from myxobacteria. *ChemBioChem* 2006, 7, 678–683. [CrossRef]
222. Sasse, F.; Steinmetz, H.; Heil, J.; Höfle, G.; Reichenbach, H. Tubulysins, New Cytostatic Peptides from Myxobacteria Acting on Microtubuli. Production, Isolation, Physico-chemical and Biological Properties. *J. Antibiot.* 2000, 53, 879–885. [CrossRef] [PubMed]
223. Cheng, K.L.; Bradley, T.; Budman, D.R. Novel microtubule-targeting agents—The epothilones. *Biol. Targets Ther.* 2008, 2, 789–811.
224. Fumoleau, P.; Coudert, B.; Isambert, N.; Ferrant, E. Novel tubulin-targeting agents:anticancer activity and pharmacologic profile of epothilones and related analogues. *Ann. Oncol.* 2007, 18, 9–15. [CrossRef]
225. Steinmetz, H.; Glaser, N.; Herdtweck, E.; Sasse, F.; Reichenbach, H.; Höfle, G. Isolation, crystal and solution structure determination, and biosynthesis of tubulysins-powerful inhibitors of tubulin polymerization from myxobacteria. *Angew. Chem. Int. Ed. Engl.* 2004, 43, 4888–4892. [CrossRef]
226. Patterson, A.W.; Peltier, H.M.; Sasse, F.; Ellman, J.A. Design, synthesis, and biological properties of highly potent tubulysin D analogues. *Chemistry* 2007, 13, 9534–9541. [CrossRef]
227. Kaur, G.; Hollingshead, M.; Holbeck, S.; Schauer-Vukasinovic, V.; Camalier, R.F.; Domling, A.; Agarwal, S. Biological evaluation of tubulysin A: A potential anticancer and antiangiogenic natural product. *Biochem. J.* 2006, 396, 235–242. [CrossRef]
228. Beckers, A.; Organe, S.; Timmermans, L.; Scheys, K.; Peeters, A.; Brusselmans, K.; Verhoeven, G.; Swinnen, J.V. Chemical inhibition of acetyl-CoA carboxylase induces growth arrest and cytotoxicity selectively in cancer cells. *Cancer Res.* 2007, 67, 8180–8187. [CrossRef]
229. Rosenberg, E.; Varon, M. Antibiotics and Lytic Enzymes. In *Myxobacteria*; Rosenberg, E., Ed.; Springer Series in Molecular Biology; Springer: New York, NY, USA, 1984.
230. Hill, D.S.; Stein, J.I.; Torkewitz, N.R.; Morse, A.M.; Howell, C.R.; Pachlatko, J.P.; Becker, J.O.; Ligon, J.M. Cloning of genes involved in the synthesis of pyrrolnitrin from *Pseudomonas fluorescens* and role of pyrrolnitrin synthesis in biological control of plant disease *Appl. Environ. Microb.* 1994, 60, 78–85. [CrossRef] [PubMed]
231. Hocking, D.; Cook, F.D. Myxobacteria exert partial control of damping-off and root disease in container-grown tree seedlings. *Can. J. Microbiol.* 1972, 18, 1557–1560. [CrossRef]
232. Homma, Y. Perforation and lysis of hyphae of *Rhizoctonia solani* and conidia of *Cochliobolus miyabeanus* by soil myxobacteria. *Agris.* 1984, 74, 1234–1239.
233. Norén, B.; Odham, G. Antagonistic effects of *Myxococcus xanthus* on fungi: II. Isolation and characterization of inhibitory lipid factors. *Lipids* 1973, 8, 573–583. [CrossRef] [PubMed]
234. Lautru, S.; Deeth, R.J.; Bailey, L.M.; Challis, G.L. Discovery of a new peptide natural product by *Streptomyces coelicolor* genome mining. *Nature Chem. Biol.* 2005, 1, 265–269. [CrossRef]
235. Bode, H.B.; Bethe, B.; Höfs, R.; Zeeck, A. Big effects from small changes: Possible ways to explore nature's chemical diversity. *ChemBioChem.* 2002, 3, 619–627. [CrossRef]
236. Christian, O.E.; Compton, J.; Christian, K.R.; Mooberry, S.L.; Valeriote, F.A.; Crews, P. Using jasplakinolide to turn on pathways that enable the isolation of new chaetoglobosins from *Phomopsis asparagi*. *J. Nat. Prod.* 2005, 68, 1592–1597. [CrossRef] [PubMed]
237. Bergmann, S.; Schümann, J.; Scherlach, K.; Lange, C.; Brakhage, A.; Hertweck, C. Genomics-driven discovery of PKS-NRPS hybrid metabolites from *Aspergillus nidulans*. *Nat. Chem. Biol.* 2007, 3, 213–217. [CrossRef]
238. Sandmann, A.; Frank, B.; Müller, R. A transposon-based strategy to scale up myxothiazol production in myxobacterial cell factories. *J. Biotechnol.* 2008, 135, 255–261. [CrossRef]
239. Julien, B.; Tian, Z.Q.; Reid, R.; Reeves, C.D. Analysis of the ambruticin and jerangolid gene clusters of Sorangium cellulosum reveals unusual mechanisms of polyketide biosynthesis. *Chem. Biol.* 2006, 13, 1277–1286. [CrossRef]
240. Weissman, K.J.; Müller, R. A brief tour of myxobacterial secondary metabolism. *Bioorg. Med. Chem.* 2009, 17, 2121–2136. [CrossRef]
241. Sandmann, A.; Dickschat, J.; Jenke-Kodama, H.; Kunze, B.; Dittmann, E.; Müller, R. A Type II Polyketide Synthase from the Gram-Negative Bacterium *Stigmatella aurantiaca* Is Involved in Aurachin Alkaloid Biosynthesis. *Angew. Chem. Int. Ed.* 2007, 46, 2712–2716. [CrossRef] [PubMed]
242. Carvalho, R.; Reid, R.; Viswanathan, N.; Gramajo, H.; Julien, B. The biosynthetic genes for disorazoles, potent cytotoxic compounds that disrupt microtubule formation. *Gene* 2005, 359, 91–98. [CrossRef]
243. Sandmann, A.; Sasse, F.; Müller, R. Identification and analysis of the core biosynthetic machinery of tubulysin, a potent cytotoxin with potential anticancer activity. *Chem. Biol.* 2004, 11, 1071–1079. [CrossRef]
244. Rachid, S.; Sasse, F.; Beyer, S.; Müller, R. Identification of StiR, the first regulator of secondary metabolite formation in the myxobacterium *Cystobacter fuscus* Cb f17.1. *J. Biotechnol.* 2006, 121, 429–441. [CrossRef] [PubMed]
245. Rachid, S.; Gerth, K.; Kochems, I.; Müller, R. Deciphering regulatory mechanisms for secondary metabolite production in the myxobacterium *Sorangium cellulosum* So ce56. *Molecul. Microbiol.* 2007, 63, 1783–1796. [CrossRef] [PubMed]
246. Silakowski, B.; Kunze, B.; Nordsiek, G.; Blöcker, H.; Höfle, G.; Müller, R. The myxochelin iron transport regulon of the myxobacterium *Stigmatella aurantiaca* Sg a15. *Eur. J. Biochem.* 2000, 267, 6476–6485. [CrossRef]

247. Wenzel, S.; Kunze, B.; Höfle, G.; Silakowski, B.; Scharfe, M.; Blöcker, H.; Müller, R. Structure and Biosynthesis of Myxochromides S1-3 in *Stigmatella aurantiaca*: Evidence for an Iterative Bacterial Type I Polyketide Synthase and for Module Skipping in Nonribosomal Peptide Biosynthesis. *ChemBioChem.* **2005**, *6*, 375–385. [CrossRef]
248. Ostash, B.; Saghatelian, A.; Walker, S. A streamlined metabolic pathway for the biosynthesis of moenomycin A. *Chem. Biol.* **2007**, *14*, 257–267. [CrossRef]
249. Ostash, B.; Campbell, J.; Luzhetskyy, A.; Walker, S. MoeH5: A natural glycorandomizer from the moenomycin biosynthetic pathway. *Mol. Microbiol.* **2013**, *90*, 1324–1338. [CrossRef] [PubMed]
250. Kodumal, S.; Patel, K.; Reid, R.; Menzella, H.; Welch, M.; Santi, D. Total synthesis of long DNA sequences: Synthesis of a contiguous 32-kb polyketide synthase gene cluster. *Proc. Nat. Acad. Sci. USA* **2004**, *101*, 15573–15578. [CrossRef] [PubMed]
251. Julien, B.; Shah, S. Heterologous expression of epothilone biosynthetic genes in *Myxococcus xanthus*. *Antimicrob. Agents Chemother.* **2002**, *46*, 2772–2778. [CrossRef] [PubMed]
252. Tang, L.; Shah, S.; Chung, L.; Carney, J.; Katz, L.; Khosla, C.; Julien, B. Cloning and heterologous expression of the epothilone gene cluster. *Science* **2000**, *287*, 640–642. [CrossRef]
253. Mutka, S.C.; Carney, J.R.; Liu, Y.; Kennedy, J. Heterologous production of epothilone C and D in *Escherichia coli*. *Biochemistry* **2006**, *45*, 1321–1330. [CrossRef]
254. Fu, J.; Wenzel, S.C.; Perlova, O.; Wang, J.; Gross, F.; Tang, Z.; Yin, Y.; Stewart, A.F.; Müller, R.; Zhang, Y. Efficient transfer of two large secondary metabolite pathway gene clusters into heterologous hosts by transposition. *Nucleic Acids Res.* **2008**, *36*, e113. [CrossRef]
255. Zirkle, R.; Ligon, J.M.; Molnár, I. Heterologous production of the antifungal polyketide antibiotic soraphen A of *Sorangium cellulosum* So ce26 in *Streptomyces lividans*. *Microbiology* **2004**, *150*, 2761–2774. [CrossRef]
256. Perlova, O.; Fu, J.; Kuhlmann, S.; Krug, D.; Stewart, A.; Zhang, Y.; Müller, R. Reconstitution of the Myxothiazol Biosynthetic Gene Cluster by Red/ET Recombination and Heterologous Expression in *Myxococcus xanthus*. *Appl. Environ. Microbiol.* **2007**, *72*, 7485–7494. [CrossRef] [PubMed]
257. Gross, F.; Luniak, N.; Perlova, O.; Gaitatzis, N.; Jenke-Kodama, H.; Gerth, K.; Gottschalk, D.; Dittmann, E.; Müller, R. Bacterial type III polyketide synthases: Phylogenetic analysis and potential for the production of novel secondary metabolites by heterologous expression in pseudomonads. *Arch. Microbiol.* **2006**, *185*, 28–38. [CrossRef]
258. Zhang, Y.; Buchholz, F.; Muyrers, J.P.; Stewart, A.F. A new logic for DNA engineering using recombination in *Escherichia coli*. *Nat. Genet.* **1998**, *20*, 123–128. [CrossRef] [PubMed]
259. Weissman, K.J.; Leadlay, P.F. Combinatorial biosynthesis of reduced polyketides. *Nat. Rev. Microbiol.* **2005**, *3*, 925–936. [CrossRef] [PubMed]

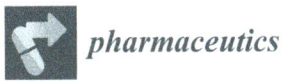

Article

Inhibition of Indigoidine Synthesis as a High-Throughput Colourimetric Screen for Antibiotics Targeting the Essential *Mycobacterium tuberculosis* Phosphopantetheinyl Transferase PptT

Alistair S. Brown [1,2,3], Jeremy G. Owen [1,2,3], James Jung [3,4,†], Edward N. Baker [3,4] and David F. Ackerley [1,2,3,*]

1. School of Biological Sciences, Victoria University of Wellington, Wellington 6012, New Zealand; alistair.brown@vuw.ac.nz (A.S.B.); jeremy.owen@vuw.ac.nz (J.G.O.)
2. Centre for Biodiscovery, Victoria University of Wellington, Wellington 6012, New Zealand
3. Maurice Wilkins Centre for Molecular Biodiscovery, Auckland 1142, New Zealand; jjung@genzentrum.lmu.de (J.J.); en.baker@auckland.ac.nz (E.N.B.)
4. School of Biological Sciences, University of Auckland, Auckland 1142, New Zealand
* Correspondence: david.ackerley@vuw.ac.nz; Tel.: +64-4-4635576
† Current address: Gene Center and Department of Biochemistry, Ludwig-Maximilians-Universität München, 81377 Munich, Germany.

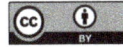

Citation: Brown, A.S.; Owen, J.G.; Jung, J.; Baker, E.N.; Ackerley, D.F. Inhibition of Indigoidine Synthesis as a High-Throughput Colourimetric Screen for Antibiotics Targeting the Essential *Mycobacterium tuberculosis* Phosphopantetheinyl Transferase PptT. *Pharmaceutics* **2021**, *13*, 1066. https://doi.org/10.3390/pharmaceutics13071066

Academic Editors: Corneliu Tanase, Aura Rusu and Valentina Uivarosi

Received: 2 June 2021
Accepted: 9 July 2021
Published: 12 July 2021

Publisher's Note: MDPI stays neutral with regard to jurisdictional claims in published maps and institutional affiliations.

Copyright: © 2021 by the authors. Licensee MDPI, Basel, Switzerland. This article is an open access article distributed under the terms and conditions of the Creative Commons Attribution (CC BY) license (https://creativecommons.org/licenses/by/4.0/).

Abstract: A recently-validated and underexplored drug target in *Mycobacterium tuberculosis* is PptT, an essential phosphopantetheinyl transferase (PPTase) that plays a critical role in activating enzymes for both primary and secondary metabolism. PptT possesses a deep binding pocket that does not readily accept labelled coenzyme A analogues that have previously been used to screen for PPTase inhibitors. Here we report on the development of a high throughput, colourimetric screen that monitors the PptT-mediated activation of the non-ribosomal peptide synthetase BpsA to a blue pigment (indigoidine) synthesising form in vitro. This screen uses unadulterated coenzyme A, avoiding analogues that may interfere with inhibitor binding, and requires only a single-endpoint measurement. We benchmark the screen using the well-characterised Library of Pharmaceutically Active Compounds (LOPAC[1280]) collection and show that it is both sensitive and able to distinguish weak from strong inhibitors. We further show that the BpsA assay can be applied to quantify the level of inhibition and generate consistent EC_{50} data. We anticipate these tools will facilitate both the screening of established chemical collections to identify new anti-mycobacterial drug leads and to guide the exploration of structure-activity landscapes to improve existing PPTase inhibitors.

Keywords: PPTase; NRPS; indigoidine; PptT; antibiotic screening

1. Introduction

Despite diminishing rates of infection, the disease burden of *Mycobacterium tuberculosis* remains high, with 2019 seeing approximately 10 million people infected and 1.4 million deaths worldwide [1]. The emergence of drug-resistant strains of *M. tuberculosis* coupled with long treatment times has resulted in a pressing need for new therapeutics [2]. *M. tuberculosis* is difficult to treat effectively, in part due to its lipid-rich cell wall and envelope, which contain a diversity of unusual lipids that help it to survive and evade the host immune system [3–5]. Mega-synthetases, including the fatty acid synthetase (FAS) I and II systems and polyketide synthetases (PKSs), play crucial roles in the biosynthesis of these lipids [6]. A further mega-synthetase family, the non-ribosomal peptide synthetases (NRPSs), is required to produce the important virulence factor mycobactin [7]. Each of these mega-synthetases requires the attachment of a phosphopantetheinyl (Ppant) arm to one or more carrier protein (CP) domain(s) to convert them from an inactive *apo* to an active *holo* form, a post-translational modification that is essential for functionality [8].

The attachment of the Ppant arm is catalysed by an enzyme superfamily called the 4′-phosphopantetheinyl transferases (PPTases), which in prokaryotes fall into two broad classes that differ in their structure and substrate specificity [8]. Type I (or AcpS type) PPTases are homotrimers that have a narrow substrate specificity and typically recognise acyl carrier protein (ACP) domains present in the FAS-I and FAS-II systems. Type II (or Sfp type) PPTases tend to be pseudodimers, have a much broader substrate specificity and typically activate ACP, peptidyl carrier protein (PCP) and aryl carrier protein (ArCP) domains present in PKSs and NRPSs [8]. Due to their lynchpin roles in both primary and secondary metabolism, many PPTases are essential [8] and have been identified as promising drug targets [9].

M. tuberculosis possesses both a Type I PPTase (AcpS) and a Type II PPTase (PptT) [10]. Although it activates the FAS-1 system [11], the essential nature of AcpS has not been confirmed in *M. tuberculosis* [10,12]. Conversely, PptT, which governs the activation of at least 18 PKSs [13], three NRPSs involved in the biosynthesis of the siderophore mycobactin [14] and AcpM (the standalone CP in the FAS-II system [11]), has been confirmed as essential for *M. tuberculosis* growth in vitro [12,13] and in murine models [13]. Importantly for drug targeting, even partial inhibition of PptT can be enough to kill *M. tuberculosis* [13]. This is likely because a Ppant hydrolase (PptH) that removes the Ppant from carrier proteins is expressed in the same operon as PptT, thereby restricting the ability of *M. tuberculosis* to upregulate PptT without also increasing PptH to detrimental levels [15]. PptT is a pseudodimer and has a broadly similar α/β fold to other crystallised Type-II PPTases with some minor variations, one of the most significant being that the Ppant arm extends into a deep hydrophobic pocket in the binding pocket [16,17]. By way of contrast, in the crystal structure of the well-characterised Type II PPTase, Sfp from *Bacillus subtilis*, the Ppant arm directs into the solvent [18] (Figure 1A).

Several high throughput screens to identify bacterial PPTase inhibitors have been developed that monitor the binding of fluorescently labelled coenzyme A (CoA) to a carrier protein or peptide, using either fluorescent polarisation or FRET-based detection [9,19–21]. However, rather than directly targeting the PPTase of a pathogenic species, these screens have all employed the canonical PPTase Sfp from *B. subtilis* as a surrogate. This is problematic for discovering inhibitors of *M. tuberculosis* PptT, as it does not accept fluorescent CoA analogues as readily as Sfp [13], due to its deeper binding pocket (Figure 1A) [16,17]. It is also noteworthy that 8918, a promising PptT inhibitor that was recently identified in a whole-organism screen against *M. tuberculosis*, binds to the PptT active site, close to the Ppant arm [15]. Fluorescent analogues of CoA, which are substantially bulkier than native CoA, may therefore exclude otherwise promising inhibitors from the active site. With this in mind, we considered it important to develop a cost-effective direct screen against PptT that uses unadulterated CoA as a substrate.

We have previously shown that the NRPS BpsA (blue pigment synthetase A) could be used to assess the relative levels of inhibition of Sfp and two *Pseudomonas* Type II bacterial PPTases by the generic inhibitor 6-nitroso-1,2-benzopyrone [22]. BpsA is a single-module NRPS that in vitro can convert two molecules of L-glutamine into the blue pigment indigoidine, provided it can been activated to the *holo* form by a co-incubated PPTase (Figure 1B) [23]. Here we demonstrate that recombinant BpsA purified in the *apo* form can be used to provide a robust and high-throughput screen for compounds that inhibit PptT from activating BpsA.

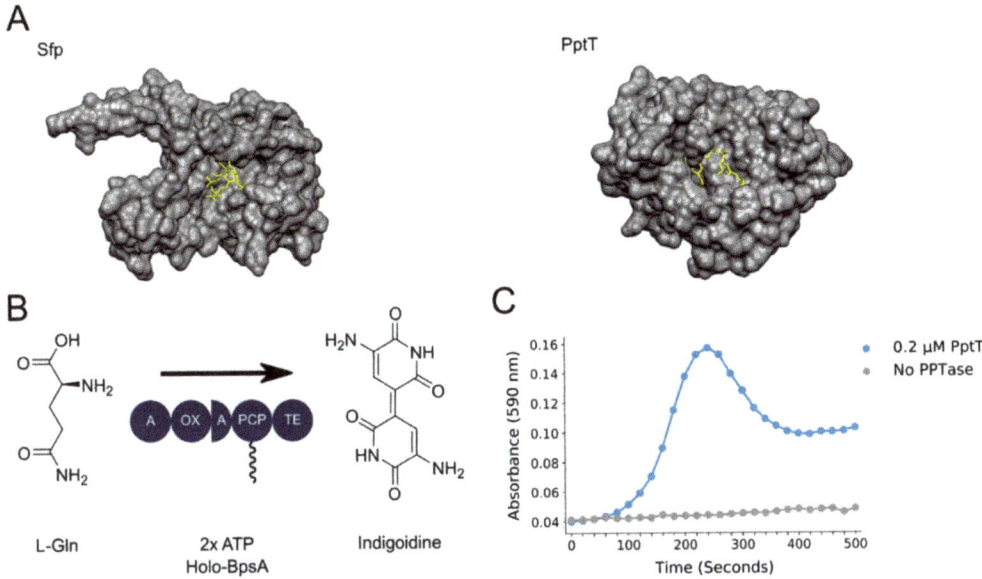

Figure 1. (**A**) Crystal structures of Sfp and PptT, highlighting the orientation of CoA: CoA (yellow) is orientated towards the solvent in the crystal structure of Sfp (PDB: 1QR0), while in our structure of PptT (PDB:4QVH), it is encapsulated by the binding pocket. Visualisation was performed using Chimera [24]. (**B**) Schematic showing biosynthesis of indigoidine by *holo*-BpsA: *Holo*-BpsA synthesises indigoidine from two molecules of L-glutamine in an ATP powered reaction. When indigoidine is solubilised in DMSO, it has a characteristic deep blue colouring that can readily be detected by monitoring absorbance at 590 nm. (**C**) Characteristic curve of indigoidine biosynthesis during the activation of *apo*-BpsA by PptT: Indigoidine production in an aqueous solution yields a sigmoidal curve of absorbance at 590 nm until it reaches saturation and precipitates, after which the A_{590} drops.

2. Materials and Methods

2.1. Materials and Reagents

Unless otherwise stated, chemicals, media and reagents used in this study were supplied by Sigma-Aldrich (St Louis, MO, USA), Thermo Fisher Scientific (Waltham, MA, USA), Duchefa Biochemie (BH Haarlem, Netherlands) or New England Biolabs (Ipswich, MA, USA). Sanguinarine chloride for kinetic screening was supplied by Sapphire Biosciences (Redfern, NSW, Australia).

2.2. Plasmid Construction

Construction of the BpsA expression plasmid pCDFDUET1::*bpsA* was described previously [22]. Construction of NOHISPET::*pcpS*, which expresses an untagged version of the broad-spectrum PPTase PcpS to covert *apo*-BpsA to *holo*-BpsA and not co-purify during Ni-NTA chromatography, was as previously described [25]. pET28a(+)::*pptT* was constructed by amplifying *pptT* from *M. tuberculosis* H37Ra genomic DNA using the primers CCCCCATATGGACGGTAGGCACGCTG and CCCCCTCGAGTCATAGCACGATCGCGGT (restriction sites underlined). The amplified gene was ligated into pET28a(+) between the NdeI and XhoI restriction sites.

2.3. Protein Expression

All protein expression used *E. coli* BL21(DE3) Δ*entD* [26] as an expression strain. Cultures were grown in lysogeny broth (LB) with plasmid appropriate antibiotics (spectinomycin 100 μg/mL, kanamycin 50 μg/mL). Fresh 400 mL expression cultures were inoculated to an A_{600} of 0.1 overnight and incubated at 37 °C, 200 rpm until an A_{600} of between 0.6 and 0.8 was obtained. The cultures were then chilled on ice for approximately 30 min. Protein expression was induced with the addition of IPTG to a final concentration of 0.5 mM. The cultures were then incubated for 24 h at 18 °C, 200 rpm before harvesting by centrifugation (2700× g, 20 min, 4 °C). The cell pellets were then stored at −80 °C until needed.

2.4. Protein Purification

PPTases were purified using standard Tris-Cl Ni-NTA chromatography buffers with the following modification: the bind, wash and elute buffers were supplemented with 25% v/v glycerol to enhance protein stability. The eluted PPTases were then desalted using a HiTrap desalting column (Cytiva, Marlborough, MA, USA) with a desalting buffer of 50 mM Tris-Cl (pH 7.8) and 12.5% glycerol (v/v). The buffer composition was then adjusted to a final concentration of 40% (v/v) glycerol, and aliquots were stored at −80 °C until needed. *Apo* and *holo*-BpsA were purified as previously described [25].

2.5. Optimisation of Enzyme Concentrations

To determine the optimal concentration of BpsA for the detection of PptT inhibition, 30 µL of reaction mix comprising 50 mM Tris-Cl (pH 8.0), 10 mM $MgCl_2$ and 5 mM ATP was added to individual wells of a standard 96 well plate. Next, 10 µL *holo*-BpsA (purified and activated as previously described [25]) was added to each well to give a range of final concentrations (0–1 µM). To initiate indigoidine synthesis, 10 µL of 5 mM L-glutamine was added to each well. The plate was then shaken at 1000 rpm for 10 s and incubated at room temperature for 1 h. The indigoidine was then resolubilised by the addition of 200 µL DMSO and then incubated at 37 °C with shaking at 200 rpm for 0.5 h. A Perkin Elmer Enspire Plate reader was then used to record the absorbance readings at 590 nm.

To determine the optimal concentration of PptT for the detection of inhibitors, 10 µL of PPTase mix comprising 50 mM Tris-Cl (pH 8.0) and PptT at a range of concentrations (0–0.5 µM) was added to individual wells of a standard 96 well plate. To initiate indigoidine synthesis, 40 µL of a reaction mix comprising 50 mM Tris-Cl (pH 8.0), 10 mM $MgCl_2$, 5 mM ATP, 5 mM L-glutamine, 10 µM CoA and 0.6 µM *apo*-BpsA was added to each well. The plate was then shaken at 1000 rpm for 10 s and incubated at room temperature for 1 h. The indigoidine was then resolubilised by the addition of 200 µL DMSO and incubated at 37 °C with shaking at 200 rpm for 0.5 h. A Perkin Elmer Enspire plate reader was then used to record the absorbance of each well at 590 nm.

2.6. Z-Factor Calculation

To determine the Z-factor of the screen, 80 reactions were established in columns 2–11 of a standard 96 well-plate. Each was prepared from 30 µL of reaction mix comprising 50 mM Tris-Cl (pH 8.0), 0.01% (v/v) Triton-X, 10 mM $MgCl_2$, 5 mM ATP, 5 mM L-glutamine and 10 µM CoA. Next, 10 µL PPTase mix containing either 0.4 µM PptT and 50 mM Tris-Cl (pH 8.0) (or else unadulterated 50 mM Tris-Cl (pH 8.0) as a negative control) was added to each well. To initiate indigoidine synthesis, 10 µL of 0.6 µM *apo*-BpsA in 50 mM Tris-Cl (pH 8.0) was added to each well. The plate was then shaken at 1000 rpm for 10 s and incubated at room temperature for 1 h. The indigoidine was then resolubilised by the addition of 200 µL DMSO and incubated at 37 °C with shaking at 200 rpm for 0.5 h. A Perkin Elmer Enspire plate reader was then used to record the absorbance readings at 590 nm. To calculate the Z-factor, the following equation was used (derived from the method of Zhang et al. [27]), with σ representing the standard deviation, µ representing the means and ρ representing the positive and n the negative control.

$$Z\,factor = 1 - \frac{3(\sigma_\rho + \sigma_n)}{|\mu_\rho - \mu_n|}$$

2.7. Screening of the LOPAC^{1280} Collection and EC$_{50}$ Calculations

The Sigma-Aldrich LOPAC^{1280} collection was first diluted to a working stock of 500 mM per compound. To screen the collection, 88 reactions at a time were established in columns 1–11 of a standard 96 well-plate. Each was prepared from 30 µL of reaction mix comprising 50 mM Tris-Cl (pH 8.0), 0.01% (v/v) Triton-X, 10 mM MgCl$_2$, 5 mM ATP, 5 mM L-glutamine and 10 µM CoA. Next, a CyBio liquid handler was used to pin 2 µL of compound into columns 2–11 and 2 µL of DMSO into column 1. To screen for PptT inhibitors, 10 µL of PPTase mix comprising a freshly-prepared stock of 0.4 µM PptT and 50 mM Tris-Cl (pH 8.0) was added to wells A1–C1 and columns 2–11 (see Supplementary Figure S1). To initiate indigoidine synthesis, 10 µL of 0.6 µM *apo*-BpsA in 50 mM Tris-Cl (pH 8.0) was added to each well. To screen for *holo*-BpsA inhibitors, an equivalent screening format was established only using 0.6 µM *holo*-BpsA and with no PPTase mix added. Each plate was then shaken at 1000 rpm for 10 s and incubated at room temperature for 1 h. Indigoidine was then resolubilised by the addition of 200 µL DMSO and incubation at 37 °C with shaking at 200 rpm for 0.5 h. A Perkin Elmer Enspire plate reader was then used to record the absorbance readings at 590 nm. The Python package Pandas [28] was used to process the data, which was then visualised using the Python package Seaborn [29].

To calculate the EC$_{50}$ values of inhibitors, a two-fold serial dilution between 40 µM and 0.625 µM of each compound was established in 30 µL reaction mixes comprising 50 mM Tris-Cl (pH 8.0), triton-X 0.01% (v/v), 10 mM MgCl$_2$, 5 mM ATP, 5 mM L-glutamine and 10 µM CoA in replicate rows of a 96 well plate. To screen for PptT inhibitors, 10 µL of PPTase mix comprising a freshly-thawed stock of 0.4 µM PptT in 50 mM Tris-Cl (pH 8.0) was added. To initiate indigoidine synthesis, 10 µL of 0.6 µM *apo*-BpsA in 50 mM Tris-Cl (pH 8.0) was added to each well. The plate was then shaken at 1000 rpm for 10 s and incubated at room temperature for 1 h. Indigoidine was resolubilised by the addition of 200 µL DMSO and incubation at 37 °C with shaking at 200 rpm for 0.5 h. A Perkin Elmer Enspire plate reader was then used to record the absorbance readings at 590 nm. The percentage inhibition at each compound concentration was then compared to a DMSO only control, and GraphPad Prism 9.0 was used to fit a four parameter dose–response curve.

2.8. Kinetic Analysis of PptT Inhibition

To calculate the inhibition of PptT by 6-nitroso-1,2-benzopyrone and sanguinarine chloride, a serial dilution between 200 µM and 0.2 µM was established for each compound in 30 µL 50 mM Tris-Cl (pH 8.0) and Triton-X 0.01% (v/v) across individual rows of a standard 96 well plate. Next, 35 µL of a PPTase mix comprising a freshly-thawed stock of 0.4 µM PptT, 50 mM Tris-Cl (pH 8.0) and Triton-X 0.01% (v/v) was added to each well. To initiate indigoidine synthesis, a 35 µL reaction mix comprising 0.01% (v/v) Triton-X, 50 mM Tris-Cl (pH 8.0), 10 mM MgCl$_2$, 5 mM ATP, 5 mM L-glutamine, 10 µM CoA and 0.6 µM apo-BpsA was added to each well. The plate was then shaken at 1000 rpm for 10 s, and absorbance readings at 590 nm were read every 20 s. To determine the EC$_{50}$ values, the maximum indigoidine synthesis velocities were determined as described previously [22], and four-parameter dose–response curves were fitted using GraphPad Prism version 9.0.

3. Results

To determine whether BpsA could be used to screen for inhibitors of PptT, it was first necessary to show that PptT is capable of activating BpsA from the inactive *apo* to active *holo* form. BpsA was purified in the *apo* form from the Type II PPTase null *E. coli* strain BL21 ΔentD [26] and co-incubated with purified PptT. We and others [16,17,30] have found PptT to be quite unstable in aqueous solutions, with it rapidly aggregating and losing activity. This necessitated freshly thawed PptT (purified and stored on glycerol at −80 °C) to be used for each assay. Nonetheless, PptT was capable of rapidly activating *apo*-BpsA in vitro, yielding a typical indigoidine synthesis curve that reflects an initial burst of indigoidine synthesis followed by subsequent indigoidine precipitation [22] (Figure 1C).

In our previous demonstration that BpsA could be used to quantify the strength of PPTase inhibition by the broad-specificity PPTase inhibitor 6-nitroso-1,2-benzopyrone, we monitored the change in velocity of indigoidine synthesis via continuous kinetic measurements [22]. We have since developed BpsA as a biosensor to measure glutamine [25] and ATP [31] and in so doing observed that end-point measurements post-solubilisation of the total indigoidine in 80% DMSO yielded more consistent data. To implement a similar approach here to quantify inhibition of PptT, we first assayed pre-activated *holo*-BpsA at a concentration range from 0 to 1 μM in 50 μL reactions. This enabled us to identify 0.6 μM BpsA as an enzyme concentration that could provide a robust signal within the linear range of the assay, in a volume that could accommodate the addition of DMSO to 80% (v/v) without exceeding the well capacity of a standard 96-well plate (Figure 2A). We then identified 0.4 μM PptT as a suitable concentration of target PPTase that, in the absence of inhibitor, induced a strong indigoidine synthesis signal when co-incubated with 0.6 μM *apo*-BpsA (Figure 2B).

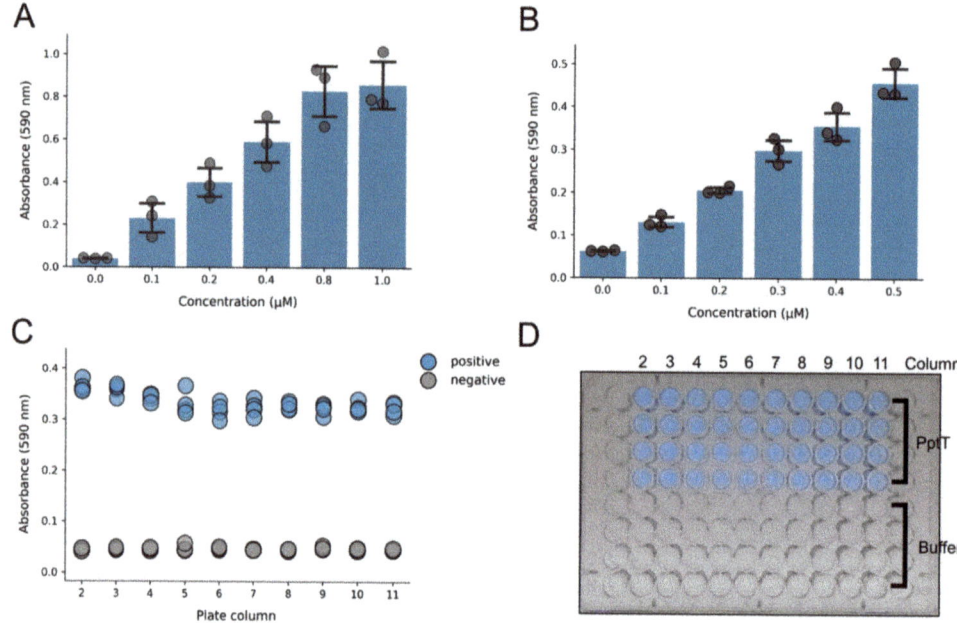

Figure 2. Optimisation of assay parameters: (**A**) increasing concentrations of *holo*-BpsA were added to a reaction mix containing 10 mM MgCl$_2$, 5 mM ATP and 50 mM Tris-Cl (pH 8.0). The reaction was then initiated by addition of 5 mM L-glutamine and incubated for 1 h. The indigoidine was then resolubilised by the addition of DMSO, which gave a linear increase in absorbance until the assay began to saturate at an A$_{590}$ of approximately 1.0. Data are the averages of three independent replicates and error bars represent one standard deviation. (**B**) Increasing concentrations of PptT were added to a reaction mix containing 10 mM MgCl$_2$, 5 mM ATP, 5 mM L-glutamine, 0.6 μM apo-BpsA and 10 μM CoA. The reaction was incubated for 1 h and then resolubilised by the addition of DMSO, and A$_{590}$ values were recorded. A higher concentration of PptT resulted in an increased absorbance reading, indicating that a single endpoint assay can be used to detect inhibition. Data are the averages of three independent replicates, and error bars represent one standard deviation. (**C**) To determine the Z' factor of the screen, a reaction mix was established in columns 2–11 comprising 0.01% triton X, 50 mM Tris-Cl (pH 8.0), 10 mM MgCl$_2$, 5 mM ATP, 5 mM L-glutamine and 10 μM CoA. Next, PptT (to a final concentration of 0.4 μM) and buffer were added to rows 1–4, while only buffer was added to rows 5–8. To initiate each reaction, 0.6 μM *apo*-BpsA was added. The A$_{590}$ values for rows containing PptT (blue, positive) and the buffer controls (grey, negative) were recorded following a 1 h incubation and subsequent solubilisation with DMSO. (**D**) A photo of the plate from the experiment described for panel C following solubilisation by DMSO. The plate was placed on a light box prior to taking the photo.

To validate the performance of the assay under conditions similar to a high throughput screen, we compared 80 reactions in a 96 well plate. A screening master mix comprising buffer, all requisite substrates (CoA, ATP and L-glutamine) and 0.01% Triton X-100 (to minimise nonspecific inhibitory activity from compounds that induce protein aggregation [32]) was aliquoted into each well. Next, PptT was added to 40 of the wells (to a final concentration of 0.4 µM), while the other 40 wells received only buffer to simulate reactions in which PptT had been completely inhibited. Finally, apo-BpsA was added to each well (to a final concentration of 0.6 µM) to initiate indigoidine synthesis, where possible. Following incubation for 1 h at room temperature, each 50 µL reaction was stopped by the addition of 200 µL of DMSO to solubilise the indigoidine, after which the A_{590} was measured (Figure 2C). The calculated Z'-factor for the assay was 0.77. This is a key measure of quality for high-throughput screens that derives from the separation of positive and negative control data; a Z'-factor above 0.5 represents 12 standard deviations of separation between the controls and hence a highly robust screen [27].

Having established the assay parameters, we then screened 1280 drug-like compounds from the Sigma-Aldrich library of pharmacologically active compounds (LOPAC^{1280}) to identify inhibitors of PptT (a schematic of the complete high-throughput screening procedure is presented in Figure S3A). The LOPAC^{1280} collection is widely used for screen validation studies and has previously been found to contain a diverse range of inhibitors of B. subtilis Sfp [19], giving us confidence that it was likely to contain a diversity of PptT inhibitors also. Each screening plate contained 80 compounds arrayed in columns 2–11. Three no-inhibitor positive controls and three negative controls lacking PptT were arrayed in column 1 of the screening plate, while column 12 was left empty (Supplementary Figure S1). The percentage activity for each well was then calculated relative to the average of the three positive controls located on each plate, revealing that 21 compounds caused ≥50% reduction in indigoidine levels (Figure 3B). Position effects were evident, owing to the instability of PptT upon addition to the aqueous reaction mix (in a row-by-row fashion using a multi-well pipette), which yielded a wave-like pattern of A_{590} readings from row to row (Supplementary Figure S2A). This phenomenon was not observed in a counter-screen that was conducted using pre-activated holo-BpsA, to eliminate any compounds that were inhibiting BpsA rather than PptT (Supplementary Figure S2B). While it is possible that variation in the levels of soluble PptT may have confounded identification of some weak PptT inhibitors, most of the 21 "hits" yielded data that were clearly separated from the baseline (Figure 3B, dashed line).

In counter-screening the LOPAC^{1280} collection against pre-activated holo-BpsA (Supplementary Figure S3B), four compounds were identified as inhibiting indigoidine synthesis rather than being PptT-specific: ebselen, suramin hexasodium, chlorprothixene hydrochloride and 4-chloromercuribenzoic acid. Chlorprothixene hydrochloride did not register as an inhibitor of PptT and may have been a false positive in this counter-screen, while the other three were discarded from further consideration as likely pan assay interference compounds (PAINS) [33].

We next quantified the inhibition conferred by each of the 18 remaining compounds, using two-fold serial dilutions (40 µM to 0.3 µM) of each compound added to a PptT/apo-BpsA reaction mix to generate EC_{50} values (Supplementary Figure S3). In one case (8-hydroxy-DPAT hydrobromide), no inhibitory activity was observed, indicating this was likely a false positive from our initial screen, while for nine of the remaining cases, the level of inhibition was insufficient to calculate meaningful EC_{50} values. Ultimately, we were able to confirm and quantify eight effective inhibitors of PptT (Table 1). Other than tyrphostin AG 537 and tyrphostin AG 538, all of these compounds had previously been reported as inhibitors of the canonical PPTase Sfp from B. subtilis [32].

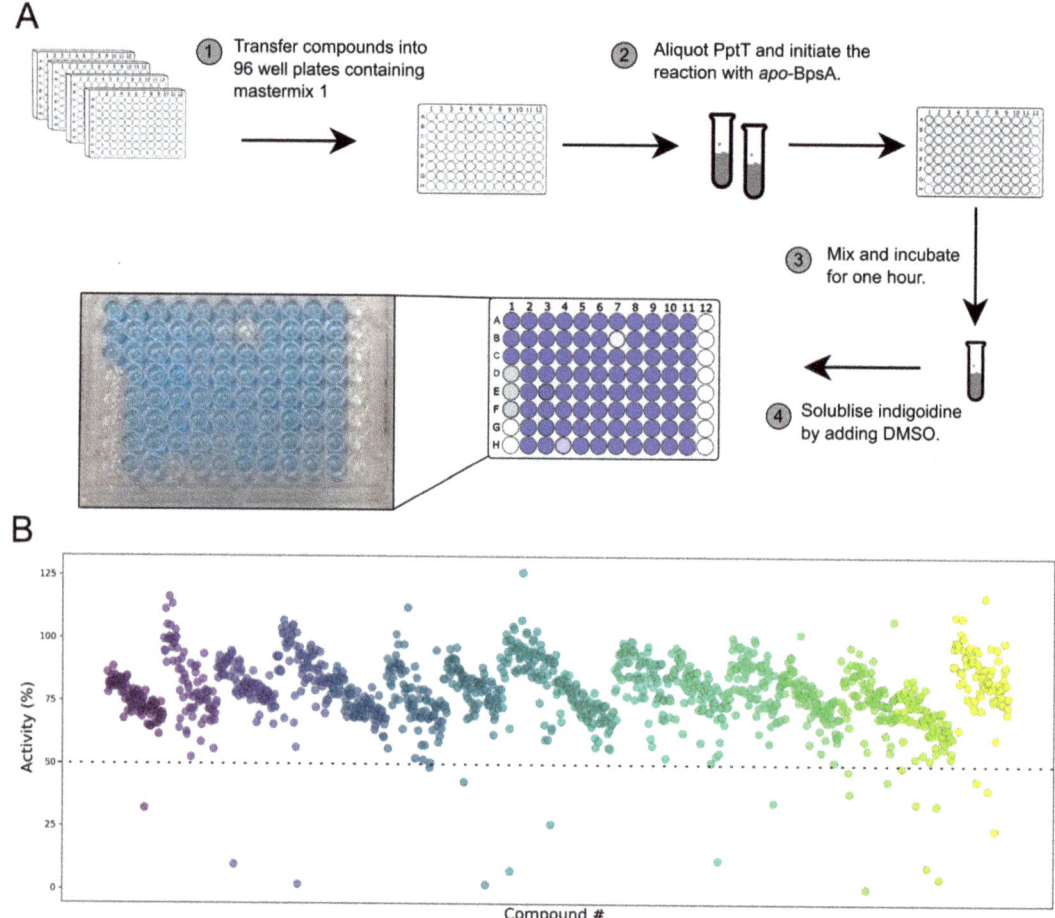

Figure 3. High-throughput screening of the LOPAC^{1280} library: (**A**) schematic diagram illustrating the screening process; (**B**) percentage activity of each compound in the library, with data derived from distinct 96 well plates presented in different colours.

Table 1. PptT inhibitors recovered from BpsA screen. Names and descriptions were derived from the LOPAC[1280] manifest. EC_{50} averages were calculated from three independent replicates ± standard error.

Name	Known Drug Activities	% Activity in PptT Screen	EC_{50} (µM)
Aurintricarboxylic acid	DNA topoisomerase II inhibitor	32	4.8 ± 0.9
SCH-202676 hydrobromide	Allosteric agonist and antagonist of GPCRs	0.7	5.9 ± 0.1
Tyrphostin AG 537	EGFR protein tyrosine kinase inhibitor	35	5.9 ± 0.5
Disulfiram	Alcohol dehydrogenase inhibitor	9	6.0 ± 1.5
Tyrphostin AG 538	(IGF-1) receptor protein tyrosine kinase inhibitor	24	6.4 ± 0.7
Bay 11-7085	Inhibitor of NFκB	10	7.4 ± 0.4
U-73122	Phospholipase C and A2 inhibitor	44	8.1 ± 0.5
6-Nitroso-1,2-benzopyrone	Poly(ADP-ribose) ligand	12	8.3 ± 1.7
6-Hydroxy-DL-DOPA	Precursor of the catecholaminergic neurotoxin	26	N.D.[1]
Tyrphostin AG 808	Protein tyrosine kinase inhibitor	34	N.D.[1]
I-OMe-Tyrphostin AG 538	(IGF-1) receptor protein tyrosine kinase inhibitor	40	N.D.[1]
Reactive Blue 2	P2Y receptor antagonist	38	N.D.[1]
GW5074	cRaf1 kinase inhibitor	43	N.D.[1]
PD 404, 182	KDO-8-P synthase inhibitor	35	N.D.[1]
Sanguinarine chloride	Inhibitor of ATPase	44	N.D.[1]
7,7-Dimethyl-(5z,8z)-eicosadienoic acid	Phospholipase A2 and lipoxygenase inhibitor	49	N.D.[1]
Rottlerin	PKC and CaM kinase III inhibitor	48	N.D.[1]

[1] N.D. = not determined, i.e., binding was insufficiently strong to permit a robust curve to be fitted to determine an EC_{50} value.

In other work, we recently screened the LOPAC[1280] collection against the SARS-CoV-2 protease using a FRET-based reporter and noticed that 8 of our 17 candidate PptT inhibitors (PD 404, 182, Disulfiram, U-73122, 6-nitroso-1,2-benzopyrone, aurintricarboxylic acid, sanguinarine chloride, Bay 11-7085 and 6-hydroxyl-DL-DOPA) also gave hits as strong protease inhibitors [34]. This suggested to us that many of these compounds may be generic enzyme inhibitors rather than specific for PptT. To further probe the specificity of hit compounds for PptT, we re-screened each for inhibition of *holo*-BpsA at a higher concentration of 40 µM (Supplementary Figure S4). In this higher-concentration counter-screen, SCH 202626, previously identified as a broad-spectrum PPTase inhibitor [19], became noticeably inhibitory of *holo*-BpsA. Only five compounds exhibited less than 15% inhibition of *holo*-BpsA: 6-nitroso-1,2-benzopyrone, 6-hydroxy-DL-DOPA, 7,7-dimethyl-(5Z,8Z)-eicosadienoic acid, disulfiram and sanguinarine chloride.

We next sought to benchmark our DMSO-resolubilisation end-point assay against the kinetic assay we had previously described [22]. For this, we selected two compounds with different inhibition profiles, namely 6-nitroso-1,2-benzopyrone, which has been shown to have activity in vitro against numerous PPTases [19,22,35] and in vivo against the fungus *Aspergillus fumigatus* in a PPTase dependant manner [36], and the weaker inhibitor sanguinarine chloride, which has been previously reported as an inhibitor of both Sfp from *B. subtilis* [21] and *M. tuberculosis* PptT [16]. We used identical enzymatic concentrations across both assays to permit a direct comparison. In the kinetic assay, we derived an EC_{50} value of 4.4 ± 1.2 µM for 6-nitroso-1,2-benzopyrone (Supplementary Figure S5A), which is similar to the EC_{50} value of 8.3 µM we calculated from our endpoint assay. However, the kinetic assay data for sanguinarine chloride was more variable (Supplementary Figure S5B), and GraphPad Prism 9.0 was unable to fit a robust curve. Based on this, we conclude that the endpoint assay is more sensitive and reproducible than the kinetic assay, at least at the tested enzyme concentrations.

4. Discussion

Here, we report on the development, optimisation and validation of a simple high-throughput assay to rapidly identify inhibitors of the promising antibiotic target PptT from *M. tuberculosis*. We validated the assay by screening the LOPAC[1280] collection from Sigma-Aldrich. To the best of our knowledge, this is the first reported direct chemical library screen for inhibitors of PptT. From this screen we identified 18 inhibitors, but further investigation indicated that ten of these were non-specific compounds that also inhibited *holo*-BpsA when added at higher concentrations. Of the remaining eight, two were novel

PPTase inhibitors that may be specific for PptT, while six had previously been identified as inhibitors of the *B. subtilis* canonical Type II PPTase Sfp, providing evidence by association for the efficacy of our screen. Finally, we compared our optimised end-point assay against a kinetic BpsA assay we had employed earlier [22] and concluded that the optimised assay is more amenable to high-throughput screening.

Two other assays have been developed to evaluate possible inhibitors of PptT. The first uses a scintillation proximity assay that is substantially more complex than our simple colourimetric BpsA assay, requiring radiolabelled CoA and a scintillation counting machine, and validation against PPTase inhibitors has not yet been reported [13]. The second assay uses rhodamine-labelled CoA to provide a more accessible fluorometric output [16]. This assay has been tested against a small panel of PptT inhibitors, but it is unclear if it would be able to detect inhibitors such as 8918. While 8918 is the best PptT inhibitor reported to date [15], it binds immediately alongside CoA in the active site and might be precluded from binding by a conjugated rhodamine at that position. As our screen uses unadulterated CoA, this would not be a concern.

PPTases have been discussed in the literature as promising drug targets for almost two decades [37]. Despite this, limited progress has been made on progressing inhibitors through drug development pipelines. Thus far the two most promising PPTase inhibitor drug candidates are ML-267, which was identified after high-throughput screening of approximately 330,000 compounds against *B. subtilis* Sfp [38], but has not yet had efficacy reported against other PPTases; and 8918, which was identified from a whole-cell screen of *M. tuberculosis* HR7Rv against approximately 90,000 small molecules, with PptT subsequently identified as the drug target [15]. While whole cell screens offer the major advantage that biological activity is guaranteed, at least under the assay conditions employed, target identification is often far more difficult, and high-proportions of time-wasting promiscuous "nuisance compounds" are frequently recovered [39]. Moreover, for mycobacterial screens it has been reported that variations in media can substantially alter the spectrum of inhibitors identified from a given chemical collection, raising concerns as to how well host-relevant physicochemical conditions are represented [40]. Conversely, target-based screens for *M. tuberculosis* offer substantial promise in enabling selection of a suitable target upfront [41] and facilitating rational exploration of structure–activity relationships [42]. Our assay therefore meets a need for a simple high-throughput assay that can be applied to directly screen for inhibitors of PptT or other Type II PPTases, or to guide the development of next-generation drug leads based on promising scaffolds such as ML-267 and 8918. Recently, we have also shown that the PCP-domain of BpsA can be rapidly evolved using error-prone mutagenesis to be recognised by other Type II PPTases that initially cannot activate BpsA [35]. This provides a platform to enable the rapid integration of multiple PPTases for inhibitory activity, or to counter-screen the endogenous human PPTase to eliminate drug candidates likely to have undesirable off-target effects. Collectively, we hope this toolbox will prove useful in guiding future medicinal chemistry efforts to design or identify broad spectrum PPTase inhibitors.

Supplementary Materials: The following are available online at https://www.mdpi.com/article/10.3390/pharmaceutics13071066/s1, Figure S1: LOPAC1280 screening plate layout, Figure S2: Raw values absorbance values of the LOPAC1280 collection, Figure S3: EC50 values for top compounds, Figure S4: Inhibition of *holo*-BpsA at an inhibitor concentration of 40 µM, Figure S5: Kinetic determination of EC_{50} values.

Author Contributions: Conceptualization, A.S.B., E.N.B. and D.F.A.; Data curation, A.S.B.; Formal analysis, A.S.B.; Funding acquisition, D.F.A.; Investigation, A.S.B.; Methodology, A.S.B., J.G.O. and D.F.A.; Project administration, D.F.A.; Resources, J.G.O. and J.J.; Supervision, E.N.B. and D.F.A.; Validation, A.S.B. and J.G.O.; Writing—original draft, A.S.B. and D.F.A.; Writing—review and editing, A.S.B., J.J., E.N.B. and D.F.A. All authors have read and agreed to the published version of the manuscript.

Funding: This research was funded by the Royal Society of New Zealand Marsden Fund (Contract VUW0901 to D.F.A.). A.S.B. was supported by a VUW postgraduate scholarship.

Institutional Review Board Statement: Not applicable.

Informed Consent Statement: Not applicable.

Data Availability Statement: The data presented in this study are available on request from the corresponding author.

Conflicts of Interest: The authors declare no conflict of interest. The funders had no role in the design of the study; in the collection, analyses or interpretation of data; in the writing of the manuscript; or in the decision to publish the results.

References

1. Global Tuberculosis Report. 2020. Available online: https://www.who.int/publications-detail-redirect/9789240013131 (accessed on 5 May 2021).
2. Shetye, G.S.; Franzblau, S.G.; Cho, S. New tuberculosis drug targets, their inhibitors, and potential therapeutic impact. *Transl. Res.* **2020**, *220*, 68–97. [CrossRef] [PubMed]
3. Neyrolles, O.; Guilhot, C. Recent advances in deciphering the contribution of *Mycobacterium tuberculosis* lipids to pathogenesis. *Tuberculosis* **2011**, *91*, 187–195. [CrossRef] [PubMed]
4. Daffé, M. The cell envelope of tubercle bacilli. *Tuberculosis* **2015**, *95*, S155–S158. [CrossRef] [PubMed]
5. Karakousis, P.C.; Bishai, W.R.; Dorman, S.E. *Mycobacterium tuberculosis* cell envelope lipids and the host immune response. *Cell. Microbiol.* **2004**, *6*, 105–116. [CrossRef]
6. Gokhale, R.S.; Saxena, P.; Chopra, T.; Mohanty, D. Versatile polyketide enzymatic machinery for the biosynthesis of complex mycobacterial lipids. *Nat. Prod. Rep.* **2007**, *24*, 267–277. [CrossRef]
7. McMahon, M.D.; Rush, J.S.; Thomas, M.G. Analyses of MbtB, MbtE, and MbtF Suggest Revisions to the Mycobactin Biosynthesis Pathway in *Mycobacterium tuberculosis*. *J. Bacteriol.* **2012**, *194*, 2809–2818. [CrossRef]
8. Beld, J.; Sonnenschein, E.; Vickery, C.R.; Noel, J.P.; Burkart, M.D. The phosphopantetheinyl transferases: Catalysis of a post-translational modification crucial for life. *Nat. Prod. Rep.* **2014**, *31*, 61–108. [CrossRef]
9. Foley, T.L.; Young, B.S.; Burkart, M.D. Phosphopantetheinyl transferase inhibition and secondary metabolism. *FEBS J.* **2009**, *276*, 7134–7145. [CrossRef]
10. Chalut, C.; Botella, L.; de Sousa-D'Auria, C.; Houssin, C.; Guilhot, C. The nonredundant roles of two 4′-phosphopantetheinyl transferases in vital processes of *Mycobacteria*. *Proc. Natl. Acad. Sci. USA* **2006**, *103*, 8511–8516. [CrossRef] [PubMed]
11. Zimhony, O.; Schwarz, A.; Raitses-Gurevich, M.; Peleg, Y.; Dym, O.; Albeck, S.; Burstein, Y.; Shakked, Z. AcpM, the Meromycolate Extension Acyl Carrier Protein of *Mycobacterium tuberculosis*, Is Activated by the 4′-Phosphopantetheinyl Transferase PptT, a Potential Target of the Multistep Mycolic Acid Biosynthesis. *Biochemistry* **2015**, *54*, 2360–2371. [CrossRef] [PubMed]
12. Sassetti, C.M.; Boyd, D.H.; Rubin, E.J. Comprehensive identification of conditionally essential genes in mycobacteria. *Proc. Natl. Acad. Sci. USA* **2001**, *98*, 12712–12717. [CrossRef]
13. Leblanc, C.; Prudhomme, T.; Tabouret, G.; Ray, A.; Burbaud, S.; Cabantous, S.; Mourey, L.; Guilhot, C.; Chalut, C. 4′-Phosphopantetheinyl Transferase PptT, a New Drug Target Required for *Mycobacterium tuberculosis* Growth and Persistence In Vivo. *PLOS Pathog.* **2012**, *8*, e1003097. [CrossRef] [PubMed]
14. Quadri, L.E.; Sello, J.; Keating, T.A.; Weinreb, P.; Walsh, C.T. Identification of a *Mycobacterium tuberculosis* gene cluster encoding the biosynthetic enzymes for assembly of the virulence-conferring siderophore mycobactin. *Chem. Biol.* **1998**, *5*, 631–645. [CrossRef]
15. Ballinger, E.; Mosior, J.; Hartman, T.; Burns-Huang, K.; Gold, B.; Morris, R.; Goullieux, L.; Blanc, I.; Vaubourgeix, J.; Lagrange, S.; et al. Opposing reactions in coenzyme A metabolism sensitize *Mycobacterium tuberculosis* to enzyme inhibition. *Science* **2019**, *363*, eaau8959. [CrossRef] [PubMed]
16. Vickery, C.R.; Kosa, N.M.; Casavant, E.P.; Duan, S.; Noel, J.P.; Burkart, M.D. Structure, Biochemistry, and Inhibition of Essential 4′-Phosphopantetheinyl Transferases from Two Species of *Mycobacteria*. *ACS Chem. Biol.* **2014**, *9*, 1939–1944. [CrossRef]
17. Jung, J.; Bashiri, G.; Johnston, J.M.; Brown, A.S.; Ackerley, D.F.; Baker, E.N. Crystal structure of the essential *Mycobacterium tuberculosis* phosphopantetheinyl transferase PptT, solved as a fusion protein with maltose binding protein. *J. Struct. Biol.* **2014**, *188*, 274–278. [CrossRef] [PubMed]
18. Reuter, K.; Mofid, M.R.; Marahiel, M.A.; Ficner, R. Crystal structure of the surfactin synthetase-activating enzyme Sfp: A prototype of the 4′-phosphopantetheinyl transferase superfamily. *EMBO J.* **1999**, *18*, 6823–6831. [CrossRef]
19. Yasgar, A.; Foley, T.L.; Jadhav, A.; Inglese, J.; Burkart, M.D.; Simeonov, A. A strategy to discover inhibitors of *Bacillus subtilis* surfactin-type phosphopantetheinyl transferase. *Mol. BioSyst.* **2009**, *6*, 365–375. [CrossRef]
20. Duckworth, B.P.; Aldrich, C.C. Development of a high-throughput fluorescence polarization assay for the discovery of phosphopantetheinyl transferase inhibitors. *Anal. Biochem.* **2010**, *403*, 13–19. [CrossRef]
21. Kosa, N.M.; Foley, T.L.; Burkart, M.D. Fluorescent techniques for discovery and characterization of phosphopantetheinyl transferase inhibitors. *J. Antibiot.* **2013**, *67*, 113–120. [CrossRef]

22. Owen, J.G.; Copp, J.N.; Ackerley, D.F. Rapid and flexible biochemical assays for evaluating 4′-phosphopantetheinyl transferase activity. *Biochem. J.* **2011**, *436*, 709–717. [CrossRef]
23. Takahashi, H.; Kumagai, T.; Kitani, K.; Mori, M.; Matoba, Y.; Sugiyama, M. Cloning and Characterization of a Streptomyces Single Module Type Non-ribosomal Peptide Synthetase Catalyzing a Blue Pigment Synthesis. *J. Biol. Chem.* **2007**, *282*, 9073–9081. [CrossRef]
24. Pettersen, E.F.; Goddard, T.D.; Huang, C.C.; Couch, G.S.; Greenblatt, D.M.; Meng, E.C.; Ferrin, T.E. UCSF Chimera—A visualization system for exploratory research and analysis. *J. Comput. Chem.* **2004**, *25*, 1605–1612. [CrossRef]
25. Brown, A.S.; Robins, K.; Ackerley, D.F. A sensitive single-enzyme assay system using the non-ribosomal peptide synthetase BpsA for measurement of L-glutamine in biological samples. *Sci. Rep.* **2017**, *7*, srep41745. [CrossRef]
26. Owen, J.G.; Robins, K.; Parachin, N.; Ackerley, D.F. A functional screen for recovery of 4′-phosphopantetheinyl transferase and associated natural product biosynthesis genes from metagenome libraries. *Environ. Microbiol.* **2012**, *14*, 1198–1209. [CrossRef] [PubMed]
27. Zhang, J.-H.; Chung, T.D.Y.; Oldenburg, K.R. A Simple Statistical Parameter for Use in Evaluation and Validation of High Throughput Screening Assays. *J. Biomol. Screen.* **1999**, *4*, 67–73. [CrossRef] [PubMed]
28. The Pandas Development Team. Pandas-Dev/Pandas: Pandas 1.2.4. *Zenodo* **2021**. [CrossRef]
29. Waskom, M.L. seaborn: Statistical data visualization. *J. Open Source Softw.* **2021**, *6*, 3021. [CrossRef]
30. Rottier, K.; Faille, A.; Prudhomme, T.; Leblanc, C.; Chalut, C.; Cabantous, S.; Guilhot, C.; Mourey, L.; Pedelacq, J.-D. Detection of soluble co-factor dependent protein expression in vivo: Application to the 4′-phosphopantetheinyl transferase PptT from Mycobacterium tuberculosis. *J. Struct. Biol.* **2013**, *183*, 320–328. [CrossRef] [PubMed]
31. Brown, A.S.; Calcott, M.J.; Collins, V.M.; Owen, J.G.; Ackerley, D.F. The indigoidine synthetase BpsA provides a colorimetric ATP assay that can be adapted to quantify the substrate preferences of other NRPS enzymes. *Biotechnol. Lett.* **2020**, *42*, 2665–2671. [CrossRef]
32. Feng, B.Y.; Shoichet, B.K. A detergent-based assay for the detection of promiscuous inhibitors. *Nat. Protoc.* **2006**, *1*, 550–553. [CrossRef]
33. Baell, J.B.; Nissink, J.W.M. Seven Year Itch: Pan-Assay Interference Compounds (PAINS) in 2017—Utility and Limitations. *ACS Chem. Biol.* **2018**, *13*, 36–44. [CrossRef] [PubMed]
34. Brown, A.S.; Ackerley, D.F.; Calcott, M.J. High-Throughput Screening for Inhibitors of the SARS-CoV-2 Protease Using a FRET-Biosensor. *Molecules* **2020**, *25*, 4666. [CrossRef] [PubMed]
35. Brown, A.S.; Sissons, J.A.; Owen, J.G.; Ackerley, D.F. Directed Evolution of the Nonribosomal Peptide Synthetase BpsA to Enable Recognition by the Human Phosphopantetheinyl Transferases for Counter-Screening Antibiotic Candidates. *ACS Infect. Dis.* **2020**, *6*, 2879–2886. [CrossRef] [PubMed]
36. Johns, A.; Scharf, D.; Gsaller, F.; Schmidt, H.; Heinekamp, T.; Straßburger, M.; Oliver, J.D.; Birch, M.; Beckmann, N.; Dobb, K.S.; et al. A Nonredundant Phosphopantetheinyl Transferase, PptA, Is a Novel Antifungal Target That Directs Secondary Metabolite, Siderophore, and Lysine Biosynthesis in *Aspergillus fumigatus* and Is Critical for Pathogenicity. *mBio* **2017**, *8*, e01504-16. [CrossRef] [PubMed]
37. Gilbert, A.M.; Kirisits, M.; Toy, P.; Nunn, D.S.; Failli, A.; Dushin, E.G.; Novikova, E.; Petersen, P.J.; Joseph-McCarthy, D.; McFadyen, I.; et al. Anthranilate 4H-oxazol-5-ones: Novel small molecule antibacterial acyl carrier protein synthase (AcpS) inhibitors. *Bioorg. Med. Chem. Lett.* **2004**, *14*, 37–41. [CrossRef]
38. Foley, T.L.; Rai, G.; Yasgar, A.; Daniel, T.; Baker, H.L.; Attene-Ramos, M.; Kosa, N.M.; Leister, W.; Burkart, M.D.; Jadhav, A.; et al. 4-(3-Chloro-5-(trifluoromethyl)pyridin-2-yl)-N-(4-methoxypyridin-2-yl)piperazine-1-carbothioamide (ML267), a Potent Inhibitor of Bacterial Phosphopantetheinyl Transferase That Attenuates Secondary Metabolism and Thwarts Bacterial Growth. *J. Med. Chem.* **2014**, *57*, 1063–1078. [CrossRef]
39. Matano, L.M.; Morris, H.G.; Wood, B.M.; Meredith, T.C.; Walker, S. Accelerating the discovery of antibacterial compounds using pathway-directed whole cell screening. *Bioorg. Med. Chem.* **2016**, *24*, 6307–6314. [CrossRef] [PubMed]
40. Miller, C.H.; Nisa, S.; Dempsey, S.; Jack, C.; O'Toole, R. Modifying Culture Conditions in Chemical Library Screening Identifies Alternative Inhibitors of Mycobacteria. *Antimicrob. Agents Chemother.* **2009**, *53*, 5279–5283. [CrossRef]
41. Abrahams, K.A.; Besra, G.S. Mycobacterial drug discovery. *RSC Med. Chem.* **2020**, *11*, 1354–1365. [CrossRef]
42. Kana, B.D.; Karakousis, P.C.; Parish, T.; Dick, T. Future target-based drug discovery for tuberculosis? *Tuberculosis* **2014**, *94*, 551–556. [CrossRef] [PubMed]

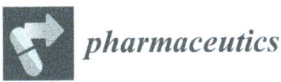

Article

Development of Novel Peptides for the Antimicrobial Combination Therapy against Carbapenem-Resistant *Acinetobacter baumannii* Infection

Joonhyeok Choi [1], Ahjin Jang [1], Young Kyung Yoon [2] and Yangmee Kim [1,*]

[1] Department of Bioscience and Biotechnology, Konkuk University, Seoul 05029, Korea; jun9688@konkuk.ac.kr (J.C.); ajin931017@konkuk.ac.kr (A.J.)
[2] Division of Infectious Diseases, Department of Internal Medicine, Korea University College of Medicine, Seoul 02841, Korea; young7912@korea.ac.kr
* Correspondence: ymkim@konkuk.ac.kr; Tel.: +822-450-3421; Fax: +822-447-5987

Citation: Choi, J.; Jang, A.; Yoon, Y.K.; Kim, Y. Development of Novel Peptides for the Antimicrobial Combination Therapy against Carbapenem-Resistant *Acinetobacter baumannii* Infection. *Pharmaceutics* **2021**, *13*, 1800. https://doi.org/10.3390/pharmaceutics13111800

Academic Editor: Clive Prestidge

Received: 31 August 2021
Accepted: 25 October 2021
Published: 27 October 2021

Publisher's Note: MDPI stays neutral with regard to jurisdictional claims in published maps and institutional affiliations.

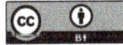

Copyright: © 2021 by the authors. Licensee MDPI, Basel, Switzerland. This article is an open access article distributed under the terms and conditions of the Creative Commons Attribution (CC BY) license (https://creativecommons.org/licenses/by/4.0/).

Abstract: Carbapenem-resistant *Acinetobacter baumannii* (CRAB) infection has a high mortality rate, making the development of novel effective antibiotic therapeutic strategies highly critical. Antimicrobial peptides can outperform conventional antibiotics regarding drug resistance and broad-spectrum activity. PapMA, an 18-residue hybrid peptide, containing N-terminal residues of papiliocin and magainin 2, has previously demonstrated potent antibacterial activity. In this study, PapMA analogs were designed by substituting Ala[15] or Phe[18] with Ala, Phe, and Trp. PapMA-3 with Trp[18] showed the highest bacterial selectivity against CRAB, alongside low cytotoxicity. Biophysical studies revealed that PapMA-3 permeabilizes CRAB membrane via strong binding to LPS. To reduce toxicity via reduced antibiotic doses, while preventing the emergence of multi-drug resistant bacteria, the efficacy of PapMA-3 in combination with six selected antibiotics was evaluated against clinical CRAB isolates (C1–C5). At 25% of the minimum inhibition concentration, PapMA-3 partially depolarized the CRAB membrane and caused sufficient morphological changes, facilitating the entry of antibiotics into the bacterial cell. Combining PapMA-3 with rifampin significantly and synergistically inhibited CRAB C4 (FICI = 0.13). Meanwhile, combining PapMA-3 with vancomycin or erythromycin, both potent against Gram-positive bacteria, demonstrated remarkable synergistic antibiofilm activity against Gram-negative CRAB. This study could aid in the development of combination therapeutic approaches against CRAB.

Keywords: antimicrobial peptides; antibiotics; synergistic effect; CRAB

1. Introduction

The emergence of multi-drug resistant (MDR) bacteria, combined with the failure of most antibiotic candidates in clinical trials, poses a serious threat to global public health [1–3]. In particular, diseases caused by Gram-negative bacteria, such as postoperative wound infection, urinary tract infection, hospital-acquired pneumonia, catheter-associated bloodstream infection, meningitis, and sepsis [4,5], have high mortality. Carbapenems such as doripenem, imipenem, and meropenem are generally considered to be the final choice of treatment for MDR Gram-negative bacteria; however, these bacteria have recently begun to show increased resistance to these drugs. MDR bacterial infections featuring carbapenem-resistant *Acinetobacter baumannii* (CRAB) are at the top of the World Health Organization (WHO) priority list for the development of new antibiotics [6–8]. Therefore, there is a need to accelerate the development of new antibiotic therapeutic strategies.

As antibiotic resistance develops rapidly after the introduction of new antimicrobial agents, it is necessary to develop antimicrobial compounds with novel mechanisms that differ from those of conventional antibiotics. Antimicrobial peptides (AMPs) are diverse, and they are produced by various living organisms [9,10], where they are known to participate in the organism's innate immunity [11–13]. Unlike conventional antibiotics, most AMPs have amphiphilic structures, and they exhibit antibacterial activity primarily through interactions with the negatively charged bacterial membrane, making it difficult for the bacteria to develop resistance [14]. In addition, their rapid and broad-spectrum antimicrobial activity make them potential therapeutic alternative to antibiotics [15].

In the clinical setting, different antibiotics are often used in combination therapy to broaden the antimicrobial spectra. The main advantage of combination antibiotic therapy is that it can prevent the emergence of MDR bacteria. Antibiotics can exhibit side effects such as diarrhea, rash, nausea, liver damage, and kidney damage; therefore, decreasing drug toxicity through lowering the doses is beneficial [16–18]. A few novel AMPs exhibit synergistic effects with known antibiotics against MDR bacteria. (p-BthTX-I)$_2$ and LL-37 in combination with florfenicol and thiamphenicol exert antimicrobial activity against *Citrobacter freundii* [19]. Melittin in combination with clindamycin has shown antimicrobial activity against methicillin-resistant *Staphylococcus aureus* [20]. AMPs have also been combined with antibiotics such as T3, T4 with ampicillin and oxacillin [21], WW304 with ciprofloxacin [22], and G3KL with erythromycin and vancomycin [23]. As carbapenem is the most used front-line antibiotic for treating Gram-negative bacterial infections, the accelerating appearance of CRAB seriously threatens global public health [6–8]. Antimicrobial activity against MDR-Gram-negative bacteria has been improved through the synergistic effects of SET-M33 [24] or melittin [25] with antibiotics; however, such synergistic combinations with antibiotics to combat CRAB infections remains challenging to develop. AMPs have thus demonstrated some potential regarding combination therapy with conventional antibiotics. Additionally, to overcome drug resistance, AMPs can be easily manipulated to design potent novel AMPs by substituting their amino acid residues. Therefore, the development of AMPs that have synergistic effects with antibiotics against MDR Gram-negative bacteria, and especially clinical CRAB isolates, is important but challenging.

AMPs with improved antimicrobial activities include a series of hybrid peptides that were designed by combining the active regions of two AMPs. For example, cecropin A-magainin 2 (CAMA) and cecropin A-melittin (CAME) hybrid peptides have previously been reported to demonstrate high antimicrobial and antitumor activities [26–28]. A hybrid peptide with a broad spectrum of antimicrobial activity (PapMA) was discovered by connecting the N-termini of papiliocin and magainin 2, joined by a proline (Pro) hinge [29]. The structure of PapMA was investigated using nuclear magnetic resonance (NMR) spectroscopy, revealing that it had an N-terminal α-helix from Lys^3 to Lys^7 and a C-terminal α-helix from Lys^{10} to Lys^{17}, with a Pro^9 hinge in between. PapMA showed potent antibacterial activity against both Gram-negative and Gram-positive bacteria.

In this study, we aimed to design a novel PapMA analog with increased anti-CRAB activity, while maintaining low cytotoxicity. Its synergistic antibacterial activities against CRAB were then investigated when combined with conventional antibiotics, and the inhibition of biofilm formation was also assessed. In total, six analogs of PapMA were designed by substituting Ala^{15} or Phe^{18} with Ala, Phe, and Trp at the C-terminus. Among the six analogs, we chose PapMA-3 as a candidate for further investigation, as it showed potent anti-CRAB activity with low cytotoxicity. PapMA-3 was found to depolarize CRAB cell membranes, which disrupted biofilm formation and increased susceptibility to the conventional antibiotics. Therefore, in this study, the key mechanism of action underlying this AMP activity was elucidated, suggesting that they are valuable as an adjuvant pharmaceutical to overcome Gram-negative bacterial resistance and represents a good starting point for the development of new antibiotics against CRAB infection.

2. Materials and Methods

2.1. Peptides and Materials

All peptides were synthesized through N-(9-fluorenyl) methoxycarbonyl solid-phase synthesis and were purified using reversed-phase high-performance liquid chromatography (RP-HPLC, YL9100, Younglin, Korea). Peptide purities were over 95%, as evaluated using an analytical HPLC (C18 column, 4.6 × 250 mm) with two different linear gradients of 0.05% aqueous trifluoroacetic acid (TFA, eluent A) and 0.05% TFA in CH_3CN (eluent B) at a flow rate of 1.5 mL per min at 25 °C. The molecular masses of the peptides (Table 1) were determined using Axima (Shimadzu Scientific Instruments, Kyoto, Japan) matrix-assisted laser-desorption ionization-time of flight mass spectrometry at the Korea Basic Science Institute (KBSI, Ochang, Korea). The conventional antibiotics (purity over 95%) were purchased as follows: imipenem, meropenem, erythromycin, and rifampin from Sigma-Aldrich (St. Louis, MO, USA), vancomycin from BIO BASIC (Markham, Ontario, Canada), and linezolid from Pharmacia & Upjohn Company (Kalamazoo, MI, USA).

2.2. Antimicrobial Activity

The Gram-negative bacterial strain *Escherichia coli* (KCTC 1682) and Gram-positive bacterial strain *Staphylococcus aureus* (KCTC 1621) were purchased from the Korean Collection for Type Cultures (Jeongeup, Korea). *Acinetobacter baumannii* (KCCM 40203) were purchased from Korea Culture Center of Microorganisms (Seoul, Korea). Additionally, five carbapenem-resistant *Acinetobacter baumanii* C1–C5 (CRAB C1–C5), which have the OXA-23 gene with carbapenem-resistance were collected from the patients with CRAB bacteremia, who presented symptoms and signs of infection at Korea University Anam Hospital (Seoul, Korea) (IRB registration no. 2020AN0157). The minimum inhibitory concentrations (MIC) of the AMP and antibiotics against the various bacterial strains were assessed using the serial dilution method on Muller–Hinton (MH) media, as described previously [30]. In brief, the peptides at 128 µg·mL^{-1} and antibiotics at 512 µg·mL^{-1} were serially diluted to 1/2 and incubated with a bacterial suspension of 2×10^5 CFU·mL^{-1} in MH media at 37 °C for 16 h. Absorbance at 600 nm was measured using a SpectraMAX microplate reader (Molecular Devices, San Jose, CA, USA).

2.3. Peptide-LPS Binding Assay

The capacity of PapMA series peptides to bind with LPS was analyzed using a fluorescent probe, BODIPY-TR cadaverine (BC) (Thermo Fisher Scientific, MA, USA), as described previously [31]. The probe complex was prepared by incubating LPS (50 µg·mL^{-1}) with BC (5 µg·mL^{-1}) in a 50 mM Tris buffer (pH 7.4) for 6 h at 25 °C. Varying concentrations of peptides (1–64 µg·mL^{-1}) were added to a 96-well, dark fluorescence plate and allowed to interact with the LPS–BC complex for 30 min. The fluorescence intensity was recorded at an excitation wavelength of 580 nm and emission wavelength of 620 nm using a SpectraMAX Gemini^{TM} fluorescence microplate reader (Molecular Devices). The %ΔF (A.U.) was calculated using Equation (1):

$$\%\Delta F\ (A.U.) = [(F_{obs} - F_0) / (F_{100} - F_0)] \times 100 \quad (1)$$

F_{obs} is the observed fluorescence due to the peptide. F_0 is the fluorescence without the addition of the peptide. F_{100} is the fluorescence value measured using LL 37, a control peptide with outstanding LPS-neutralizing properties [32].

2.4. Membrane Depolarization

The membrane depolarization activity of each AMPs at varying concentrations (1–16 µg·mL^{-1}) against CRAB C1 intact cells were measured using 3,3′-dipropylthiadicarbocyanine iodide (diSC$_3$-5). CRAB C1 was washed two times in washing buffer (5 mM HEPES, 20 mM glucose, pH 7.4), the experiment buffer was changed (5 mM HEPES, 20 mM glucose, 0.1 M KCl, pH 7.4), and diSC$_3$-5 dye was added. As a control, 100% depolarization was obtained by treating CRAB C1 with 1% triton X-100 [33]. Spheroplast cells were prepared by the osmotic shock, as previously described [34]. Melittin, which exhibits strong membrane permeabilization, was used for the control treatment at varying concentrations (1–16 µg·mL^{-1}). The corresponding fluorescent were measured using RF-6000PC fluorescent spectrophotometer (Shimadzu Scientific Instruments, Kyoto, Japan).

2.5. Time-Dependent Permeabilization of the Outer Membrane

Time-dependent outer membrane permeabilization activity of PapMA-3 in CRAB C1 intact cells was evaluated using fluorescence-based 1-N-phenylnaphthylamine (NPN). Melittin was used as the control. CRAB C1 cells were washed twice with buffer (5 mM HEPES, 20 mM glucose, pH 7.4) and diluted to $OD_{600} = 0.05$; 1 µM NPN was added to the cells. Time-dependent NPN uptake was monitored following treatment with PapMA-3 for 30 min. PapMA-3, at varying concentrations (4–32 µg·mL^{-1}), was added to the cells, and the fluorescence was measured using the RF-6000PC fluorescent spectrophotometer (Shimadzu Scientific Instruments).

2.6. Cell Cytotoxicity

Human embryonic kidney (HEK)-293 cells, purchased from Korean cell line bank (Seoul, Korea) were cultured in Dulbecco's modified Eagle's medium (DMEM) (Welgene, Gyeong-san, Korea) with 10% fetal bovine serum, 1% penicillin-streptomycin at 37 °C in a humidified 5% CO_2 incubator as described previously [30]. The cytotoxicity of the six PapMA peptides and melittin was determined using WST-8 Cell Proliferation Assay Kit (Biomax Co., Ltd., Seoul, Korea), according to the manufacturer's instructions. The effects of the most potent peptide, PapMA-3, on mammalian cells were evaluated by measuring the cell activity of HEK-293 cells and human keratinocyte HaCaT cells (Korean cell line bank, Seoul, Korea) after 24 h and 48 h of treatment. The absorbance was measured at 450 nm using a SpectraMAX microplate reader (Molecular Devices).

2.7. Stability of PapMA-3 Compared to Melittin in Human Serum

Serum stability of PapMA-3 was assessed by comparing its activity with that of melittin, based on the effects on E. coli, A. baumannii, and CRAB C1. MIC was measured in the presence of 50% human serum (Sigma-Aldrich) in the MH medium, in comparison to that of melittin, as described in Section 2.1. Antibacterial activity of PapMA-3 in combination with imipenem was measured against CRAB C1 in the presence of 50% human serum. The treated cells were incubated for 16 h at 37 °C, and the absorbance at 600 nm was measured using a SpectraMAX microplate reader (Molecular Devices).

2.8. Hemolytic Activity

The hemolytic activity of PapMA series peptides was determined against Sheep red blood cells (sRBC) (KisanBio, Seoul, Korea). Fresh sRBC were washed at least three times with phosphate-buffered saline (PBS), followed by centrifugation for 5 min at $1000 \times g$ at 4 °C. PapMA series peptides (0.25–256 µg·mL^{-1}) dilute in PBS were incubated with 4% (v/v) sRBC for 1 h at 37 °C. The contents were then centrifuged at 4 °C for 5 min at $1000 \times g$. After transferring the supernatant, absorbance was measured at 405 nm using SpectraMAX microplate reader (Molecular Devices). As a control, 100% hemolysis was obtained by treating sRBC with 1% triton X-100.

2.9. Checkerboard Assays

The synergistic effects of AMPs and antibiotics were measured using checkerboard assays [35]. Serial dilutions of PapMA-3 and antibiotics were performed from 1 to $\frac{1}{2}$ of the MIC. Samples were then cross-mixed and cultured in MH medium with 2×10^5 CFU·ml^{-1} bacteria. Results were recorded after 16 h of incubation at 37 °C. The fractional inhibitory concentration index (FICI) was calculated according to the European Committee on Antimicrobial Susceptibility (EUCAST) [36]. The FICI was calculated using Equation (2):

$$\text{FICI} = \frac{(\text{MIC of PapMA-3 in combination})}{(\text{MIC of PapMA-3 alone})} + \frac{(\text{MIC of antibiotic in combination})}{(\text{MIC of antibiotic alone})} \quad (2)$$

where FICI ≤ 0.5 indicates synergism, $0.5 <$ FICI < 1 indicates an additive effect, $1 <$ FICI ≤ 4 represents indifference, and FICI > 4 shows antagonism [37].

2.10. Time Killing Assay

CRAB C1 cells at 2×10^5 CFU·mL^{-1} were incubated with selected concentrations of AMP or antibiotic at 37 °C. At 5, 10, 15, 30, and 40 min and 1, 2, and 4 h, a ten-fold serially diluted suspensions with MH media were spread on an LB agar plate and incubated at 37 °C for 12 h; the number of colonies was counted.

2.11. Scanning Electron Microscope Analysis

Membrane damage of CRAB C1 was visualized using a field emission scanning electron microscope (FE-SEM), as described previously [38,39], to confirm that the peptides or antibiotics specifically targeted the bacterial membrane. CRAB C1 cells were washed and diluted in PBS to an OD_{600} of 0.2 and incubated with either PapMA-3 or erythromycin or with a combination of 4 µg·mL^{-1} PapMA-3 and 128 µg·mL^{-1} erythromycin for 15 min or 30 min at 37 °C. The cells were washed using PBS, fixed in 1% osmium tetroxide for 1 h, and dehydrated using a graded ethanol series. After dehydration, ethanol contents in the sample were replaced with varying ratio (2:1, 1:1, 1:2, 0:1 v/v) of ethanol–isoamyl acetate mixture. The cells were fixed on a glass slide with hexamethyldisilzane, dried under reduced pressure, and platinum-coated; they were visualized using an FE-SEM (SU8020; Hitachi, Tokyo, Japan).

2.12. Biofilm Inhibition

Biofilm inhibition activity of PapMA-3 and antibiotics was measured against CRAB C1, as described previously [30]. CRAB C1 cells (2×10^5 CFU·mL^{-1}) were incubated with PapMA-3 and antibiotics in a tissue-culture well plate in MH medium containing 0.2% glucose for 16 h at 37 °C. The cells were stained with 0.1% (w/v) crystal violet in 0.25% (v/v) acetic acid for 1 h at room temperature; the dye complex was dissolved with ethanol. Absorbance at 595 nm was measured using SpectraMAX microplate reader (Molecular Devices) to quantify the biofilm formation.

2.13. Isothermal Titration Calorimetry (ITC)

Binding affinity was measured using MicroCal Auto-iTC200 (Malvern Panalytical, Malvern, UK) at the KBSI (Ochang, Korea). Each peptide (0.2 mM; 370 µL) was added to 0.025 mM of LPS (E. coli O111:B4, Sigma-Aldrich) in Dulbecco's phosphate-buffered saline (DPBS, pH 7.0); the injection duration was 2s, the spacing was 150 s, and the temperature was 37 °C. ITC data were analyzed using MicroCal Origin 2020b software (MicroCal origin, MA, USA).

2.14. Saturation Transfer Difference (STD)-NMR

STD-NMR experiments were performed at 25 °C on a Bruker 900 MHz spectrometer at KBSI (Ochang, Korea). The STD-NMR spectra were obtained using selective saturation of 15 µM LPS (E. coli O111:B4, Sigma-Aldrich, St. Louis, MO, USA) resonances at −1.0 ppm (40 ppm for reference spectra). Peptide was dissolved in 10mM sodium phosphate (pH 6.8, D_2O) to a concentration of 0.5 mM. For all STD-NMR experiments, a cascade of 40 selective gaussian-shaped pulses of 50 ms duration were used with a total saturation time of 2 s. Difference spectrum was obtained by subtraction of the two spectra (on resonance-off resonance), which shows signals arising from the saturation transfer.

2.15. Statistical Analysis

Measurements were taken at least three times, and all statistical analyses were performed using the GraphPad Prism software 8.0 for windows (GraphPad Software, CA, USA). The values are expressed as mean ± standard deviation (SD). Statistical significance ($p < 0.05$) was determined using one-way or two-way ANOVA with Dunnett's test.

3. Results

3.1. Design of PapMA and Its Analogs

The cationicity and amphiphilicity of antimicrobial peptides are important regarding their binding to bacterial cell membranes via electrostatic interactions with phospholipid head groups, as well as via hydrophobic interactions with membrane lipids [40]. Papiliocin is a 37-residue AMP that was isolated from the swallowtail butterfly (Papilio xuthus) [41]; magainin 2 is a 23-residue AMP isolated from the skin of the African clawed frog (Xenopus laevis) [42,43]. These two peptides are highly cationic, have amphipathic α-helical structures, and have low cytotoxic effects against mammalian cells. Papiliocin has demonstrated high antibacterial activity against Gram-negative bacteria through bacterial membrane disruption, while magainin 2 has displayed high antimicrobial activity against both Gram-negative and Gram-positive bacteria. An 18-residue hybrid peptide (PapMA) was developed by incorporating N-terminal residues 1–8 of papiliocin and N-terminal residues 4–12 of magainin 2, joined by a proline (Pro) hinge [29]. However, the antibacterial activity of PapMA is not potent enough for it to function as a peptide antibiotic.

Table 1. Peptides and their physicochemical properties.

Peptides	Sequence	Length	Molecular Weight	Hydrophobicity <H> [1]	Net Charge [2]
papiliocin	RWKIFKKIE-KVGRNVRDGIIKAGPAVAVVGQAAT-VVK-NH$_2$	37	4002.8	0.300	7
Magainin 2	GIGKFLHSAKKFGKAFVGEIMNS	23	2466.9	0.373	3
PapMA	RWKIFKKIPKFLHSAKKF-NH$_2$	18	2302.1	0.394	7
PapMA-2	RWKIFKKIPKFLHSAKKA-NH$_2$	18	2225.5	0.312	7
PapMA-3	RWKIFKKIPKFLHSAKKW-NH$_2$	18	2340.6	0.419	7
PapMA-4	RWKIFKKIPKFLHSFKKF-NH$_2$	18	2377.5	0.476	7
PapMA-5	RWKIFKKIPKFLHSWKKF-NH$_2$	18	2416.4	0.502	7
PapMA-6	RWKIFKKIPKFLHSWKKW-NH$_2$	18	2455.6	0.527	7

[1] Hydrophobicity <H> was calculated using http://heliquest.ipmc.cnrs.fr/cgi-bin/ComputParams.py (accessed on 17 August 2021) [44]. Bold letters in sequence represent substituted residues. [2] HeliQuest calculates the net charge at pH = 7.4.

To improve and optimize the balance between its antibacterial activity and cytotoxicity, here, analogs were designed by changing the hydrophobicity but maintaining the cationicity. A previous study demonstrated that Trp^2 and Phe^5 in the N-terminus of papiliocin play important roles in its antibacterial activity. Therefore, new analogs of PapMA were designed here by substituting Ala^{15} or Phe^{18} with Ala, Phe, or Trp at the C-terminus of PapMA to optimize the hydrophobicity and membrane permeabilizing activity, while achieving low cytotoxicity (Table 1). To investigate the role of Phe^{18} at the C-terminus, Phe^{18} was substituted with Ala or Trp (PapMA-2 and PapMA-3, respectively). To increase the hydrophobicity, Ala^{15} was substituted with Phe or Trp (PapMA-4 and PapMA-5, respectively). For PapMA-6, both residues were substituted by Trp. PapMA-2, which had Ala at both positions, exhibited the lowest hydrophobicity (0.312), while PapMa-6, which had Trp at both positions, showed the highest hydrophobicity (0.527; Table 1). The hydrophobic moment of the C-terminal helix was highest in PapMA-6 (0.834), with an order of: PapMA-2 < PapMA < PapMA-3 < PapMA-4 < PapMA-5 < PapMA-6, as shown in Figure 1. The antimicrobial activities and cytotoxicities of peptides were also compared to the parent hybrid peptide, PapMA.

3.2. Antimicrobial Activities of PapMA Analogs

Measurement of the minimum inhibitory concentrations (MIC) was conducted to determine the effect of the hydrophobicity of each antimicrobial peptide on its antimicrobial activity. MIC was defined as the minimum concentration that killed more than 99% of bacteria; it was measured against two standard Gram-negative bacteria (*E. coli* and *A. baumanii*), five clinically isolated CRAB (C1–C5), and one Gram-positive bacteria (*S. aureus*). The antimicrobial activities of PapMA and its analogs are listed in Table 2.

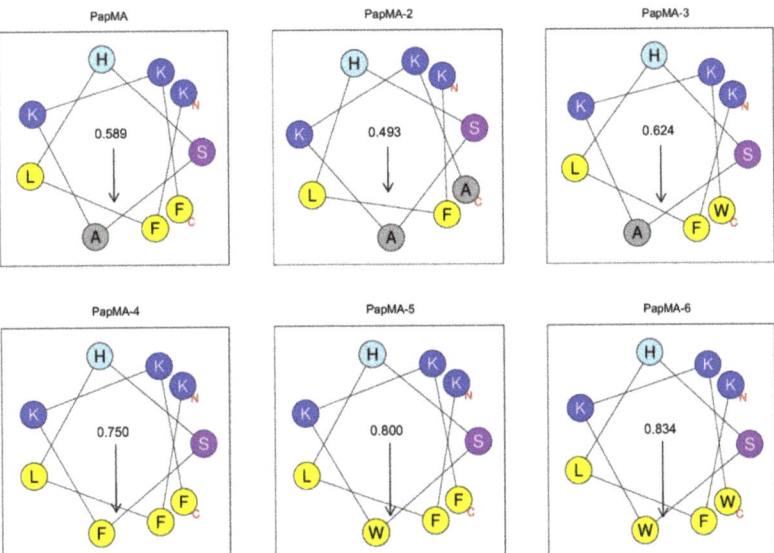

Figure 1. Helical wheel diagram of C-terminal helix from 10th to 18th residue of PapMA and its analogs after Pro hinge generated using HeliQuest at pH 7.4 [44]. Residues at the N-terminus and C-terminus of C-terminal helix are marked as N and C in the figure. Hydrophilic residues are shown in blue. Hydrophobic residues are shown in yellow. Uncharged His is shown in cyan, and Ser is shown in purple. The arrows represent the helical hydrophobic moment.

Table 2. Antibacterial activities of antimicrobial peptides and antibiotics against microorganisms.

Peptides	Minimum Inhibitory Concentration ($\mu g \cdot mL^{-1}$)								Gram-Positive Bacteria
	Gram-Negative Bacteria								
	E. coli	A. baumanii	CRAB C1	CRAB C2	CRAB C3	CRAB C4	CRAB C5	GM [1]	S.aureus
PapMA	32	32	32	32	16	64	32	34	64
PapMA-2	64	128	128	>128	64	>128	128	146	>128
PapMA-3	16	16	16	16	16	32	16	18	32
PapMA-4	16	8	8	8	8	16	8	10	32
PapMA-5	16	16	16	16	16	32	16	18	32
PapMA-6	16	8	8	8	8	16	16	11	32
melittin	8	16	16	16	16	8	16	14	16
Antibiotics									
Imipenem	0.25	0.25	64	64	64	64	64	46	1
Meropenem	0.25	0.25	128	64	64	128	64	64	1
Rifampin	2	4	128	64	128	128	256	101	1
Erythromycin	16	32	>512	512	512	>512	>512	592	0.25
Vancomycin	128	256	256	256	256	512	256	274	0.5
Linezolid	256	256	256	256	256	512	512	329	1

[1] The geometric means (GMs) are the mean minimum inhibitory concentration (MIC) values of Gram-negative bacterial strains. The GMs were assumed to be 256 $\mu g \cdot mL^{-1}$ for MIC > 128 $\mu g \cdot mL^{-1}$ and 1024 $\mu g \cdot mL^{-1}$ for MIC > 512 $\mu g \cdot mL^{-1}$.

In this study, six conventional antibiotics were selected for analysis. Imipenem and meropenem are carbapenem antibiotics that have demonstrated potency against Gram-negative bacteria; they inhibit cell wall synthesis [45]. They have very strong antibacterial activity against *E. coli* and *A. baumanii*; however, their antibacterial activity against carbapenem-resistant CRAB strains is very low. Rifampin has been shown to be potent against *Mycobacterium* and *S. aureus*; it inhibits bacterial deoxyribonucleic acid (DNA)-dependent ribonucleic acid (RNA) polymerase [46]. The antibiotic vancomycin is only potent against Gram-positive bacteria; it inhibits cell wall peptidoglycan synthesis [47]. Erythromycin and linezolid, meanwhile, can bind to 50s ribosome RNA, causing Gram-positive bacterial death through the inhibition of protein synthesis [48]. Compared to PapMA, PapMA-2, which had a lower hydrophobicity due to substitution with Ala, showed a reduced antimicrobial activity. However, PapMA-3, -4, -5, and -6, which exhibited increased hydrophobicities, demonstrated enhanced antimicrobial activities. PapMA and its analogs showed more potent antibacterial activity against Gram-negative bacteria than against Gram-positive bacteria.

Geometric means (GM) were calculated to compare the relative antimicrobial activities of the analogs against Gram-negative bacteria. The GM values were in the order of PapMA-4 < PapMA-6 < PapMA-5 < PapMA-3 < PapMA < PapMA-2, confirming the improved activities of the analogs compared to PapMA (except for PapMA-2). These results suggest that the increased hydrophobicity had a positive effect on the antimicrobial activity. CRAB C1–C5 are carbapenem-resistant to imipenem and meropenem. In contrast, erythromycin [49], vancomycin [50], and linezolid have shown potent antibacterial activity against Gram-positive bacteria, but much lower antimicrobial activity against Gram-negative bacteria. Next, the antibacterial mechanisms of peptides were investigated.

3.3. Antibacterial Mechanisms of PapMA Analogs against CRAB

3.3.1. Binding Assay of LPS-PapMA Analogs

LPS is a major component of the outer membrane of Gram-negative bacteria. It is the permeability barrier of conventional antibiotics, and results in the complication of antibiotic development. Therefore, it is useful to design AMPs that can perturb the bacterial membrane by interacting with LPS. To confirm the antibacterial mechanisms of the developed PapMA analogs against Gram-negative bacteria, the LPS binding mechanisms of the PapMA analogs were investigated using the BC displacement assay (Figure 2). LL-37, which is well-known as the most efficient LPS-neutralizing peptide, was used as a control; its fluorescence intensity at 64 $\mu g \cdot mL^{-1}$ of LL-37 was selected as 100% for comparison. The activity was compared to that of polymyxin B, which is also a well-known LPS-neutralizing peptide [51]. As a result of incubating the LPS-BC complex and the peptides together, all the peptides produced stronger dose-dependent enhancements in fluorescence intensity. All the PapMA analogs showed higher LPS binding interactions than that of polymyxin B. The results showed that LPS interaction increased following the substitution of Ala with Phe or Trp at the C-terminus. Comparing the interactions of PapMA and PapMA-3, LPS interactions increased slightly when Phe^{18} was replaced with Trp. LPS interactions with PapMA-4, -5, and -6 with two aromatic rings at the C-terminus were slightly higher compared to those of PapMA, PapMA-2, and -3.

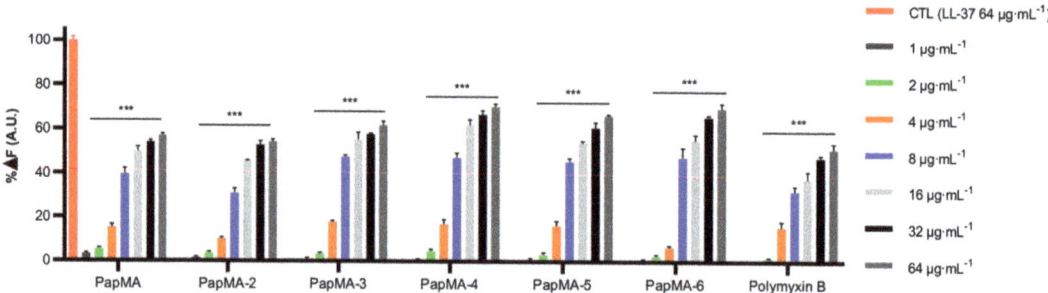

Figure 2. LPS interaction of PapMA analogs. Binding affinity of PapMA derivatives and polymyxin B to LPS based on displacement assays with BODIPY-TR-cadaverine fluorescent dye. Statistical analysis was performed using two-way ANOVA with Dunnett's comparison test. The values are expressed as the mean ± SEM of three independent experiments and are statistically significant at ***$p < 0.001$; ns, not significant.

3.3.2. Depolarization of PapMA and Its Analogs against CRAB C1

To elucidate the antibacterial mechanisms of the PapMA analogs on the CRAB C1 membrane, depolarization experiments were performed using intact CRAB C1, as well as CRAB C1 spheroplasts that were created by removing LPS and peptidoglycan; melittin was used as a control. Figure 3A shows that, at a concentration of 8 µg·mL^{-1}, the depolarization of PapMA analogs and melittin occurred close to the maximum. At 4 µg·mL^{-1} (i.e., half of the concentration of maximum depolarization), depolarization values of 70.7, 57.6, 75.7, 76.5%, 73.2, 70.5, and 86.4% were achieved, respectively. Melittin showed the highest depolarization, while PapMA-2, which had the lowest hydrophobicity, showed the lowest depolarization among all peptides. Interestingly, the PapMA analogs induced bacterial membrane damage even at concentrations much lower than their MICs. When LPS was removed from the CRAB C1 membrane, all peptides displayed approximately 30–40% lower depolarization for CRAB C1 spheroplasts than for the intact membrane (Figure 3B). These results, along with those from the BC displacement assays, indicate that PapMA and its analogs interacted with LPS, major outer membrane component of CRAB, implying that the PapMA peptides targeted and disrupted the outer bacterial membrane more efficiently than the inner membrane.

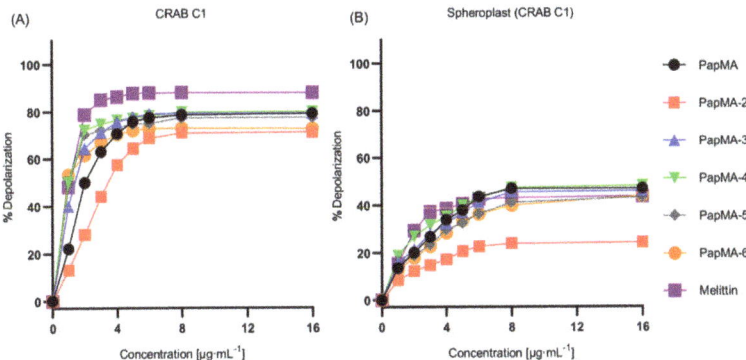

Figure 3. CRAB C1 membrane destruction caused by PapMA analogs. The concentration dependent depolarization of (**A**) intact CRAB C1 and its (**B**) spheroplast induced by PapMA and its analogs, determined using the membrane potential-sensitive fluorescent dye diSC$_3$-5. Dye release was monitored by measuring fluorescence, at an excitation wavelength of 654 nm and an emission wavelength of 670 nm.

3.4. Cytotoxicities of PapMA Analogs

To utilize AMPs as therapeutic agents, they should exhibit low toxicity against mammalian cells [15]. Antibiotics could cause kidney damage; polymyxins, the last-resort antibiotics to treat Gram-negative bacterial infections, have limited use due to its nephrotoxicity [52]. Therefore, to assess the cytotoxicity and to select safe candidates, the cytotoxicities of PapMA and its analogs were investigated against the HEK-293 cell line (Figure 4A). PapMA, PapMA-2, and PapMA-3 showed 100% survival rates at concentrations below 64 µg·mL^{-1}, whereas PapMA-4, PapMA-5, and PapMA-6 showed survival rates of 32.1, 21.4, and 34.8%, respectively, at 64 µg·mL^{-1}. These results show that cytotoxicity increased proportional to increasing hydrophobicity.

PapMA, PapMA-2, and PapMA-3 showed 100% survival rates at concentrations below 64 µg·mL^{-1}, whereas PapMA-4, PapMA-5, and PapMA-6 showed survival rates of 32.1, 21.4, and 34.8%, respectively, at 64 µg·mL^{-1}. These results show that cytotoxicity increased proportional to increasing hydrophobicity.

The hemolytic activity was analyzed against sheep red blood cells (sRBC; Figure 4B). The incubation of sRBC with 256 µg·mL^{-1} for PapMA-4, -5, and -6 induced 1.4, 2.2, and 3.8% hemolysis, respectively. However, PapMA, -2, and -3 caused almost no hemolysis (much lower than 1%). In contrast, melittin exhibited more than 90% hemolysis at 32 µg·mL^{-1}. These results also confirmed that increases in hydrophobicity led to increases in toxicity, through strong hydrophobic interactions occurred between the aromatic residues of peptides and phospholipids in the mammalian cell membranes (which have higher compositions of neutral phospholipids). Among all six peptides studied, PapMA-3 exhibited the highest bacterial cell selectivity, with a GM of 18.3 and a 100% survival rate at 64 µg·mL^{-1} in HEK-293 cells. Even though PapMA-4, -5, and -6 showed potent antibacterial activities, with GMs of 10.3–18.3, they showed severe cytotoxicity (<35% survival rates at 64 µg·mL^{-1} in HEK-293 cells). Therefore, PapMA-3 was selected as a candidate therapeutic peptide for further investigation.

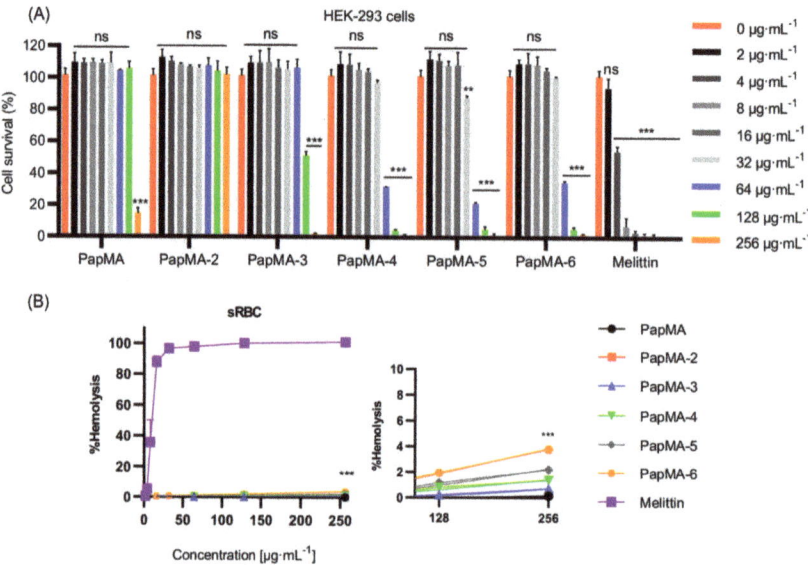

Figure 4. Cytotoxicity of PapMA analogs. (**A**) Cytotoxicity of PapMA and its analogs against HEK-293 cell. The peptide was serially diluted and incubated with cells for 24 h. (**B**) Hemolysis activity of PapMA analogs against sRBC. The peptide was serially diluted and incubated with sRBC for 1 h with melittin as a control. Statistical analysis was performed using two-way ANOVA with Dunnett's comparison test. The values are expressed as the mean ± SEM of three independent experiments and are statistically significant at ** $p < 0.01$; and *** $p < 0.001$. ns, not significant.

3.5. Synergistic Effects of PapMA-3 with Antibiotics against Five CRAB

The appearance of CRAB has accelerated the usage of combination therapy as a new therapeutic approach for its treatment [53–55]. As PapMA-3 was selected as a candidate peptide antibiotic, the synergistic effects of PapMA-3 with conventional antibiotics were investigated using checkerboard assays against five clinically isolated CRAB (C1–C5) [35,56]. Regarding the combinations with front-line conventional antibiotics, imipenem and meropenem were used for Gram-negative infections. The synergistic effects of PapMA-3 were also investigated with rifampin, erythromycin, vancomycin, and linezolid, which are well-known antibiotics that are potent against Gram-positive bacteria.

The ability of PapMA-3 to facilitate these antibiotics in penetrating the bacterial membranes of Gram-negative bacteria was investigated. Each peptide was serially diluted to 1/16 from 1 MIC; the experiment was carried out by cross-mixing them. As shown in Figure 5 and Figure S1, the checkerboard assays revealed that PapMA-3 displayed an outstanding synergistic effect with all antibiotics against CRAB C1. PapMA-3 at 4 µg·mL^{-1} (1/4 MIC) displayed synergistic effects towards CRAB C1, exhibiting FICI values lower than 0.50 when combined with all six antibiotics (Table 3). PapMA-3 also showed synergistic effects against CRAB C2 with imipenem (0.38), rifampin (0.25), vancomycin (0.25), and linezolid (0.50; Figure S2). For CRAB C3, PapMA-3 only showed a synergistic effect when combined with rifampin (FICI = 0.38; Figure S3). Among all cases, the combination of PapMA-3 (1 µg·mL^{-1}) and rifampin (16 µg·mL^{-1}) showed the most effective synergistic effect against CRAB C4, with a FICI value of 0.16 (Figure S4). Figure S5 shows that PapMA-3 demonstrated synergistic effects against CRAB C5 with rifampin, vancomycin, erythromycin, and linezolid; the FICI value was 0.5, respectively. Interestingly, combining PapMA-3 at 2 µg·mL^{-1} (1/8 MIC) and vancomycin at 32 µg·mL^{-1} (1/8 MIC) demonstrated an effective synergistic effect (FICI = 0.25) against both CRAB C1 and C2 (Figure S2). Antibiotics potent for Gram-positive bacteria, such as erythromycin, vancomycin, and linezolid, cannot pass the outer membrane barriers of Gram-negative bacteria; they only demonstrate antibacterial activity against Gram-positive bacteria. Combining PapMA-3 with these antibiotics demonstrated significant antibacterial effects on CRAB, confirming that the interaction of PapMA-3 with the Gram-negative CRAB membrane allowed these antibiotics to penetrate it.

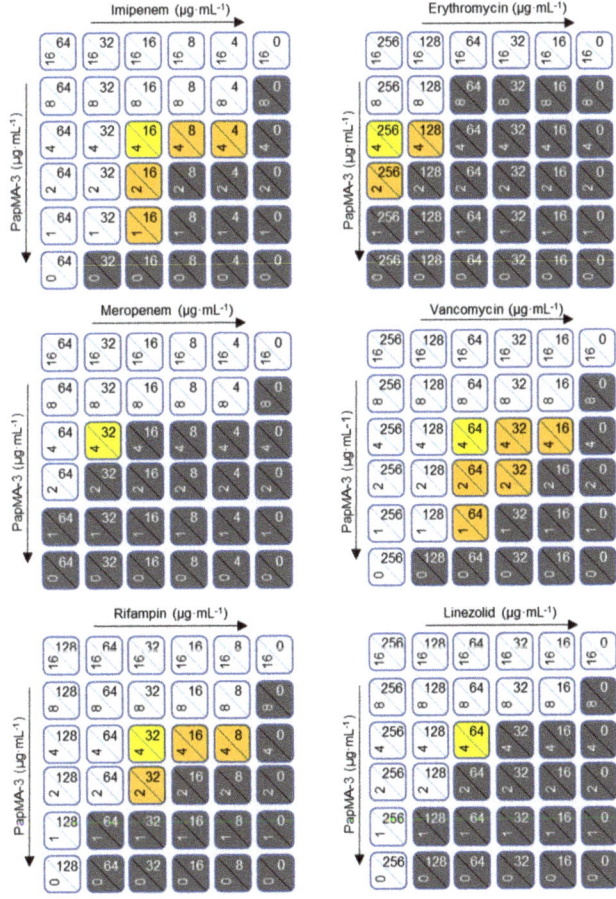

Figure 5. Checkerboard assays of PapMA-3 in combination with six conventional antibiotics against CRAB C1. PapMA-3 and antibiotics were subjected to 1/2 dilution vertically and horizontally from the MIC concentration at the upper left corner. White (0.5 < FICI < 2) indicates a partial synergistic effect, yellow (FICI = 0.5) and orange (FICI < 0.5) indicate a synergistic effect, and gray indicates growth of bacteria. We defined MIC that inhibits completely over 99% of CRAB C1 bacterial growth.

Table 3. FICI for the synergistic effect of PapMA-3 in combination with antibiotics against CRABs.

PapMA-3 with Antibiotics	Strain	MIC (µg·mL^{-1})		MIC in Combination (µg·mL^{-1})		FICI [#]
		PapMA-3	Antibiotics	PapMA-3	Antibiotics	
PapMA-3 + Imipenem	CRAB C1	16	64	4.0	4.0	0.31 *
	CRAB C2	16	64	4.0	8.0	0.38
	CRAB C3	16	64	8.0	1.0	0.52
	CRAB C4	32	64	8.0	8.0	0.38
	CRAB C5	16	64	8.0	16	0.75
PapMA-3 + Meropenem	CRAB C1	16	128	4.0	32	0.50
	CRAB C2	16	64	8.0	32	1.00
	CRAB C3	16	64	8.0	16	0.75
	CRAB C4	32	128	8.0	32	0.50
	CRAB C5	16	64	8.0	16	0.75
PapMA-3 + Rifampin	CRAB C1	16	128	4.0	8.0	0.31
	CRAB C2	16	64	2.0	8.0	0.25
	CRAB C3	16	128	4.0	16	0.38
	CRAB C4	32	128	2.0(8.0)	8.0(4.0)	0.13(0.27)
	CRAB C5	16	256	4.0	64	0.50
PapMA-3 + Erythromycin	CRAB C1	16	>512	4.0	128	0.38
	CRAB C2	16	512	8.0	128	0.75
	CRAB C3	16	512	8.0	64	0.63
	CRAB C4	32	>512	4.0(8.0)	64(16)	0.19(0.27)
	CRAB C5	16	>512	4.0	256	0.50
PapMA-3 + Vancomycin	CRAB C1	16	256	2.0(4.0)	32(16)	0.25(0.31)
	CRAB C2	16	256	2.0	32	0.25
	CRAB C3	16	256	8.0	4.0	0.52
	CRAB C4	32	512	4.0(8.0)	64(16)	0.25(0.28)
	CRAB C5	16	256	4.0	64	0.50
PapMA-3 + Linezolid	CRAB C1	16	256	4.0	64	0.50
	CRAB C2	16	256	4.0	64	0.50
	CRAB C3	16	256	8.0	128	1.00
	CRAB C4	32	512	8.0	64	0.38
	CRAB C5	16	512	4.0	128	0.50

[#] The fractional inhibitory concentration index (FICI) was calculated according to Equation (1). If the MIC value was not obtained at the highest concentration measured due to poor antibacterial activity, the FICI was considered to be twice the value of the measurement limit. * Combinations that showed synergistic effects are shaded in gray. Where there were multiple sets of combinations with low FICI values, they are listed in parentheses.

3.6. Mechanism of Synergistic Activity of PapMA-3 with Antibiotics against CRAB

3.6.1. Confirmation of Synergistic Effects between PapMA-3 and Antibiotics through Time Killing Assays

Time-killing assays of PapMA-3 alone or in combination with antibiotics against CRAB C1 were performed at those concentrations that showed synergistic effects (FICI < 0.5) in the checkerboard assay. As shown in Figure 6, at the MIC of PapMA-3 (16 µg·mL^{-1}), peptide treatment completely killed CRAB C1 strains. At a PapMA-3 concentration of 4 µg·mL^{-1}, for which most combined treatments showed synergistic effects in checkboard assays, the peptide-only treatment did not show any bacterial killing for 4 h. However, when the six antibiotics were incubated at synergistic concentrations in combination with PapMA-3 at 4 µg·mL^{-1} (Table 3, Figure S1), meropenem (32 µg·mL^{-1}) exhibited the most synergistic effect—all bacteria were killed within 1 h. Erythromycin (128 µg·mL^{-1}), rifampin (8 µg·mL^{-1}), and vancomycin (16 µg·mL^{-1}) killed all bacteria within 2 h, while imipenem (4 µg·mL^{-1}) and linezolid (64 µg·mL^{-1}) killed all bacteria within 4 h. Therefore, these antibiotics, when combined with PapMA-3 (4 µg·mL^{-1}), could completely and rapidly kill CRAB C1 in a synergistic manner (Figure 6).

3.6.2. Visualization of CRAB C1 Membrane Disruption by PapMA-3 in Combination with Antibiotics Using a Field Emission Scanning Electron Microscope (FE-SEM)

To elucidate the antibacterial mechanism and synergistic effect, the membrane disruption of CRAB by PapMA-3, in combination with antibiotics at concentrations showing synergistic effects, were investigated using an FE-SEM. The changes in the membrane morphology of CRAB C1 were investigated either with PapMA-3 treatment alone or in combination with erythromycin. Figure 7A shows the intact CRAB C1 membrane, revealing that the morphology was maintained at a steady state of membrane integrity, with a smooth surface. As shown in Figure 7B–I, CRAB C1 gradually lost its membrane integrity after 30 min and 1 h as the PapMA-3 concentration increased (4–32 µg·mL^{-1}). PapMA-3 treatment caused the CRAB membrane surface to become severely roughened and wrinkled, in proportion to the concentration of peptide (Figure 7C–I). Peptide treatment at its MIC (16 μg·mL^{-1}) after 1 h caused severe damage, supporting the antibacterial mechanism of PapMA-3 via the membrane disruption of CRAB C1.

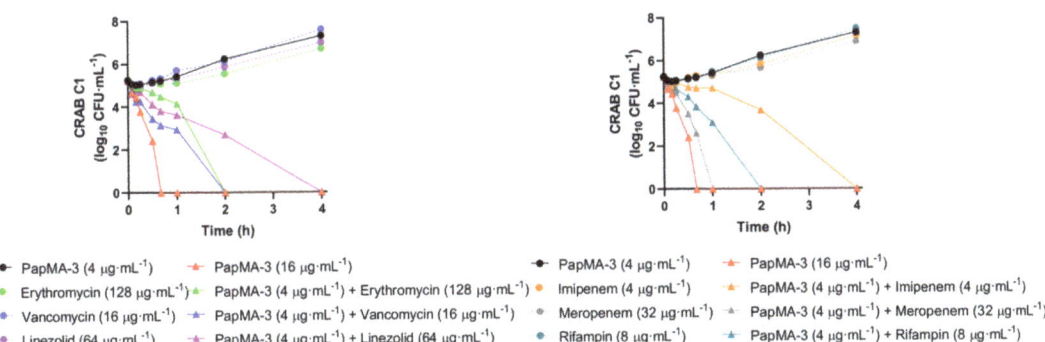

Figure 6. Time-killing curve of PapMA-3 and antibiotics at synergistic concentration against CRAB C1. Y-axis indicates CFU in log scale.

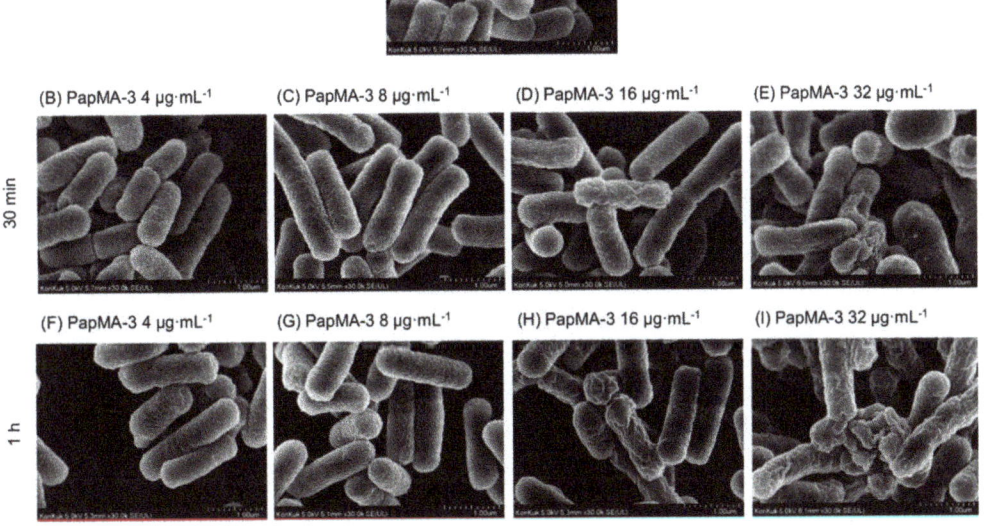

Figure 7. FE-SEM images of CRAB C1 treated with PapMA-3. (**A**) Only CRAB C1. (**B–E**) after incubation for 30 min with PapMA-3 at 4 (1/4 MIC), 8 (1/2 MIC), 16 (1 MIC), and 32 μg·mL^{-1} (2 MIC), respectively. (**F–I**) same experiments after incubation for 1 h, respectively.

The membrane integrity of CRAB C1 was not altered by erythromycin itself (128 μg·mL^{-1}), which was lower than the MIC (Figure 8A,C). However, when CRAB C1 was co-treated with 4 μg·mL^{-1} PapMA-3 and 128 μg·mL^{-1} erythromycin, severe membrane disruption was observed at 2 h (Figure 8B,D). Therefore, PapMA-3 helped in the entry of antibiotics through the cell membrane by sufficiently changing the morphology of the membrane. In addition, a combination of PapMA-3 and antibiotics resulted in more efficient membrane damage. These results agree with the result obtained from time killing assay (Figure 6).

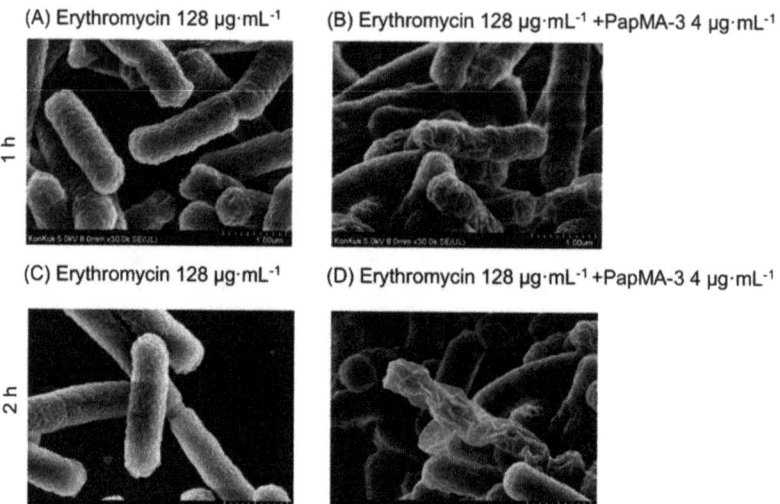

Figure 8. FE-SEM images of CRAB C1 treated with erythromycin and PapMA-3. (**A**) after incubation for 1 h with erythromcyin (128 µg·mL^{-1}; synergistic concentration) and (**B**) with erythromycin (128 µg·mL^{-1}) + PapMA-3 (4 µg·mL^{-1}). (**C**) After incubation for 2 h with erythromcyin (128 µg·mL^{-1}; synergistic concentration) and (**D**) with erythromycin (128 µg·mL^{-1}) + PapMA-3 (4 µg·mL^{-1}).

To confirm the time-dependent outer membrane permeabilization by PapMA-3, we investigated the time required by PapMA-3 for the membrane permeabilization of outer membrane of CRAB C1 by monitoring NPN uptake at 4, 8, 16, and 32 µg·mL^{-1} of PapMA-3 (Figure S6). Destabilization of the outer membrane by PapMA-3 caused the dye to enter the damaged CRAB C1 membrane, and fluorescence was increased rapidly in a concentration-dependent manner and saturated after 10 min, confirming that PapMA-3 disrupted rapidly outer membrane of CRAB.

3.7. Synergistic Effects of PapMA-3 on Biofilm Inhibition

Biofilms confer resistance to bacteria against their environment [57,58]. Biofilm formation can occur on an assortment of surfaces, including living tissues such as wounds and infected skin, as well as on prosthetic implants and various abiotic surfaces [59,60]. The rate of formation of biofilms is high in the case of *A. baumannii*, which is found in urinary catheter, bronchial epithelial cells, as well as abiotic surfaces [61]. Bacterial biofilms confer antibiotic resistance and reduce antibiotic penetrance [62].

Biofilm formation in CRAB C1 was inhibited by PapMA-3 combined with antibiotics (Figure 9). PapMA-3 exhibited a significantly superior biofilm inhibition activity against CRAB C1 compared with that of the other tested antibiotics, in a concentration-dependent manner. Biofilm inhibition was quantified by measuring the absorbance at 595 nm of the crystal violet-stained biofilms. Absorbance treated with 32 µg·mL of PapMA-3, imipenem, meropenem, rifampin, erythromycin, vancomycin, and linezolid were 0.15, 0.19, 0.27, 0.28, 0.74, 0.35, and 1.07, respectively (Figure 9A). The absorbance of biofilm formed by CRAB C1 without peptide or antibiotics served as control was 1.11. The percentage of biofilm inhibition caused by these antibiotics at 32 µg·mL^{-1} was 98.5, 88.9, 79.2, 77.5, 37.7, 77.2, and 4.4%, respectively, compared to the control (Figure 9B).

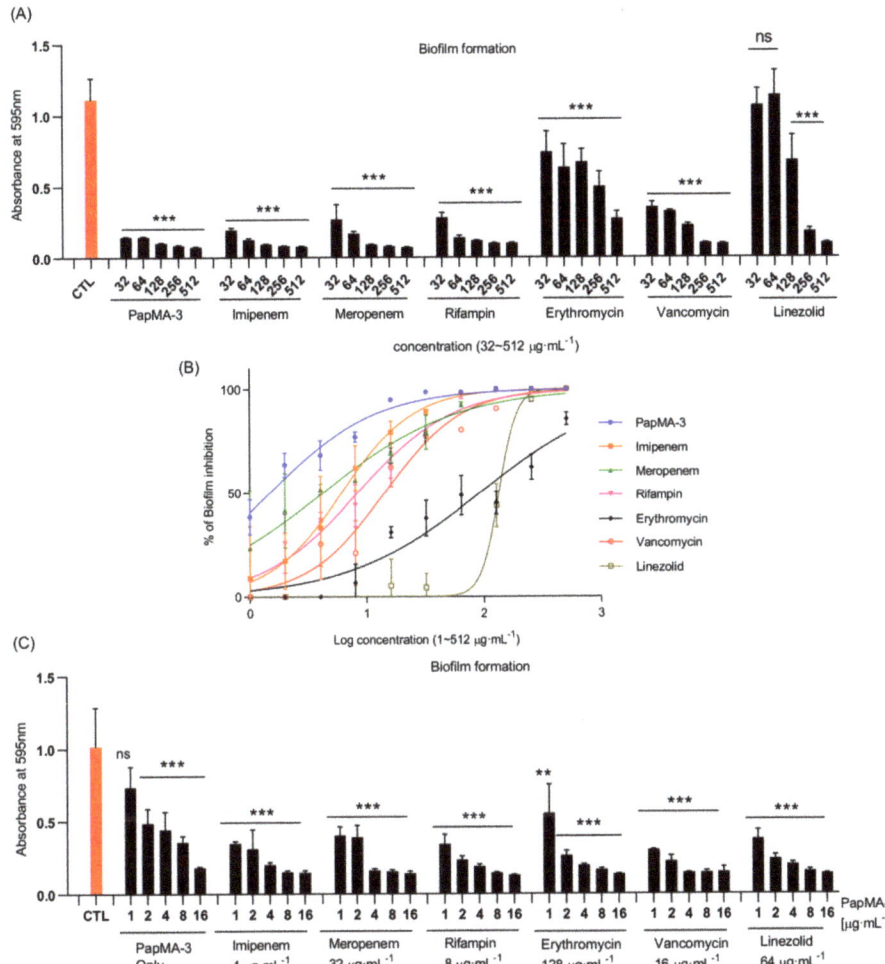

Figure 9. Anti-biofilm activity of PapMA-3 in combination with antibiotics. Biofilms were quantified by staining with crystal violet. (**A**) Absorbance of crystal violet-stained biofilms with treatment of PapMA-3 and antibiotics at a concentration range of 32 to 512 μg·mL^{-1}, assessed at 595 nm. (**B**) Confirmation of anti-biofilm activity against CRAB C1 at log scale concentrations (from 1 to 512 μg·mL^{-1}) of PapMA-3 and antibiotics, comparative calculation result with CTL of 0% without peptide or antibiotics. (**C**) Synergistic anti-biofilm activities of PapMA-3 and antibiotics against CRAB C1, assessed based on absorbance at 595 nm. CRAB C1 without peptides or antibiotics served as the control (red). Statistical analysis was performed using two-way ANOVA with Dunnett's comparison test. The values are expressed as the mean ± SEM of three independent experiments and are statistically significant at ** $p < 0.01$ and *** $p < 0.001$. ns, not significant.

However, co-treatments comprising 4 μg·mL^{-1} PapMA-3 with antibiotics (4 μg·mL^{-1} imipenem, 32 μg·mL^{-1} meropenem, 8 μg·mL^{-1} rifampin, 128 μg·mL^{-1} erythromycin, 16 μg·mL^{-1} vancomycin, or 64 μg·mL^{-1} linezolid) showed synergistic effects (Table 3); the absorbance at 595 nm for these co-treatments were less than 0.20. Thus, it can be concluded that combining PapMA-3 with antibiotics can deliver superior therapeutic effects compared to using antibiotics alone, regarding the inhibition of biofilm formation. This occurred due to the effect of PapMA-3 on inducing the permeabilization of the bacterial membrane (Figure 9C).

3.8. Stability and Effects of PapMA-3 on Mammalian Cells Compared to That of Melittin

3.8.1. Stability of PapMA-3 Compared to That of Melittin in the Presence of Human Serum

High stability is necessary for the in vivo efficacy of peptides. Peptides are degraded by proteases and other components in the serum; therefore, we measured the stability of PapMA-3 alone or in combination with imipenem in human serum to confirm its potential as an AMP candidate [25]. The antibacterial activity of PapMA-3 was reduced four-fold in the presence of 50% human serum in MH media (Table 4), while melittin lost antibacterial activity considerably. Checkerboard assays revealed that 4 µg·mL^{-1} PapMA-3 displayed an outstanding synergistic effect with 4 µg·mL^{-1} imipenem, exhibiting FICI value of 0.31 against CRAB C1 (Table 3). PapMA-3 in combination with 16 µg·mL^{-1} imipenem retained its antibacterial activity at 16 µg·mL^{-1}, even in the presence of 50% serum (Table 4). Even though PapMA-3 contains all L-amino acids in the sequence, these results ascertain the potential of PapMA-3 for therapeutic applications and combinational therapy can compensate the problems caused by the instability of peptide antibiotics in the serum.

Table 4. Measurement of serum stability of PapMA-3 and melittin against *E.coli*, *A.baumannii*, and CRAB C1.

Microorganisms	Minimum Inhibitory Concentration (µg·mL^{-1})							
	PapMA-3		Melittin		Imipenem		PapMA-3 + Imipenem	
	MH Media	+ Serum (50%)	MH Media	+ Serum (50%)	MH Media	+ Serum (50%)	MH Media	+ Serum (50%)
E. coli	16	64	8	256				
A. baumannii	16	64	16	128				
CRAB C1	16	64	16	256	64	64	4 + 4	16 + 16

3.8.2. Effects of PapMA-3 Compared to That of Melittin on Mammalian Cells

We investigated the effect of PapMA-3 on the mammalian cells, HEK-293, and HaCaT for 48 h to evaluate its cytotoxicity (Figure 10). Cell activities were monitored at 24 h and 48 h following the peptide treatment. At 32 µg·mL^{-1}, the cell proliferation and viability remained unaltered at 24 h and 48 h compared to that of the blank control. Even at 64 µg·mL^{-1}, viability was reduced to less than 20% at 24 h and at 48 h compared to the control. In contrast, treatment with melittin caused severe toxicity and significantly reduced viability at 24 h and 48 h, even at its MIC. Therefore, PapMA-3 could be a potent antibiotic peptide.

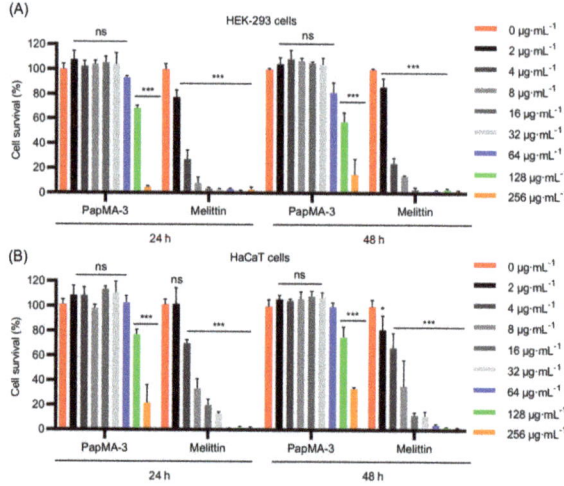

Figure 10. Cytotoxicity of PapMA-3 (**A**) Cytotoxicity of PapMA-3 against HEK-293 cells at 24 h and 48 h. (**B**) Cytotoxicity of PapMA-3 against HaCaT cell at 24 h and 48 h. Statistical analysis was performed

using two-way ANOVA with Dunnett's comparison test. The values are expressed as the mean ± SEM of three independent experiments and are statistically significant at * $p < 0.05$; *** $p < 0.001$; ns, not significant.

3.9. Binding Interactions of PapMA-3 with LPS as Studied by STD-NMR Spectroscopy and ITC

STD NMR experiments were conducted to clarify the antibacterial mechanism of PapMA-3. To determine which residues in PapMA-3 were the most favorable to LPS binding, they were compared to ^{1}D ^{1}H NMR spectra of PapMA-2 (with Ala^{18}) and PapMA-3 (with Trp^{18}); a previously obtained spectrum of PapMA was also used [63]. The STD effect was determined using the spectral differences; it primarily constituted resonances belonging to peptide protons bound to LPS. Significant STD effects were identified in the aromatic ring region for Trp^2, Phe^5, and Trp^{18} (in the region of 7.8–7.4 ppm). This confirmed that all aromatic residues at both the N- and C-termini had direct molecular interactions with LPS (Figure 11A,B). Furthermore, protons in aliphatic regions also showed an STD effect with LPS, confirming that PapMA-3 enacted antibacterial activity via strong LPS interactions, resulting in disruption of CRAB bacterial membrane.

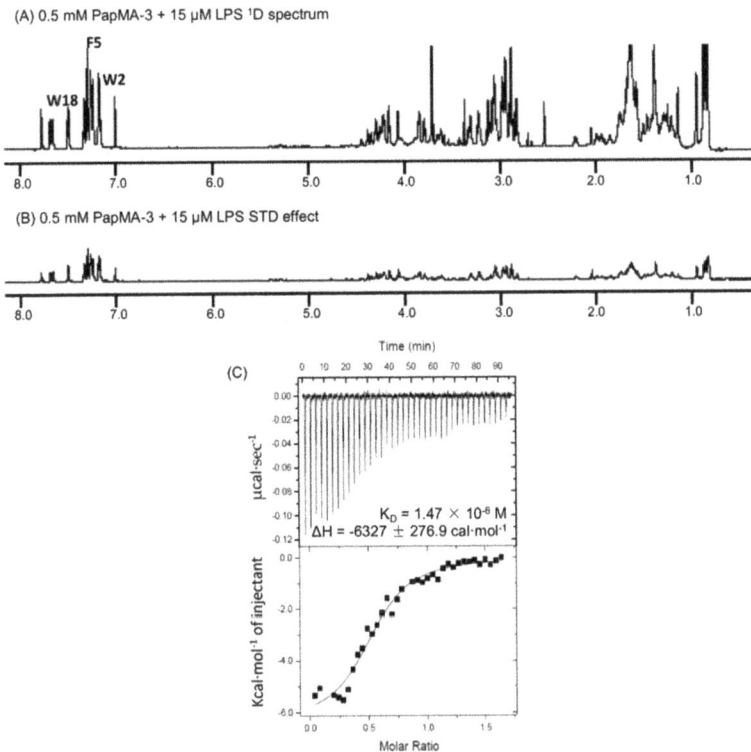

Figure 11. Binding interaction of PapMA-3 with LPS. Saturation transfer difference (STD) NMR analysis of interaction between PapMA-3 and LPS in D$_2$O at 298 K. (**A**) ^{1}D ^{1}H NMR spectra of 0.5 mM PapMA-3 plus 15 μM LPS (sample A), (**B**) STD NMR spectrum obtained on sample A at 298 K. (**C**) Isothermal titration calorimetry (ITC) measurement showing the binding affinity of 0.2 mM PapMA-3 to 0.025 mM LPS from E. coli O55:B5.

The binding affinity of PapMA-3 to LPS was further investigated using ITC, revealing that an exothermic process with strong electrostatic interactions occurred between PapMA-3 and LPS, with a binding affinity of 1.47×10^{-6} M at 37 °C (Figure 11C). The

STD-NMR spectroscopy and ITC results together confirmed that PapMA-3 exhibited antibacterial activity via its strong interaction with LPS; thereby, it can enhance the membrane permeability of conventional antibiotics.

4. Discussion

The discovery and advancement of antibiotics initially seemed to have effectively combated diseases caused by bacterial infections; however, the overuse of antibiotics has led to the emergence of MDR bacterial strains. As a countermeasure against resistant strains, multiple antibiotics can be used in combination. In clinical settings, this strategy is advantageous, as it can broaden the target spectra against pathogens and prevent the development of drug resistance by reducing the amounts of antibiotics used. Furthermore, combination therapy can decrease the toxicity by allowing lower doses of the combined harmful drugs to be used. Combination therapies for antibiotics that have recently been approved by the US Food and Drug Administration (FDA) include ceftolozane/tazobactam, ceftazidime/avibactam, and meropenem/vaborbactam; furthermore, imipenem/relebactam and aztreonam/avibactam remain under clinical research [64].

Many studies have explored the combination of AMPs and antibiotics. The emergence of resistant strains to carbapenem, which is an important antibiotic against Gram-negative bacteria, has intensified the need for new alternatives for the treatment of CRAB pathogens classified as critical MDR bacteria by WHO [2]. However, few studies have synergistically investigated the combined effects of AMPs and antibiotics against Gram-negative bacteria, due to complications posed by the bacterial membranes. For example, Ω76 has been studied regarding its synergistic effects on CRAB; an FICI value of 0.56 was obtained with colistin [54], demonstrating a partial synergistic effect via a synergistic mechanism that enhanced the membrane permeability of antibiotics. The combination of melittin and doripenem has also shown a very good synergistic combination, achieving a FICI value of <0.1 against CRAB, whereas melittin was found not to exhibit a synergistic effect with doxycycline and colistin [25]. However, the severe toxicity of melittin can limit the clinical application. SET-M33 has showed synergistic effects with aztreonam, meropenem, rifampin, and tobramycin against CRAB strain [24].

In clinical trials, combinations of colistin and conventional antibiotics are mainly used to treat MDR Gram-negative bacteria [65,66]. Although colistin itself has excellent antibacterial activities, its high nephrotoxicity is a factor that limits its use alone; the appearance of colistin-resistant bacteria also limits its usage. For example, a randomized clinical trial of colistin in combination with meropenem is currently ongoing in Europe and the United States (ClinicalTrials.gov IDs NCT01732250 and NCT01597973) [67]. Additionally, clinical trials of colistin and rifampin in Korea have confirmed the presence of a partial synergistic effect (NCT03622918) [68]. However, in these studies, the combination treatments have not been shown to be superior to colistin monotherapy, as no similar or significant differences have been obtained [65,66].

Mechanisms of antibiotic resistance in bacteria include thickening the membrane to lower the permeability of antibiotics, creating an efflux pump to re-release antibiotics, modifying the target of antibiotics, and inactivating antibiotics by decomposing them [69]. Carbapenem antibiotics are members of β-lactam antibiotics, which inhibit synthesis of bacterial cell wall by binding to penicillin-binding proteins. Furthermore, carbapenem resistance mechanisms have been described in *A. baumannii*, including the alteration or loss of outer membrane proteins and efflux modifications [70]. Among many carbapenem-hydrolyzing oxacillinase-encoding genes, OXA-23 is widespread in Korea, and the number of antibiotics available to treat CRAB are decreasing [71]. The present study aimed to find an efficient treatment method for CRAB infections using combinational therapy of the newly designed PapMA-3 and six conventional antibiotics, which included antibiotics that are potent against Gram-negative or Gram-positive bacteria. PapMA-3-antibiotic combinations were assessed against five clinical isolates, OXA-23-producing CRAB (C1–C5), and the underlying mechanism was explored.

To facilitate the uptake of antibiotics through the LPS outer membrane, PapMA-3 showed strong interactions with LPS and depolarized the CRAB outer membrane, while demonstrating low cytotoxicity. Its binding interactions with LPS were investigated using BC displacement assays, ITC, and STD-NMR experiments, confirming that membrane permeabilization via strong binding to LPS was the major antibacterial mechanism. PapMA-3 showed a superior BC displacement to a well-known LPS-neutralizing peptide, polymyxin B, by binding the core part of LPS, lipid A [72,73]. The therapeutic potential of PapMA-3 against CRAB was examined in combination with imipenem and meropenem, which are effective against Gram-negative bacteria. Furthermore, PapMA-3 was also combined with four antibiotics that have demonstrated antibacterial activity against Gram-positive bacteria. Outstanding synergistic effects (FICI < 0.5) between PapMA-3 and all six antibiotics were confirmed against both CRAB C1 and C4 clinical isolates. In particular, combining PapMA-3 with rifampin, vancomycin, and erythromycin achieved efficient synergistic effects against CRAB C4, with FICI values of <0.25, implying that PapMA-3 disrupted the membrane integrity of CRAB, allowing the antibiotics that are effective against Gram-positive bacteria to enter and reach their intracellular targets in the CRAB cells. Additionally, PapMA-3 might help imipenem and meropenem to overcome the CRAB membrane; however, underlying mechanism is not yet clearly understood.

Biofilm formation by MDR bacteria aids antibiotic resistance; it needs to be overcome due to its effects in causing pneumonia, meningitis, bacteremia, wounds, and soft-tissue infections [74]. PapMA-3 itself was able to suppress biofilm formation at its MIC, but it was also able to suppress sufficiently biofilm formation at lower concentrations when combined with antibiotics. This implies that combinational therapies constituting PapMA-3 and conventional antibiotics could be applied clinically. FE-SEM images suggested that PapMA-3 destabilized the morphology of the bacterial membrane even at concentrations below the MIC. Importantly, the CRAB membrane was destroyed when PapMA-3 was applied in combination with erythromycin, which alone are only effective against Gram-positive bacteria. Time killing assays suggested that the combinations of PapMA-3 with meropenem or erythromycin completely and rapidly killed CRAB C1 (within 1 h). Therefore, this combinational therapy could be applied to the enable the usage of potent antibiotics against both Gram-negative and Gram-positive bacteria by facilitating membrane permeability.

However, several problems persist that need to be addressed in future studies. First, the resistance to protease needs to be improved in our peptides by introducing D-amino acids, non-natural amino acids, or cyclization [75–77]. Additionally, these synergistic effects need to be confirmed by in vivo animal experiments before this combinational therapy can be applied clinically. Additionally, underlying mechanisms for synergistic effect on combination therapy should be investigated further in our future studies.

5. Conclusions

In this study, PapMA-3, a novel peptide, was designed and demonstrated potent anti-microbial activity against CRAB without notable cytotoxicity against mammalian cells. PapMA-3 was shown to target the outer bacterial membrane of CRAB via a strong interaction with LPS. At synergistic concentrations, PapMA-3 was found to cause the partial depolarization of the CRAB membrane, which changed the membrane morphology sufficiently to allow the antibiotics to penetrate intracellularly. This synergistic usage of PapMA-3 with well-known antibiotics resulted in the killing of CRAB and the inhibition of their biofilm formation. This was even achieved when the antibiotics used had previously only demonstrated potency against Gram-positive bacteria. This study may provide insights regarding the development of alternative therapies that utilize novel peptide antibiotics in combination with classical antibiotics to treat CRAB infections.

6. Patents

Patent applications for these peptides have been registered in Korea (101875057). These peptides have given rise to patent number PCT/KR2017/006650, and patent applications have been completed in United State (SOP114552US) and China (201780039278.1).

Supplementary Materials: The following are available online at https://www.mdpi.com/article/10.3390/pharmaceutics13111800/s1, Figure S1: PapMA-3 and antibiotic checkboard assay results, showing fractional inhibitory concentration index (FICI) calculated against CRAB C1 according to Equation (1), Figure S2: PapMA-3 and antibiotic checkboard assay results, showing FICI calculated against CRAB C2., Figure S3: PapMA-3 and antibiotic checkboard assay results, showing FICI calculated against CRAB C3, Figure S4: PapMA-3 and antibiotic checkboard assay results, showing FICI calculated against CRAB C4, Figure S5: PapMA-3 and antibiotic checkboard assay results, showing FICI calculated against CRAB C5.

Author Contributions: Conceptualization, Y.K.; methodology, J.C. and Y.K.; data analysis, J.C. and A.J.; resources, Y.K.Y.; writing—original draft preparation, J.C. and Y.K.; writing—review and editing, J.C. and Y.K.; visualization, J.C. and A.J.; supervision, Y.K.; project administration, Y.K. All authors have read and agreed to the published version of the manuscript.

Funding: This work was supported by the National Research Foundation of Korea (NRF) grant funded by the Korea government (MSIT) (No. 2020R1A2C2005338).

Institutional Review Board Statement: Not applicable.

Informed Consent Statement: Not applicable.

Data Availability Statement: Not applicable.

Conflicts of Interest: The authors declare no conflict of interest.

References

1. Neu, H.C. Infections due to gram-negative bacteria: An overview. *Rev. Infect. Dis.* **1985**, *7* (Suppl. 4), S778–S782. [CrossRef] [PubMed]
2. Tacconelli, E.; Carrara, E.; Savoldi, A.; Harbarth, S.; Mendelson, M.; Monnet, D.L.; Pulcini, C.; Kahlmeter, G.; Kluytmans, J.; Carmeli, Y.; et al. Discovery, research, and development of new antibiotics: The WHO priority list of antibiotic-resistant bacteria and tuberculosis. *Lancet Infect. Dis.* **2018**, *18*, 318–327. [CrossRef]
3. Vasoo, S.; Barreto, J.N.; Tosh, P.K. Emerging issues in gram-negative bacterial resistance: An update for the practicing clinician. *Mayo Clin. Proc.* **2015**, *90*, 395–403. [CrossRef]
4. Deelen, J.W.T.; Rottier, W.C.; van Werkhoven, C.H.; Woudt, S.H.S.; Buiting, A.G.M.; Dorigo-Zetsma, J.W.; Kluytmans, J.; van der Linden, P.D.; Thijsen, S.F.T.; Vlaminckx, B.J.M.; et al. The burden of bacteremic and non-bacteremic Gram-negative infections: A prospective multicenter cohort study in a low-resistance country. *J. Infect.* **2020**, *81*, 895–901. [CrossRef] [PubMed]
5. Lien, C.Y.; Lee, J.J.; Tsai, W.C.; Chen, S.Y.; Huang, C.R.; Chien, C.C.; Lu, C.H.; Chang, W.N. The clinical characteristics of spontaneous Gram-negative bacterial meningitis in adults: A hospital-based study. *J. Clin. Neurosci.* **2019**, *64*, 101–105. [CrossRef] [PubMed]
6. World Health Organization. *Guidelines for the Prevention and Control of Carbapenem-Resistant Enterobacteriaceae, Acinetobacter baumannii and Pseudomonas aeruginosa in Health Care Facilities*; World Health Organization: Geneva, Switzerland, 2017.
7. Shrivastava, S.R.; Shrivastava, P.S.; Ramasamy, J. World health organization releases global priority list of antibiotic-resistant bacteria to guide research, discovery, and development of new antibiotics. *J. Med Soc.* **2018**, *32*, 76. [CrossRef]
8. Sleiman, A.; Fayad, A.G.A.; Banna, H.; Matar, G.M. Prevalence and molecular epidemiology of carbapenem-resistant Gram-negative bacilli and their resistance determinants in the Eastern Mediterranean Region over the last decade. *J. Glob. Antimicrob. Resist.* **2021**, *25*, 209–221. [CrossRef]
9. Zasloff, M. Antimicrobial peptides of multicellular organisms. *Nature* **2002**, *415*, 389–395. [CrossRef] [PubMed]
10. Wu, Q.; Patocka, J.; Kuca, K. Insect Antimicrobial Peptides, a Mini Review. *Toxins* **2018**, *10*, 461. [CrossRef] [PubMed]
11. Diamond, G.; Beckloff, N.; Weinberg, A.; Kisich, K.O. The roles of antimicrobial peptides in innate host defense. *Curr. Pharm. Des.* **2009**, *15*, 2377–2392. [CrossRef] [PubMed]
12. Mookherjee, N.; Anderson, M.A.; Haagsman, H.P.; Davidson, D.J. Antimicrobial host defence peptides: Functions and clinical potential. *Nat. Rev. Drug Discov.* **2020**, *19*, 311–332. [CrossRef]
13. Narayana, J.L.; Chen, J.Y. Antimicrobial peptides: Possible anti-infective agents. *Peptides* **2015**, *72*, 88–94. [CrossRef] [PubMed]
14. Fjell, C.D.; Hiss, J.A.; Hancock, R.E.; Schneider, G. Designing antimicrobial peptides: Form follows function. *Nat. Rev. Drug Discov.* **2011**, *11*, 37–51. [CrossRef]

15. Datta, S.; Roy, A. Antimicrobial Peptides as Potential Therapeutic Agents: A Review. *Int. J. Pept. Res. Ther.* **2021**, *27*, 555–577. [CrossRef]
16. Kim, M.K.; Lee, T.G.; Jung, M.; Park, K.H.; Chong, Y. In Vitro Synergism and Anti-biofilm Activity of Quercetin-Pivaloxymethyl Conjugate against Staphylococcus aureus and Enterococcus Species. *Chem. Pharm. Bull.* **2018**, *66*, 1019–1022. [CrossRef]
17. Pachon-Ibanez, M.E.; Docobo-Perez, F.; Lopez-Rojas, R.; Dominguez-Herrera, J.; Jimenez-Mejias, M.E.; Garcia-Curiel, A.; Pichardo, C.; Jimenez, L.; Pachon, J. Efficacy of rifampin and its combinations with imipenem, sulbactam, and colistin in experimental models of infection caused by imipenem-resistant *Acinetobacter baumannii*. *Antimicrob. Agents Chemother.* **2010**, *54*, 1165–1172. [CrossRef]
18. Mgbeahuruike, E.E.; Stalnacke, M.; Vuorela, H.; Holm, Y. Antimicrobial and Synergistic Effects of Commercial Piperine and Piperlongumine in Combination with Conventional Antimicrobials. *Antibiotics* **2019**, *8*, 55. [CrossRef]
19. Assane, I.M.; Santos-Filho, N.A.; de Sousa, E.L.; de Arruda Brasil, M.C.O.; Cilli, E.M.; Pilarski, F. Cytotoxicity and antimicrobial activity of synthetic peptides alone or in combination with conventional antimicrobials against fish pathogenic bacteria. *J. Appl. Microbiol.* **2021**, *131*, 1762–1774. [CrossRef] [PubMed]
20. Mahmoudi, H.; Alikhani, M.Y.; Imani Fooladi, A.A. Synergistic antimicrobial activity of melittin with clindamycin on the expression of encoding exfoliative toxin in Staphylococcus aureus. *Toxicon* **2020**, *183*, 11–19. [CrossRef] [PubMed]
21. Rishi, P.; Vij, S.; Maurya, I.K.; Kaur, U.J.; Bharati, S.; Tewari, R. Peptides as adjuvants for ampicillin and oxacillin against methicillin-resistant Staphylococcus aureus (MRSA). *Microb. Pathog.* **2018**, *124*, 11–20. [CrossRef] [PubMed]
22. Shi, J.; Chen, C.; Wang, D.; Tong, Z.; Wang, Z.; Liu, Y. Amphipathic Peptide Antibiotics with Potent Activity against Multidrug-Resistant Pathogens. *Pharmaceutics* **2021**, *13*, 438. [CrossRef] [PubMed]
23. Gan, B.H.; Cai, X.; Javor, S.; Kohler, T.; Reymond, J.L. Synergistic Effect of Propidium Iodide and Small Molecule Antibiotics with the Antimicrobial Peptide Dendrimer G3KL against Gram-Negative Bacteria. *Molecules* **2020**, *25*, 5643. [CrossRef] [PubMed]
24. Pollini, S.; Brunetti, J.; Sennati, S.; Rossolini, G.M.; Bracci, L.; Pini, A.; Falciani, C. Synergistic activity profile of an antimicrobial peptide against multidrug-resistant and extensively drug-resistant strains of Gram-negative bacterial pathogens. *J. Pept. Sci.* **2017**, *23*, 329–333. [CrossRef] [PubMed]
25. Akbari, R.; Hakemi-Vala, M.; Pashaie, F.; Bevalian, P.; Hashemi, A.; Pooshang Bagheri, K. Highly Synergistic Effects of Melittin with Conventional Antibiotics Against Multidrug-Resistant Isolates of Acinetobacter baumannii and Pseudomonas aeruginosa. *Microb. Drug Resist.* **2019**, *25*, 193–202. [CrossRef]
26. Shin, S.Y.; Kang, J.H.; Lee, M.K.; Kim, S.Y.; Kim, Y.; Hahm, K.S. Cecropin A—magainin 2 hybrid peptides having potent antimicrobial activity with low hemolytic effect. *Biochem. Mol. Biol. Int.* **1998**, *44*, 1119–1126. [CrossRef] [PubMed]
27. Shin, S.Y.; Lee, M.K.; Kim, K.L.; Hahm, K.S. Structure-antitumor and hemolytic activity relationships of synthetic peptides derived from cecropin A-magainin 2 and cecropin A-melittin hybrid peptides. *J. Pept. Res.* **1997**, *50*, 279–285. [CrossRef] [PubMed]
28. Oh, D.; Shin, S.Y.; Kang, J.H.; Hahm, K.S.; Kim, K.L.; Kim, Y. NMR structural characterization of cecropin A(1-8)—magainin 2(1-12) and cecropin A (1-8)—melittin (1-12) hybrid peptides. *J. Pept. Res.* **1999**, *53*, 578–589. [CrossRef] [PubMed]
29. Shin, A.; Lee, E.; Jeon, D.; Park, Y.G.; Bang, J.K.; Park, Y.S.; Shin, S.Y.; Kim, Y. Peptoid-Substituted Hybrid Antimicrobial Peptide Derived from Papiliocin and Magainin 2 with Enhanced Bacterial Selectivity and Anti-inflammatory Activity. *Biochemistry* **2015**, *54*, 3921–3931. [CrossRef] [PubMed]
30. Krishnan, M.; Choi, J.; Jang, A.; Kim, Y. A Novel Peptide Antibiotic, Pro10-1D, Designed from Insect Defensin Shows Antibacterial and Anti-Inflammatory Activities in Sepsis Models. *Int. J. Mol. Sci.* **2020**, *21*, 6216. [CrossRef]
31. Krishnan, M.; Choi, J.; Choi, S.; Kim, Y. Anti-Endotoxin 9-Meric Peptide with Therapeutic Potential for the Treatment of Endotoxemia. *J. Microbiol. Biotechnol.* **2021**, *31*, 25–32. [CrossRef]
32. Golec, M. Cathelicidin LL-37: LPS-neutralizing, pleiotropic peptide. *Ann. Agric. Environ. Med.* **2007**, *14*, 1–4. [PubMed]
33. Jeon, D.; Jacob, B.; Kwak, C.; Kim, Y. Short Antimicrobial Peptides Exhibiting Antibacterial and Anti-Inflammatory Activities Derived from the N-Terminal Helix of Papiliocin. *Bull. Korean Chem. Soc.* **2017**, *38*, 1260–1268. [CrossRef]
34. Lee, E.; Kim, J.K.; Jeon, D.; Jeong, K.W.; Shin, A.; Kim, Y. Functional Roles of Aromatic Residues and Helices of Papiliocin in its Antimicrobial and Anti-inflammatory Activities. *Sci. Rep.* **2015**, *5*, 12048. [CrossRef] [PubMed]
35. Bonapace, C.R.; Bosso, J.A.; Friedrich, L.V.; White, R.L. Comparison of methods of interpretation of checkerboard synergy testing. *Diagn. Microbiol. Infect. Dis.* **2002**, *44*, 363–366. [CrossRef]
36. European Committee for Antimicrobial Susceptibility Testing (EUCAST) of the European Society of Clinical Microbiology and Infectious Diseases (ESCMID). Terminology relating to methods for the determination of susceptibility of bacteria to antimicrobial agents. *Clin. Microbiol. Infect.* **2000**, *6*, 503–508. [CrossRef] [PubMed]
37. Kumar, S.D.; Shin, S.Y. Antimicrobial and anti-inflammatory activities of short dodecapeptides derived from duck cathelicidin: Plausible mechanism of bactericidal action and endotoxin neutralization. *Eur. J. Med. Chem.* **2020**, *204*, 112580. [CrossRef]
38. Kim, J.; Jacob, B.; Jang, M.; Kwak, C.; Lee, Y.; Son, K.; Lee, S.; Jung, I.D.; Jeong, M.S.; Kwon, S.H.; et al. Development of a novel short 12-meric papiliocin-derived peptide that is effective against Gram-negative sepsis. *Sci. Rep.* **2019**, *9*, 3817. [CrossRef] [PubMed]
39. Jang, M.; Kim, J.; Choi, Y.; Bang, J.; Kim, Y. Antiseptic Effect of Ps-K18: Mechanism of Its Antibacterial and Anti-Inflammatory Activities. *Int. J. Mol. Sci.* **2019**, *20*, 4895. [CrossRef] [PubMed]
40. Giangaspero, A.; Sandri, L.; Tossi, A. Amphipathic alpha helical antimicrobial peptides. *Eur. J. Biochem.* **2001**, *268*, 5589–5600. [CrossRef] [PubMed]

41. Kim, S.R.; Hong, M.Y.; Park, S.W.; Choi, K.H.; Yun, E.Y.; Goo, T.W.; Kang, S.W.; Suh, H.J.; Kim, I.; Hwang, J.S. Characterization and cDNA cloning of a cecropin-like antimicrobial peptide, papiliocin, from the swallowtail butterfly, Papilio xuthus. *Mol. Cells* **2010**, *29*, 419–423. [CrossRef] [PubMed]
42. Zasloff, M. Magainins, a class of antimicrobial peptides from Xenopus skin: Isolation, characterization of two active forms, and partial cDNA sequence of a precursor. *Proc. Natl. Acad. Sci. USA* **1987**, *84*, 5449–5453. [CrossRef]
43. Maloy, W.L.; Kari, U.P. Structure-activity studies on magainins and other host defense peptides. *Biopolymers* **1995**, *37*, 105–122. [CrossRef] [PubMed]
44. Gautier, R.; Douguet, D.; Antonny, B.; Drin, G. HELIQUEST: A web server to screen sequences with specific alpha-helical properties. *Bioinformatics* **2008**, *24*, 2101–2102. [CrossRef] [PubMed]
45. Zhanel, G.G.; Simor, A.E.; Vercaigne, L.; Mandell, L.; Canadian Carbapenem Discussion Group. Imipenem and meropenem: Comparison of in vitro activity, pharmacokinetics, clinical trials and adverse effects. *Can. J. Infect. Dis.* **1998**, *9*, 215–228. [CrossRef] [PubMed]
46. Campbell, E.A.; Korzheva, N.; Mustaev, A.; Murakami, K.; Nair, S.; Goldfarb, A.; Darst, S.A. Structural mechanism for rifampicin inhibition of bacterial rna polymerase. *Cell* **2001**, *104*, 901–912. [CrossRef]
47. Nagarajan, R. Antibacterial activities and modes of action of vancomycin and related glycopeptides. *Antimicrob. Agents Chemother.* **1991**, *35*, 605–609. [CrossRef] [PubMed]
48. Papich, M.G. *Saunders Handbook of Veterinary Drugs: Small and Large Animal*, 4th ed.; Elsevier: St. Louis, MO, USA, 2016; p. 24. 900p.
49. Mao, J.C.; Putterman, M. Accumulation in gram-postive and gram-negative bacteria as a mechanism of resistance to erythromycin. *J. Bacteriol.* **1968**, *95*, 1111–1117. [CrossRef]
50. Watanakunakorn, C. Mode of action and in-vitro activity of vancomycin. *J. Antimicrob. Chemother.* **1984**, *14* (Suppl. D), 7–18. [CrossRef] [PubMed]
51. Ferrari, D.; Pizzirani, C.; Adinolfi, E.; Forchap, S.; Sitta, B.; Turchet, L.; Falzoni, S.; Minelli, M.; Baricordi, R.; Di Virgilio, F. The antibiotic polymyxin B modulates P2X7 receptor function. *J. Immunol.* **2004**, *173*, 4652–4660. [CrossRef] [PubMed]
52. Nation, R.L.; Rigatto, M.H.P.; Falci, D.R.; Zavascki, A.P. Polymyxin Acute Kidney Injury: Dosing and Other Strategies to Reduce Toxicity. *Antibiotics* **2019**, *8*, 24. [CrossRef] [PubMed]
53. Nageeb, W.; Metwally, L.; Kamel, M.; Zakaria, S. In vitro antimicrobial synergy studies of carbapenem-resistant Acinetobacter baumannii isolated from intensive care units of a tertiary care hospital in Egypt. *J. Infect. Public Health* **2015**, *8*, 593–602. [CrossRef]
54. Nagarajan, D.; Roy, N.; Kulkarni, O.; Nanajkar, N.; Datey, A.; Ravichandran, S.; Thakur, C.; Sandeep, T.; Aprameya, I.V.; Sarma, S.P.; et al. Omega76: A designed antimicrobial peptide to combat carbapenem- and tigecycline-resistant Acinetobacter baumannii. *Sci. Adv.* **2019**, *5*, eaax1946. [CrossRef]
55. Bozkurt-Guzel, C.; Inci, G.; Oyardi, O.; Savage, P.B. Synergistic Activity of Ceragenins Against Carbapenem-Resistant Acinetobacter baumannii Strains in Both Checkerboard and Dynamic Time-Kill Assays. *Curr. Microbiol.* **2020**, *77*, 1419–1428. [CrossRef] [PubMed]
56. Bonapace, C.R.; White, R.L.; Friedrich, L.V.; Bosso, J.A. Evaluation of antibiotic synergy against Acinetobacter baumannii: A comparison with Etest, time-kill, and checkerboard methods. *Diagn. Microbiol. Infect. Dis.* **2000**, *38*, 43–50. [CrossRef]
57. Lee, C.R.; Lee, J.H.; Park, M.; Park, K.S.; Bae, I.K.; Kim, Y.B.; Cha, C.J.; Jeong, B.C.; Lee, S.H. Biology of Acinetobacter baumannii: Pathogenesis, Antibiotic Resistance Mechanisms, and Prospective Treatment Options. *Front. Cell Infect. Microbiol.* **2017**, *7*, 55. [CrossRef] [PubMed]
58. Al-Shamiri, M.M.; Zhang, S.; Mi, P.; Liu, Y.; Xun, M.; Yang, E.; Ai, L.; Han, L.; Chen, Y. Phenotypic and genotypic characteristics of Acinetobacter baumannii enrolled in the relationship among antibiotic resistance, biofilm formation and motility. *Microb. Pathog.* **2021**, *155*, 104922. [CrossRef] [PubMed]
59. Ashrafi, M.; Novak-Frazer, L.; Bates, M.; Baguneid, M.; Alonso-Rasgado, T.; Xia, G.; Rautemaa-Richardson, R.; Bayat, A. Validation of biofilm formation on human skin wound models and demonstration of clinically translatable bacteria-specific volatile signatures. *Sci. Rep.* **2018**, *8*, 9431. [CrossRef] [PubMed]
60. Abdallah, M.; Benoliel, C.; Drider, D.; Dhulster, P.; Chihib, N.E. Biofilm formation and persistence on abiotic surfaces in the context of food and medical environments. *Arch. Microbiol.* **2014**, *196*, 453–472. [CrossRef] [PubMed]
61. Longo, F.; Vuotto, C.; Donelli, G. Biofilm formation in Acinetobacter baumannii. *New Microbiol.* **2014**, *37*, 119–127.
62. Hall, C.W.; Mah, T.F. Molecular mechanisms of biofilm-based antibiotic resistance and tolerance in pathogenic bacteria. *FEMS Microbiol. Rev.* **2017**, *41*, 276–301. [CrossRef]
63. Kim, J.K.; Lee, E.; Shin, S.; Jeong, K.W.; Lee, J.Y.; Bae, S.Y.; Kim, S.H.; Lee, J.; Kim, S.R.; Lee, D.G.; et al. Structure and function of papiliocin with antimicrobial and anti-inflammatory activities isolated from the swallowtail butterfly, Papilio xuthus. *J. Biol. Chem.* **2011**, *286*, 41296–41311. [CrossRef]
64. Wright, H.; Bonomo, R.A.; Paterson, D.L. New agents for the treatment of infections with Gram-negative bacteria: Restoring the miracle or false dawn? *Clin. Microbiol. Infect.* **2017**, *23*, 704–712. [CrossRef] [PubMed]
65. Piperaki, E.T.; Tzouvelekis, L.S.; Miriagou, V.; Daikos, G.L. Carbapenem-resistant Acinetobacter baumannii: In pursuit of an effective treatment. *Clin. Microbiol. Infect.* **2019**, *25*, 951–957. [CrossRef] [PubMed]
66. Viehman, J.A.; Nguyen, M.H.; Doi, Y. Treatment options for carbapenem-resistant and extensively drug-resistant Acinetobacter baumannii infections. *Drugs* **2014**, *74*, 1315–1333. [CrossRef] [PubMed]

67. Lenhard, J.R.; Nation, R.L.; Tsuji, B.T. Synergistic combinations of polymyxins. *Int. J. Antimicrob. Agents* **2016**, *48*, 607–613. [CrossRef] [PubMed]
68. Park, H.J.; Cho, J.H.; Kim, H.J.; Han, S.H.; Jeong, S.H.; Byun, M.K. Colistin monotherapy versus colistin/rifampicin combination therapy in pneumonia caused by colistin-resistant Acinetobacter baumannii: A randomised controlled trial. *J. Glob. Antimicrob. Resist.* **2019**, *17*, 66–71. [CrossRef] [PubMed]
69. Reygaert, W.C. An overview of the antimicrobial resistance mechanisms of bacteria. *AIMS Microbiol.* **2018**, *4*, 482–501. [CrossRef] [PubMed]
70. Hamidian, M.; Nigro, S.J. Emergence, molecular mechanisms and global spread of carbapenem-resistant Acinetobacter baumannii. *Microb. Genomics* **2019**, *5*, e000306. [CrossRef] [PubMed]
71. Wong, M.H.; Chan, B.K.; Chan, E.W.; Chen, S. Over-Expression of ISAba1-Linked Intrinsic and Exogenously Acquired OXA Type Carbapenem-Hydrolyzing-Class D-ss-Lactamase-Encoding Genes Is Key Mechanism Underlying Carbapenem Resistance in Acinetobacter baumannii. *Front. Microbiol.* **2019**, *10*, 2809. [CrossRef] [PubMed]
72. Pristovsek, P.; Kidric, J. Solution structure of polymyxins B and E and effect of binding to lipopolysaccharide: An NMR and molecular modeling study. *J. Med. Chem.* **1999**, *42*, 4604–4613. [CrossRef]
73. Mares, J.; Kumaran, S.; Gobbo, M.; Zerbe, O. Interactions of lipopolysaccharide and polymyxin studied by NMR spectroscopy. *J. Biol. Chem.* **2009**, *284*, 11498–11506. [CrossRef]
74. Sahoo, A.; Swain, S.S.; Behera, A.; Sahoo, G.; Mahapatra, P.K.; Panda, S.K. Antimicrobial Peptides Derived From Insects Offer a Novel Therapeutic Option to Combat Biofilm: A Review. *Front. Microbiol.* **2021**, *12*, 661195. [CrossRef] [PubMed]
75. Kapil, S.; Sharma, V. d-Amino acids in antimicrobial peptides: A potential approach to treat and combat antimicrobial resistance. *Can. J. Microbiol.* **2021**, *67*, 119–137. [CrossRef] [PubMed]
76. Hicks, R.P.; Abercrombie, J.J.; Wong, R.K.; Leung, K.P. Antimicrobial peptides containing unnatural amino acid exhibit potent bactericidal activity against ESKAPE pathogens. *Bioorg. Med. Chem.* **2013**, *21*, 205–214. [CrossRef] [PubMed]
77. Falanga, A.; Nigro, E.; De Biasi, M.G.; Daniele, A.; Morelli, G.; Galdiero, S.; Scudiero, O. Cyclic Peptides as Novel Therapeutic Microbicides: Engineering of Human Defensin Mimetics. *Molecules* **2017**, *22*, 1217. [CrossRef] [PubMed]

MDPI
St. Alban-Anlage 66
4052 Basel
Switzerland
Tel. +41 61 683 77 34
Fax +41 61 302 89 18
www.mdpi.com

Pharmaceutics Editorial Office
E-mail: pharmaceutics@mdpi.com
www.mdpi.com/journal/pharmaceutics

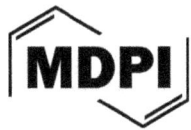